Cardiac Metabolism

Cardiac Metabolism

Edited by

Angela J. Drake-Holland

Department of Medicine 1,
St George's Hospital Medical School,
London, UK

and

Mark I. M. Noble

Midhurst Medical Research Institute,
Midhurst, West Sussex, UK

A Wiley-Interscience Publication

JOHN WILEY & SONS

Chichester · New York · Brisbane · Toronto · Singapore

Library of Congress Cataloging in Publication Data:
Main entry under title:
Cardiac metabolism.
    (Developments in cardiopulmonary research; v. 1)
    'A Wiley–Interscience publication.'
    Includes index.
    1. Heart—Muscle.   2. Metabolism.
    I. Drake-Holland, Angela J.   II. Noble, Mark I. M.
    III. Series.
    [DNLM: 1. Myocardium—Metabolism. W1 DE997VMC
    v. 1/WG 220 C26504]
    QP113.2.C367   1983   612'.173   82-16127

ISBN 0 471 10249 0

British Library Cataloguing in Publication Data:
Cardiac metabolism.
    1. Cardiology
    I. Drake-Holland, Angela J.   II. Noble, Mark I. M.
    III. Series
    612'.17   QP111.4

ISBN 0 471 10249 0

Filmset and Printed in Northern Ireland at
The Universities Press (Belfast) Ltd
Bound at the Pitman Press Ltd., Bath, Avon

Contributors

H. Van Belle Department of Biochemistry, Janssen Pharmaceutica Research Laboratories, B-2340 Beerse, Belgium

L. Blayney Department of Cardiology, Welsh National School of Medicine, Heath Park, Cardiff CF4 4XN, UK

R. G. Butcher Midhurst Medical Research Institute, Midhurst, West Sussex GU29 0BL, UK

J. B. Chapman Department of Physiology, Monash University, Clayton, Victoria 3168, Australia

R. A. Chapman Department of Physiology, University of Berne, Bühlplatz 5, 3012 Berne, Switzerland

A. Coray Department of Physiology, University of Berne, Bühlplatz 5, 3012 Berne, Switzerland

M. J. Dawson Department of Physiology, University College London, Gower Street, London WC1E 6BT, UK

A. J. Drake-Holland Department of Medicine 1, Jenner Wing, St George's Hospital Medical School, London SW17, UK

G. Elzinga Department of Physiology, Free University, Amsterdam, The Netherlands

P. J. England Department of Biochemistry, University of Bristol Medical School, Bristol BS8 1TD, UK

M. Fillenz University Laboratory of Physiology, Oxford OX1 3PT, UK

S. S. Galhotra Division of Biological Science and Pritzker School of Medicine, 950 East 59th Street, Chicago, Illinois 60637, USA

H. E. D. J. ter Keurs Department of Experimental Cardiology, Academisch Ziekenhuis, Leiden, The Netherlands

J. D. Laird Department of Physiology and Physiological Physics, University of Leiden, The Netherlands

B. Lewartowski Medical Centre of Postgraduate Education, Marymonka 99, 01-813 Warsaw, Poland

H. Lüllmann Department of Pharmacology, University of Kiel, 2300 Kiel, West Germany

J. A. S. McGuigan Department of Physiology, University of Berne, Bühlplatz 5, 3012 Berne, Switzerland

J. Nauman   *Medical Centre for Postgraduate Education, Marymonka 99, 01-813 Warsaw, Poland*

M. I. M. Noble   *Midhurst Medical Research Institute, Midhurst, West Sussex GU29 0BL, UK*

R. A. Olsson   *Suncoast Cardiovascular Research Laboratory, Department of Internal Medicine, University of South Florida College of Medicine, Tampa, Florida 33612, USA*

L. H. Opie   *Department of Medicine, University of Cape Town, Observatory 7925, Cape Town, South Africa*

T. Peters   *Department of Pharmacology, University of Kiel, 2300 Kiel, West Germany*

J. Preuner   *Department of Pharmacology, University of Kiel, 2300 Kiel, West Germany*

R. S. Reneman   *Department of Physiology, Biomedical Centre, University of Limburg, Maastricht, The Netherlands*

G. J. van der Vusse *Department of Physiology, Biomedical Centre, University of Limburg, Maastricht, The Netherlands*

A. Williams   *Cardiothoracic Institute, 2 Beaumont Street, London W1N 2DX, UK*

R. Zak   *Division of Biological Science and Pritzker School of Medicine, 950 East 59th Street, Chicago, Illinois 60637, USA*

Contents

Preface

The idea of a book on Cardiac Metabolism which represented current ideas and theories based on recent experimental evidence was an appealing, if somewhat daunting, task. The concept of Cardiac Metabolism covers a vast area, every aspect of which is important in its own right. There has been such an advance in techniques and thinking over the last few years that it is not possible for any one person (or laboratory) to be able to cope with research into all the aspects of cardiac metabolism. We have, therefore, produced a multi-author book. This has the advantage of bringing a spectrum of approaches and opinions together. Where overlap of subject matter has occurred, we have retained the material where different chapter authors have different opinions. We have tried to introduce some newer personalities in the field whose views deserve consideration. Many of the ideas presented are unconventional, and are intended to stimulate thought and argument.

It has been necessary to make many omissions of important subjects in cardiac metabolism. We have concentrated on various aspects of calcium metabolism and energy utilization, but also included some relatively neglected subjects and interesting methodological approaches (NMR and histochemistry). We failed to persuade anyone to write about membrane protein phosphorylation. This would have made a real gap in view of the inclusion of other chapters on cyclic AMP, contractile protein phosphorylation and catecholamines. We have therefore written such a chapter based on our literature reading and thank Drs. Tsien and England for their help with this.

The presentation of the book is to offer to the reader many aspects of cardiac metabolism, beginning with the handling of calcium ions, through biochemical reactions, to the metabolic factors concerning blood flow and performance. The heart is not an isolated organ: it is surrounded by a changing environment. Each chapter may be read on its own as a source of information relevant to the particular subject of interest, though the reader will find himself gently directed to other chapters that we feel should be considered as well. It is hoped that each reader, be they teacher or research worker of any discipline, will find interesting and provoking reading, in or related to their own subject.

ix

One or both of us have been privileged at one time or another to visit, or to have visit us, many of the authors in this book. To visit other laboratories is stimulating and extremely worthwhile; it benefits both the visitor and host. Our thanks go particularly to Professors Lewartowski, Lüllman, Elzinga, Laird, and Drs. ter Keurs, van der Vusse, Reneman and Nauman for their generosity and hospitality during our 'invasion' of their laboratories. Of the remaining authors we thank those who have visited us and/or for stimulating discussions.

Our interest in cardiac metabolism stems from two main sources. Firstly one of us was basically trained in Biochemistry (when privileged to work with Professor Opie) and though having now 'changed courses' to Physiology, retains a fondness for the subject. The other has been persuaded (over the years) that though the mechanics are interesting, metabolism is more fundamentally important.

The invitation to compile this book arose from conversations between representatives of John Wiley from nearby Chichester and Professor G. Cumming, Director of the Midhurst Medical Research Institute.

We are indebted to our colleagues who put up with the trials of trying to meet deadlines, and our laboratory colleagues who put up with us during the writing and editing of this book. We are also grateful to the many typists who helped with the manuscripts.

ANGELA J. DRAKE-HOLLAND
MARK I. M. NOBLE

Cardiac Metabolism
Edited by A. J. Drake-Holland and M. I. M. Noble
© 1983 John Wiley & Sons Ltd

CHAPTER 1

Role of the Plasmalemma for Calcium Homeostasis and for Excitation–Contraction Coupling in Cardiac Muscle

Heinz Lüllmann, Thies Peters, and Jürgen Preuner

Department of Pharmacology, University of Kiel, 2300 Kiel, West Germany

INTRODUCTION

Abundant efforts have been made in the past to elucidate the mechanisms involved in the calcium homeostasis and in the excitation–contraction (EC) coupling process of mammalian heart muscle cells. For a pharmacologist it is of more than academic interest to resolve these problems: these mechanisms are fundamental to the molecular basis of drug action.

In skeletal muscle, depolarization of the plasmalemma is conducted to the transverse tubules from where it spreads to the terminal cisternae of the sarcoplasmic reticulum (SR), whence it is thought to release Ca ions (Ca^{++}). These Ca^{++} diffuse to the nearby Z-lines of the sarcomeric units and activate contraction. Contraction is terminated by an active, ATP-driven calcium sequestration into the longitudinal tubules of the sarcoplasmic reticulum from whence it is translocated back to the terminal cisternae. This hypothesis is far from being proven.

In cardiac muscle, it is necessary to postulate essential modifications as far as the mechanism of Ca^{++} release is concerned. By means of voltage clamp experiments it could be demonstrated that some calcium enters the cell during depolarization: slow, inward directed calcium current. Initially, it was suggested that the amount of calcium invading the cell during depolarization would suffice to activate contraction. Yet the amount turned out to be too small (of the order of up to 1×10^{-6} mol per kilogram of cell per beat). As a consequence, a calcium-triggered calcium-release mechanism from the SR was postulated (also called regenerative calcium release). At the time of writing, a mechanism of this kind has not been proven under physiological conditions. Recently, by using isolated cells, which are deprived of their glycocalyx, Isenberg and Klöckner, (1980) demonstrated a much more pronounced influx of Ca^{++} into the cardiac cell which would be able to activate contraction *per se*. The physiological relevance of this finding remains unclear, since the permeability of these cells does not appear to agree completely with that observed in intact cells (see below as regards the rate of radio-calcium entry and exchange). Moreover, it has been difficult to visualize the ability of cardiac sarcoplasmic reticulum to terminate contraction or induce relaxation by actively pumping back calcium from the cytosol. Both the paucity of cardiac SR and its affinity constant for calcium with respect to the Ca^{++} concentration present in the cytosol during and after contraction do not seem to allow a significant contribution to relaxation (Mullins, 1981). From experiments conducted on mechanically skinned cardiac fibres of different sections of the heart muscle it was claimed that the SR does contribute to contraction and relaxation (for a review see Fabiato and Fabiato, 1979). However, the property of a preparation of this kind to display spontaneous contraction and relaxation does not necessarily reflect what happens in intact tissue; especially as these skinned fibres require loading at rather high calcium concentrations.

We propose a mechanism of excitation–contraction coupling in heart muscle of a completely different type. Before this hypothesis is outlined below, we discuss several essential aspects of the movements and distribution of calcium in heart muscle; these are prerequisites for further consideration of the problem.

Ca MOVEMENTS UNDER VARIOUS CONDITIONS

Resting Heart Muscle

When cardiac tissues are not beating for a while, all intracellular Ca compartments are in equilibrium with an extremely low cytosolic Ca^{++} concentration ($<10^{-7}$ M); only the outer layer of the plasmalemma is in equilibrium with the extracellular Ca^{++} concentration ($\sim 10^{-3}$ M Ca^{++}, see Figure 1.1). Net movements of Ca do not occur under this condition. The Ca leaking along the high gradient into the cell is counterbalanced by the plasmalemmal Ca pump. Studying Ca movements under this condition by means of radio-Ca reveals that ^{45}Ca is initially rapidly taken up; but the rate declines with time, attaining its final equilibrium not before 30–60 min of exposure. Thus the ^{45}Ca uptake process does not obey an exponential function, but rather reflects the exchange of ^{45}Ca with Ca bound at differing dissociation rate constants or reflects different accessibilities (deep compartments). The reverse experiment, namely the efflux of ^{45}Ca from a heart muscle previously equilibrated with radio-Ca, yields mirror-like curves: again initially a rapid loss of ^{45}Ca followed by a declining process of exchange. From this type of experiment it can be concluded that even in resting heart muscle a high turnover of Ca proceeds within (and through) the plasmalemma as indicated by the initial rate, which soon slows down since the amount of rapidly exchangeable binding sites is limited It should be kept in mind that the freely exchangeable Ca^{++} present in the cytosol amount only to about 6×10^{-8} mol. kg^{-1} w.w. and is thus quantitatively negligible with respect to exchange processes at a tissue Ca

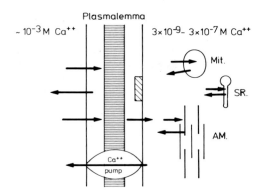

Figure 1.1 Schematic presentation of Ca movement in resting heart muscle. Under this condition only Ca exchange processes will occur (black arrows). The extracullular Ca^{++} concentration ($\sim 10^{-3}$ M) is in equilibrium with the Ca bound to the outer leaflet of the plasmalemma. The barrier between the high extracellular and low intracellular Ca^{++} concentrations is posed by the highly hydrophobic middle layer of the unit membrane (horizontally hatched area). The Ca bound to or stored by intracellular organelles is in equilibrium with the low cytosolic Ca^{++} concentration. Mit = mitochondria, SR = sarcoplasmic reticulum, AM = actomyosin, $\rightarrow$ = exchange. The plasmalemmal Ca pump compensates for the leak of Ca along the extemely steep gradient. The high affinity potential-dependent binding sites are marked by a hatched box at the inner membrane surface

content of about 1.2×10^{-3} mol. kg^{-1} w.w. (at an extracellular Ca^{++} concentration of about 1.0 mM).

The initial ^{45}Ca uptake rate can be considered – though with reservation – to reflect the turnover rate of Ca in the plasmalemma. Since a heart muscle preparation is always a multicellular system with complex geometry, the rate of disposition of ^{45}Ca might, however, become rate-limiting. This applies particularly to resting muscles whereas strongly beating preparations might accelerate the diffusion and therewith the disposition of ^{45}Ca. If this consideration holds true for the present case the initial uptake (and release) rate of ^{45}Ca provides an underestimate of the initial exchange rate, which therefore should be even faster than experimentally determined. (For further studies, see Lewartowski, Chapter 5 in this volume). In conclusion, in resting heart muscles net Ca movements do not occur but a vigorous Ca exchange proceeds at rates varying over a wide range, according to the dissociation of Ca from different binding sites.

Net Movements after Raising the Extracellular Ca Concentration

A sudden rise of the Ca^{++} concentration is followed by a rapid increase of contractile force of beating preparations. Its time course depends on the rate of disposition of Ca^{++}, in perfused preparations (Langendorff hearts) at about $t_{1/2} = 10$ s and in superfused preparations at about $t_{1/2} = 20-30$ s. This observation suggests that alterations of the extracellular Ca^{++} concentration are almost immediately transferred to the cardiac cells and are available for EC coupling. Which net Ca movements occur in resting preparations, a simpler situation than that of contracting muscles?

The increased Ca^{++} concentration has to approach the cell surface by diffusion. As shown in experiments with guinea-pig and cat atrial and ventricular muscles, a sudden increase of the Ca^{++} concentration in the bath up to about 8 mM does not alter the resting tension. This indicates that the cytosolic Ca^{++} concentration remains below the threshold concentration as regards the activation of actomyosin ($\sim 3 \times 10^{-7}$ M), but a pronounced net uptake of Ca results, which depends upon the degree of increase of the extracellular Ca. The muscles require 15–20 min to attain the new equilibrium (Körnich and Lüllman, 1970). From recent experiments on guinea-pig atria, the initial rate of net uptake could be calculated because of a proper time resolution within the first minutes, after raising the Ca^{++} concentration from 0.9 to 3.6 mM. The initial net uptake rate amounted to 5×10^{-7} mol kg^{-1} s^{-1} (H. Lüllmann and A. Ziegler, unpublished). This figure lies in the same range as the electrogenic Ca flux determined for the plateau phase of the action potential ($\sim 6 \times 10^{-7}$ mol kg^{-1}), which is considered to carry part of the inward current necessary to keep the membrane depolarized. In contrast, no depolarization whatsoever occurs when a heart muscle is suddenly exposed to higher Ca^{++} concentrations, a condition under which a correspondingly high net uptake proceeds. This indicates strongly that Ca taken up does not cross the plasmalemma as an ion but becomes primarily bound to the outer leaflet of the plasmalemma, i.e. the net uptake appears to be non-electrogenic.

From the outer leaflet Ca will, according to the higher gradient, increasingly leak into the cytosol, slightly raise the free Ca^{++} concentration (but still less than 3×10^{-7} M), and supply all intracellular compartments which slowly adapt to the new level within 10–15 min. The cell's outward directed Ca pump supposedly participates in keeping the cytosolic Ca^{++} concentration low. In contrast to ventricular muscles of guinea-pigs and cats, rat ventricular muscles possess a Ca pump of only minor potency (Olbrich and Preuner, 1982). In this species a stepwise increase of extracellular Ca results in an increase in resting tension.

What has been outlined for the resting heart muscle is also applicable for contracting muscles after raising the Ca^{++} concentration: the diastolic tension remains unaltered over a wide range of stepwise increases (guinea-pig, cat) and the net uptake of Ca is also non-electrogenic.

In conclusion, a rise in extracellular Ca^{++} concentration results in a corresponding net uptake of Ca which is non-electrogenic, i.e. the Ca becomes primarily bound to the plasmalemma and is slowly distributed to intracellular binding sites via a cytosolic Ca^{++} concentration still below threshold with respect to the actomyosin.

Excitation-dependent Ca Movements

During depolarization two events take place: (a) a Ca^{++} influx through a specialized pore (slow inward current); (b) a release of Ca^{++} from high affinity, potential-dependent binding sites. From their location at the inner surface of the plasmalemma, Ca^{++} ions diffuse into the cytosol and activate the contractile apparatus in a concentration-dependent way.

As outlined above the slow inward current is not sufficient to supply the amount of Ca^{++} required to activate the contractile system. Nevertheless it provides a net cellular uptake of Ca which eventually has to be counterbalanced by the Ca pump. Comparing the initial ^{45}Ca exchange rates of resting and beating atrial tissue, an extra Ca exchange of 0.5 μM kg^{-1} per beat can be calculated which is in good agreement with the estimates of Ca^{++} flux during the plateau.

The depolarization-dependent release of Ca^{++} from high affinity binding sites located at the inner surface of the plasmalemma is a cellular event and does not primarily involve extracellular Ca. These binding sites are thought to possess the following properties: a high affinity for Ca if the plasmalemma is polarized, a low affinity during depolarization of the membrane, and a capacity sufficient to supply Ca^{++} in excess for activation of the contractile system.

The requirements are met by an array of phosphatidylserine (PS) molecules which are part of the Na, K-ATPase and are integrated into the inner leaflet of the plasmalemma.

At low proton concentrations present in the polarized membrane due to the strong electric field across the plasmalemma, PS complexes Ca with high affinity. When the membrane depolarizes the proton activity drastically increases within the membrane, approaching the bulk pH because the transmembrane field has collapsed. This results in protonation of the PS amino groups and a loss of affinity for Ca (Lüllmann and Peters, 1977; 1979). PS is an essential constituent of cardiac plasmalemma, it can be calculated to amount to about 2% of membrane wet weight and is clustered around the protein moiety of the Na,K-ATPase (Figure 1.2) (Zwaal *et al.*, 1973). The total capacity of PS to bind Ca is of the order of 2×10^{-4} M kg^{-1} cell. At a 2:1 ratio, the maximum Ca binding capacity of plasmalemmal PS would amount to about 10^{-4} M kg^{-1}, a store thus large enough to activate the contractile system even upon partial release.

During the plateau phase the intracellular structures such as the actomyosin system, the mitochondria, and the sarcoplasmic reticulum will face an increasing Ca^{++} concentration. The actomyosin displaying a K_{DCa} of about 1×10^{-6} M will react correspondingly, whereas the mitochondria having a K_{DCa} of about 1×10^{-4} M will hardly participate in sequestering Ca.

Ca Movement During and after Repolarization

Beginning in phase 4 of the action potential, the electric field across the plasmalemma is built up again with increasing polarization and therewith the

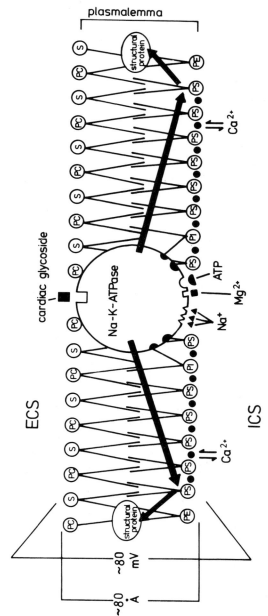

Figure 1.2 Schematic drawing of the plasmalemma including one Na,K-ATPase molecule and the associated Ca binding phospholipids, the acidic lipids representing an essential part of the Na,K pump. The actual array of the phospholipids and structural proteins is controlled by the functional state of the ATPase protein (indicated by black arrows). The voltage of $\sim$80 mV across the unit membrane ($\sim$8 nm) creates an electric field in the order of 10 kV mm^{-1}. The affinity of Ca to the acidic phospholipids depends on the existence of the electric field (for details see text). PC = phosphatidylcholine; S = sphingomyelin; PE = phosphatidylethanolamine; PS = phosphatidylserine; PI = phosphatidylinositol

high affinity binding sites for Ca reoccur. Ca^{++} from the adjacent cytosolic space will become bound and the diffusion gradient within the cytosol will be reversed. Due to the high affinity of the potential-dependent binding sites the actual Ca^{++} concentration will decrease below the threshold concentration with respect to actomyosin, which accordingly relaxes with a time course determined by the diffusion of Ca^{++} directed towards the plasmalemma. After relaxation has been established, the high affinity Ca store will be refilled corresponding to the prevailing conditions (extracellular Ca^{++} concentration, end-diastolic cytosolic Ca^{++} concentration, beat frequency). Although the Ca^{++} released from the high affinity, potential-dependent binding sites will be rebound at the end of the diastole, the cardiac cell has gained some Ca by the slow inward current. It is this Ca load which has to be pumped out by the Ca,Mg-ATPase such that the Ca homeostasis is maintained. Thus, simultaneously with the refilling of the high affinity binding sites, the Ca pump will bind cytosolic Ca^{++} and translocate them against the high gradient to the outside (compensatory net transport). The plasmalemmal Ca pump possessing a K_{DCa} of 7×10^{-7} M will essentially participate in reducing the cytosolic Ca^{++} concentration below 3×10^{-7} M (for details see below).

PLASMALEMMAL Ca PUMP

The presence of an active Ca outward transport in heart muscle, similar to that described for erythrocytes by Schatzmann and Vincenzi (1969), has been postulated for a long time (Lahrtz *et al.*, 1967; Sulakhe and Dhalla, 1971; Sulakhe and St Louis, 1976) as a necessity to counterbalance the net uptake of Ca occurring both under conditions of rest and of activity. Recently, a highly active Ca,Mg-ATPase located in the plasmamembrane has been ascertained (Cielejewski *et al.*, 1980; Kliem and Preuner, 1980; Kliem 1981). One of the reasons for the difficulty to detect the plasmalemmal Ca pump in heart muscle is based on the fact that the methodical procedures which have proven successful in preparing Ca-pumping vesicles (microsomes) of sarcoplasmic reticulum of skeletal muscles have been transferred to cardiac muscle without modification. But there are two experimental pitfalls: (a) in contrast to vesicles obtained from sarcoplasmic reticulum, the vesicles derived from the plasmalemma of ventricular muscle cells with the abundant T-tubular system consist mainly of inside-out vesicles (hiding the plasmalemmal marker enzyme Na,K-ATPase!) (Lüllmann and Peters, 1976); (b) the Ca pump activity of the cardiac plasmalemma is completely lost if Ca complexing agents have been used during the preparation procedure of the vesicles, this is in contrast to vesicles obtained from sarcoplasmic reticulum. In contrast to earlier reports on the activity of the plasmalemmal calcium pump, ranging between 2 and 30 nmol Ca per milligram of protein per minute (Stam *et al.*, 1973; Lüllmann and Peters, 1976; Caroni and Carafoli, 1981a,b; Spitzer *et al.*, 1981), the activity yielded by preparing sarcolemmal microsomes in the absence of Ca chelating agents, like EDTA or EGTA, results in a pump activity between 90 and 130 nmol Ca per milligram of protein per minute at 22 °C but otherwise comparable conditions. At 37 °C the pump activity was even found to be increased up to 350–400 nmol Ca per milligram of protein per minute. This value has to be compared with the maximum pump activity reported so far by Caroni and Carafoli (1981a), who obtained a value of 31 nmol Ca per milligram of protein per minute at this temperature.

According to these considerations the existence of Ca pump activity in a microsomal fraction can no longer be accepted as a general and characteristic marker of the sarcoplasmic reticulum, as has been claimed previously (Dhalla *et al.*, 1976; Bers, 1979; Van Alstyne *et al.*, 1979). This assumption can only be made, if – by the use of special procedures of preparation and the use of Ca chelating agents – the activity of the plasmalemmal Ca pump is minimized, while the sarcoplasmic reticular Ca pump, which is rather insensitive to this treatment, is selectively preserved (Cielejewski *et al.*, 1980; Kliem and Preuner 1980; Kliem, 1981).

When plasmalemmal inside-out vesicles obtained from guinea-pig heart muscles are exposed to increasing Ca^{++} concentrations in the presence of 2.5 mM oxalate they accumulate Ca in a dose-dependent way as shown in Figures 1.3 and 1.4. At 22 °C, the half maximum saturation, K_D, was calculated to be about 7×10^{-7} M (actual calcium ion concentration). The maximum uptake rate amounted to 90–130 nmol per milligram of protein per minute and to 350–400 nmol per milligram of protein per minute at 37 °C, yielding a Q_{10} of 3.5 (22–32 °C). Recalculating the maximum accumulation rate on the basis of membrane protein yield per unit of wet weight, a transport capacity of 0.45 mmol per kilogram wet weight per minute was estimated. The efficacy of the Ca pump, therefore, easily matches the Ca load imposed on cardiac cells under physiological conditions (Preuner, 1981). The data are compiled in Table 1.1.

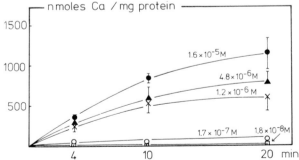

Figure 1.3 Time course of Ca accumulation by plasmalemmal microsomes (guinea-pig heart muscle) at different Ca^{++} concentrations (22 °C). Abscissa, time in minutes; ordinate, nanomoles of Ca per milligram of protein

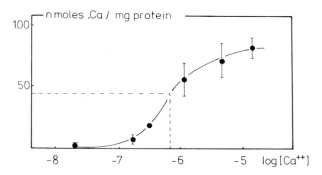

Figure 1.4 Dose–response curve of Ca uptake by plasmalemmal microsomes (guinea-pig heart muscle) at 22 °C. Abscissa, Ca^{++} concentration; ordinate, nanomoles of Ca taken up per milligram of protein at equilibrium. The K_{DCa} is indicated by a dashed line

Concerning the Ca pump, cat hearts were found to behave in a similar way to those of guinea-pigs. The maximum pump activity amounted to about 100 nmol per milligram of protein per minute at 22 °C. Plasmalemmal vesicles derived from rat hearts displayed a rather low Ca pump activity, the maximum Ca accumulation rate was as low as about 30 nmol per milligram of protein per minute at 22 °C, thus much less than the pump activity of guinea-pig and cat hearts (Olbrich and Preuner, 1982). It is known from rat hearts that their capacity to maintain the Ca homeostasis is easily overcharged: raising the extracellular Ca^{++} concentrations stepwise from 1.8 to 3.6 mM increases the end-diastolic tone of ventricular muscle preparation (under given experimental conditions) whereas guinea-pig and cat heart preparations tolerate a sudden increase of the Ca^{++} concentration up to 8 mM without an increase in tone. These findings with isolated organs seem to reflect the low Ca pump capacity of rat heart sarcolemma.

Table 1.1 Compilation of the properties of the Ca pump derived from guinea-pig ventricular muscles

V_{max}	22 °C: 90–130 nmol per milligram of protein per minute
	37 °C: 350–400 nmol per milligram of protein per minute
K_D value	7×10^{-7} M Ca^{++} (22 °C)
Optimal ATP concentration	3–5 mM ($K_{D\,Mg \cdot ATP} = 5 \times 10^{-4}$ M)
Optimal Mg concentration	5–7.5 mM ($K_{D\,Mg^{++}} = 6 \times 10^{-5}$ M)
Na^+ and K^+	>40–140 mM stimulate two- to threefold, but are exchangeable, if combined concentration is constant
Temperature dependence	$Q_{10} = 3.5$ in the range from 22 to 32 °C
pH optimum	6.7–7.1 (imidazole buffer)
No inhibition by ouabain *in vitro*	

In conclusion, guinea-pig and cat ventricular plasmalemma possess a Ca transport mechanism (Ca,Mg-ATPase) which pumps Ca from the inside to the outside at a high rate. This Ca pump cannot be inhibited directly by cardiac glycosides.

Affinity Constants of Cellular Ca Binding Sites

The cellular structures involved in metabolism of Ca display rather different affinity constants. Consequently they are saturated to different extents within the Ca^{++} concentration range occurring under physiological conditions. The contribution of the different structures is determined by their affinities and their capacities, e.g. by their proportion as related to cell volume.

The K_{DCa} values and the corresponding binding curves are schematically summarized with respect to the position on a Ca^{++} concentration scale in Figure 1.5. Actomyosin displays a central position characterized by a K_{DCa} of 10^{-6} M Ca^{++} (Ebashi and Endo, 1968; Solaro *et al.*, 1974; Chapman, 1979; Kerrick *et al.*, 1980). The activation starts above 3×10^{-7} M and attains a maximum at 3×10^{-6} M. The outward directed Ca pump exhibits a somewhat higher affinity, a K_{DCa} of 7×10^{-7} M (Preuner, 1981), thus starting its pump activity well below the activation threshold of actomyosin by Ca^{++}. According to Solaro and Briggs (1974), Kitazawa (1976), Will *et al.*, (1976a,b), Endo (1977), and Mullins (1981) the K_{DCa} of the cardiac sarcoplasmic reticulum (SR) is of the order of 3×10^{-6} M, which would yield a curve slightly shifted towards higher concentrations as compared with that of the actomyosin. In principle this would

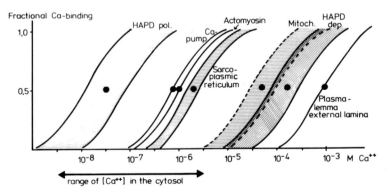

Figure 1.5 Concentration-dependent binding of Ca^{++} to cellular binding partners. Abscissa, Ca^{++} concentration; ordinate, Ca binding as a fraction of maximum attainable binding. The range over which the Ca^{++} concentration within the cytosol can oscillate under physiological conditions is indicated by a black arrow below the abscissa. The black dots point to the mean K_{DCa} as taken from the literature and according to our own experiments. HADP = high affinity potential-dependent binding sites in polarized (pol) and depolarized (dep) state

allow a Ca^{++} uptake into the SR when the actomyosin is activated (see, however, below). It appears that the mitochondria exhibiting a K_{DCa} of $\sim 10^{-4}$ M (Scarpa and Williamson, 1974; Kitazawa, 1976) do not participate in the regulation of the cytosolic Ca^{++} concentration under physiological conditions but may become involved whenever the cell is flooded with Ca (contracture, Ca paradox, metabolic inhibition, intoxication by cardiac glycosides). The lowest affinities are displayed by the inner and outer leaflet of the plasmalemma ($K_{DCa} \sim 10^{-3}$ M). The outer leaflet facing the high extracellular Ca^{++} concentration will accordingly be more or less saturated; in contrast practically no Ca will be bound to the inner leaflet because of the low intracellular Ca^{++} concentration. With respect to excitation–contraction coupling the most interesting properties seem to be displayed by potential-dependent, high affinity binding sites. In order to warrant proper relaxation, a high affinity binding site has to be postulated, the K_{DCa} of which should be of the order of 3×10^{-8} M.

Theoretically this requirement is fulfilled by acidic lipids such as phosphatidylserine which possess a comparably high Ca binding affinity under the influence of a transmembrane electric field (Lüllmann and Peters, 1977, 1979). As soon as the membrane is depolarized this particular phospholipid reduces its Ca binding affinity to a value similar to that of other lipids of the inner leaflet. The affinity in the absence of an electric field has been measured in isolated plasmalemmal preparations and yields values between 2×10^{-5} and 10^{-3} M, possibly involving two types of binding sites (Lüllmann and Peters, 1976; Preuner, 1979; Pang, 1980). Also in Figure 1.5, the possible undulation range of the cytosolic Ca^{++} concentration is indicated by a double-headed arrow below the abscissa.

Cellular Distribution of Ca

The cellular distribution of Ca is additionally determined by the 'capacity' for Ca of the different cellular structures. The capacity can clearly be defined for isolated preparations of cellular organelles as maximum binding capability per milligram of protein upon increasing the Ca^{++} concentration in the incubation medium until maximum binding or uptake is attained. However, under the aspects of intact cells only fractions of this capacity may be involved since the actual Ca^{++} concentration may be far lower than required to saturate the respective capacity. Under physiological conditions it is this fractional saturation of the capacity and the fractional size of the respective organelles in relation to the entire cell volume which determines its contribution to total cell Ca content.

From this aspect, actomyosin can maximally bind up to 10^{-4} mol Ca per kilogram of cardiac cells (Solaro *et al.*, 1974). Since this will only be achieved under the condition of maximal activation and, under physiological conditions, occurs only transiently, the contribution of the actomyosin-bound Ca to the total

Ca content will remain far below this value. In resting muscle it will add negligible amounts in spite of the fact that actomyosin makes up about 8% of the cell volume.

The amount of Ca actually bound to the Ca,Mg-ATPase can also be considered to be minor since the number of Ca pumps is so small that it would not be detectable in terms of Ca molarity.

The sarcoplasmic reticulum in heart muscle is estimated to occupy about 1% of the cell volume. Even if maximally saturated, its contribution to total cell Ca would only yield 10^{-5}–2×10^{-5} mol per kilogram of cells and thus 1% of the total cell Ca (Mullins, 1980). Since under physiological conditions the mean cytosolic Ca^{++} concentration will be far lower than the Ca^{++} concentration necessary for maximal saturation, the sarcoplasmic reticulum should contribute even less.

The mitochondria occupying a large fraction of the cell volume but displaying a low Ca affinity will contain little Ca due to the concentration range of the cytosolic Ca^{++} concentration. From a cell biological aspect it should be considered that, if the mitochondrial Ca uptake would proceed at Ca^{++} concentrations occurring during normal excitation–contraction coupling, then part of the coupling Ca^{++} for actomyosin activation would be lost during tension development and relaxation would be slowed by corresponding release of Ca^{++} by mitochondria. This process would at least in part consume energy. A participation of this kind seems unreasonable.

The outer leaflet of the plasmalemma binds Ca by means of abundant negatively charged groups provided by different classes of acidic moieties. The overall K_{DCa} ranges around 10^{-3} M. At the extracellular Ca^{++} concentration ($>10^{-3}$ M) these binding sites should be fairly saturated. Calculations of the amount bound to this structure yield values of about 1 mmol per kilogram of cells, thus contributing more than half of total cellular Ca. This tentative estimate is linked to the assumption that the plasmalemma occupies 1% of total cell volume in ventricular muscle. The inner leaflet of the plasmalemma may possess the same K_{DCa} and capacity. Since it faces the low intracellular Ca^{++} concentration, the amount bound should be far lower.

The high affinity, potential-dependent binding site is estimated to display a K_{DCa} of around 3×10^{-8} M; its capacity amounts to about 10^{-4} mol per kilogram of cells. This figure can be obtained by calculating the molarity of phosphatidylserine present in the inner leaflet and by the number of Na,K-ATPases per kilogram of cells (see above). One determining factor for the fractional saturation of this pool will be the actual Ca^{++} concentration in the cytosol. At a Ca^{++} concentration of 3×10^{-8} M half-saturation can be assumed. Upon depolarization of the plasmalemma, part of the Ca bound to these sites will be released and diffuse into the cytosol.

In conclusion most of the cellular Ca is located in the plasmalemma (outer leaflet and high affinity, potential-dependent binding site). Intracellular organelles contain only minor amounts of Ca under physiological conditions.

Rates of Ca Binding and Transport

The sections above dealt with Ca distribution under equilibrium conditions. However, when rapid changes of actual Ca^{++} concentrations occur – as is the case for a contraction cycle – then the rates of Ca binding and transport are the essential determinants for the amount removed from the cytosol per unit of time. The adsorption to and desorption from binding sites at the plasmalemma and at the actomyosin are simple physicochemical events which proceed immediately and are only governed by the diffusion rates of Ca^{++} within the cytosol. In contrast, the plasmalemma, the mitochondria, and the sarcoplasmic reticulum possess Ca ATPases, the activity of which can become rate limiting. The rates of Ca transport are dependent on the Ca^{++} concentration. These rates have been determined *in vitro* and amount to 10^{-5} mol per kilogram of cells per second for the plasmalemmal Ca pump, 5×10^{-7} mol per kilogram of cells per second for sarcoplasmic reticulum, and 1.2×10^{-7} mol per kilogram of cells per second for the mitochondria at a Ca^{++} concentration of 10^{-6} M; this lies in the range of the possible Ca^{++} concentration during a contraction cycle which exists only transiently. From this it can be taken that the contribution of these structures to the actual regulation during the contractile cycle can only be minor. Under pathological conditions when the cytosolic Ca^{++} concentration may be excessively increased, these systems become involved in keeping the end-diastolic Ca^{++} concentration as low as possible. The highest efficiency will be displayed by the plasmalemmal Ca pump which extrudes Ca into the extracellular space, thus exhibiting an unlimited capacity, and by the mitochondria because of their large fractional volume which is, of course, limited.

Regulation of Contractile Force

The contractile force of a beat will be determined mainly by the amount of Ca^{++} released from the high affinity, potential-dependent Ca binding sites, the slow Ca^{++} inward current adding another 10–20%. The filling of this store will equilibrate with the end-diastolic cytosol Ca^{++} concentration which – as far as is known – varies over a wide range, i.e. 3×10^{-7}–3×10^{-9} M Ca^{++}. This implies that the Ca amount present in the high affinity store varies according to its adsorption isotherm. It is not only the amount of Ca present in the store but the fraction of it which is actually released by an action potential which determines the contractile force. Thus the contractile force is finally determined by (a) the size of the Ca store; (b) the Ca fraction actually releasable; (c) the Ca^{++} inward current.

Whereas the amount of Ca within the store depends upon the end-diastolic cytosol Ca^{++} concentration, the releasability will be a function of the actual state of the plasmalemma. The higher the order and the smaller the kinetic energy of the membrane constituents the more tightly Ca will become bound to the

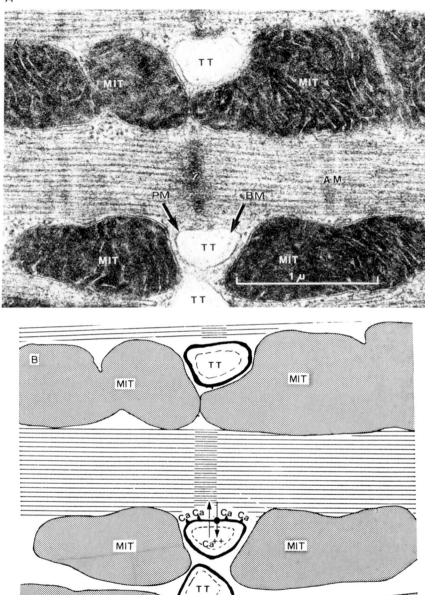

Figure 1.6 Ca movements in resting, excited, and repolarizing heart muscle. (A) Electron micrograph of guinea-pig ventricular muscle showing the intimate relation between transverse tubules (TT) and I bands of the sarcomere. MIT = mitochondria; AM = actomyosin; Z = Z-line, PM = plasmamembrane; BM = basement membrane. (B), (C) and (D) Schematic reproduction of electron micrograph A demonstrating Ca movements during rest (B), excitation (C), and repolarization (D). (B) Passive Ca leak and active compensation by the plasmalemmal Ca pump. (C) Ca^{++} release from

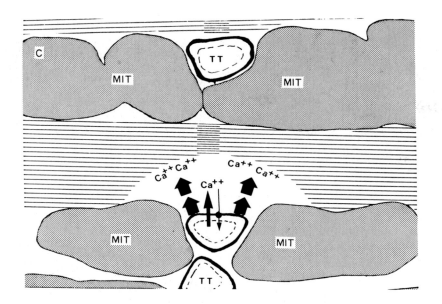

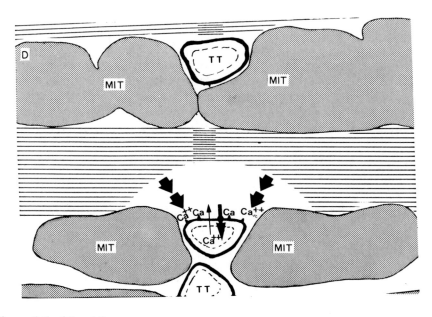

Figure 1.6 (*Cont'd*)

the high affinity, potential-dependent binding sites and the electrogenic slow Ca^{++} inward current. (D) Rebinding of Ca^{++} to the high affinity, potential-dependent binding site and active outward transport of Ca by the Ca,MgATPase. [Electron micrograph reproduced by courtesy of Dr Renate Lüllmann-Rauch, Department of Anatomy, University of Kiel] phospholipids, resulting in a reduced releasability, and vice versa. Any intervention which increases the kinetic disturbances of the plasmalemma, such as frequent depolarizations and a high turnover rate of the Na,K-ATPase, will augment the releasable fraction. The opposite will occur when the membrane constituents rearrange to attain a state of lower kinetic energy (low beat frequency), or if amphiphilic drugs intercalate between the polar lipids of the membrane, or if general anaesthetics alter the physicochemical state of the apolar membrane phase. The negative inotropic effect of interventions of this kind may be the result of one common mechanism, the reduced releasability of Ca^{++} from the high affinity store ('coupling insufficiency').

SUMMARY

Different cellular calcium pools are discussed with respect to their calcium binding and calcium pump ability at rest and during the contractile cycle of cardiac muscle. By means of calculations based on their affinity constant for Ca, on their relative size in proportion to cell volume, their capacity, and their rate of calcium binding or transport *in vitro*, the following picture arises: The predominant proportion of cellular calcium is located in the outer leaflet of the plasmalemma which is in equilibrium with the high extracellular Ca^{++} concentration. Only minor fractions are stored in mitochondria or in the sarcoplasmic reticulum, the pump activities of which are governed by the low intracellular Ca^{++} concentration. There exists ample evidence that even under the condition of cardiac activity the contribution of these 'stores' to sequester or to release Ca^{++} remains minor. From these aspects a high affinity, polarization-dependent binding site at the inner surface of the plasmalemma, which releases Ca^{++} upon depolarization and binds Ca^{++} upon repolarization, gains even more plausibility. The essentials of the mechanism outlined above are summarized schematically in Figure 1.6 on the basis of cardiac ultrastructure.

REFERENCES

Bers, D. M. (1979). Isolation and characterization of cardiac sarcolemma. *Biochim. Biophys. Acta.* **555**, 131–146.

Caroni, P., and Carafoli, E. (1981a). The Ca^{2+}-pumping ATPase of heart sarcolemma. Characterization, calmodulin dependence, and partial purification. *J. Biol. Chem.*, **236**, 3263–3270.

Caroni, P., and Carafoli, E. (1981b). Regulation of Ca^{2+}-pumping ATPase of heart sarcolemma by a phosphorylation–dephosphorylation process. *J. Biol. Chem.*, **256**, 9371–9373.

Chapman, R. A. (1979). Excitation–contraction coupling in cardiac muscle. *Prog. Biophys. Mol. Biol.*, **35**, 1–52.

Cielejewski, B., Lell, R., Preuner, J., and Rauch, U. (1980). Demonstration of an ouabain sensitive active Ca-extrusion mechanism in cardiac sarcolemma. *Naunyn-Schmiedeberg's Arch. Pharmacol.*, **311**, R40.

Ebashi, S., and Endo, M. (1968). Calcium ion and muscle contraction. *Prog. Biophys. Mol. Biol.*, **18**, 123–184.

Endo, M. (1977). Calcium release from the sarcoplasmic reticulum. *Phys. Rev.*, **57**, 71–108.

Fabiato, A., and Fabiato, F. (1979). Calcium and cardiac excitation–contraction coupling. *Annu. Rev. Physiol.*, **39**, 201–220.

Hui, E. C., Drummond, G. I., and Drummond, M. (1975). Isolation and characterization of plasma membrane-enriched fractions from guinea pig heart. *Advanc. Cyclic Nucleotide Res.*, **5**, 839.

Isenberg, G., and Klöckner, U. (1980). Glycocalyx is not required for slow inward calcium current in isolated rat heart myocytes. *Nature*, **234**, 358–360.

Kerrick, W. G. L., Malencik, D. A., Hoar, P. E., Potter, J. D., Coby, R. L., Pocinwong, S., and Fischer, E. H. (1980). Ca^{2+} and Sr^{2+} activation: comparison of cardiac and skeletal muscle contraction models. *Pflügers Arch. Europ. J. Physiol.*, **386**, 207–213.

Kitazawa, T. (1976). Physiological significance of Ca uptake by mitochondria in the heart in comparison with that of cardiac sarcoplasmic reticulum. *J. Biochem.*, **80**, 1129–1147.

Kliem, V. (1981). Preparation of an active Ca-pump in cardiac sarcolemma: experimental conditions for preservation of its functional state during isolation *Naunyn-Schmiedeberg's Arch. Pharmacol.*, **316**, R29.

Kliem, V., and Preuner, J. (1980). Inhibition of an active calcium transport system in cardiac sarcolemma by ouabain: involvement of sodium and potassium. *Naunyn-Schmiedeberg's Arch. Pharmacol.*, **313**, R41.

Körnich, H., and Lüllmann, H. (1970). The adaptation of the Ca content of cardiac muscle to altered external Ca concentration under various conditions. *Ärze. Forsch.*, **24**, 144–148.

Lahrtz, H. G., Lüllmann, H., and Van Zwieten, P. A. (1967). Calcium transport in isolated guinea-pig atria during metabolic inhibition. *Biochim. Biophys. Acta*, **135**, 701–709.

Lüllmann, H., and Peters, T., (1976). On the sarcolemmal site of action of cardiac glycosides. In *Recent Advanc. Stud. Cardiac Struct. Metab.*, **9**, 311–328.

Lüllmann, H., and Peters, T. (1977). Plasmalemmal calcium in cardiac excitation–contraction coupling. *Clin. Exp. Pharmacol. Physiol.*, **4**, 49–57.

Lüllmann, H., and Peters, T. (1979). Action of cardiac glycosides on the excitation–contraction coupling in heart muscle. *Prog. Pharmacol.*, **2**, 1–57.

Mullins, L. J. (1981). *Ion Transport in Heart*, Raven Press, New York.

Olbrich, H. G., and Preuner, J. (1982). The *in vivo* preformed effects of ouabain on the activity of the cardiac plasmalemmal Ca-pump of different species. *Naunyn-Schmiedeberg's Arch. Pharmacol.*, **319**, R41.

Pang, D. C. (1980). Effect of inotropic agents on the calcium binding to isolated sarcolemma. *Biochim. Biophys. Acta*, **598**, 528–542.

Preuner, J. (1979). Cardiac glycoside-induced changes of the Ca-binding in guinea pig plasmalemma. *Naunyn-Schmiedeberg's Arch. Pharmacol.*, **307**, R36.

Preuner, J. (1981). Ca-homeostasis in cardiac muscle cell: an active Ca-pump and its functional dependence on plasmamembrane bound Ca. *Naunyn-Schmiedeberg's Arch. Pharmacol.*, **316**, R30.

Scarpa, A., and Williamson, J. R. (1974). Calcium binding and calcium transport by subcellular fractions of heart. In *Calcium Binding Proteins* (eds W. Drabikowski, H. Strzelecka-Gobaszewska, and E. Carafoli), PWN, Warsaw, pp. 547–585.

Schatzmann, A. J., and Vincenzi, F. J. (1969). Calcium movements across the membrane of human red cells. *J. Physiol. (Lond.)*, **201**, 369–395.

Solaro, R. J., and Briggs, F. N. (1974). Estimating the functional capabilities of sarcoplasmic reticulum in cardiac muscle. *Circulation Res.*, **34,** 531–540.

Solaro, R. J., Wise, R. M., Shiner, J. S., and Briggs, F. N., (1974). Calcium requirement for cardiac myofibrillar activation. *Circulation Res.*, **34,** 525–530.

Spitzer, E., Grosse, R., Kuprinajov, V., and Preobrazhensky, A. (1981). Demonstration of a digitalis-sensitive sarcolemmal Ca^{2+}-pump functionally coupled with a membrane associated creatine phosphokinase. *Acta Biol. Med. Germ.*, **40,** 1111–1122.

Stam, A. C., Jr, Weglicki, W. B., Gertz, E. W., and Sonnenblick, E. H. (1973). A calcium-stimulated, ouabain-inhibited ATPase in a myocardial fraction enriched with sarcolemma. *Biochim. Biophys. Acta*, **298,** 927–931.

Sulakhe, P. V., and Dhalla, N. S. (1971). Excitation–contraction coupling in heart. VI. Demonstration of calcium activated ATPase in dog heart sarcolemma. *Life Sci.*, **10,** 185–191.

Sulakhe, P. V., and St Louis, P. J. (1976). Membrane phosphorylation and calcium transport in cardiac and skeletal muscle membranes. *Gen. Pharmacol.*, **7,** 313–319.

Van Alstyne, E., Bartschat, D. K., Wellsmith, N. V., Poe, S. L., Schilling, W. P., and Lindenmayer, G. E. (1979). Isolation of a highly enriched sarcolemma membrane fraction from canine heart. *Biochim. Biophys. Acta*, **553,** 388–395.

Zwaal, R. F. A., Roelofsen, B., and Colley, C. M. (1973). Localization of red cell membrane constituents. *Biochim. Biophys. Acta*, **300,** 159–182.

Cardiac Metabolism
Edited by A. J. Drake-Holland and M. I. M. Noble
© 1983 John Wiley & Sons Ltd

CHAPTER 2

Cardiac Sarcoplasmic Reticulum.

Lynda Blayney

*Department of Cardiology, Welsh National School of Medicine, Heath Park,
Cardiff CF4 4XN, UK*

INTRODUCTION

The sarcoplasmic reticulum (SR) is a discrete intracellular network of tubules surrounding the myofilaments which are found in all mammalian and many non-mammalian muscle types (Porter and Palade, 1957; Peachey, 1965). Its ascribed function is to regulate cytosolic calcium concentrations by sequestering calcium to effect relaxation and subsequently releasing it to contract the myofilaments. This was deduced from *in vitro* experimental evidence that microsomal fractions could relax isolated myofibrillar bundles (Marsh, 1951; Bendall, 1952; Weber, 1971; Ebashi, 1958) by removing calcium from the medium in the presence of magnesium and adenosine triphosphate (ATP) (Ebashi, 1961; Hasselbach and Makinose, 1961). These calcium-accumulating microsomal fractions were concluded to be membrane vesicles derived from the SR (Porter, 1961). These observations were made on skeletal muscle preparations; there are some reservations about a strictly analagous role for cardiac SR, see Lüllmann *et al.*, Chapter 1 and Drake-Holland and Nobel, Chapter 17, in this volume.

MORPHOLOGY

The SR consists of tubules, the membranes of which surround a discrete lumen that is not connected to either the extracellular space nor to the cytoplasm. From its ultrastructural appearance the SR can be roughly divided into two categories, junctional SR and longitudinal (free) SR. Junctional SR is associated with either the sarcolemma, where it forms peripheral couplings (subsarcolemmal cisternae), or the T-tubules, where it forms internal couplings (terminal cisternae). The SR membrane that forms the junctional couplings has junctional processes (feet) protruding from it, which sometimes appear to be attached to the sarcolemma or T-tubule

19

Table 2.1 Major proteins isolated from skeletal and cardiac SR

Protein	Location	Function	Morphological feature	Cardiac molecular weight (daltons)	Skeletal molecular weight (daltons)	References
Ca ATPase	Spans SR membrane	Active transport of Ca into lumen	4 nm particles on membrane surface in negative staining; 9 nm particles of internal membrane revealed by freeze fracture	100 000	100 000	MacLennan, 1975; Ikemoto et al., 1968; Inesi and Scales, 1974; Deamer and Baskin, 1969
Calsequestrin	SR lumen	Ca binding and storage	Electron dense granules in lumen	55 000?	46 000–65 000	MacLennan, 1975; Jones and Cala, 1981
Phospholamban	Cytoplasmic leaflet of membrane	Regulation (by cAMP and protein-kinase phosphorylation of Ca-ATPase activity	—	22–24 000	Absent	Tada et al., 1975a; Bidlack and Shamoo, 1980

6000 dalton protein		Phosphorylated by cAMP and protein-kinase	—	6000	Absent	Tada et al., 1975a; Jones et al., 1978b
High affinity Ca binding protein	Luminal leaflet of membrane	Unknown; Ca binding and storage	—		55 000	MacLennan 1975
50 000–55 000 dalton protein	—	Unknown	—	50–55 000	?	Campbell et al., 1980
34 000–33 000 dalton protein	Outer surface of junctional SR	Apparent connection of SR T-tubule or SR and SL	Junctional processes or feet		34 000–38 000	Campbell et al., 1980
30 000–33 000 dalton protein	Junctional SR intrinsic membrane protein associated with feet				30 000–33 000	Campbell et al., 1980
Proteolipid(s)	Hydrophobic interior of membrane	Coupling factor for ATPase and Ca transport/structural aid during assembly/ionophone for Ca release			12 000, 13 600, 11 900	MacLennan, 1975; Sarzala et al., 1975; Knowles et al., 1980; Racker and Eytan, 1975

membranes (Sommer and Waugh, 1976; Scales, 1981). Junctional SR represents about 20% of total SR volume in both rabbit and rat (Page, 1978).

Longitudinal SR forms a tight network around the myofibrils, which form a collar at the M-rete, which may be a specialization to increase the surface area (Scales, 1981). Structural features are the 4 nm particles which are observed on the outer face of the longitudinal SR by negative staining and are part of the calcium pump protein (Ikemoto *et al.*, 1968; Inesi and Scales, 1974). It is a matter of some debate whether the calcium pump functions as a monomer or in oligomeric form (Ikemoto *et al.*, 1981).

A number of observations suggest a constant proportionality between SR and myofibrillar volume density in relation to age in adult rat (Page *et al.*, 1974), in developing rabbit heart (Page and Beucker, 1981), and in comparison of right ventricle and left ventricle of rat heart (Page and Surdyk-Droske, 1979).

Isolated SR Preparations

In vitro preparations of SR from homogenates of muscle are shown to be vesicles bounded by the SR membrane. In cardiac muscle, it is extremely difficult to obtain pure fractions of SR vesicles. In particular SR preparations contain contaminating sarcolemma vesicles (Jones *et al.*, 1978b) and some derived from mitochondria (Lighty and Bertrand, 1979; Blayney *et al.*, 1978). Loading vesicles with calcium oxalate (Levitsky *et al.*, 1976; Jones *et al.*, 1979) or phosphate (Bonnet *et al.*, 1978) to increase their density and then separation by sucrose density gradient centrifugation is possible, but as few as 10% of vesicles take up oxalate and subsequent study of the kinetics of calcium movement with such loaded vesicles is difficult. In spite of this two types of cardiac SR vesicle have been described (Jones and Cala, 1981). These are distinguished by their ability to take up oxalate. Sucrose density gradient centrifugation has been used to separate SR from sarcolemma but it is a lengthy procedure (Jaqua-Stewart *et al.*, 1979; Lighty and Bertrand, 1979).

SR Molecular Structure

The molecular structure of the cardiac SR has not been studied as extensively as that of skeletal muscle. The proteins (Table 2.1) have been isolated and identified. The major component (30–35% in cardiac SR), is the calcium pump (Shigekawa *et al.*, 1976; Suko and Hasselbach, 1976). The 4 nm particles on the cytoplasmic leaflet of the membrane can be removed by digestion with trypsin and this also eliminates calcium-activated magnesium ATPase activity. The particles contain the active site for ATP hydrolysis, since the presence of ATP protects the vesicles from inactivation by sulphydryl agents. Progressive digestion of SR vesicles with trypsin yields initially 40 000 and 55 000 dalton active fragments of the calcium pump protein. A 20 000 dalton fragment has been identified as the ionophoric component of the calcium pump protein. It is thought that the ATPase section of the molecule with specific calcium binding sites confers selectivity for the transport of calcium (Tada *et al.*, 1978b). The proteolipid component of SR membranes is also associated with the calcium pump activity and when added to reconstituted systems greatly improves the transport ratio, and has thus been assigned as a coupling factor (Racker and Eytan, 1975).

The SR membrane is physically traversed by the calcium pump and functionally by calcium; however, the actual mechanisms by which calcium makes this passage into and out of the SR lumen are still speculative. A number of models have been proposed for active calcium transport. The rotary carrier model suggests the calcium pump molecule physically rotating through the membrane. The mobile pore model predicts a conformational change in the calcium pump molecule to open and close a calcium channel. The fixed pore model suggests a number of carrier molecules which successively alter in affinity and thus pass calcium down a fixed transmembrane channel (Tada *et al.*, 1978b).

Both calsequestrin and the high affinity calcium binding protein are extrinsic proteins, i.e. loosely associated with the SR membrane and thus easily removed by washing with mild detergent. They differ in the quantity of calcium they can bind and in the affinity of their binding sites. Calsequestrin has 43 binding sites and the high affinity calcium-binding protein about half that number (Ostwald and MacLennan, 1974). They are located within the lumen of the SR and are thought to serve as calcium storage sites, and in so doing lower the luminal free calcium concentration.

Phospholipids represent about 80% of the total lipid and all but 5% of the other 20% is cholesterol. The predominant phospholipid is phosphatidylcholine, up to 70% of the total, and between 12 and 19% of the remainder is phosphatidylethanolamine; the remaining 10–12% is phosphatidylinositol, phosphatidylserine, sphingomyelin, and cardiolipin. Thirty molecules of lipid are found to interact directly with the calcium pump molecule, although a total of 90 are associated with each molecule. Calcium pump activity can be reconstituted by adding phosphatidylcholine alone, although maximum activity requires phosphatidylethanolamine as well (Tada *et al.*, 1978b).

ENZYME MECHANISM OF CALCIUM ACCUMULATION

The way in which ATP hydrolysis is coupled to calcium transport by the calcium-activated magnesium ATPase (calcium pump) has been extensively studied in skeletal muscle. For every molecule of ATP hydrolysed, two molecules of calcium are transported across the membrane into the SR lumen. The stoicheiometry is $1\,ATP:2\,Ca^{++}$; the transport ratio is 2. Two molecules of Ca^{++}, one of ATP, and one of Mg^{++} (Kanazawa *et al.*, 1971) bind in random sequence to specific binding sites on the calcium pump at the cytoplasmic side of the SR vesicle (Tada *et al.*, 1978b):

$$
\begin{array}{c}
\text{Mg-ATP} \\
| \\
E
\end{array}
\tag{2.1}
$$

The next step is a transition of the enzyme binding both $2\,Ca^{++}$ and ATP to form a high energy phosphorylated (acyl phosphate) intermediate (termed EP) with the resultant loss of ADP to the cytoplasm. A minimal reaction sequence for the calcium pump has been proposed (Makinose, 1971):

$$
\tag{2.2}
$$

where E represents the enzyme (calcium-activated magnesium-ATPase), E^* represents a different conformational and/or energetic form of E, Ca_o is calcium outside the SR lumen, Ca_i is calcium inside the SR lumen, and $E\sim P$ represents a high energy acyl phosphate bond.

EP decomposition requires magnesium (Kanazawa *et al.*, 1971) and is the step which dissociates calcium into the lumen of the SR. Magnesium binds to EP and there is a resultant dramatic decrease in the affinity for calcium. Phosphate is released to the cytoplasm. It is the dissociation of EP that is the rate-limiting step of calcium accumulation (Cheisi and Inesi, 1979):

$$
\begin{array}{c}
P \\
| \\
E \\
\diagup\;\diagdown \\
Ca \quad\; Ca
\end{array}
+ Mg^{++} \rightleftharpoons
\begin{array}{c}
E \\
| \\
Mg^{++}
\end{array}
+ P_i + 2Ca^{++}
\tag{2.3}
$$

This series of reactions is fully reversible (Makinose, 1971) and under conditions where there is high calcium concentration in the vesicles, and a low magnesium concentration, and when ADP (together with EGTA to lower the external calcium concentration) is added, ATP can be formed via EP (Kanazawa *et al.*, 1970, 1971). EP formation precedes calcium translocation and once saturated reaches a steady state of formation and decomposition. This steady state rate of calcium pump activity can be stimulated by increasing ATP concentrations (Kanazawa *et al.*, 1971; Yamamoto and Tonomura, 1967), a process thought to involve the rapid transition between two E–ATP complexes according to the equation

$$E + ATP \leftrightharpoons E\text{–}ATP \underset{\underset{\text{stimulated by ATP}}{\uparrow}}{\rightharpoonup} E^*\text{–}ATP \leftrightharpoons EP + ADP \qquad (2.4)$$

The internal calcium concentration of the vesicle also controls calcium pump activity, such that high concentrations decrease the rate (Weber, 1971). It was proposed that the enzymic basis of this observation was the inhibition of magnesium-dependent EP decomposition by calcium (Yamada and Tonomura, 1972). Stimulation of calcium pump activity by potassium has been reported. It was proposed that potassium was a countertransport ion of the ATPase (Kanazawa *et al.*, 1971).

Early work on the preparations of vesicles isolated from cardiac muscle and labelled as SR preparations demonstrated that these too could accumulate calcium and possessed calcium 'activated' magnesium ATPase activity. However, calcium accumulation even in the presence of oxalate was slower, and expressed as calcium accumulated per milligram of protein was quantitatively less than that observed in skeletal muscle (Baskin and Deamer, 1969). Calcium-'activated' magnesium ATPase activity had to be measured against a comparatively high 'basic' or magnesium ATPase activity, which seems characteristic of cardiac muscle preparations, particularly the rat (Hollingworth and England, 1978; Penpargkul, 1979). The stoicheiometry of calcium accumulation is usually much less than 2 (Jones and Besch, 1979), although some workers report the value 2 (Tada *et al.*, 1974, 1979). Calcium accumulation measured in the absence of oxalate was termed calcium binding and in its presence calcium uptake (Harigaya and Schwartz, 1969). Based on kinetic differences between calcium binding and uptake and other distinguishing features of the two preparations fundamental differences between calcium accumulation in cardiac and skeletal SR preparations have been postulated by the group of Dr. A. Schwartz.

More recent work, along the lines of that on skeletal muscle, unequivocally demonstrated that the calcium pump in the two tissues is essentially the same. The formation of EP is common to both and experiments on EP formation and decomposition (Shigekawa *et al.*, 1976) have shown that the turnover of the calcium pump is similar in both tissues, but that in cardiac muscle the affinity for the calcium binding sites is lower and the pump density on the membrane is less. This accounts for the comparatively 3.5 times slower rate of calcium transport in cardiac muscle. EP formation is slower in cardiac (Sumida *et al.*, 1978) than skeletal muscle. EP decomposition is the rate-limiting step of calcium pump activity in both cardiac and skeletal muscle. It is subject to allosteric control by Mg-ATP, Mg^{++}, and K^+ (Jones *et al.*, 1978a). K^+ has been implicated in the stimulation of the calcium pump by several workers (Jones *et al.*, 1978a; Briggs *et al.*, 1978; Jones, 1979) and may, in addition to accelerating EP decomposition, increase its rate of formation (Briggs *et al.*, 1978). Examination of nucleoside triphosphate (NTP/P_i) exchange reactions in SR prepared from canine ventricle yield results that are entirely compatible with Makinose's reaction sequence for calcium pump activity (Plank *et al.*, 1979); see equation (2.2).

Some differences between the two systems have been reported. It has been demonstrated that unlike skeletal muscle, cardiac SR cannot use GTP as a substitute for ATP in calcium translocation. However, GTP is hydrolysed, but this is not coupled to EP formation (Van Winkle *et al.*, 1981). Small differences in the action of potassium and ADP on the transient state kinetics of the calcium pump have been noted for rabbit skeletal and dog cardiac muscle (Wang *et al.*, 1981). Immunological studies of cross-reactivity of antibodies to rabbit skeletal and cardiac calcium pump proteins have shown them to be different (Defloor *et al.*, 1980). Comparing the capacity of isolated vesicles (of presumed similar volume) to sequester calcium may not be a true comparison of the *in vivo* calcium-sequestering ability of skeletal and cardiac SR.

REGULATIONS OF SARCOPLASMIC RETICULUM FUNCTION

Adrenergic agonists enhance contractility and the ability of heart muscle to relax (Graham and Lamb, 1968; Morad and Rolett, 1972). The beta-adrenergic system is thought to exert its influence intracellularly via adenylate cyclase, which produces cyclic AMP (cAMP). Cyclic AMP activates the enzyme protein kinase which phosphorylates a serine residue of a 22 000 dalton protein called phospholamban (Tada *et al.*, 1975a). Phospholamban can be dephosphorylated by phosphoprotein phosphatase (Tada *et al.*, 1975b). An outline of cardiac SR in the overall control of intracellular calcium concentrations is given in Figure 2.1. Further consideration is given in other chapters in this volume – cAMP by Van Belle (Chapter 18) and phosphorylation of SR membrane protein by Drake-Holland and Noble (Chapter 17).

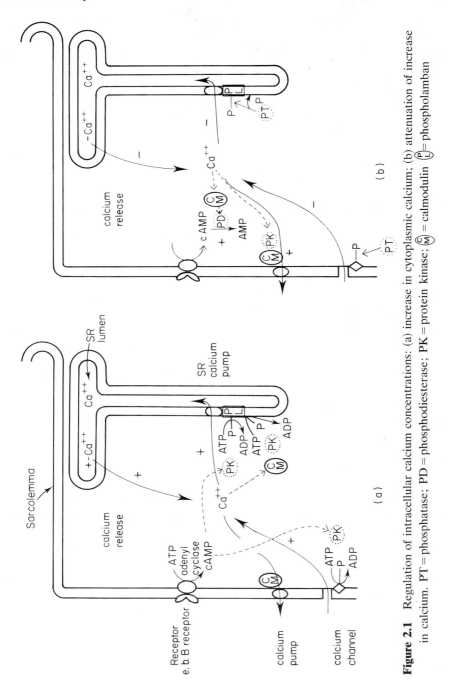

Figure 2.1 Regulation of intracellular calcium concentrations: (a) increase in cytoplasmic calcium; (b) attenuation of increase in calcium. PT = phosphatase; PD = phosphodiesterase; PK = protein kinase; Ⓒ = calmodulin ⓁⒼ = phospholamban

PHYSIOLOGICAL IMPORTANCE OF SR CALCIUM
REGULATION

Cyclic AMP-mediated regulation of calcium transport by cardiac SR is generally accepted to be one of the important routes by which catecholamines exert their influence on cardiac muscle (see Figure 2.1). The binding of catecholamines (such as noradrenaline) to the beta-receptor on the exterior of the sarcolemma stimulates adenylate cyclase leading to cAMP production. This in turn activates protein kinase, which phosphorylates phospholamban, which in turn increases turnover of the calcium pump. This accelerates relaxation and has its physiological equivalent in the abbreviation of systole. If the result of increased uptake of calcium into the SR is that a greater fraction of calcium is subsequently available for release at the next beat, contractility is enhanced (Drake-Holland and Noble, Chapter 17 in this volume).

The effects of calmodulin are less easy to understand. It has been demonstrated that *in vitro* the effects of calmodulin are additive to or even essential for cAMP stimulation of calcium uptake into the SR. Following work on red blood cells it has been postulated that the role for calmodulin is both to mediate (cf. troponin-C) and to terminate the effects of calcium on intracellular activity, thus providing a 'fail safe' mechanism to prevent over-activity (Vincenzi and Larsen, 1980). This interpretation could be extended to cardiac muscle on the assumption that the effects observed on isolated SR preparations are due to the action of calmodulin on contaminating sarcolemma (Figure 2.1). A calcium pump has been demonstrated in cardiac sarcolemma (as in red blood cell plasmalemma) which is stimulated by a calmodulin-dependent protein kinase (see Chapter 1 in this volume). It is useful to reflect that it has always been the dilemma of biochemists that 'test-tube' phenomena may need careful interpretation for a plausible physiological role to be postulated. (For further discussion see Drake-Holland and Noble, Chapter 17 in this volume.)

CALCIUM RELEASE

In skeletal muscle calcium is pumped into the SR and stored there to effect relaxation, but calcium is probably also the sole source of calcium for contraction. Cardiac muscle, is absolutely dependent upon extracellular calcium for contraction and indeed the strength of contraction is related to the extracellular calcium concentration (Nobel, Chapter 3, and Lewartowski, Chapter 5 in this volume).

Calcium is thought to be released from the SR in response to depolarization of the sarcolemma and T-system. The mechanisms postulated to bring this about are controversial, and no definite proof in favour of any currently holds sway. The two mechanisms currently under debate are depolarization-induced calcium release and calcium-induced calcium release. Both have been demonstrated in cardiac and skeletal muscle.

Calcium-induced Calcium Release

This phenomenon was first demonstrated in skeletal muscle by Ford and Podolsky (1970) (for a review see Endo, 1977), and in cardiac muscle by Fabiato and Fabiato (1975a). It was shown using 'skinned' fibres (i.e. fibres whose sarcolemma has been rendered permeable to ions by chemical or mechanical means) that the addition of small increments of calcium, them-selves insufficient to cause contraction, could evoke a contractile response by releasing calcium from internal stores – the SR. The characteristics of this type of release are that it is progressively inhibited by magnesium. The lower the magnesium concentration, the lower the concentration of calcium necessary to induce release. There was also a loading threshold below which calcium cannot be released; this threshold could be lowered by increasing the stimulating calcium concentration or by decreasing the magnesium. The amount of calcium released was increased by increasing the level of calcium loading (Fabiato and Fabiato, 1979).

The relationship between and magnitude of loading and/or subsequent calcium-induced release is affected by pH, cAMP/protein kinase phosphory-lation, caffeine, and local anaesthetics (Fabiato and Fabiato, 1975a, 1978a). It was shown that the calcium content of the SR had to reach a particular threshold level between contractions before calcium-induced calcium release could be triggered (Fabiato and Fabiato, 1979). So it was argued that such release could be a graded process where the amount of calcium entering the calcium stores dictated the quantity available for release at the next beat, and was also responsive to changes in amount of 'trigger' calcium entering during the calcium current. The calcium concentration in skeletal muscle that is necessary to induce release is as high as that required to saturate the myofilaments (Endo, 1977), i.e. too high to be a physiological trigger. However, in heart the threshold for release was within the necessary physiological range (10^{-7} M); in rat in particular the threshold was much lower than in dog, cat, rabbit, human, or frog (Fabiato and Fabiato, 1978b).

Studies on the rate of calcium efflux from isolated SR vesicles from skeletal muscle (Katz *et al.*, 1977a,b) when loaded with calcium oxalate or calcium phosphate have shown that the concentration of calcium ions across the SR membrane can radically alter the permeability of the SR membrane and the rate of calcium efflux from the vesicles. A 3000-fold change in the $[Ca]_i : [Ca]_o$ ratio resulted in a 1000-fold difference in permeability of skeletal SR vesicle membranes, with a maximum rate of calcium efflux of

10^{-10} mol cm^{-2} s^{-1} ($[Ca]_o$ 0.1–3.3 μM, $[Ca]_i$ 4–750 μM). This was approximately one order of magnitude smaller than that calculated to be necessary to match the rate of tension development in skeletal muscle (Ashley and Ridgway, 1970). Similar experiments also suggested that the rate of calcium transport was linked to the rate of subsequent calcium efflux (Katz *et al.*, 1977a). This supported the findings in skinned muscle fibres of the relationship between uptake and release, although the *in vitro* experiments did not match skinned fibre rates.

Where is the site of calcium efflux and what is the mechanism bringing it about? The calcium pump has been implicated as the protein involved in calcium release by experiments incorporating this into lipid bilayer, where its presence increased the passive permeability for calcium (and nonselectively that of other anions and cations); however, a further 1000-fold increase would have been necessary to match physiological rates of efflux (Jilka *et al.*, 1975). The appearance of calcium-induced calcium release in developing rat hearts has been found to coincide with the appearance of increased calcium pump activity that appears around birth (Martonosi, 1975; Nayler and Fassold, 1977). It was found that passive efflux was greater in light (longitudinal SR) than heavy vesicles (junctional SR) and concluded that this was because there was a greater concentration of calcium pump protein in these light vesicles (Louis *et al.*, 1980). Both spontaneous calcium release and calcium uptake have been shown to have a similar calcium dependence (Katz *et al.*, 1980) and the rate of spontaneous calcium release is related to calcium uptake (Katz *et al.*, 1977b).

Depolarization-induced Calcium Release

It has been proposed that the SR membrane can itself be depolarized, which alters the permeability for stored calcium and promotes rapid release. Evidence for depolarization has come from a number of sources.

A slowly penetrating anion such as propionate or methanosulphate, or a cation such as Na$^+$, Tris$^+$, choline$^+$, or Li$^+$, was substituted for a more rapidly penetrating anion (such as Cl$^-$) or cation (such as K$^+$). Calcium release resulted in both skinned muscle fibres (Endo and Nakajima, 1973) and isolated SR vesicles (Kasai and Miyamoto, 1973; Inesi and Malan, 1976). The concentrations of ions required for the latter are greater than those required for skinned fibres; there is some dispute that the osmotic effects of changing the ionic environment might be the cause of calcium release in isolated preparations.

Some workers have tried to demonstrate the existence of a membrane potential across the SR membrane. Birefringence studies – which had been shown to coincide with membrane potential changes in nerve (Cohen *et al.*,

1971) – detected three temporal components following electrical stimulation of skeletal muscle. The first corresponded to the action potential, the second was thought to reflect a potential change in the SR, and the third to conformational changes of the contractile proteins. Based on known values for the potential change across the sarcolemma, it was calculated that the change in membrane potential across the SR was 135 mV (Baylor and Oetliker, 1975). Intracellular electrodes have detected potential changes in response to local stimulation (Strickholm, 1974) or propagated contractions (Natori, 1975). These experiments have all been done on skeletal muscle.

If a useful potential difference exists across the SR then it must be of the order of 100 mV (Endo, 1977). The only ion pump in the membrane is the Ca-ATPase, but this would have to be extremely efficient to produce an important membrane potential and would have to be electrogenic. An inside positive potential has been measured by Beeler (1980). Membrane potentials altered both calcium transport and ATP hydrolysis. An electrogenic model of calcium transport has been proposed (Zimniak and Racker, 1978) and evidence has been obtained (from measurement of light scattering) for osmotic change with calcium accumulation (Kometani and Kasai, 1980). A cotransport model of calcium exchange may be necessary to explain K stimulation effects (Chiu and Haynes, 1980). Experiments on the distribution of ions across the SR membrane between the cytoplasm and SR lumen have shown an equal distribution except for calcium being higher in the SR lumen in relaxed muscle (Somlyo *et al.*, 1977).

Protons may be important to control of calcium release, it has been shown that protons can diffuse freely through the SR memebrane during calcium transport (Meissner and Young, 1980) and indeed protons are suggested as the countertransport ion to calcium (Chiesi and Inesi, 1980) – with a burst of proton ejection with the initial phase of calcium transport (Madeira, 1980). A model has been proposed where the proton gradient so generated controls a calcium release channel (Shoshan *et al.*, 1981). Dissipation of the proton gradient (by some mechanism related to excitation – as yet unknown) opens up the channel and high cytoplasmic calcium closes it (negative feedback).

There is much recent evidence for a monovalent cation channel in SR (Miller and Rosenberg, 1979). The number of these channels is thought to be 1% of the total calcium pump molecules, but the transport rate for K^+ was four times greater than the turnover rate of the pump. Potassium ions could therefore flow as quickly as calcium was transported (Labarca *et al.*, 1980). It is argued that the role of the channel is to maintain electroneutrality; measurement of the Donnan potential of vesicles using a fluorescent cyanine dye has shown no significant variation during calcium transport (Yamamoto and Kasai, 1980). Acid pH and calcium binding block the channel (Miller and Rosenberg, 1979; Bennett and Dupont, 1981). Gating by calcium in this way may regulate the channel via the cytoplasmic calcium concentrations.

The mechanism by which the depolarization of the T-tubule brings about calcium release from the SR is uncertain, the specialized junctions seem suitable sites for the 'message' promoting release to be transferred. Indeed, junctional SR rather than longitudinal SR may be the site of calcium release in skeletal muscle (Winegrad, 1965). A correlation has also been found between the number of junctional couplings and the threshold for calcium-induced calcium release (Page and Surdyk-Droske, 1979). The passage of a depolarizing current across the junction to depolarize the SR is thought to be incompatible with the morphological appearance. A coupling of low resistance where the current could run directly from the T-tubule to SR requires close proximity of the membranes, but the gap (containing the feet) is 30 nm, and therefore too wide. Capacitive coupling, where the charge on the sarcolemma induces a charge on the SR would require the junction to have material (i.e. the feet) of high dielectric constant, and would need a greater total area of contact between sarcolemma and SR than that observed (Franzini-Armstrong, 1980). While Schneider and Chandler (1973) proposed that the depolarization of the T-tubule created a voltage-related charge transfer, Chiu *et al.* (1980) (again using skeletal muscle) isolated heavy vesicles that possibly corresponded to junctional SR and proposed calcium as the trigger for charge movement. Can this mechanism reconcile the two theories of calcium or depolarization induced calcium release by being common to both?

COMPARATIVE STUDIES OF SR FUNCTION

Comparison of different muscle types and different species have contributed much to our understanding of the way in which biochemical mechanisms govern mechanical performance. Heart rate generally increases as the body weight of a species decreases as compensation for a relatively greater requirement for cardiac output in small animals (Holt *et al.*, 1968; Whyte *et al.*, 1978). The faster the heart rate, the greater the rates of contraction and relaxation (Henderson *et al.*, 1970).

Species differences in the contribution of extracellular calcium to the cytosolic ('contractile') calcium required for tension development have been suggested. Rat, in particular, differs from species with slower heart rates in having no plateau phase to its action potential. The plateau is partly associated with the slow inward calcium current, and the rat also possesses a negative frequency staircase, which indicates that increasing frequency of contraction depletes the internal (SR) stores of calcium. These facts suggest that rat relies more heavily on the release from SR for its 'contractile' calcium than other species (Langer *et al.*, 1975): A correlation between contractility and calcium binding to the sarcolemma has been shown in isolated sarcolemmal vesicles from hearts of rabbit, neonatal rat, and frog, which did not hold for adult rat or rabbit atrium. The data was interpreted on the lines of a correlation between calcium binding and calcium influx, the calcium influx being largely responisible for the 'contractile' calcium in rabbit, neonatal rat, and frog. However, adult rat and rabbit atrium are postulated to rely more heavily on calcium-induced calcium release from the SR (Bers *et al.*, 1981). In support of this is the finding that adult rat SR has a much lower threshold for such release (although this is not so for neonatal rat where such release cannot be detected; Fabiato and Fabiato, 1978b), and more junctional couplings than other species (Page and Surdyk-Droske, 1979) – these couplings being the putative sites of triggering calcium release from the SR.

The rate of calcium accumulation by isolated SR vesicles has also been shown to correlate with heart rate comparing rat, guinea-pig, rabbit, and sheep (Table 2.2). This is the exponential rate constant for calcium accumulation (without oxalate) measured with dual wavelength spectrophotometry and the indicator arsenazo III. Similar species differences for guinea-pig, rabbit, and rat have been described using the indicator murexide (Nayler *et al.*, 1975). The exponential rate constant is essentially a filling time for the isolated SR vesicles. Since vesicle size (surface to volume ratio) was not species variable (Table 2.2) the observed differences in rate constant might reflect the intrinsic rate of the calcium pump. It has been suggested that different pump rates may result from species differences in the lipid environment of the ATPase molecule (Chiesi and Inesi, 1979). Alternatively, differences in calcium pump density in the SR membrane may be important because the number of internal membrane particles correlates with relaxation speed in different muscle (Franzini-Armstrong, 1980; Heilmann *et al.*, 1980).

The exponential rate constant for calcium accumulation is expressed independent of SR vesicle protein. The lack of correlation with heart rate of the other measurements of calcium pump activity might be due to methodological problems, (Blayney *et al.*, 1977). Of interest is the correlation of basic magnesium-ATPase activity with heart rate. The unusually high basic activity in rat heart has been noted before (Hollingworth and England, 1978; Penpargkul, 1979), and a histochemical study suggests that its origin is the sarcolemma (Malouf and Meissner, 1980). Also the basic ATPase activity could have come from contaminating contractile or mitochondrial proteins, (Blayney *et al.*, 1978).

The yield of SR protein also correlates with heart rate. This could have reflected ease of recovery, but collagen content (hydroxyproline) did not show a concomitant correlation. There is no evidence that SR volume

Table 2.2 Species differences in myocardial SR properties and hydroxyproline content

	Sheep	Rabbit	Guinea-pig	Rat	Significant differences†	Significant correlation ($P < 0.001$) with natural heart rate (r value)
Yield of SR (mg protein per gram wet weight of ventricle)	0.358±0.03 (6)	0.923±0.087 (12)	0.940±0.113 (12)	1.582±0.101 (18)	1, 2, 3, 5, 6	0.813
Basic ATPase (nmol ATP per milligram of SR protein per minute)	153±14.7 (6)	516±41 (12)	787±157 (12)	1260±161 (12)	1, 2, 3, 5, 6	0.772
Ca-ATPase at 60 µM Ca (nmol ATP per milligram of SR protein per minute)	77±11 (6)	318±37 (12)	268±22 (12)	152±43 (12)	1, 2, 5, 6	—

Ca accumulated (without oxalate) (nmol Ca per milligram of SR protein)	29.3±8.6 (5)	36.1±4.1 (9)	23.0±2.0 (6)	25.0±1.5 (6)	1, 4, 5	—
Rate constant of Ca accumulated (without oxalate), $t_{1/2}$ (s)	46.7±6.3 (5)	24.8±2.2 (9)	23.7±2.4 (6)	17.5±1.6 (6)	1, 2, 3, 5, 6	0.729
Ca accumulated (with oxalate) (nmol Ca per milligram of SR protein) — at 1 min	167±34 (6)	328±33 (6)	1239±112 (6)	256±36 (6)	1, 2, 4, 6	—
at 10 min	567±65 (6)	987±77 (6)	1842±106 (6)	1159±168 (6)	1, 2, 3, 4, 6	—
Hydroxyproline (μg per milligram of wet weight ventricle)	1.01±0.05 (6)	0.88±0.04 (6)	0.50±0.05 (7)	0.75±0.02 (7)	2, 3, 4, 5, 6	—
Natural heart rate (beats min[1])	75*	227±6.9 (5)§	277±14 (6)§	443±6 (6)§	—	—
Surface:volume ratio	0.866±0.07 (5)	0.828±0.08 (5)	0.756±0.04 (5)	0.784±0.01 (5)	NS	—

Mean ± S.E.M. values are shown; the values in parentheses indicated the number of samples.
† Significant ($P < 0.05$) differences between sheep and rabbit (1), and sheep and pig (2), sheep and rat (3), rabbit and guinea-pig (4), rabbit and rat (5), and guinea-pig and rat (6). NS = not significant.
§ See Henderson *et al.* (1970).
* See Swenson in Dukes Physiology of Domestic Animals (Cornstock, 1977).

density is species variable, so the reason for the yield correlation with heart rates is unknown.

PATHOLOGY AND SR FUNCTION

SR function is altered in a variety of pathological conditions; it is not known whether this is compensatory or the prime cause. Most of the observed changes are in animal models designed to mimic a particular human condition.

All models of heart failure have shown a decreased activity of the SR calcium pump (e.g. Harigaya and Schwartz, 1969; Suko *et al.*, 1970; Mead *et al.*, 1971; Sordahl *et al.*, 1973; Ito *et al.*, 1974), as one study of compensated hypertrophy (Ito *et al.*, 1974) but not in another (Swynghedauw *et al.*, 1973). Indeed, increased activity of the calcium pump in 'mild' cardiac hypertrophy has been reported (Limas *et al.*, 1980) and the activity attributed to increased pump density. There are indications that SR function may begin to decline before the stage of heart failure (Ito *et al.*, 1974). It has been shown by the author's own group, using pulmonary artery banding in sheep to produce compensated cardiac hypertrophy, that SR function is impaired when myosin isoenzyme content and mitochondrial respiratory function are normal. This suggests that decline of SR function may provide the earliest detectable biochemical disturbance characteristic of compensated hypertrophy. This may possibly be a contributory factor in the process of decomposition. Changes in SR function in mechanical overload induced hypertrophy and the differences reported may well relate to the duration, severity, and animal model chosen. SR function is enhanced in rats following a swimming regime (Penpargkul *et al.*, 1977) and following physical training by running (Penpargkul *et al.*, 1980).

Hyper- and hypothyroidism result in opposite effects on SR calcium pump activity (Nayler *et al.*, 1971a; Suko, 1971, 1973; Limas, 1978). One exception to the observations was a very long term study of thyroxin administration to dogs (Conway *et al.*, 1976). The rate of pump turnover was unaffected (Limas, 1980a) but there was an increased affinity for calcium (Limas, 1978). Changes in cardiac membrane lipid (Limas, 1978, 1980a) have been suggested to alter calcium pump activity by altering the fluidity of the membrane (Chiesi, 1979). Coincident with the changes in the calcium pump activity was an increase in the quantity of endogenous protein kinase (Newcomb *et al.*, 1978; Limas, 1978) and resultant phosphorylation of phospholamban (Limas, 1978) and an increase in beta-receptor numbers (Ciaralidi and Martinetti, 1977; Limas, 1980b).

Spontaneously hypertensive rats (SHR) show a gradually increasing hypertrophy with age, starting at around 4 weeks (Bhalla and Ashley, 1978). SR calcium pump activity is reduced (Aoki *et al.*, 1974; Limas and Cohn,

1977; Heilmann *et al.*, 1980), as is the number of internal membrane particles (Heilmann *et al.*, 1980). Interestingly, hypertrophy produced by the two methods (hypertension and hyperthyroidism) have opposite features. In that in SHR the number of beta-receptors is reduced (Limas, 1978), as are adenylate cyclase (Bhalla and Ashley, 1978) and protein kinase levels (Limas and Cohn, 1977; Bhalla *et al.*, 1982). Increased sympathetic activity may be a contributory factor in SHR, and this is noted for a 'turn-down' in the responsiveness to catecholamine stimulation due to the reduction in beta-receptor numbers (Mukherjee *et al.*, 1975).

A notable feature of isoprenaline-treated animals is necrotic areas of tissue (Rona *et al.*, 1959). The cause of the necrosis is thought to be calcium overload, due to massive influx of calcium (Fleckenstein, 1971) with reduced calcium pump activity and swelling of the SR has been observed following isoprenaline administration with severe swelling and disruption in necrotic cells. Again the decline in SR function is accompanied by a decrease in beta-receptor numbers, adenylate cyclase activity, and protein kinase activity, and an increase in phosphodiesterase (Tse *et al.*, 1978, 1979). Chronic isoprenaline administration resulted in increased soluble protein kinase that returned to normal when the hypertrophy stabilized (Horwood and Singhal, 1976).

Decline of SR function in various models of ischaemia have been reported, although the degree depends very much upon the duration of the ligation (Lee *et al.*, 1967) or perfusion (Nayler *et al.*, 1971b; Hess *et al.*, 1979; Feher *et al.*, 1980). In addition, ultrastructural studies have shown swollen and disrupted SR (McCallister *et al.*, 1978). Ischaemia results in intracellular acidosis which could depress SR calcium pump function (Mandel *et al.*, 1982). Acidosis has been shown to depress calcium-induced calcium release in skinned cells (Fabiato and Fabiato, 1978a). Long chain fatty acids which also accumulate during ischaemia have been shown to alter SR function (Adams *et al.*, 1979; Messineo *et al.*, 1980). As well as perfusion experiments to produce ischaemia, perfusion without calcium followed by reperfusion with calcium showed reduced SR calcium pump activity (Alto and Dhalla, 1981). This leads to the suggestion that this could be a feature of the damage associated with the 'calcium paradox'. Perfusion with substrate-depleted medium also reduced SR calcium pump activity (Muir *et al.*, 1970).

SR calcium pump activity is progressively reduced with age in cardiomyopathy of the Syrian hampster (McCollum *et al.*, 1970; Gertz *et al.*, 1970; Alpert *et al.*, 1976), and in turkeys with a cardiomyopathy termed 'round-heart disease' (Staley *et al.*, 1981). In addition, diabetes can be associated with a specific cardiomyopathy and rats which were treated with streptozotocin to produce diabetes had depressed calcium pump function (Penpargkul *et al.*, 1981).

In summary it appears that declined SR function is a feature of nearly every pathological condition associated with heart, but is not implicated as the prime cause of any one of them.

ACKNOWLEDGEMENTS

I would like to thank Dr A. K. Campbell (Department of Medical Biochemistry, Welsh National School of Medicine) and Dr P. England (Department of Biochemistry, University of Bristol Medical School) for helpful discussion during the preparation; also Professor A. H. Henderson for his encouragement.

REFERENCES

Adams, R. J., Cohen, D. W., Gupte, S., Johnson, J. D., Wallick, E. T., Wang, T., and Schwartz, A. (1979). *In vitro* effects of palmitylcarnitine on cardiac plasma membrane Na,K ATPase and sarcoplasmic reticulum Ca^{2+} ATPase and Ca^{2+} transport. *J. Biol. Chem.*, **254**, 12404–12410.

Alpert, A. W., Welty, T. D., and Peterson, M. B. (1976). Change in sarcolemmal and sarcoplasmic reticulum ATPase activities with age in the cardiomyopathic Syrian hampster. *J. Mol. Cell. Cardiol.*, **8**, 901–907.

Alto, L. E., and Dhalla, N. S. (1981). Role of changes in microsomal calcium uptake in the effects of reperfusion of Ca^{2+}-deprived rat hearts. *Circulation Res.*, **48**, 17–24.

Aoki, K., Ireda, N., Yamashita, K., and Hotta, K. (1974). ATPase activity and Ca^{2+} interaction of myofibrils and sarcoplasmic reticulum isolated from hearts of spontaneously hypertensive rats. *Europ. Heart J.*, **15**, 475–481.

Ashley, C. C., and Ridgway, F. B. (1970). On the relationship between membrane potential, calcium transient and tension in single barnacle muscle fibres. *J. Physiol. (Lond.)*, **209**, 105–130.

Baskin, R. J., and Deamer, D. W. (1969). Comparative ultrastructure and calcium transport in heart and skeletal muscle microsomes. *J. Cell Biol.*, **43**, 610–617.

Baylor, S. M., and Oetliker, H. (1975). Birefringence experiments on isolated skeletal muscle fibres suggest a possible signal from the sarcoplasmic reticulum. *Nature*, **253**, 97–101.

Beeler, T. J. (1980). Calcium uptake and membrane potential in SR vesicles. *J. Biol. Chem.*, **255**, 9156–9161.

Bendall, J. R. (1952). Effect of the 'Marsh factor' on the shortening of muscle fibre models in the presence of adenosine triphosphate. *Nature*, **170**, 1058–1060.

Bennett, N., and Dupont, Y. (1981). Evidence for a calcium-gated cation channel in SR vesicles. *FEBS Lett.*, **128**, 269–274.

Bers, D. M., Philipson, K. D., and Langer, G. A. (1981). Cardiac contractility and sarcolemmal Ca binding in several cardiac muscle preparations. *Amer. J. Physiol.*, **240**, H576–H583.

Bhalla, R. C., and Ashley, T. (1978). Altered function of adenylate cyclase in hypertensive rat. *Biochem. Pharmacol.*, **27**, 1967–1971.

Bhalla, R. C., Gupta, R. C., and Sharma, R. V. (1982). Ditribution and properties of cAMP-dependent protein kinase isoenzymes in the myocardium of spontaneously hypertensive rat. *J. Mol. Cell. Cardiol.*, **14**, 33–39.

Bidlack, J. M., and Shamoo, A. E. (1980). Adenosine-3,5-monosphate-dependent phosphorylation of a 6,000 and 22,000 dalton protein from cardiac sarcoplasmic reticulum. *Biochim. Biophys. Acta*, **632**, 310–325.

Blayney, L. M., Thomas, H., Muir, J., and Henderson, A. H. (1977). Critical re-evaluation of murexide technique in the measurement of calcium transport by cardiac sarcoplasmic reticulum. *Biochim. Biophys. Acta*, **70**, 128–133.

Blayney, L. M., Thomas, H., Muir, J., and Henderson, A. H. (1978). Action of caffeine on calcium transport by isolated fractions of myofibrils, mitochondria and sarcoplasmic reticulum from rabbit heart. *Circulation Res.*, **43**, 520–526.

Bonnet, J. P., Galante, M., Brethes, D., Dedieu, J. C., and Chevallier, J. (1978). Purification of sarcoplasmic reticulum vesicles through their loading with calcium phosphate. *Arch. Biochem. Biophys.*, **191**, 32–41.

Briggs, F. N., Wise, R. M., and Hearn, J. A. (1978). The effect of lithium and potassium on the transient state kinetics of the (Ca + Mg)-ATPase of cardiac sarcoplasmic reticulum. *J. Biol. Chem.*, **253**, 5884–5885.

Campbell, K. P., Franzini-Armstrong, C., and Shamoo, A. E. (1980). Further characterization of light and heavy sarcoplasmic reticulum vesicles. Identification of the sarcoplasmic reticulum feet associated with heavy sarcoplasmic reticulum vesicles. *Biochem. Biophys. Res. Commun.*, **602**, 97–116.

Chiesi, M. (1979). Temperature dependency of the functional activities of dog cardiac sarcoplasmic reticulum. A comparison with sarcoplasmic reticulum from rabbit and lobster muscle. *J. Mol. Cell. Cardiol.*, **11**, 245–259.

Chiesi, M., and Inesi, G. (1979). The use of quench reagents for resolution of single transport cycles in sarcoplasmic reticulum. *J. Biol. Chem.*, **254**, 10370–10377.

Chiesi, M., and Inesi, G. (1980). Adenosine-5′-triphosphate-dependent fluxes of manganese and hydrogen ions in SR vesicles. *Biochemistry*, **19**, 2912–2918.

Chiu, V. C., and Haynes, D. H. (1980a). Rapid kinetic study of the passive permeability of a Ca^{2+} ATPase-rich fraction of the sarcoplasmic reticulum. *J. Membr. Biol.*, **56**, 203–218.

Chiu, V. C., Mouring, D., Watson, B. D., and Haynes, D. H. (1980). Measurement of surface potential and surface charge densities of sarcoplasmic reticulum membranes. *J. Membr. Biol.*, **56**, 121–132.

Ciaraldi, T., and Marinetti, G. V. (1977). Thyroxine and propylthiouracil effects *in vitro* on alpha and beta adrenergic receptors in rat heart. *Biochem. Biophys. Res. Commun.*, **74**, 984–991.

Cohen, L. B., Hille, B., Keynes, R. D., Landowne, D., and Rojas, E. (1971). Analysis of the potential dependent changes in optical retardation in the squid giant axon. *J. Physiol. (Lond.)*, **218**, 205–237.

Conway, G., Heazlitt, R. A., Fowler, N. O., Gabel, M., Green, S. (1976). The effect of hyperthyroidism on the sarcoplasmic reticulum and myosin ATPase of dog hearts. *J. Mol. Cell. Cardiol.*, **8**, 39–51.

Deamer, D. W., and Baskin, R. J. (1969). Ultrastructure of sarcoplasmic reticulum preparations. *J. Cell Biol.*, **42**, 296–307.

Defloor, P. H., Levitsky, D., Biryukova, T., and Fleischer, S. (1980). Immunological dissimilarity of the calcium pump protein of skeletal and cardiac muscle sarcoplasmic reticulum. *Arch. Biochem. Biophys.*, **200**, 196–205.

Ebashi, I. (1961). Calcium binding activity of vesicular relaxing factor. *J. Biochem.*, **50**, 236–244.

Ebashi, S. (1958). A granule-bound relaxation factor in skeletal muscle. *Arch. Biochem. Biophys.*, **76**, 410–423.

Endo, M. (1977). Calcium release from the sarcoplasmic reticulum. *Physiol. Rvs*, **57**, 71–108.

Endo, H., and Nakajima, Y. (1973). Release of calcium induced by depolarization of the sarcoplasmic reticulum membrane. *Nature New Biol.*, **246**, 216–218.

Fabiato, A., and Fabiato, F. (1975a). Contractions induced by calcium triggered release of calcium from the SR of single skinned cardiac cells. *J. Physiol. (Lond.)*, **249**, 469–495.

Fabiato, A., and Fabiato, F. (1975b). Relaxing and inotropic effects of cyclic AMP on skinned cardiac cells. *Nature*, **253**, 556–558.

Fabiato, A., and Fabiato, F. (1978a). Effects of pH on the myofilaments and sarcoplasmic reticulum of skinned cells from cardiac and skeletal muscles. *J. Physiol. (Lond.)*, **276**, 233–255.

Fabiato, A., and Fabiato, F. (1978b). Calcium-induced release of calcium from the sarcoplasmic reticulum of skinned cells from adult human, dog, cat, rabbit, rat and frog hearts and from fetal and newborn rat ventricles. *Ann. N.Y. Acad. Sci.*, **307**, 491–522.

Fabiato, A., and Fabiato, F. (1979). Use of chlorotetracycline fluorescence to demonstrate Ca^{2+} induced release of Ca^{2+} from the sarcoplasmic reticulum of skinned cardiac cells. *Nature*, **281**, 146–148.

Feher, J. J., Briggs, F. N., and Hess, H. L. (1980). Characterization of cardiac sarcoplasmic reticulum from ischaemic myocardium: comparison of isolated sarcoplasmic reticulum with unfractionated homogenates. *J. Mol. Cell. Cardiol.*, **12**, 427–432.

Fleckenstein, A. (1971). Specific inhibitors and promotors of calcium action in the excitation contraction coupling of heart muscle and their role in the prevention or production of myocardial lesions 1. In *Calcium and the Heart* (P. Harris and L. R. Opie, eds), Academic Press, London, pp. 135–182.

Ford, L. E., and Podolsky, R. J. (1970). Regenerative calcium release within muscle cells. *Science*, **167**, 58–59.

Franzini-Armstrong, C. (1980). Structure of sarcoplasmic reticulum. *Fed. Proc.*, **39**, 2403–2409.

Gertz, F. W., Stam, A. C., and Sonnenblick, E. H. (1970). A quantitative and qualitative defect in the sarcoplasmic reticulum in the hereditary cardiomyopathy of the Syrian hampster. *Biochem. Biophys. Res. Commun.*, **40**, 746–753.

Graham, J. A., and Lamb, J. F. (1968). The effect of adrenaline on the tension developed in contractures and twitches of the frog. *J. Physiol. (Lond.)*, **197**, 479–509.

Harigaya, S., and Schwartz, A. (1969). Rate of calcium binding and uptake in normal animal and failing human cardiac muscle membrane vesicles (relaxing system), and mitochondria. *Circulation Res.*, **25**, 781–794.

Hasselbach, W., and Makinose, M. (1961). Die Calciumpumpe der 'Erschlaffungsgrana' des Muskels und 1 hre Abhangigkeit van der ATP-Spattung. *Biochem. Z.*, **33**, 518–528.

Heilmann, C., Linol, T., Muller, W., and Pette, D. (1980). Characterization of cardiac microsomes from spontaneously hypertensive rats. *Basic Res. Cardiol.*, **75**, 92–96.

Henderson, A. H., Craig, R. J., Sonnenblick, E., and Urschel, C. W. (1970). Species differences in intrinsic myocardial contractility. *Proc. Soc. Exp. Biol. Med.*, **134**, 930–932.

Hess, M. L., Barnhart, G., Crute, S., Krause, S., Komwatana, P., and Greenfield, L. J. (1979). Mechanical and biochemical effects of transient ischaemic arrest. *Surg. Res.*, **26,** 175–184.

Hollingworth, D. N., and England, P. J. (1978). The stimulation of calcium uptake into sarcoplasmic reticulum vesicles from rat heart by adenosine $3',5'$-phosphate dependent protein kinase. *Biochem. Soc. Trans.*, **6,** 573–575.

Holt, T. P., Rhode, F. A., and Kines, H. (1968). Ventricular volumes and body weight in mammals. *Amer. J. Physiol.*, **215,** 704–715.

Horwood, D. M., and Singhal, R. L. (1976). Myocardial protein kinase II. Isoproterenol induced changes in the activity of soluble and membrane bound enzymes of rat left ventricle. *J. Mol. Cell. Cardiol.*, **8,** 29–38.

Ikemoto, N., Sreter, F. A., and Nakamura, A. (1968). Tryptic digestion and localization of calcium uptake and ATPase activity in fragments of sarcoplasmic reticulum. *J. Ultrastruct. Res.*, **23,** 216–222.

Ikemoto, N., Miyao, A., and Kurobe, Y. (1981). Further evidence for an oligomeric calcium pump by sarcoplasmic reticulum. *J. Biol. Chem.*, **256,** 10809–10814.

Inesi, G., and Malan, N. (1976). Mechanisms of calcium release in sarcoplasmic reticulum. Minireview. *Life Sci.*, **18,** 773–779.

Inesi, G., and Scales, D. (1974). Tryptic cleavage of sarcoplasmic reticulum protein. *Biochemistry*, **13,** 3298–3306.

Ito, Y., Suko, J., and Chidsey, C. A. (1974). Intracellular calcium and myocardial contractility V. Calcium uptake of sarcoplasmic reticulum fractions in hypertrophied and failing rabbit hearts. *J. Mol. Cell. Cardiol.*, **6,** 237–247.

Jaqua-Stewart, M. J., Read, W. O., and Steffen, R. P. (1979). Isolation of pure myocardial subcellular organelles. *Analyt. Biochem.*, **96,** 293–297.

Jilka, R. L., Martonosi, A. M., and Tillack, T. W. (1975). Effect of purified $(Mg^{2+}+Ca^{2+})$ activated ATPase of sarcoplasmic reticulum upon the passive Ca^{2+} permeability and ultrastructure of phospholipid vesicles. *J. Biol. Chem.*, **250,** 7511–7524.

Jones, L. R. (1979). Mg^{2+} and ATP effects on K^+ activation of the Ca^{2+}-transport ATPase of cardiac SR. *Biochim. Biophys. Acta*, **557,** 230–242.

Jones, L. R., and Besch, H. R. (1979). Calcium handling by cardiac sarcoplasmic reticulum. *Texas Rep. Biol. Med.*, **39,** 19–35.

Jones, L. R., Besch, H. R., Flemming, J. W., McConnaughey, M. M., and Watanabe, A. M. (1979). Separation of vesicles of cardiac sarcolemma of vesicles of cardiac sarcolemma from vesicles of cardiac sarcoplasmic reticulum. *J. Biol. Chem.*, **254,** 530–539.

Jones, L. R., Besch, H. R., and Watanabe, A. M. (1978a). Regulation of the calcium pump of cardiac sarcoplasmic reticulum. Interactive roles of potassium and ATP on the phosphoprotein intermediate of the K^+, Ca^{2+} ATPase. *J. Biol. Chem.*, **253,** 1643–1653.

Jones, L. R., and Cala, S. E. (1981). Biochemical evidence for functional heterogeneity of cardiac sarcoplasmic reticulum vesicles. *J. Biol. Chem.*, **256,** 11809–11818.

Jones, L. R., Phan, S. H., and Besch, H. R. (1978b). Cell electrophoretic and density gradient analysis of the K^+ and Ca^{2+} ATPase and the Na^+ and K^+ ATPase activities of cardiac membrane vesicles. *Biochim. Biophys. Acta*, **514,** 294–309.

Kanazawa, T., Yamada, S., and Tonomura, Y. (1970). ATP formation from ADP and a phosphorylated intermediate of Ca^{2+}-dependent ATPase in fragmented sarcoplasmic reticulum. *J. Biochem.*, **68,** 593–595.

Kanazawa, T., Yamada, S., Yamamoto, T., and Tonomura, Y. (1971). Reaction mechanism of the Ca^{2+} dependent ATPase of sarcoplasmic reticulum from skeletal muscle. V. Vectorial requirements for calcium and magnesium ions of three partial reactions of ATPase formation and decomposition of a phosphorylated intermediate and ATP formation from ADP and the intermediate. *J. Biochem.*, **70,** 95–123.

Kasai, M., and Miyamoto, H. (1973). Depolarization induced calcium release from sarcoplasmic reticulum membrane fragments by changing ionic environment. *FEBS Letters*, **34,** 299–301.

Katz, A. M., Repke, D. I., Dunnet, J., and Hasselbach, W. (1977a). Dependence of calcium permeability of sarcoplasmic reticulum vesicles on external and internal calcium ion concentrations. *J. Biol. Chem.*, **252,** 1950–1956.

Katz, A. M., Repke, D. I., and Hasselbach, W. (1977b). Dependence of ionophore and caffeine-induced calcium release from sarcoplasmic reticulum vesicles on external and internal calcium ion concentrations. *J. Biol. Chem.*, **252,** 1938–1949.

Katz, A. M., Louis, C. F., Repke, D. I., Fudymag, G., Nash-Alder, P., Kupsaw, R., and Shigekawa, M. (1980). Time dependent changes of calcium influx and efflux rates in rabbit skeletal muscle sarcoplasmic reticulum. *Biochim. Biophys. Acta*, **596,** 94–107.

Knowles, A., Zimniak, P., Alfonzo, M., Zimniak, A., and Racker, E. (1980). Isolation and characterization of proteolipids from sarcoplasmic reticulum. *J. Membr. Biol.*, **55,** 233–239.

Kometani, T., and Kasai, M. (1980). Ion movement accompanied by calcium uptake of sarcoplasmic reticulum vesicles studied through the osmotic volume change by the light scattering method. *J. Membr. Biol.*, **56,** 159–168.

Labarca, P., Coronado, R., and Miller, C. (1980). Thermodynamic and kinetic studies of the gating behaviour of a K^+ selective channel from the sarcoplasmic reticulum membrane. *J. Gen. Physiol.*, **76,** 397–424.

Langer, G. A., Brady, A. J., Tan, S. T., and Serena, S. D. (1975). Correlation of the glycoside response, the force staircase and the action potential configuration in the neonatal rat heart. *Circulation Res.*, **36,** 744–752.

Lee, K. S., Ladinsky, H., and Stuckey, J. H. (1967). Decreased Ca^{2+} uptake of sarcoplasmic reticulum after coronary artery occlusion for 60 and 90 minutes. *Arc. Res.*, **20,** 477–484.

Levitsky, D. O., Aliev, M. K., Kuzmin, A. V., Levchenko, T. S., Smirnov, V. N., and Chazov, E. I. (1976). Isolation of calcium pump system and purification of calcium ion-dependent ATPase from heart muscle. *Biochim. Biophys. Acta*, **443,** 468–484.

Lighty, G. W., and Bertrand, H. A. (1979). Cardiac sarcoplasmic reticulum isolation from slaughter house beef heart. *Analyt. Biochem.*, **99,** 41–52.

Limas, C. J. (1978). Enhanced phosphorylation of myocardial sarcoplasmic reticulum in experimental hyperthyroidism. *Amer. J. Physiol.*, **234,** H426–H431.

Limas, C. J. (1980a). Increased phospholipid methylation in the myocardium of hyperthyroid rats. *Biochim. Biophys. Acta*, **632,** 254–259.

Limas, C. J. (1980b). Effect of phospholipid methylation on beta-adrenergic receptors on the normal and hypertrophied rat myocardium. *Circulation Res.*, **47,** 536–541.

Limas, C. J., and Cohn, J. N. (1977). Defective calcium transport by cardiac sarcoplasmic reticulum in spontaneously hypertensive rats. *Circulation Res.*, **40,** Suppl. 1, 62–69.

Limas, C. J., Spier, S. S., and Kahlon, J. (1980). Enhanced calcium transport by sarcoplasmic reticulum in mild cardiac hypertrophy. *J. Mol. Cell. Cardiol.*, **12,**

1103–1116.

Louis, C. F., Nash-Alder, P. A., Fudyma, G., Sigerawa, M., Akowitz, A., and Katz, A. M. (1980). A comparison of vesicles derived from terminal cisternae and longitudinal tubules of sarcoplasmic reticulum isolated from rabbit skeletal muscle. *Europ. J. Biochem.*, **111**, 1–9.

McCallister, L. P., Daiello, D. C., and Tyers, G. F. O. (1978). Morphometric observations of the effects of normothermic ischaemic arrest on dog myocardial ultrastructure. *J. Mol. Cell. Cardiol.*, **10**, 67–80.

McCollum, B., Crow, C., Harigaya, S., Bajusz, E., and Schwartz, A. (1970). Calcium binding by cardiac relaxing system isolated from myopathic Syrian hampsters (strain 14.6.82.62, and 40.54). *J. Mol. Cell. Cardiol.*, **1**, 445–457.

MacLennan, D. H. (1975). Resolution of the calcium transport system of sarcoplasmic reticulum. *Canad. J. Biochem.*, **53**, 251–261.

Madeira, V. M. (1980). Proton movements across the membranes of sarcoplasmic reticulum during the uptake of calcium ions. *Arch. Biochem. Biophys.*, **200**, 319–325.

Makinose, M. (1971). Calcium efflux dependent formation of ATP from ADP and orthophosphate by membranes of the sarcoplasmic vesicles. *FEBS Lett.*, **12**, 269–270.

Malouf, N. N., and Meissner, G. (1980). Cyctochemical localization of a 'basic' ATPase to canine myocardial surface membrane. *J. Histochem. Cytochem.*, **28**, 1286–1294.

Mandel, F., Kranias, E. G., and Grassi De Gende, A. (1982). The effect of pH on the transport-state kinetics of Ca^{2+}–Mg^{2+} ATPase of cardiac sarcoplasmic reticulum. A comparison with skeletal sarcoplasmic reticulum. *Circulation Res.*, **50**, 310–317.

Marsh, B. B. (1951). A factor modifying muscle fibre synaeresis. *Nature*, **167**, 1065–1066.

Martonosi, A. (1975). Membrane transport during development in animals. *Biochim. Biophys. Acta.* **415**, 311–333.

Mead, R. J., Peterson, M. B., and Welty, J. D. (1971). Sarcolemmal and sarcoplasmic reticular ATPase activities in the failing canine heart. *Circulation Res.*, **29**, 14–20.

Meissner, G., and Young, R. C. (1980). Proton permeability of sarcoplasmic reticulum vesicles. *J. Biol. Chem.*, **255**, 6814–6819.

Messineo, F. C., Pinto, P. B., and Katz, A. M. (1980). Palmitic acid enhances calcium sequestration by isolated sarcoplasmic reticulum. *J. Mol. Cell. Cardiol.*, **12**, 725–732.

Miller, C., and Rosenberg, R. L. (1979). A voltage-gated cation conductance channel from fragmented sarcoplasmic reticulum. Effect of transition metal ions. *Biochemistry*, **18**, 1138–1145.

Morad, M., and Rolett, E. L. (1972). Relaxing effects of catecholamines on mammalian heart. *J. Physiol.* (*Lond.*), **224**, 537–558.

Muir, J. R., Dhalla, N. S., Ortega, J. F., and Olson, R. E. (1970). Energy linked calcium transport in subcellular fractions of the failing rat heart. *Circulation Res.*, **26**, 429–438.

Mukherjee, C., Caron, M. G., and Lefkowitz, R. J. (1975). Catecholamines induced subsensitivity of adenylate cyclase associated with loss of beta adrenergic receptors. *Proc. Natl. Acad. Sci.*, **72**, 1945–1949.

Natori, R. (1975). The electrical potential change of internal membrane during propagation of contraction in skinned fibre of toad skeletal muscle. *Jpn. J. Physiol.*, **25,** 51–63.

Nayler, W. G., and Fassold, E. (1977). Calcium accumulating and ATPase activity of cardiac sarcoplasmic reticulum before and after birth. *Cardiovasc. Res.*, **11,** 231–237.

Nayler, W. G., Merrilees, N. C. R., Chipperfield, D., and Kurtz, J. B. (1971a). Influence of hyperthyroidism on the uptake and binding by cardiac microsomal fractions. *Cardiovasc. Res.*, **5,** 469–482.

Nayler, W. G., Stone, J., Carson, V., and Chipperfield, D. (1971b). Effect of ischaemia on cardiac contractility and calcium exchange ability. *J. Mol. Cell. Cardiol.*, **2,** 125–143.

Nayler, W. G., Dunnet, J., and Burian, W. (1975). Further observations on species determined differences in the calcium accumulating activity of cardiac microsomal fractions. *J. Mol. Cell. Cardiol.*, **7,** 663–675.

Newcomb, M., Gibson, K., and Harris, P. (1978). Effect of 3,5,3'-tri-iodothyronine induced cardiac hypertrophy on cytosolic protein kinase. *Biochem. Biophys. Res. Commun.*, **81,** 596–601.

Ostwald, T. I., and MacLennan, D. H. (1974). Isolation of a high affinity calcium-binding protein from sarcoplasmic reticulum. *J. Biol. Chem.*, **249,** 974–979.

Page, E. (1978). Quantitative ultrastructural analysis in cardiac membrane physiology. *Amer. J. Physiol.*, **235,** C147–C158.

Page, E., and Buecker, J. L. (1981). Development of dyadic junctional complexes between sarcoplasmic reticulum and plasmalemma in rabbit left ventricular myocardial cells. Morphometric analysis. *Circulation Res.*, **48,** 519–522.

Page, E., and Surdyk-Droske, H. (1979). Distribution, surface density and membrane area of diadic junctional contacts between plasma membrane and terminal cisterns in mammalian ventricle. *Circulation Res.*, **45,** 260–267.

Page, E., Earley, J., and Power, B. (1974). Normal growth of ultrastructures in rat left ventricular myocardial cells. *Circulation Res.*, **34/35,** Suppl. II, 12–16.

Peachey, L. D. (1965). The sarcoplasmic reticulum and transverse tubules of the frog's sartorius. *J. Cell Biol.*, **25,** 209–231.

Penpargkul, S. (1979). Effects of adenine nucleotides on calcium binding by rat heart sarcoplasmic reticulum. *Cardiovasc. Res.*, **13,** 243–253.

Penpargkul, S., Repke, D. I., Katz, A. M., and Scheuer, J. (1977). Effect of physical training on calcium transport by rat cardiac sarcoplasmic reticulum. *Circulation Res.*, **40,** 134–137.

Penpargkul, S., Malhotra, A., Schaible, T., and Scheuer, J. (1980). Cardiac contractile proteins and sarcoplasmic reticulum in hearts of rats trained by running. *J. Appl. Physiol.*, **48,** 409–413.

Penpargkul, S., Fein, F., Sonnenblick, E. H., and Scheuer, J. (1981). Depressed cardiac sarcoplasmic reticular function from diabetic rats. *J. Mol. Cell. Cardiol.*, **13,** 303–309.

Plank, B., Hellmann, G., Punzengrubber, C., and Suko, J. (1979). ATP-Pi and ITP-Pi exchange by cardiac sarcoplasmic reticulum. *Biochim. Biophys. Acta*, **550,** 259–268.

Porter, K. R. (1961). The sarcoplasmic reticulum. Its recent history and present status. *J. Biophys. Biochem. Cytol.*, Suppl. 10, 219–226.

Porter, K. R., and Palade, G. E. (1957). Studies on the endoplasmic reticulum III. Its form and distribution in striated muscle cells. *J. Biophys. Biochem. Cytol.*, **3,** 269–299.

Racker, E., and Eytan, E. (1975). A coupling factor from sarcoplasmic reticulum required for the translocation of Ca^{2+} ions in a reconstituted Ca^{2+} ATPase pump. *J. Biol. Chem.*, **250,** 7533.

Rona, G., Chappell, C. I., Balazs, T., and Gaudry, R. (1959). An infarct like myocardial lesion and other toxic manifestiations produced by isoproterenol in the rat. *Arch. Pathol.*, **67,** 433–455.

Sarzala, M. G., Pilaska, M., Zubrzyka, E., and Michalak, M. (1975). Changes in the structure, composition and function of sarcoplasmic reticulum membrane during development. *Europ. J. Biochem.*, **57,** 25.

Scales, D. J. (1981). Aspects of mammalian by freeze fracture electron microscopy. *J. Mol. Cell. Cardiol.*, **13,** 373–380.

Schneider, M. F., and Chandler, W. K. (1973). Voltage dependent charge movement in skeletal muscle: a possible step in excitation contraction coupling. *Nature*, **242,** 244–246.

Shigekawa, M., Finegan, J. M., and Katz, A. M. (1976). Calcium transport ATPase of canine cardiac sarcoplasmic reticulum. A comparison with that of rabbit fast skeletal muscle sarcoplasmic reticulum. *J. Biol. Chem.*, **251,** 6894–6900.

Shoshan, V., MacLennan, D. H., and Wood, D. S. (1981). A proton gradient controls a calcium-release channel in sarcoplasmic reticulum. *Proc. Natl Acad. Sci.*, **78,** 4828–4832.

Somlyo, A. V., Shuman, H., and Somlyo, A. P. (1977). Elemental distribution in striated muscle and the effects of hypertonicity. Electron probe analysis of cryo sections. *J. Cell Biol.*, **74,** 828–857.

Sommer, J. R., and Waugh, R. A. (1976). The ultrastructure of the mammalian cardiac muscle cell – with special emphasis on the tubular membrane systems. *Amer. J. Pathol.*, **82,** 192–232.

Sordahl, L. A., McCollum, W. B., Wood, W. G., and Schwartz, A. (1973). Mitochondria and sarcoplasmic reticulum function in cardiac hypertrophy and failure. *Amer. J. Physiol.*, **224,** 497–502.

Staley, N. A., Noren, G. R., and Einzig, S. (1981). Early alterations in the function of sarcoplasmic reticulum in a naturally occurring model of congestive cardiomyopathy. *Cardiovasc. Res.*, **15,** 276–281.

Strickholm, A. (1974). Intracellular generated potentials during excitation–contraction coupling in muscle. *J. Neurobiol.*, **5,** 161–187.

Suko, J. (1971). Alterations in Ca^{2+} uptake and Ca^{2+} activated ATPase of cardiac sarcoplasmic reticulum in hyper and hypothyroidism. *Biochim. Biophys. Acta*, **252,** 324–327.

Suko, J. (1973). The calcium pump of cardiac sarcoplasmic reticulum functional alterations at different levels of thyroid state in rabbits. *J. Physiol. (Lond.)*, **228,** 563–582.

Suko, J., and Hasselbach, W. (1976). Characterization of cardiac sarcoplasmic reticulum ATP–ADP phosphate exchange and phosphorylation of the calcium transport adenosine triphosphatase. *Europ. J. Biochem.*, **64,** 123–130.

Suko, J., Vogel, H. K., and Chidsey, C. A. (1970). Intracellular calcium and myocardial activity III. Reduced calcium uptake and ATPase of the sarcoplasmic reticular fraction prepared from chronically failing calf hearts. *Circulation Res.*, **27,** 235–247.

Sumida, M., Wang, T., Mandel, F., Froehlich, J., and Schwartz, A. (1978). Transient kinetics of Ca^{2+} transport of sarcoplasmic reticulum. A comparison of cardiac and skeletal muscle. *J. Biol. Chem.*, **253,** 8772–8777.

Swynghedauw, B., Bourveret, P., and Hatt, P. Y. (1973). New fractionation scheme for preparation of heart particles. ATPase activity of purified myofibrils in chronic aortic insufficiency in the rabbit. *J. Mol. Cell. Cardiol.*, **5**, 441–459.

Tada, M., Kirchberger, M. A., Repke, D. I., and Katz, A. H. (1974). The stimulation of calcium transport in cardiac sarcoplasmic reticulum by adenosine 3′,5′-monophosphate-dependent protein kinase. *J. Biol. Chem.*, **249**, 6174–6180.

Tada, M., Kirchberger, M. A., and Katz, A. M. (1975a). Phosphorylation of a 22,000 dalton component of the cardiac sarcoplasmic reticulum by adenosine 3′:5′-monophosphate dependent protein kinase. *J. Biol. Chem.*, **250**, 2640–2647.

Tada, M., Kirchberger, M. A., and Li, H. (1975b). Phosphoprotein phosphatase-catalysed dephosphorylation of the 22,000 dalton phosphoprotein of cardiac sarcoplasmic reticulum. *J. Cyclic Nucleotide Res.*, **1**, 329–338.

Tada, M., Yamamoto, T., and Tonomura, Y. (1978b). Molecular mechanism of active calcium transport by sarcoplasmic reticulum. *Physiol. Rev.*, **58**, 1–79.

Tada, M., Ohmori, F., Yamada, M., and Abe, H. (1979). Mechanism of the stimulation of Ca^{2+} dependent ATPase of cardiac sarcoplasmic reticulum by adenosine 3′,5-monophosphate dependent protein kinase. Role of the 22,000 dalton protein. *J. Biol. Chem.*, **254**, 319–326.

Tse, J., Brackett, N. L., Kuo, J. F. (1978). Alterations in activities of cyclic nuelcotide systems and in B-adrenergic receptor mediated activation of cyclic AMP-dependent protein kinase during progression and regression of isoproterenol-induced cardiac hypertrophy. *Biochem. Biophys. Res. Commun.*, **542**, 399–411.

Tse, J., Powell, J. R., Baste, C. A., Priest, R. E., and Kuo, J. F. (1979). Isoproterenol-induced cardiac hypertrophy: modifications in characteristics of B adrenegic receptor, adenylate cyclase and ventricular contraction. *Endocrinology*, **105**, 246–255.

Van Winkle, W. B., Tate, C. A., Bick, R. J., and Entman, H. L. (1981). Nucleotide triphosphate utilization by cardiac and skeletal muscle sarcoplasmic reticulum. Evidence for a hydrolysis cycle not coupled to intermediate acyl phosphate formation and calcium translocation. *J. Biol. Chem.*, **286**, 2268–2274.

Vincenzi, F. F., and Larsen, F. L. (1980). The plasma membrane calcium pump regulation by a soluble Ca^{2+} binding protein. *Fed. Proc.*, **39**, 2427–2431.

Wang, T., Grassi De Gende, A. O., Tsai, L. I., and Schwartz, A. (1981). Influence of monovalent cations on the Ca^{2+} ATPase of sarcoplasmic reticulum isolated from rabbit skeletal and dog cardiac muscles. An interpretation of transient-state kinetic data. *Biochim. Biophys. Acta*, **637**, 523–529.

Weber, A. (1971). Regulatory mechanisms of the calcium transport system of fragmented rabbit sarcoplasmic reticulum 1. The effect of accumulated calcium on transport and adenosine triphosphate hydrolysis. *J. Gen. Physiol.*, **57**, 50–63.

Whyte, L., Haines, H., and Adams, T. (1978). Cardiac output related to body weight in small animals. *Comp. Biochem. Physiol.*, **27**, 559–565.

Winegrad, S. (1965). Autoradiographic studies of intracellular calcium in frog skeletal muscle. *J. Gen. Physiol.*, **48**, 455–479.

Yamada, S., and Tonomura, Y. (1972). Reaction mechanism of the Ca^{2+} dependent ATPase of sarcoplasmic reticulum from skeletal muscle. VII. Recognition and release of Ca^{2+} ions. *J. Biochem.*, **72**, 417–425.

Yamamoto, N., and Kasai, M. (1980). Donnan potential in sarcoplasmic reticulum vesicles measured using a fluorescent cyanine dye. *J. Biochem.*, **88**, 1425–1435.

Yamamoto, T., and Tonomura, Y. (1967). Reaction mechanism of the Ca^{2+} dependent ATPase of sarcoplasmic reticulum from skeletal muscle. 1. Kinetic studies. *J. Biochem.*, **62,** 558–575.

Zimniak, P., and Racker, E. (1978). Electrogenicity of Ca^{2+} transport catalysed by the Ca^{2+} ATPase from sarcoplasmic reticulum. *J. Biol. Chem.*, **253,** 4631–4637.

Cardiac Metabolism
Edited by A. J. Drake-Holland and M. I. M. Noble
© 1983 John Wiley & Sons Ltd

CHAPTER 3

Excitation–Contraction Coupling

M. I. M. Noble

Midhurst Medical Research Institute, Midhurst, Sussex, UK

INTRODUCTION

It is generally accepted that muscle contraction occurs as the result of an interaction between actin and myosin (the contractile proteins), adenosine triphosphate (ATP), and calcium ions (Ca^{++}); the reaction is modulated by the regulatory proteins troponin and tropomyosin. In heart muscle, the contractile system is not saturated with Ca^{++} and therefore the intensity of the reaction, as measured by ATP splitting or contractile tension, is a function of Ca^{++} concentration in the vicinity of the myosin ATPase sites. If tension is postulated to be a function of Ca^{++} released to the contractile proteins, a working hypothesis involving functional compartments of intracellular Ca^{++} is necessary to explain the behaviour of intact cardiac muscle (see review by Wohlfart and Noble, 1982).

If this model proves useful, it will then be necessary to define the site and metabolism of the calcium-handling processes. It is not possible at present to form a firm opinion on the latter because of lack of definitive information. In this chapter, therefore, the model will first be described, based on physiological behaviour. An attempt will then be made to indicate the current state of knowledge concerning the sites and metabolism of calcium handling processes that might be involved in the rapid changes of the excitation–contraction cycle.

MODEL OF CALCIUM HANDLING DURING THE EXCITATION–CONTRACTION CYCLE

The behaviour of cardiac muscle can be thought of to a large extent in terms of a model (Figure 3.1). No generally agreed allocation of functions to the various elements of the ultrastructure of the cell is possible at this time. Thus the compartments depicted in Figure 3.1 are functional compartments only and have no firm anatomical counterparts at the present stage of development of the model (see below). We know that the contractile

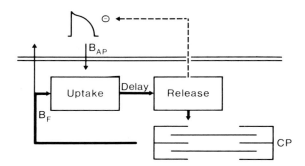

Figure 3.1 Model of calcium handling by the myocardial cell. Only the main pathways are indicated. CP = contractile proteins. B_{AP} is a coefficient relating calcium inflow to action potential duration. B_F is a coefficient relating recirculating calcium (arrow into uptake compartment) to total calcium coming from the contractile proteins during relaxation. Dashed line indicates negative feedback control of the calcium conductance of the cell membrane

proteins are an anatomical entity but all the other components of the model could reside in the same structure, e.g. plasma membrane. Similar models of the excitation–contraction mechanism have been proposed before (Wood *et al.*, 1969; Beeler and Reuter, 1970a,b; Wussling and Szymanski, 1972; Morad and Goldman, 1973; Kaufmann *et al.*, 1974; Allen *et al.*, 1976; Edman and Johannsson, 1976; Langer *et al.*, 1976; Antoni, 1977; Jewell, 1977).

Calcium is liberated from a release compartment into the myofibrillar space leading to the contractile activation of the cell. The amount of calcium released is a function of the contents of the release compartment and determines force production. Relaxation occurs as calcium is removed from the contractile proteins. A fraction of this calcium fills the uptake compartment. Another fraction is ultimately extruded from the cell. This could be by sequestration of cytosolic calcium by some intracellular structure which binds calcium and extrudes it later, or it could be pumped out of the cell continuously during contraction and relaxation; the effect is the same as far as the model is concerned.

The calcium that enters the cell during the plateau phase of the action potential is assumed to go to the uptake compartment. An important feature of the model is that calcium in the uptake compartment must undergo a delay before coming into a releasable state (represented by a separate release compartment). This delay is responsible for the time taken to 'refill' the release compartment between excitations as reflected externally by the phenomenon of mechanical restitution (Figure 3.2) (Bautovich *et al.*, 1962; Edman and Johannsson, 1976; Anderson *et al.*, 1977; Pidgeon *et al.*, 1980).

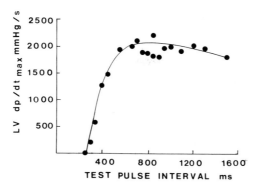

Figure 3.2 Contractility as a function of interval preceding the beat. Evidence for the delay between uptake and release in the model (Figure 3.1)

The decay of the restitution curve follows from a slow calcium efflux from the release compartment (Figure 3.2; Bass, 1976).

The system must reach an equilibrium both in the absence and in the presence of excitation–contraction cycles. The rested state contraction is a contraction that occurs after a very long pause (Koch-Weser and Blinks, 1963). This contraction is by definition independent of the preceding stimulation history. It represents the equilibrium or steady state condition in the absence of excitation–contraction cycles. Such a postulate implies that there can be a change of calcium between excitations which is small in comparison to the movements indicated by arrows in Figure 3.1. There may also be a late component of calcium entry during the action potential leading to direct activation of the contractile proteins in a rested state contraction. This has been excluded from the model because it is likely to be small in a steady state in the presence of excitation–contraction cycles.

The calcium influx during the action potential is thought to be inversely determined by the amount of intracellular calcium (Braveny and Sumbera, 1970; Isenberg, 1975; Bassingthwaighte *et al.*, 1976; Kass and Tsien, 1976; Simurda *et al.*, 1976). In the model, this is a negative feedback (inverse) control of calcium conductance by the amount of Ca^{++} in the release compartment (dashed line in Figure 3.1). Since the filling of the release compartment is assumed to be a function of the interval between excitations, this will make calcium influx during the action potential dependent on the excitation interval. Such interval-induced changes in calcium influx will only be accompanied by concomitant changes in action potential duration when repolarization is determined by decay of the slow inward (Ca^{++}) current during the plateau. A number of studies have shown that action potential duration varies with steady state stimulation interval (Trautwein and Dudel, 1954; Gibbs and Johnson, 1961; Edmands *et al.*, 1968; Reiter and Stickel, 1968; Miller *et al.*, 1971; Bass, 1975; Anderson and Johnson, 1976; Boyett and Jewell, 1980), but this may be due to factors other than intracellular calcium (Drake *et al.*, 1981a).

The presence of negative feedback control of calcium entry by the release compartment ensures and stabilizes a steady state during steady excitation–contraction cycles so that calcium entry and exit are equal (Noble, 1979).

Determinants of Contractility

In experiments on isolated papillary muscles from rabbits (Wohlfart, 1979), five factors were found to correlate with peak contractile force in a given contraction. These correlations will be discussed below in relation to the model.

(1) *The interval since the last excitation (preceding excitation interval)* When the one interval preceding a test contraction (test pulse interval) is varied, contractility rises with interval to an optimum at between 800 ms and 1 s (optimum test pulse interval) and then declines (Figure 3.2; Allen *et al.*, 1976; Edman and Johannsson, 1976). The contractility at the optimum interval is called the optimum contractile response (Edman and Johannsson, 1976; Pidgeon *et al.*, 1980). The curve depicted in Figure 3.2 is also referred to as the mechanical restitution curve; this curve arises because Ca^{++} which entered the store during the preceding excitation–contraction cycle changes with time from a non-releasable into a releasable state. This is represented in the model as two functional compartments – uptake and release with a delay in the transfer of Ca^{++} from the uptake to the release compartment (Figure 3.1).

(2) *The duration of the concomitant action potential* A prolongation of the action potential causes a longer lasting release of calcium leading to a longer time to peak force and therefore a greater amplitude of the contraction (Braveny and Sumbera, 1968; Morad and Trautwein, 1968). This factor is completely obscured in intact animals by the opening of the aortic valve and ejection, which prevents peak isometric force from being reached.

(3) *Action potential duration of the preceding excitation–contraction cycle* The amount of calcium entering the cell during the action potential is to some extent determined by the duration of the influx. An increased duration of the action potential will therefore be associated with a greater calcium uptake. Greater calcium uptake during the action potential will also occur through increased intensity of calcium inflow (greater conductance of calcium channels), but this cannot be detected in many of the preparations in which behaviour can be predicted by the model. The calcium entering is not released until the next excitation, i.e. contractility depends on the calcium entry during the action potential of the preceding beat (Figure 3.3; Antoni, *et al.* 1969; Wohlfart, 1979; Drake *et al.*, 1981b).

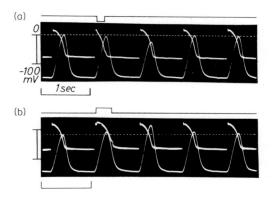

Figure 3.3 (a) Second action potential shortened leading to diminished contractility on beat 3. (b) Second action potential prolonged leading to enhanced contractility on beat 3. [Reproduced with permission from Antoni *et al.*, *Pflügers Arch. Ges. Physiol.*, **306**, 37 (1969), Fig. 1.]

(4) *Contractility of the preceding contraction* Recirculation of calcium between beats was postulated by Morad and Goldman (1973). Data compatible with this has been obtained from rabbit papillary muscle (Wohlfart, 1979) and intact dog (Elzinga *et al.*, 1981). One manifestation of this is that if there is a depression of contractility produced by a long diastole, contractility of a subsequent beat at the optimum interval is higher, returning towards the steady state value. Another manifestation is that if contractility is potentiated by a single extrasystole, the second post-extrasystolic beat is also potentiated as contractility returns towards the steady state value.

If the contractility of all beats following an optimum interval is plotted against that of the preceding beat (providing that that is also preceded by an optimum or longer interval), a continuous linear function is obtained including depressed beats, steady state beats and potentiated beats (Figure 3.4). According to the model, the slope of this line is the recirculated fraction of calcium. It is, of course, a matter for conjecture whether this really relates to recirculated calcium until the latter can be measured directly.

The influence of factors (3) and (4) can be described quantitatively by the equation

$$F(n) = B_{AP}AP(n-1) + B_F F(n-1) + A, \tag{3.1}$$

where $F(n)$ is the amplitude of a contraction designated (n) elicited at the optimum interval of factor (1) (above). The amplitude of the preceding contraction, $F(n-1)$ and the duration of the corresponding action potential, $AP(n-1)$ can be altered by earlier interventions. B_{AP} and B_F are constants expressing the influence of factors (3) and (4) respectively. These constants are assumed to reflect the inotropic state of the ventricular muscle, being

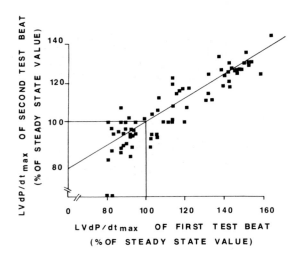

Figure 3.4 Relationship of contractility to that of the preceding beat. 100% = steady state. The slope of the line is the recirculation fraction (B_F) in the model (Figure 3.1). Intact dog data

measures of the influx during the action potential and the recirculation of calcium between beats respectively (Figure 3.1). It is interesting to note that B_F is 0.61 in the intact rabbit heart as compared to 0.21 in the isolated papilary muscle of the rabbit (Wohlfart and Elzinga, 1982). The higher value indicated a greater recirculation of calcium in the intact animal and hence a higher inotropic state (Reichel, 1976).

(5) *The interval between the preceding contraction and the pre-preceding contraction (pre-preceding excitation interval)*   This factor is of importance for post-extrasystolic potentiation (Hoffman *et al.*, 1956). Contraction 1 in Figure 3.5 is enhanced as a result of the short interval before the premature contraction, ES. The short interval causes a depression of ES (according to factor (1) above). The calcium that is not released in ES is, according to the model, located in the uptake compartment. This calcium will have reached the release compartment by the time of beat 1, adding to the calcium released and causing potentiation.

There is also another explanation of factor (5) given by the model, i.e. that the calcium influx during the action potential of beat 1 was increased because of the negative feedback control of conductance by calcium in the release compartment (Figure 3.1). The short interval before ES allows insufficient time for filling of the release compartment. The inhibition of the calcium influx by the amount of calcium in the release compartment (which is small under these circumstances) will therefore be reduced. That there is an increase of slow inward current in a premature excitation and greater

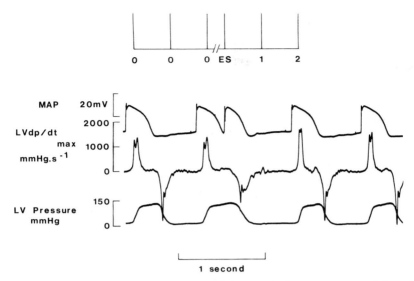

Figure 3.5 Monophasic action potential, left ventricular pressure and LV d*p*/d*t* recorded in man during the inducement of post-extrasystolic potentiation (pacing protocol at top)

uptake of calcium in a premature contraction is suggested by the studies of Hiraoka and Sano (1976) and Edmands *et al.* (1972).

The accompanying changes in action potential duration vary with species. In dog heart there is a shorter duration of the action potential in association with a premature beat (Figure 3.5). In this species, increased calcium inward current appears to be associated with earlier depolarization. By contrast in the rabbit, a premature beat is associated with a longer action potential (Wohlfart, 1979), so that in this species action potential duration reflects calcium influx. Nevertheless, the model applies to both species because the release compartment (Figure 3.1) is postulated to control calcium conductance. Thus, the model predicts increased calcium intake with the action potential of the premature beat in both species.

The percentage potentiation of beat 1 is less in the intact heart than in the isolated papillary muscle. As discussed under factor (4) above, isolation of tissue leads to lower recirculation of calcium from one beat to another and a lowered inotropic state in which the calcium content of the release compartment is abnormally low. Thus, assuming that the potentiation of calcium influx in a premature beat is maximal in both preparations so that the amount added to the system is the same in absolute quantity, the precentage increase will be much less in the case where the calcium content is already high.

Decay of Post-extrasystolic Potentiation

After potentiation of contractility by an intervention such as extra beats, there is a decay of the potentiated state which is dependent on the presence or absence of contractions. The decay depends on the number of beats and takes a much longer time when there are no contractions. The presence of contraction is thus likely to lead to an outflow of calcium. The model postulates two different kinds of outflow of calcium. The first and most important in the short term is the exit arrow at the left of Figure 3.1. This is the *beat-dependent outflow*. The other outflow is the slow continuous efflux from the release compartment.

The decay of post-extrasystolic potentiation in the intact dog is much slower than in rabbit papillary muscle. This again indicates a greater recirculation of calcium in the intact dog as compared to the isolated tissue. The decay is also more rapid if a high frequency of beating is present during the decay period; contractility decays with beat number and not with time.

Application of the Model to the Intact Dog Heart

The contractility (maximum rate of rise of left ventricular pressure, (LV dP/dt_{max}) and action potential duration were measured by Drake *et al.* (1982a,b) in intact closed-chest anaesthetized dogs with atrioventricular dissociation and beta-adrenergic blockade. The measurements were confined to two test beats (as in Figure 3.5), each following a 1 s interval (to allow for mechanical restitution, i.e. factor 1, Figure 3.2). Prior to the test intervals (priming period) a variety of potentiating stimulus trains were introduced.

When the frequency of stimulation was increased in the priming period, the decay of potentiation between test beats 1 and 2 increased. From the preceding section this might lead one to conclude that there was a reduced recirculation of calcium following higher frequency stimulation. However, linear regression of contractility of test beat 2 (DP_2) on contractility of test beat 1 (DP_1), as in Figure 3.4, yielded relationships with the same slopes for 1 Hz and 2 Hz priming frequency. The line for 2 Hz was shifted downwards and in parallel in comparison with the 1 Hz line (Figure 3.6). According to the model this would mean that the proportion of calcium recirculated was the same, but that other sources of calcium are reduced. Of these, the principle one is the calcium entering on the preceding action potential (factor (3)).

It was found that an increased priming frequency shortens the action potential duration of test beat 1. The reason for this is obscure (Attwell *et al.*, 1981; Drake *et al.*, 1982a), but it is evidently not due to increased calcium in the release compartment because there is no correlation between the action potential duration and contractility of test beat 1 (Drake *et al.*,

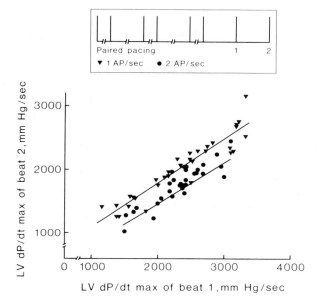

Figure 3.6. The relationship of contractility to that of the previous beat at two different frequencies (pacing protocol at top)

1981a, 1982a). The shortening of action potential with increased priming frequency is the most obvious explanation for the result shown in Figure 3.6, since a shorter action potential on test beat 1 will allow less calcium into the system to add to recirculated calcium and to appear on test beat 2. The total data of Drake *et al.* (1982b) is compatible with this aspect of the model because it is fitted by equation (3.1) when $F(n) = $ LV dP/dt_{max} of test beat 2, $AP(n-1) = $ action potential duration of test beat 1, and $F(n-1) = $ LV dP/dt_{max} of test beat 1.

Force-Frequency Relationships and the Model

Transient effects of increased stimulation frequency on force and action potential duration of rabbit papillary muscle are shown in Figure 3.7 (Wohlfart and Noble, 1982). The model provides an explanation for these characteristic responses to frequency of stimulation. Since a large series of different aspects of the model come into play sequentially as one scans from left to right through this record, they will be listed as a beat-dependent series of events below:

(1) The first contraction elicited after a shortened interval (step up in frequency of contraction) is reduced in amplitude because of incomplete

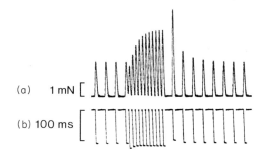

(a)   1 mN [

(b) 100 ms [

Figure 3.7 Response of rabbit papillary muscle to a brief train of high frequency stimulation and its recovery: (a) tension; (b) action potential duration (output of an analogue analyser). Reproduced with permission from Wohlfart and Noble, *Pharm. Therapeut,* 1982

replenishment of the calcium content of the release compartment. This is incomplete mechanical restitution.

(2) This first short interval also causes an increased calcium uptake during the first excitation following the step up in frequency, because the reduced filling of the release compartment (short interval) results in less inhibition of calcium entry through the negative feedback influence of that compartment on calcium conductance. In this preparation, the increased calcium entry is associated with a prolonged action potential. (This association is very useful in the rabbit for illustrating the calcium influx changes of the force–frequency phenomena. It would not be shown in the dog where the action potential duration changes are opposite in direction.)

(3) The calcium intake is also intensified during the next following beats with shortened intervals, yielding contractile potentiation during the period of increased frequency of stimulation.

(4) The increased contractility leads to an increase in the calcium levels in both compartments. This leads to a somewhat reduced calcium intake and therefore to a shortening of the action potential.

(5) The increment of force with each beat becomes less until a steady level is attained. For the steady state to be reached, if we assume the same fraction of recirculated calcium, B_F, beat-dependent calcium efflux increases until it equals the increased calcium influx.

(6) With the first beat after the excitation interval is prolonged again (step down in frequency), a high force is recorded. This results from transfer of calcium from the uptake to the release compartment for a longer time during the longer interval so that there is greater filling of the release compartment, greater calcium release, greater contractility.

(7) A second consequence of this longer interval is greater filling of the membrane compartment resulting in reduced calcium intake and reflected in Figure 3.7 by the shortened action potential.

(8) The reduced calcium intake reduces the contractility of subsequent beats until the beat dependent calcium efflux also declines to become equal to influx and re-establish a steady state.

(9) As contractility declines as a consequence of beat dependent efflux, the calcium content of both compartments declines including that of the release compartment which then exerts less inhibition of calcium influx. This is reflected in the gradual increase in action potential duration towards the original value.

Inotropic Effects and the Model

The model for calcium handling during the excitation–contraction cycle (Figure 3.1) suggests some general modes of action of interventions having a positive inotropic effect on myocardium:

(1) An increased recirculation of calcium between beats (increased B_F). According to the model this means that there is a smaller outflow of calcium in association with each contraction.

(2) An increased calcium intake with excitation. This may show up as an increased duration of the action potential and/or increased voltage of the plateau of the intracellularly recorded action potential (depending on species).

(3) An increased rate of transfer of calcium from uptake to release compartment, i.e. shortened time for sequestered calcium to become releasable again. This type of action would produce a positive inotropic response at high frequencies of stimulation but not at low.

(4) A change in the equilibrium conditions between the release compartment and the extracellular space such that a shift of calcium ions occurred from outside the cell into the release compartment. This inward shift of calcium ions would occur as a result of the action of substances interfering with the cell membrane. The result of this change is to prolong the optimum test pulse interval. Digitalis in high doses prolongs the optimum test pulse interval markedly (Wohlfart and Edman, 1979). An inotropic effect of this type is manifest with steady stimulation when low frequency stimulation is used but not at high frequencies, i.e. the opposite kind of frequency-dependent inotropic effect to that described in (3) above.

(5) A longer lasting release of calcium from the release compartment leading to the release of a greater proportion of the calcium stored in that compartment. The same result, i.e. greater proportionate release, could be achieved in the same time with a more rapid release rate.

(6) An inhibition of the uptake of calcium from the contractile proteins. This would probably be accompanied by a slowing of the relaxation of the ventricular muscle. This is seen with caffeine where the later and slower

relaxation results in a longer time to peak tension and therefore to a higher peak tension (caffeine also has other effects). The same type of effect on relaxation is seen at low temperature.

(7) An increased sensitivity of the contractile proteins to released calcium. There is evidence that decreased sensitivity occurs with adrenaline, probably as the result of a change in the degree of phosphorylation of the regulatory proteins brought about by changes in the cyclic AMPconcentration in the cell (Herzig *et al.*, 1981). This mechanism would cause adrenaline to have a negative inotropic effect if it were not masked by the positive inotropic effect due to increased calcium intake (mechanism (2) above).

CALCIUM ENTRY TO THE CELL VIA THE CELL MEMBRANE

I pass now from consideration of the model to the possible structural, functional, and metabolic components of the real system. The cell membrane (sarcolemma, plasma membrane) is a lipid bilayer which covers the cell surface (Figure 3.8), and allows calcium ions into the cell during the plateau phase of the action potential; this plateau follows the initial upstroke of the action potential (Figures 3.3, 3.5). These two phases of depolarization are thought to be due to two currents: a rapid inward current carried by Na^+ ions which causes the initial rapid depolarization and a slow inward current carried by Ca^{++} which causes the plateau.

Is the amount of calcium entering during the action potential enough to activate contraction? There are uncertainties because of lack of direct methods of measuring calcium influx. The problem is discussed in detail in Lewartowski's chapter (Chapter 5 in this volume). The most direct observations to my knowledge come from experiments from Lewartowski's group which he describes there. His conclusion is that enough calcium does enter during excitation to activate contraction. This might imply that no calcium recirculates. However, the recirculated fraction of calcium (by model analyses) in isolated tissue is extremely low, e.g. 20% or less (Wohlfart and Elzinga, 1982). If this was the case in Lewartowski's experiments, his result does not necessarily disprove the model presented here. According to the model, 80% of released calcium enters per action potential in rabbit papillary muscle while only 40% enters in the intact rabbit (Wohlfart and Elzinga, 1982). According to Lewartowski's scheme, C_3 would be the internal store and C_2 the influxing Ca^{++} in the model presented here.

In the experiments of Simurda *et al.* (1976), following the introduction of a series of equal voltage clamp depolarizations, the force of each induced contraction increased, climbing to a steady level; this response is referred to as 'positive staircase'. As the force rose, the slow inward current declined even though the voltage of each successive clamp was made identical. If the

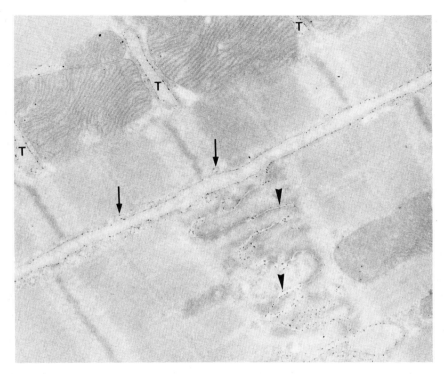

Figure 3.8 Calcium distribution in a dog left ventricular myocardial cell fixed in a relaxed state. Cytochemical localization is assessed with a combined phosphate–pyroantimonate method. The Ca^{++} deposits are lining the cytoplasmic leaflet of the sarcolemma, sarcolemma-derived vesicles (arrows), T-tubules (T), and intercalated disc (arrow head). ×18 500. [Photograph kindly provided and reproduced by courtesy of M. Borgers, Department of Cell Biology, Janssen Pharmaceutica, Beerse, Belgium.]

rising force indicates an increase in the amount of Ca^{++} in an intracellular store, the gradient of calcium between the extracellular fluid and the store is decreasing. It would seem that this gradient is determining the driving force of the slow inward current since both gradient and current are declining progressively with the build-up of the staircase phenomenon, i.e. the amount of calcium bound in this store has a negative feedback stabilizing control on the amount of calcium influx. A similar conclusion emerges from the studies of Lewartowski (see Chapter 5 in this volume).

CALCIUM BINDING AND STORAGE

The cell membrane can also bind calcium (Figure 3.8). There are invaginations of the cell membrane which form the transverse tubular system. The lumens of the transverse T-tubules contain extracellular fluid. They penetrate the cell to run alongside the Z discs separating each sarcomere from its longitudinal neighbour; they can also run longitudinally between sarcomeres. The T-tubules conduct the signal of excitation–contraction coupling into the cell interior. Calcium ions entering during the plateau phase of the action potential can also pass from the tubule lumen (extracellular space) into the depths of the cell interior. The T-tubule system is so extensive that it can be calculated from electron micrographs that the surface of plasma membrane in the T-tubules is about seven times that of the cell surface. Outside the plasma membrane there is an extracellular protein–polysaccharide coating (the glycocalyx), which can also store Ca^{++} (Langer, 1978).

The plasmalemma is an obvious candidate for an intracellular Ca^{++} store. The system of excitation–contraction coupling which has been outlined could be achieved by release of bound calcium from the plasma membrane during depolarization, and rebinding of calcium could take place on repolarization (Lüllmann and Peters, 1977). Another idea is to suppose that calcium bound on the outer surface of the cell membrane is the important calcium in excitation–contraction coupling (Langer, 1978). However, this idea seems to be giving way to that of a membrane-bound store (Lewartowski, Chapter 5, and Lüllmann *et al.*, Chapter 1, in this volume).

An alternative school of thought regards the sarcoplasmic reticulum as the store of activator Ca^{++} (Fabiato and Fabiato, 1977). The sarcoplasmic reticulum has a lace-like network of tubules which is wrapped around the myofibrils. The intimate anatomical relationship with the contractile proteins has led most students of excitation–contraction coupling to postulate that the sarcoplasmic reticulum is responsible for removing calcium ions from the contractile proteins during relaxation. The mechanism for this process is discussed by Drake-Holland and Noble (Chapter 17 in this volume).

These concepts are not necessarily mutually exclusive. It is possible that the relative importance of one or the other store may vary between different preparations. This would explain differences in behaviour found by various authors. On the other hand, mitochondria are not now thought to participate in beat to beat control of calcium (Carafoli, 1982).

EVIDENCE THAT CALCIUM SWITCHES ON THE CONTRACTILE PROTEINS

The system of contractile proteins (actin and myosin filaments) can be activated *in vitro* by calcium ions in the presence of ATP to cause splitting of the ATP by the enzymatic ATPase portion of the system – the heavy meromyosin. This activation causes contraction. The question arises, 'Are calcium ions the activator in the intact cell?' There is considerable evidence that this is the case:

(1) In skinned muscle cells (Fabiato and Fabiato, 1975a), the calcium ion concentration of the fluid bathing the preparation must be kept extremely low in order to keep it relaxed. As the calcium ion concentration rises, the preparation develops tension and reaches full tension at concentrations above 10^{-5} M (see ter Keurs, Chapter 4 in this volume).

(2) For heart muscle, if calcium ions are removed from the extracellular fluid, the muscle becomes non-contractile. Contractility recovers when calcium ions are restored (Ringer, 1883).

(3) Aequorin, a bioluminescent protein which emits light in the presence of calcium ions, can be injected intracellularly into a muscle cell (Ashley and Ridgeway, 1970; Blinks *et al.*, 1978). Allen and Kurihara (1980) have recently obtained signals with this method from frog atrium and cat papillary muscle by injecting many cells. In all these preparations, the light signal obtained from aequorin follows the action potential and precedes the development of tension.

(4) If calcium causes the contraction, it must be removed from the contractile proteins in order to produce relaxation. Isolated cardiac microsomes bind and take up calcium ions actively from the surrounding medium. That the membranes remove calcium by this process, in the muscle cell, is suggested by their close proximity to the myofilaments. Calcium uptake by the microsomes and relaxation are both accelerated by adrenaline and cyclic AMP (Weber, 1968; Fuchs, 1969; Blinks *et al.*, 1972; Kirchberger *et al.*, 1972; Morad and Rolett, 1972; Clark and Olson, 1973; Fabiato and Fabiato, 1975b; Meinertz *et al.*, 1975). These correlations again suggest that it is the calcium interaction with the myofilaments which causes them to convert chemical into mechanical energy.

CALCIUM BINDING PROTEINS

The whole process of Ca^{++} ion transport from the extracellular space to the contractile proteins is complicated by the presence of many calcium binding sites within the cell. Sites on the cell membrane, sarcoplasmic reticulum, and contractile proteins (e.g. troponin) are fixed but the calcium binding protein calmodulin (Cheung, 1980) is mobile. Thus, movements of Ca^{++} within the cell could be transported in a form in which it is bound to calmodulin; under these circumstances it will not be indicated by the light reaction with aequorin (see previous section).

The possibility that calmodulin could be involved in the rapid movement of calcium within a twitch is suggested by the mathematical model of Robertson *et al.* (1981). They took available data for cell content and metal

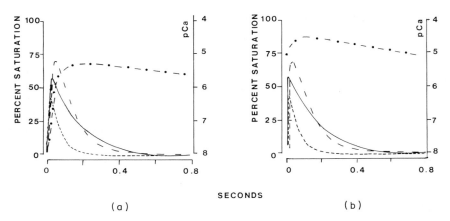

Figure 3.9 Response times of various binding sites according to the model of Roberston *et al.* (1981). —, pCa (i.e. $-\log[\mathrm{Ca}^{++}]$); -----, calmodulin; – –, Ca^{++}-specific troponin site; -·-·-, Ca^{++}, Mg^{++} troponin site. (a) Single twitch, (b) steady-state

binding capacity of calmodulin (a Ca^{++}-specific site) and the calcium-specific site of troponin. In addition the Ca^{++}–Mg^{++} binding capacities of troponin and myosin were included in the calculations. Assumptions were made about the rate constants for association and dissociation of Ca^{++}. Using these assumptions, calmodulin was found to bind and release Ca^{++} with a rapid time course during an imposed transient rise of free Ca^{++} concentration (Figure 3.9). The 'calmodulin transient' was in advance of that of troponin. Thus, calmodulin could serve the function of a transporter of activator calcium from the release compartment to the contractile proteins, assuming that the release compartment is another fixed Ca^{++} binding site elsewhere in the cell. On the other hand, Chapman *et al.* (see Chapter 6 in this volume) present data to suggest that calmodulin does not bind a sufficient amount of Ca^{++}.

It is interesting to see the model prediction for Ca^{++} binding to the Ca^{++}–Mg^{++} binding sites on the contractile proteins. The affinity of the myosin site appears to be so low that hardly any binding occurs. Considerable binding to the Ca^{++}–Mg^{++} site of troponin occurs but in a slow manner. Thus, during a twitch, this site would be expected to take up some Ca^{++} but to release it so slowly that the amount of binding increases in a steady train of twitches compared to a single twitch following rest (compare Figure 3.9(b) with Figure 3.9(a)). This site illustrates one of the Ca^{++} 'sinks' which allow the total calcium content to change slowly but which do not take part in the rapid events of the excitation–contraction cycle; the mitochondria are probably the most important of these sites (Chapter 7 in this volume).

COUPLING BETWEEN CALCIUM ENTRY
AND CONTRACTION

In the previous sections evidence was reviewed that calcium ions enter the myocardial cell during the action potential and that they activate contraction. Can these two facts be simply linked together to produce excitation–contraction coupling? It appears that this is not the case and that there is a complicated system linking the two events. The most important evidence for this is the study of Antoni *et al.* (1969) (Figure 3.3). They applied current during a single action potential in a rhythmically driven papillary muscle. The contraction resulting from the prolonged action potential was only slightly affected. Following this beat, the muscle was returned to the previous regular stimulation with normal action potentials. The beat after the one with the artificially prolonged action potential was potentiated even though the action potential of this potentiated beat was normal. This type of experiment led to the idea that activator calcium is buffered by some sort of intracellular store. Thus, the experiment of Antoni *et al.* (1969) is explained on the basis of this hypothesis by supposing that the extra calcium, which was driven into the cell during the current applied for one depolarization only, entered this intracellular store so that no effect was seen on that contraction. However, the extra calcium now in the store was released on the subsequent excitation, which triggered a potentiated contraction.

Although the action potential duration and contractility of a given beat do not have a direct relationship (above), there does seem to be a relationship between the duration of the action potential and the duration of contraction. Morad and Trautwein (1968), for instance, found an S-shaped relationship between action potential duration and time to peak isometric force. This observation can be fitted to the idea of the intracellular store by postulating that the time for release of ionic calcium from the store is controlled by the duration of the depolarization signal. Alternatively, one could postulate a double mechanism, i.e. some release from the store and some direct flow to the myofilaments. Such a hypothesis seems to be necessary to account for the behaviour of rested state contractions but is not necessary for rhythmically stimulated preparations at physiological frequencies.

With an intracellular Ca store, we would expect that if calcium entry is increased in a steady state of rhythmic beats, the filling of the store and therefore force production would both increase. This has been done by applying voltage clamp pulses of increased amplitude and duration to drive the Ca^{++} into the cell (Beeler and Reuter, 1970b; New and Trautwein, 1972; Tritthart *et al.*, 1973). Within limits, this results in greater force production. More than five depolarizations are required before a new steady state in force production is reached. This is interpreted as being due to the fact that the extra calcium coming into the cell goes into the buffer store, the filling of which has to build up to new level before a consistently higher level of calcium is released each beat. Furthermore, the contractile response to the first altered depolarization clamp in such an experiment is affected very little by the voltage of that clamp. Again this indicates that the contractile element is not directly activated by the slow inward current.

It has been shown that the membrane has to remain repolarized for about 500 ms before a complete reactivation of the contractile system can be obtained (Tritthart *et al.*, 1973). With the intracellular store hypothesis this can be explained by postulating that some time for the store to be free of depolarizing signal is required before the calcium bound there is available again for release.

MECHANISMS OF CALCIUM RELEASE FROM INTRACELLULAR SITES

Since it is probable that most contractile calcium is released from the intracellular store, there have been a number of studies of the mechanism of such release in the case of cardiac membranes and how it would be triggered by the action potential. This has been studied by using isolated membrane vesicles (microsomes) or by using the 'skinned' muscle cell without cell membrane.

There appear to be two ways of triggering calcium release in these preparations, both of which consist of a mixture of sarcoplasmic reticulum and plasma membrane. These mechanisms are depolarization-induced Ca^{++} release and Ca^{++}-induced Ca^{++} release (see Blayney, Chapter 2 in this volume.)

In intact cardiac muscle, a twitch is produced by an artificially curtailed action potential with no plateau (Morad and Trautwein, 1968). This means that internal Ca^{++} is released as a consequence of the fast Na^+ current of the initial part of the action potential. This might imply that the release of internal Ca^{++} occurs by depolarization of the cell and T-tubule membrane, and that Ca^{++} which enters the cell during the action potential plateau goes into replenishing the internal Ca^{++} store. This interpretation fits particularly well with the ideas of Lüllmann and Peters (1979) who think that the activator calcium is that calcium which binds tightly in large quantity to a lipid on the intracellular surface of the plasma membrane. Depolarization of the membrane would cause reduced binding of the calcium and release of a fraction of the calcium in the ionized form. However, the experiment with curtailed action potential (above) could be interpreted in another way: the cisternae with their intimate proximity to the cell membrane could be depolarized and release enough Ca^{++} to trigger the rest of the sarcoplasmic reticulum by the Ca^{++}-induced Ca^{++} release mechanism.

CALCIUM EFFLUX

The first and most obvious control of calcium efflux is the amount of intracellular calcium in some cellular compartment from which calcium can be extruded to the exterior. There is evidence for a calcium extrusion mechanism that exchanges intracellular Ca^{++} for extracellular sodium ions (Reuter, 1974). More recent evidence suggests that three sodium ions are involved in the exchange (Lewartowski, Chapter 5, and Chapman *et al.*, Chapter 6, in this volume) making the system electrogenic, i.e. calcium efflux by the mechanism causes an inward current tending to depolarize the cell. The sodium ions which enter the cell are presumably pumped out in exchange for K^+ by the Na^+–K^+ pump (an energy-consuming membrane ATPase) which is also electrogenic causing an *outward* current (tending to polarize the cell). If this Na^+–Ca^{++} exchange mechanism proceeds between depolarizations, its rate will presumably depend upon the intracellular content of calcium and the interval between depolarizations, i.e. it would not be beat dependent.

Calcium efflux is, however, a more complicated phenomenon. If intracellular calcium and contractility are potentiated, e.g. by post-extrasystolic potentiation, the decay of the potentiated state is much faster in the presence than in the absence of rhythmic beating (Hoffman *et al.*, 1956). Thus there is a dominant, beat-dependent calcium outflow in addition to the outflow which occurs in a quiescent fibre. Actual outflow of ^{45}Ca has also been measured (Lewartowski, Chapter 5 in this volume) and shown to be predominantly beat dependent. It is therefore important to consider by what mechanism there is an outflow of calcium in association with each excitation–contraction–relaxation cycle. During the action potential, Na^+–Ca^{++} exchange could be responsible, depending on its sensitivity to membrane potential and cytosolic calcium ion concentration. The active pump in the plasma membrane (Caroni and Carafoli, 1980) would transport Ca^{++} from the inside to the outside of the cell whenever the cytosolic Ca^{++} concentration rose, i.e. with each concentration. This seems a more effective hypothesis for the problem of maintaining a low internal calcium in all conditions.

REFERENCES

Allen, D. G., Jewell, B. R., and Wood, E. H. (1976). Studies on the contractility of mammalian myocardium at low rates of stimulation. *J. Physiol. (Lond.)*, **254**, 1–17.

Allen, D. G., and Kurihara, S. (1981). Length changes during contraction affect the intracellular Ca^{2+} of heart muscle. *J. Physiol. (Lond.)*, **310**, 75P.

Anderson, T. W., and Johnson, E. A. (1976). The repolarization phase of the cardiac action potential: a comparative study of rate-induced changes in its waveform. *J. Mol. Cell. Cardiol.*, **8**, 103–121.

Anderson, P. A. W., Manning, A., and Johnson, E. A. (1977). The force of contraction of isolated papillary muscle: a study of the interaction of its determining factors. *J. Mol. Cell. Cardiol.*, **9**, 131–150.

Antoni, H. (1977). Elementary events in excitation-contraction coupling of the mammalian myocardium. *Basic Res. Cardiol.*, **72**, 140–146.

Antoni, H., Jacob, R., and Kaufman, R. (1969). Mechanische Reaktionen des Frasch und Saugetiermyokards bei Veränderung Aktionspotential-Danez durch konstante Gleichström impulse. *Pfügers Arch. Ges. Physiol.*, **306**, 33–57.

Ashley, C. C., and Ridgeway, E. B. (1970). On the relationships between membrane potential, calcium transient and tension in single barnacle muscle fibres. *J. Physiol. (Lond.)*, **209**, 105–130.

Attwell, D., Cohen, I., and Eisner, D. A. (1981). The effects of heart rate on the action potential of guinea-pig and human ventricular muscle. *J. Physiol. (Lond.)*, **313**, 439–461.

Bass, B. G. (1975). Restitution of the action potential in cat papillary muscle. *Amer. J. Physiol.*, **228**, 1712–1724.

Bass, O. (1976). The decay of the potentiated state in sheep and calf ventricular fibres. Influences of agents acting on transmembrane Ca^{2+} flux. *Circulation Res.*, **39**, 396–399.

Bassingthwaighte, J. B., Fry, C. H., and McGuigan, J. A. S. (1976). Relationship between internal calcium and outward current in mammalian ventricular muscle: a mechanism for the control of the action potential duration? *J. Physiol. (Lond.)*, **262**, 15–37.

Bautovich, G., Gibb, D. B., and Johnson, E. A. (1962). The force of contraction of the rabbit papillary muscle preparation as a function of the frequency and pattern of stimulation. *Austral. J. Exp. Biol.*, **40**, 455–472.

Beeler, G. W., and Reuter, H. (1970a) Membrane calcium current in ventricular myocardial fibres. *J. Physiol. (Lond.)*, **207**, 191–209.

Beeler, G. W., and Reuter, H. (1970b). The relation between membrane potential, membrane currents and activation of contraction in ventricular myocardial fibres. *J. Physiol. (Lond.)*, **207**, 211–229.

Blinks, J. R., Olson, C. B., Jewell, B. R., and Braveny, P. (1972). Influence of caffeine and other methylxanthines on mechanical properties of isolated mammalian heart muscle. Evidence for a dual mechanism of action. *Circulation Res.*, **33**, 367–392.

Blinks, J. R., Rudel, R., and Taylor, S. R. (1978). Calcium transients in isolated amphibian skeletal muscle fibres: detection with aequorin. *J. Physiol. (Lond.)*, **277**, 291–323.

Boyett, M. R., and Jewell, B. R. (1980). Analysis of the effects of changes in rate and rhythm upon electrical activity in the heart. *Prog. Biophys. Mol. Biol.*, **36**, 1–52.

Braveny, P., and Sumbera, J. (1968). Relation of contraction and repolarization time in guinea pig atria and ventricles. *Scripta Medica*, **41**, 241–248.

Braveny, P., and Sumbera, J. (1970). Electromechanical correlation in the mammalian heart muscle. *Pflügers Arch. Ges. Physiol.*, **319**, 36–48.

Carafoli, E. (1982). The transport of calcium across the inner membrane of mitochondria. In *Membrane Transport of Calcium* (E. Carafoli, ed.), Academic Press, London, pp. 109–139.

Caroni, P., and Carafoli, E. (1980). An ATP-dependent Ca^{++}-pumping system in dog heart sarcolemma. *Nature*, **283**, 765–767.

Cheung, W. Y. (1980). Calmodulin plays a pivotal role in cellular regulation. *Science*, **207**, 19–27.

Clark, A., and Olson, C. B. (1973). Effects of caffeine and isoprenaline on mammalian ventricular muscle. *Brit. J. Pharmacol.*, **47**, 1–11.

Drake, A. J., Noble, M. I. M., Schouten, V., Seed, A., ter Keurs, H. E. D. J., and Wohlfart, B. (1981a). Evidence that the cardiac action potential is not inversely related to intracellular calcium. *J. Physiol. (Lond.)*, **318**, 31P.

Drake, A. J., ter Keurs, H. E. D. J., Noble, M. I. M., Pieterse, M., Seed, W. A., Schouten, V., and Wohlfart, B. (1981b). The effect of cardiac stimulus frequency on the subsequent decay of contractility. *J. Physiol. (Lond.)*, **320**, 35P.

Drake, A. J., ter Keurs, H. E. D. J., Noble, M. I. M., Schouten, V., Seed, A., and Wohlfart, B. (1982a). Is action potential duration of the dog heart related to contractility or stimulus rate? *J. Physiol. (Lond.)*, **331**, 499–510.

Drake, A. J., ter Keurs, H. E. D. J., Noble, M. I. M., Pieterse, M., Seed, W. A., Schouten, V. J. A., and Wohlfart, B. (1982b). Dependence of contractility on the excitation–contraction cycle of the previous beat in the intact dog. *Circulation Res.*, submitted for publication.

Edman, K. A. P., and Johannsson, M. (1976). The contractile state of rabbit papillary muscle in relation to stimulation frequency. *J. Physiol. (Lond.)*, **254**, 565–581.

Edmands, R. E., Greenspan, K., and Bailey, J. C. (1972). Role of the premature action potential in contractile potentiation: a study of paired stimulation. *Cardiovasc. Res.*, **6**, 368–374.

Edmands, R. E., Greenspan, K., and Fisch, C. (1968). Electrophysiological correlates of contractile change in mammalian and amphibian myocardium. *Cardiovasc. Res.*, **3**, 253–260.

Elzinga, D., Lab, M. J., Noble, M. I. M., Papadoyannis, D. E., Pidgeon, J. Seed, A., and Wohlfart, B. (1981). The action potential duration and contractile response of the intact heart related to the preceding interval and the preceding beat. *J. Physiol. (Lond.)*, **314**, 481–500.

Fabiato, A., and Fabiato, F. (1975a). Contractions induced by a calcium-triggered release of calcium from the sarcoplasmic reticulum of single skinned cardiac cells. *J. Physiol. (Lond.)*, **249**, 469–495.

Fabiato, A., and Fabiato, F. (1975b). Relaxing and inotropic effects of cyclic AMP on skinned cardiac cells. *Nature*, **253**, 556–558.

Fabiato, A., and Fabiato, F. (1977). Calcium release from the sarcoplasmic reticulum. *Circulation Res.*, **40**, 119–129.

Fuchs, F. (1969). Inhibition of sarcotubular calcium transport by caffeine: species and temperature dependence. *Biochim. Biophys. Acta*, **172**, 566–570.

Gibbs, C. L. (1978). Cardiac energetics. *Physiol. Rev.*, **58**, 174–254.

Gibbs, C. L., and Johnson, E. A. (1961). Effect of changes in frequency of stimulation upon rabbit ventricular action potential. *Circulation Res.*, **9**, 165–170.

Herzig, J. W. Kohler, G., Pfizer, G., Ruegg, J. C., and Woffle, G. (1981). Cycle AMP inhibits contractility of detergent-treated glycerol extracted cardiac muscle. *Pfluger's Arch. Europ. J. Physiol.*, **391**, 208–212.

Hiraoka, M., and Sano, T. (1976). Role of slow inward current in the genesis of ventricular arrhythmia. *Jpn. Circulation J.*, **40**, 1419–1427.

Hoffman, B. F., Bindler, E., and Suckling, B. E. (1956). Post-extrasystolic potentiation of contraction in cardiac muscle. *Amer. J. Physiol.*, **185**, 95–102.

Isenberg, G. (1975). Is potassium conductance of cardiac Purkinje fibres controlled by $[Ca_i^{2+}]$? *Nature*, **253**, 273–274.

Jewell, B. R. (1977). A re-examination of the influence of muscle length of myocardial performance. *Circulation Res.*, **40**, 221–230.

Kass, R. S., and Tsien, R. W. (1976). Control of action potential duration by calcium ions in cardiac Purkinje fibres. *J. Gen. Physiol.*, **67**, 599–617.

Kaufmann, R., Bayer, R., Fürniss, T., Krause, H., and Tritthart, H. (1974). Calcium movement controlling cardiac contractility. II. Analog computation of cardiac excitation–contraction coupling on the basis of calcium kinetics in a multi-compartment model. *J. Mol. Cell. Cardiol.*, **6**, 543–559.

Kirchberger, M. A., Tada, M., Repke, D. I., and Katz, A. M. (1972). Cyclic adenosine 3′,5′-monophosphate dependent protein kinase stimulation of calcium uptake by canine microsomes. *J. Mol. Cell. Cardiol.*, **4**, 673–680.

Koch-Weser, J., and Blinks, J. R. (1963). The influence of the interval between beats on myocardial contractility. *Pharmacol. Rev.*, **15**, 601–652.

Langer, G. A. (1978). The structure and function of the myocardial cell surface. *Amer. J. Physiol.*, **235**, H461–H468.

Langer, G. A., Frank, J. S., and Brady, A. J. (1976). The myocardium. In *MTP International Review of Physiology, Series 2*, Vol. 9, *Cardiovascular Physiology* (A. C. Guyton and A. W. Cowley, eds), University Park Press, Baltimore, pp. 191–237.

Lüllman, H., and Peters, T. (1977). Plasmalemmal calcium in cardiac excitation–contraction coupling. *Clin. Exp. Pharmacol. Physiol.*, **4**, 49–57.

Lüllman, H., and Peters, T. (1979). Action of cardiac glycosides on the excitation–contraction coupling in heart muscle. A new concept. *Prog. Pharmacol.*, **2**, 1–57.

Meinertz, T., Nawarth, H., and Scholz, H. (1975). Relaxant effects of dibutyryl cyclic AMP on mammalian cardiac muscle. *J. Cyclic Nucleotide Res.*, **1**, 31–36.

Miller, J. P., Wallace, A. G., and Feezar, M. D. (1971). A quantitative comparison of the relation between the shape of the action potential and the pattern of stimulation in canine ventricular muscle and Purkinje Fibres. *J. Mol. Cell. Cardiol.*, **2**, 3–19.

Morad, M., and Goldman, Y. (1973). Excitation–contraction coupling in heart muscle: membrane control of development of tension. *Prog. Biophys. Mol. Biol.*, **27**, 257–313.

Morad, M., and Rolett, E. L. (1972). Relaxing effects of catecholamines on mammalian heart. *J. Physiol. (Lond.)*, **224**, 537–558.

Morad, M., and Trautwein, W. (1968). The effect of the duration of the action potential on contraction in the mammalian heart muscle. *Pflügers Arch. Ges. Physiol.*, **299**, 66–82.

New, W., and Trautwein, W. (1972). Inward membrane currents in mammalian myocardium. *Pflügers Arch. Ges. Physiol.*, **335**, 1–23.

Noble, M. I. M. (1979). *The Cardiac Cycle*. Blackwell Sceintific Publications, Oxford.

Pidgeon, J., Lab, M., Seed, A., Elzinga, G., Papadoyannis, D., and Noble, M. I. M. (1980). The contractile state of cat and dog heart in relation to the interval between beats. *Circulation Res.*, **47**, 559–567.

Reichel, H. (1976). The effect of isolation on myocardial properties. *Basic Res. Cardiol.*, **71**, 1–16.

Reiter, M., and Stickel, F. J. (1968). Der Einfluss der Kontraktiono-Beguenz auf das Aktionspotential de Meerschweinschen-Papillarmuskels. *Naumyn Schmiedebergs Arch. Pharmacol.*, **260**, 342–365.

Reuter, H. (1974). Exchange of calcium ions in the mammalian myocardium. Mechanisms and physiological significance. *Circulation Res.*, **34**, 599–605.

Ringer, S. (1883). A further contribution regarding the influence of the different constituents of the blood on the contraction of the heart. *J. Physiol. (Lond.)*, **4**, 27–42.

Robertson, S. P., Johnson, J. D., and Potter, J. D. (1981). The time-course of Ca^{2+} exchange with calmodulin, troponin, parvalbumin and myosin in response to transient increases in Ca^{2+}. *Biophys. J.*, **34**, 559–569.

Simurda, J., Simurdova, M., Braveny, P., and Sumbera, J. (1976). Slow inward current and action potentials of papillary muscles under non-steady state conditions. *Pflügers Arch. Europ. J. Physiol.*, **362,** 209–218.

Trautwein, W. (1973). Membrane currents in cardiac muscle fibres. *Physiol. Rev.*, **53,** 793–835.

Trautwein, W., and Dudel, J. (1954). Aktionspotential und Mechanogramm des Warmblütesherz-Muskels als Funktion der Schlagfrequenz. *Pflügers Arch. Ges. Physiol.*, **260,** 24–39.

Tritthart, H., Kaufman, R., Volkmer, H. P., Bayer, R., and Krause, H. (1973). Ca-movement controlling myocardial contractility. *Pflügers Arch. Ges. Physiol.*, **338,** 207–234.

Weber, A., (1968). The mechanism of the action of caffeine on sarcoplasmic reticulum. *J. Gen. Physiol.*, **52,** 760–772.

Wohlfart, B. (1979). Relationships between peak force, action potential duration and stimulus interval in rabbit myocardium. *Acta Physiol. Scand.*, **106,** 395–409.

Wohlfart, B., and Edman, K. A. P. (1979). An analysis of the effects of digitalis on the excitation–contraction mechanism of mammalian myocardium. *Acta Physiol. Scand.*, *Suppl.* L173, 30.

Wohlfart, B., and Elzinga, E. (1982). Electrical and mechanical responses of the intact rabbit heart in relation to the excitation interval. A comparison with the isolated papillary muscle preparation. *Acta. Physiol. Scand.*, **115,** 331–340.

Wohlfart, B., and Noble, M. I. M. (1982). The cardiac excitation–contraction cycle. *Pharmacol. Therapeut.*, **16,** 1–43.

Wood, E. H., Heppner, R. L., and Weidmann, S. (1969). Inotropic effects of electric currents. *Circulation Res.*, **14,** 409–445.

Wussling, M., and Szymanski, G. (1972). A two-Ca-store model for potentiation phenomena on rabbit papillary muscle. *Studia Biophysica (Berlin)*, **34,** 121–130.

Cardiac Metabolism
Edited by A. J. Drake-Holland and M. I. M. Noble
© 1983 John Wiley & Sons Ltd

CHAPTER 4

Calcium and Contractility

H. E. D. J. ter Keurs

Department of Experimental Cardiology, Academisch Ziekenhuis, Leiden, The Netherlands

INTRODUCTION

In this chapter we will follow the sequence of events that result from transient elevation of the calcium ion concentration in myocardial cells during activation.

Structural Properties of a Myocyte

Figure 4.1 shows the main structures in a myocardial cell: the membranous elements; the sarcolemma that regularly invaginates the cell by its T-tubules (see previous chapters in this volume) which make contact with an intracellular tubular system; the sarcoplasmic reticulum. The membranes of T tubules and sarcoplasmic reticulum come into extremely close contact with every myofibril and form functional units with the latter. All myofibrils are accompanied by strings of mitochondria. The myofibrils are organized in a ladder-like structure of identical units: the sarcomeres. Myosin and actin (Huxley and Hanson, 1954) can slide freely alongside each other, but maximal length is restrained in mammalian heart to 2.4 μm and shortening is probably limited to 1.65 μm by the myosin molecule resisting deformation (Gordon *et al.*, 1966). The working range of 1.6 and 2.4 μm implies that over a large part, double overlap of actin filaments occurs.

Mechanical Output of the Contractile Apparatus

If the sarcomeres are flooded with calcium by the membrane systems of the cell, interaction sites between the actin and myosin filaments are activated (Endo, 1977; Ebashi, 1980). The activated actomyosin complexes become chemomechanical transducers that convert ATP rapidly to ADP in a cyclic way. Normally ATP is abundantly available to the contractile unit. The energy set free by this process is converted into force development and sliding of the filaments along each other. This whole process is rapidly

Figure 4.1 *Calcium and the contractile unit.* Myofibril and sarcomere adjacent to mitochondria next to T tubules (T) and sarcolemma. Localization of calcium with a combined phosphate–pyroantimonate method. The deposit lines the sarcolemma (arrows) and the T tubules of this myocardial cell of the left ventricle of a dog fixed in a relaxed state. The section was not counterstained. ×30 260. [Photograph kindly supplied by and reproduced by courtesy of Dr M. Borgers, Laboratory for Cell Biology, Janssen Pharmaceutica, Belgium.]

stopped in the intact cardiac contractile unit by resorption of the calcium by the membrane system. The rate of energy liberation during contraction by this process alone depends on the number of active transducers and on the rate of ATP turnover by each transducer. In studies on skeletal muscle Hill (1973) showed that the rate of energy liberation depended linearly on the load supported by the muscle. The relation between the rate of energy liberation and load is described by

$$(P+a)V = b(P_0 - P) \qquad (4.1)$$

where P is the load supported by the muscle, V is the velocity of shortening of the sarcomeres, and P_0 is the maximal load that can be supported by the sarcomeres without being stretched; a and b are constants. Rewriting the above equation as

$$(P+a)(v+b) = b(P_0 - a) \qquad (4.2)$$

shows that the relation between v and P represents a rectangular hyperbola with asymptotes $P = -a$ and $v = -b$.

Factors that influence the number of active transducers will evidently affect P_0. Some factors have been revealed, e.g. those affecting the intracellular calcium concentration and those affecting the sensitivity of the filament interaction sites.

Factors that affect the ATPase activity of the active transducers influence the maximal velocity of shortening which is determined by the cycle time and effective stroke of the transducers.

Mechanical output is determined by (a) initial length of the contractile unit through a hitherto unknown mechanism, (b) the control system of calcium handling, (c) the load supported, and (d) the passive mechanical properties of the muscle.

The determinants of mechanical performance will be discussed in more detail in the following sections.

SUBCELLULAR PROPERTIES

The Response to Ca^{++} of the Isolated Contractile Apparatus

Force versus [Ca^{++}]

Myofibrils – or bundles of them (Figure 4.1) – can be isolated functionally or physically from the membrane systems that control the movement of calcium. If appropriate precautions concerning the composition of the pseudo-intracellular solution and size of the preparation are taken, it appears that the properties of the myofibrillar apparatus are very similar to those in the cell. For a review of the techniques the reader is referred to recent publications by Fabiato (1981), Winegrad (1979), and Reuben and Wood (1979).

Force development by the myofibrils upon activation by calcium ions depends on a number of factors:

(a) The free calcium concentration $[Ca]_i$ reached during activation. If $[Ca]_i$ is controlled by the experimenter through adding calcium ions to a pseudo-intracellular solution that is strongly buffered with EGTA, the relation between force and calcium concentration appears to be a dose–response curve that reflects the binding of two calcium ions to each activated actomyosin site (see Figure 4.2; Fabiato, 1981). It is probable that calcium

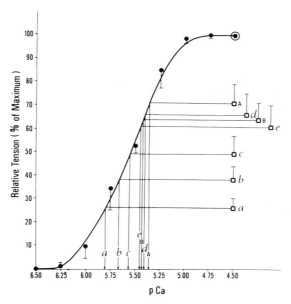

Figure 4.2 *Force versus intracellular calcium.* Rat ventricular cells: inference of the myoplasmic [free Ca^{++}] reached during the twitch of intact cells (capital letters) and the Ca^{++}-induced release of Ca^{++} from the SR of skinned cardiac cells. Each point represents the mean and each vertical bar represents the s.d. (shown in one direction only). The number of observations was seven for each data point on the twitch of intact cells, 10 for each data point on tension transients of skinned cardiac cells, and between six and nine for the tension–pCa curve in skinned cardiac cells. For the intact cells: A, twitch during regular single-pulse stimulation at $12 \, min^{-1}$ in the presence of 2.50 mM free Ca^{++}; B, twitch during paired-pulse stimulation under the same conditions as for A. For the mechanically skinned cardiac cells, the Ca^{++} transients were induced by an increase of 0.2 s of the [free Ca^{++}] from pCa 7.50 to pCa 7.00 for *a*, 6.75 for *b*, 6.50 for *c*, 6.25 for *d*, and 6.15 for *e*. [Reproduced with permission from A. Fabiato, *J. Gen. Physiol.*, **78**, 457–497 (1981).]

binds to actin and myosin at lower concentrations as well (Fabiato, 1981; Moisescu, 1976) such that a fully occupied actomyosin complex possibly contains six calcium ions.

(b) The position of the curve, i.e. pCa at 50% of peak force (the affinity of the myofilaments), depends on the composition of the intracellular solution; in other words it is shifted towards higher calcium concentrations by an increased proton concentration or by an increased magnesium ion concentration (Fabiato and Fabiato, 1978a; Donaldson *et al.*, 1978). It is likely that this reflects competitive binding of these ions to the sites which can be occupied by calcium.

(c) The affinity of the binding sites for calcium is lowered by phosphorylation of the contractile filaments (which results from activation of phosphorylases by the enzymatic cascade) that is a consequence of activation of adenylcyclase when beta-receptors bind catecholamines (McClellan and Winegrad, 1978).

(d) Force developed by the filaments in response to calcium depends on sarcomere length over the range of sarcomere lengths between 2.20 and 3.30 μm to the extent that at Ca^{++} concentrations in which partial activation of the myofilaments occurs force may rise between 2.2 and 3.1 μm. This has been observed in cardiac muscle (Endo, 1973; Nassar *et al.*, 1974; Winegrad

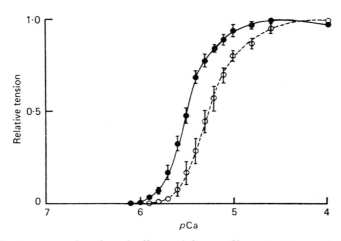

Figure 4.3 *Sarcomere length and affinity of the myofilaments.* Force–pCa curves for tonic contractions of rat trabeculae in solutions containing (in millimoles per litre): K 140, Na 30, EGTA 20, TES 50, MgATP 3, creatine phosphate 10; creatine phosphokinase was present at a concentration of 70 units ml^{-1}; ionic strength 200; pH 7.00, pMg 3.5, pCa 4–7; 20 °C. Sarcomere lengths: ○, 2.3–2.5 μm ($n=7$); ●, 1.9–2.04 μm ($n=7$). Symbols show mean tension ±S.E. of mean. Tension is expressed as a fraction of the maximum tension developed at each sarcomere length. [Reproduced with permission from M. G. Hibbert and B. R. Jewell, *J. Physiol. (Lond.)*, **292**, 30P (1979).]

et al., 1976; Fabiato and Fabiato, 1978c) and in skeletal muscle (Endo, 1973; Moisescu and Thieleczek, 1978). The mechanism of this length-dependent response is still unknown but may reflect length-dependent sensitivity of the myofilaments to calcium. It is possible that length dependence of sensitivity of the myofilaments extends over the range of sarcomere lengths even below 2.30 μm, which would be the range in which mammalian cardiac muscle operates. This is suggested by the rightward shift of the force–pCa curve (Figure 4.3) when initial sarcomere length is lowered (Hibberd and Jewell, 1979) in isolated trabeculae and papillary muscle from rat. Length dependence of sensitivity of the myofilaments is also suggested by – although less than in Hibberd's study – length-dependent force development by skinned cells at suboptimal free calcium concentration (Fabiato, 1980). At optimal concentrations of activator calcium force decreases only 20% if sarcomere length decreases from 2.3 to 1.5 μm (Fabiato and Fabiato, 1975a,b). Apparently the force-generating capacity of the myofilaments hardly depends on sarcomere length at all.

Velocity versus $[Ca^{++}]_i$

In the latter studies – near to – isometric force development has been used to assess performance of the contractile apparatus. Studies of dynamics of contraction reveal a hyperbolic relation between force and velocity of shortening in agreement with Hill's equation and with findings in intact cardiac muscle. P_0 and peak velocity of shortening at preload showed comparable dependence on the free calcium concentration (de Clerck *et al.*, 1977). It appeared that rapidly after onset of contraction the interrelations between force, length, and velocity of shortening were time-invariant. Peak velocity of shortening was 0.7 μm s^{-1}, but maximal velocity of shortening at zero load was not measured. Some evidence has been obtained that velocity of shortening at zero load also varies with the free calcium concentration and reaches maximum at lower calcium concentration than P_0, suggesting different governing mechanisms.

Control of $[Ca^{++}]_i$

Comparison of the force developed by the isolated contractile apparatus with that of the same in an intact cell (Fabiato, 1981) suggests strongly that the maximal free concentration of calcium ions in intact cells is limited to a value of 4.35 μmol l^{-1}; force is 70% of maximal force attained when the experimenter supplies calcium more generously (see Figure 4.2).

This brings us to the modus operandi of calcium ion delivery to the contractile proteins of the intact cell. This is discussed in other chapters in this volume (see Chapters 1, 3, 5, and 6).

The contraction is transient as calcium reabsorption immediately takes place in the membrane system of the sarcoplasmic reticulum. Measurements of free calcium both in intact cells and in 'skinned' cells have been performed with the aid of calcium-sensitive microelectrodes (Marban *et al.*, 1980) and by means of the light-emitting protein aequorin. Kinetics of calcium binding by aequorin and emission of light allows a reasonably (Allen *et al.*, 1977) accurate assessment of the time course of free calcium in the cell. Simultaneous study of contractions and aequorin flashes elicited by calcium-induced calcium release suggests that maximal contractile force is only related to the maximal calcium concentration that is attained following calcium release (Fabiato, 1981) and is not influenced by the rate of decrease of $[Ca]_i$. This implies that the effect of binding of calcium to the myofilament system is rapidly established and calcium dissociation occurs slowly (Allen and Kurihara, 1980). Force development in intact muscle cells is lower than in skinned cells that are maximally activated with calcium. It has been shown that calcium that enters the cell during the action potential does not contribute significantly to the concurrent contraction (see previous chapters in this volume). Thus it is likely that the amount of calcium that is released into the cell is limited by the capacity of the membranes which are responsible for calcium-induced calcium release.

Length dependence of calcium release

Release of calcium from the sarcoplasmic reticulum shows little dependence on sarcomere length, as has been shown by the use of aequorin injected in the cell (Allen and Kurihara, 1979). Figure 4.4 shows light and force recorded simultaneously in rat trabecular muscle injected with aequorin. It is clear that although force increases tenfold with increasing length, no increase in the peak of the light flash – or peak free calcium concentration – is observed. The time course of both rise and fall of light intensity seem faster at long muscle lengths than at short lengths. It could be therefore, that both the amount of calcium that is released and binding of calcium to high affinity sites in the cell is enhanced by stretch. Some length dependence of calcium release would be consistent with data derived from skinned cells in which the myosin was extracted by perfusion with solution of high ionic strength. Calcium release in these preparations, which had been brought back into solutions at normal ionic strength, was measured by spectrophotometry with arsenzao III and appeared to vary with sarcomere length (Fabiato, 1980).

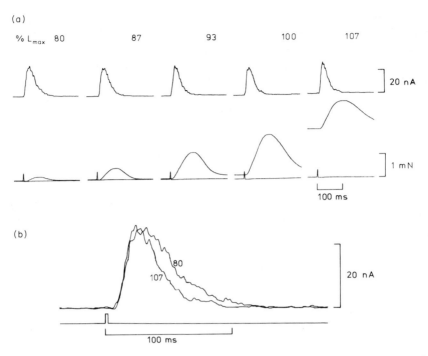

Figure 4.4 *Calcium transients versus length of rat papillary muscle.* Light and tension recorded simultaneously from an aequorin-injected rat trabecular muscle at 30 °C, stimulation rate 12 min^{-1}. Each record is the average of 64 contractions. Lengths are given as percentages of L_{max}, where L_{max} is the length at which developed tension was maximum. (a) Light (upper trace, calibration bar represents photomultiplier current) and tension (lower trace). The stimulus is shown on a line whose level represents zero tension. (b) Light records at 80 and 107% L_{max} superimposed. [Reproduced with permission from D. G. Allen and S. Kurihara, *J. Physiol. (Lond.)*, **292;** 68P–69P (1979).]

Other modulators of calcium release

Calcium release decreases with intracellular acidosis both due to depressed filling of the release sites in the sarcoplasmic reticulum and because the threshold of calcium-induced calcium release increases (Fabiato and Fabiato, 1978a). Furthermore, increase of Mg ion concentration and ADP depress calcium release (Fabiato and Fabiato, 1975a,b). Increase of the external calcium concentration from 0.5 to 8 mM in cat myocardium triples the transient rise of calcium. An increase of stimulus rate increases the maximal calcium concentration measured with aequorin even more, e.g. when cat muscle is stimulated at rates that vary between 0.0167 and 2 Hz, the transient rise of calcium varies sixfold (Allen and Kurihara, 1980).

Adrenaline causes both an increase in the concentration of calcium detected by aequorin and a more rapid decline of the calcium concentration. In high adrenaline concentration repetitive increase of calcium concentration following a single stimulus can be seen (Allen and Kurihara, 1980). As we have already seen, adrenaline also decreases the sensitivity of the myofilaments to calcium (England, Chapter 16 in this volume).

In all studies in which both aequorin flashes and force development has been studied, decline of light intensity precedes peak force. Usually peak force is reached only after the aequorin flash has subsided completely (see Figure 4.4). Only in high caffeine concentrations and during repetitive calcium peaks as a result of high concentrations of adrenaline are there exceptions. In these exceptions repetitive release of calcium is likely to have occurred. This again suggests that the dissociation of calcium from troponin or of the rate of dissociation of actomyosin complexes dominates the time course of relaxation of isometric contractions.

CELLULAR MECHANICS

Since the work of Abbott and Mommaerts (1959) muscle mechanics of the heart have been studied in preparations of papillary muscle and trabeculae dissected from the heart. Although such preparations render interpretation of mechanical behaviour much simpler than interpretation of pressure and flow data in a composite system such as the heart, the act of dissection and clamping of the preparation in the measuring apparatus creates a zone of dead elastic tissue, and damaged partially active tissue at both ends of the preparation.

Methodical Aspects

It is necessary therefore to study the central viable region of the preparation using a technique to estimate sarcomere length or an equivalent measure. Various methods have been adopted to measure length in the central region of the preparation, e.g. direct microscopy (Grimm and Wohlfart, 1974) with phase lock loop electronic analysis. Light diffraction techniques are frequently used to study properties of very thin (eg 200 μm diameter) muscles as a grating (Nassar *et al.*, 1974; Krueger and Pollack 1975; Pollack and Krueger, 1976; ter Keurs *et al.*, 1980a,b) which diffracts the incident light of a laser beam into a zero order band and multiple symmetrical higher order band pairs. The spacing (d) between the bands is related uniquely to sarcomere length given by $SL = K\lambda d$, where K is constant, and λ is the wavelength of the laser light. Rapid control of sarcomere length is possible by the use of a servosystem that adjusts overall muscle length in order to maintain sarcomere length at set-point value of the servosystem (van Heuningen *et al.*, 1982). The properties of a larger population of sarcomeres in a larger region in the specimen have been studied and controlled by the use of marker techniques (Julian *et al.*, 1976) or a magnetic field in a coil that envelops a segment of a papillary muscle (Huntsman and Stewart, 1977).

Force, transmitted by the elastic ends of the preparations, can safely be measured at the ends of the preparation if force variations are not so fast that wave propagation jeopardizes the measurement. This condition is fulfilled in most short myocardial preparations.

Contraction

The relation between force and sarcomere length

Data on the relation between force and sarcomere length (Figure 4.5) determined by various authors are largely congruent (Krueger and Pollack, 1975, Pollack and Krueger, 1976; Julian *et al.*, 1976; Gordon and Pollack, 1980; ter Keurs *et al.*, 1980a). Passive force increases with sarcomere length in rat from negligible values at about 2.00 μm to values which exceed peak active force at a sarcomere length of 2.40 μm. It is shown in Figure 4.5 that active force rises continually with sarcomere length in the range of sarcomere lengths at which cardiac muscle operates, i.e. 1.55–2.35 μm (Sonnenblick, 1968). Neither a plateau nor a descending limb is found. This contrasts with the behaviour of the isolated contractile apparatus. If the myofibrils are activated at maximal intracellular calcium concentration force at 1.50 μm sarcomere length, is only 20% less than at 2.30 μm (Fabiato and Fabiato, 1975b).

Lowering the external calcium concentration decreases force development in a length-dependent manner (Bodem *et al.*, Jewell, 1977; Huntsman and Stewart, 1977; Lakatta and Jewell, 1977; ter Keurs *et al.*, 1980a,b; Gordon and Pollack, 1980; see Figure 4.5). The effect of a decrease of $[Ca^{++}]_o$ can be fully counteracted by frequency potentiation of the preparation (ter Keurs *et al.*, 1980a,b). It is likely that calcium release depends on both $[Ca]_o$ and on the rate of stimulation. It is of interest to note here that in rat heart the recycling fraction (see Noble, Chapter 3 in this volume) of calcium can be increased to unity for up to four beats by potentiation at low $[Ca]_o$ (H. E. D. J. ter Keurs, unpublished observations). This suggests that a compartment that supplies calcium to the release compartment can contain much more calcium than the release sites.

The relation between peak force development and sarcomere length is not influenced by shortening which occurs early during contraction (Pollack and Krueger, 1976; ter Keurs *et al.*, 1980a,b; Gordon and Pollack, 1980). The

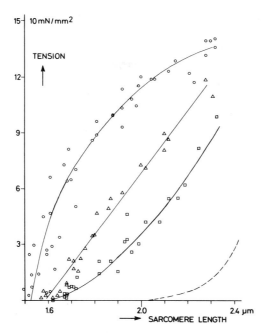

Figure 4.5 *Force versus sarcomere length.* The relation between active tension in a representative trabecula and sarcomere length measured during isometric contractions at $[Ca]_o = 2.5 \, \text{mmol} \, l^{-1}$ (open circles) and $[Ca]_o = 0.5 \, \text{mmol} \, l^{-1}$ (open triangles) and $[Ca]_o = 0.25 \, \text{mmol} \, l^{-1}$ (open squares). It is clear that the effect of an inotropic intervention depends on cell length. The relation between passive tension and sarcomere length in a representative trabecula is indicated by the dashed line. Note that the range of sarcomere lengths in which these preparations operate is 1.6–2.35 μm, which is identical to that in the intact heart

time course of force development, in contrast, is very much affected by sarcomere length changes during contractions. During isometric contractions the force rises rapidly (i.e. in 100 ms at 25 °C) towards a pseudo-plateau and this rise is followed by slow relaxation (Figure 4.6).

Force–velocity relation

Many studies of the relation between force and velocity of shortening of myocardial muscle preparation – at the level of the whole muscle – indicated that the inverse relation that was predicted by Hill (1973) holds in myocardium (Brutsaert and Sonnenblick, 1971). Considerable disagreement persists about the question whether the intercept on the velocity axis follows external influences in a similar manner as does the force intercept. This

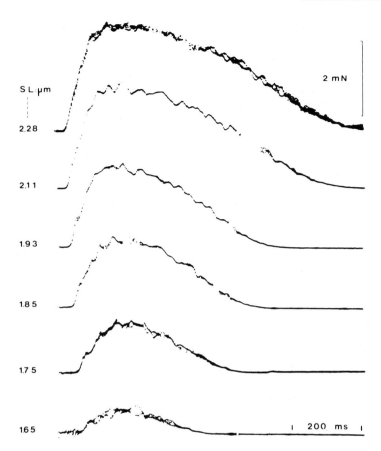

Figure 4.6   *Time course of force development versus sarcomere length.* Force development during six contractions in which sarcomere length was kept constant at values of 1.65, 1.75, 1.85, 1.93, 2.11, and 2.28 μm. Only force traces are shown. Sarcomere length at 1.75 μm and 1.65 μm was kept constant after initial shortening of the sarcomeres from slack length to set-point value. Calibrations of force and time base are depicted. [Reproduced with permission from R. van Heuningen, W. H. Rijnsburger, and H. E. D. J. ter Keurs, *Amer. J. Physiol.* **242,** H411 (1982).]

probably follows from the many experimental problems involved in the measurement of maximal velocity of shortening.

A solution to the problem is offered by the use of isovelocity releases of the muscle (Noble, 1974; Daniëls *et al.*, 1982; ter Keurs and Wohlfart, 1982). If during contractions, that start at constant initial sarcomere length, the damaged ends are released rapidly such that force falls to a desired level, shortening of the muscle at constant velocity can be permitted at such a rate that force remains at the same level. This 'isovelocity' procedure results in contractions at constant sarcomere-shortening velocity and constant force (Figure 4.7(b)). Force–velocity relations obtained from such contractions are hyperbolic and indistinguishable from those obtained from load clamps (Figure 4.7(b)). The 'isovelocity' procedure allows the measurement of the velocity of shortening of central sarcomeres in the maximally unloaded muscle by careful adjustment of the rapid and slow component of the release (Figure 4.7(a)). Figure 4.7(a) shows that the intrinsic series elastic component of the sarcomeres is very stiff, contrasting with the compliant series elastic component of the whole muscle. A decrease of sarcomere

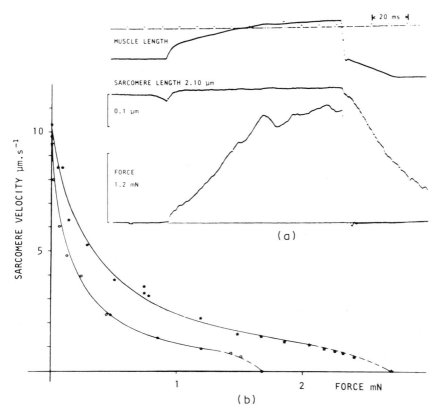

Figure 4.7 (a) *Quick release to unloaded velocity.* Force, muscle length, and sarcomere length during contraction at constant sarcomere length followed by a rapid and then controlled release of the muscle at constant velocity. (b) *Force versus velocity of sarcomere shortening.* Force–velocity relations at sarcomere lengths of 1.90 μm (circles) and 2.20 μm (asterisks) fitted by a hyperbola (drawn line). Deviation of the data above force = 85% of maximal force from the hyperbola $(P + a)v = b(P_0 - P)$ is manifest in most experiments

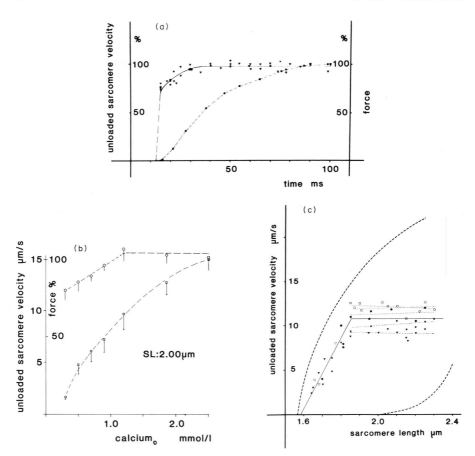

Figure 4.8 *Force and velocity versus time, sarcomere length, and* [Ca]$_o$. Maximal force at constant sarcomere length and maximal unloaded velocity of shortening at 25 °C as a function of (a) time, during a twitch at 2.10 μm sarcomere length and [Ca^{++}]$_o$ = 2.5 mM; (b) external calcium concentration, at sarcomere length 2.10 μm and 120 ms following start of a twitch; (c) sarcomere length, at 120 ms following the start of a twitch at [Ca^{++}]$_o$ = 2.5 mM

length of less than 0.5% is found during a release to zero load in 1 ms. If the release time is a fraction of a millisecond, it appears that a minimal change of sarcomere length is found: 0.25% (Delay *et al.*, 1979). This value is comparable to that found in skeletal muscle (Ford *et al.*, 1977). Velocity of shortening of unloaded sarcomeres rises much more rapidly than force at constant sarcomere length and reaches a maximum 20 ms following onset of contraction in rat (cf. 120 ms for force at constant sarcomere length) (Figure 4.8(a)). Release after 120 ms leads to lower shortening velocity, which is compatible with deactivation as a result of the rapid release (see below) (ter Keurs *et al.*, 1980a,b).

Maximal velocity of sarcomere shortening is constant at sarcomere lengths between slack length (1.85 μm) and 2.35 μm and decreases with sarcomere length below 1.85 μm to nil at 1.6 μm (see Figure 4.8(c)) while force rises with sarcomere length over the full range from 1.55 to 2.35 μm. Unloaded sarcomere shortening velocity also reaches a maximum at a calcium concentration of 1.2 mM, whereas isometric force continues to rise with $[Ca^{++}]_o$ to a maximum at 2.5 mM (at 0.2 Hz stimulus rate) (ter Keurs and Wohlfart, 1982; Figure 4.8(b)).

These observations suggest that maximal velocity depends on intracellular calcium concentration and therefore on extracellular calcium concentration and on the time following stimulation. The velocity–$[Ca^{++}]_i$ relation is shifted to the left compared to the force–$[Ca^{++}]_i$ relation as found in skinned skeletal muscle (Stephenson and Julian, 1982). It is not possible to decide yet whether the calcium dependence of velocity reflects calcium control over the activity of actomyosin ATPase that may govern the shortening velocity (Barany, 1967), or reflects the presence of internal viscosity of the activated sarcomere that presents a velocity-dependent load. The latter may add to the fall of shortening velocity at sarcomere lengths below 1.85 μm, although the amount of calcium bound to the myofilaments then probably also contributes. Forces opposing shortening that are able to restore slack length during relaxation in a cell, that has shortened to a sarcomere length below 1.85 μm, must decrease maximal velocity of shortening as well.

The influence of catecholamines that modulate the affinity of the myofilaments to calcium and additionally may change ATPase activity is to increase shortening velocity in studies on whole muscle level. However, these studies need confirmation at the level of the sarcomere.

Relaxation

Relaxation is the mechanical result of many mechanisms that cause the calcium concentration in the cell to decline. The time course of these processes is not precisely known. Full appreciation of the process of relaxation is only possible if each individual mechanism is known in detail:

(1) Calcium binding by the contractile filaments will continue initially.

(2) Calcium will be bound by the sarcoplasmic reticulum and transported by an active process into the sarcoplasmic reticulum (Katz, 1977).

(3) Calcium will be eliminated from the cytosol by a Na–Ca carrier exchange mechanism (Reuter, 1974) and by active transport mechanisms (Caroni and Carafoli, 1980, Caroni *et al.*, 1980) in the sarcolemma.

(4) Eventually dissociation of the calcium from the filaments follows these reactions.

These processes lead to a decline of mechanical output of the contractile apparatus. Shortening of the sarcomeres, on the other hand, enhances dissociation of calcium from the filaments and may affect the other processes as well. Thus the dynamics of force development and shortening during relaxation affect relaxation itself. Finally shortening of sarcomeres to below slack length (1.85–1.9 μm) will store energy in an elastic mesh that envelops the cell and the myofibrils, and will cause double overlap of thin filaments and thereby create opposing forces. Similarly storage of elastic energy will be caused by shear of cell layers in the contracting ventricle (Winegrad *et al.*, 1980).

According to such a simplified scheme we can consider a number of aspects of mechanical relaxation of cardiac muscle. In a discussion of the results of various experimental approaches it is worthwhile to mention that the term relaxation has been used both equivalent to decay of force development and indicating less or slower shortening or accelerated lengthening.

Force decay during contraction at constant sarcomere length is dependent on actual sarcomere length (Krueger and Farber, 1980; van Heuningen *et al.*, 1982). The relaxation phase of force lasts three times longer in contractions at a sarcomere length of 2.28 μm than in contractions at 1.65 μm (see Figure 4.6). This observation suggests that the dissociation rate is much slower than the rate of calcium binding. Force decay during contractions in rat myocardium at constant sarcomere length is accelerated by catecholamines (H. E. D. J. ter Keurs, unpublished observations).

Sarcomere motion, e.g. during contractions at constant muscle length, accelerates force relaxation. Quantitative studies of the effects of sarcomere length changes revealed that the enhanced force decay occurs prior to peak force of a twitch. This effect is known as deactivation and is illustrated in Figure 4.9. Dissociation of calcium from the myofilaments has been shown to result from rapid releases that induce deactivation (Gordon and Ridgway, 1977). This effect can be enhanced by introducing gross non-uniformity (Edman, 1980).

During shortening the load and changes of the load determine the time course of the relaxation process (Brutsaert *et al.*, 1978). Load dependence is specifically found in cells with an active calcium removal system, and is lost when the calcium sequestering process is slow (caffeine, hypoxia, destroyed sarcoplasmic reticulum, or atrial myocardium (Couttenye *et al.*, 1981)). Thus mechanical events influence dissociation of calcium from the myofilaments.

If passive forces are positive they will slow down lengthening during relaxation under the influence of a load (Goethals *et al.*, 1980). If the muscle shortens below slack length restoring forces, albeit small, may actually constitute the driving force for lengthening (ter Keurs *et al.*, 1980a,b).

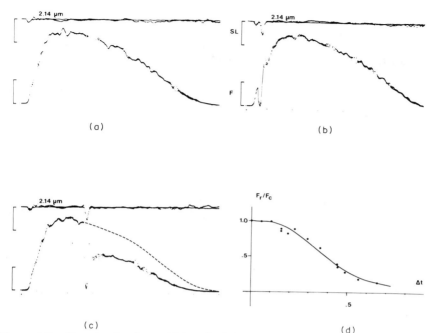

Figure 4.9 *Deactivation by rapid length changes.* Tension development at constant sarcomere length (SL = 2.14 μm) and the influence of triangular shortening functions imposed upon sarcomere length. Duration of shortening pulse was 20 ms. Velocity of shortening and stretch was 10 μm s^{-1}. The amount of shortening was 0.1 μm. Top trace in (a), (b), and (c) shows sarcomere length signals, which were measured simultaneously by the two detector systems (calibration indicates 0.2 μm); bottom trace shows force (calibration indicates 1 mN). Stimulus moment is marked by a pulse on the force trace. Timing dots are spaced 100 ms. (a) Tension development at constant sarcomere length; only an initial transient of sarcomere shortening (0–0.3 μm lasting 24 ms) is present. Tension develops to a maximum within 100 ms. Tension relaxation at this sarcomere length starts at 270 ms following onset. (b) The effect of the additional triangular shortening transient which was imposed on the muscle 20 ms following onset of contraction on tension development. Comparison with tension development shown in (a) shows no influence on the ability of the muscle to generate force. (c) The effect of a similar shortening transient, which was applied 220 ms following onset of contraction. Tension traces during the transients in (b) and (c) were retouched. Tension redevelopment upon return to SL = 2.14 μm was considerably smaller than control tension (interrupted line, copied from control contraction). (d) The relation between peak tension during tension redevelopment following a shortening transient expressed as a percentage of tension, which existed at the same moment during the control contraction, has been expressed as a function of the interval between onset of contraction and the end of the transient divided by the duration of the control contraction. [Reproduced with permission from H. E. D. J. ter Keurs, W. M. Rijnsburger and R. van Heuningen, *Europ. Heart J.*, **1**, Suppl. A, 67–80 (1980).]

LENGTH DEPENDENCE OF FORCE GENERATION

A Working Hypothesis

The properties of the contractile unit that are described above can be integrated into a model that quantitatively predicts length dependence of force generation. The basic properties of the model are as follows:

(1) The relation between force and calcium concentration near the filaments is determined by the binding of two calcium ions per force generator site.

(2) Calcium is bound so rapidly that the relation between peak force and peak calcium during a twitch of intact cells is similar to the steady state relation in skinned preparations. Calcium dissociation is slow if no sliding of the filaments occurs. The dissociation rate increases with sliding. At high velocity of sliding – or low load – calcium dissociation is rapid as well.

(3) The affinity of the filaments for calcium increases exponentially with increasing sarcomere length.

(4) The amount of calcium that is released during a twitch is assumed independent of sarcomere length. The calcium concentration that is reached in the cytosol is thus independent of sarcomere length and attains a maximal level of $4.35 \ \mu\text{mol l}^{-1}$.

(5) The sarcoplasmic calcium concentration during the twitch is proportional to the number of calcium ions that are bound to the release compartment.

(6) Calcium in the release compartment is in equilibrium with the compartments which take up calcium that enters the cell during the action potential, and which reabsorb calcium, set free during the previous contraction.

(7) Opposing forces are assumed to increase exponentially if sarcomeres shorten below $1.85 \ \mu\text{m}$, and they reach about 10% of maximal active force at a sarcomere length of $1.6 \ \mu\text{m}$.

This model is schematized in Figure 4.10. The observations by various authors made on rat myocardium (Hibberd and Jewell, 1979; Allen and Kurihara, 1979; ter Keurs *et al.*, 1980a,b; Fabiato, 1981) are incorporated in the figure.

Figure 4.10 *Force, intracellular calcium, and sarcomere length: a working hypothesis.* (a) The relations between force and intracellular calcium concentration and shift of the curves due to a change in sarcomere length. Curve C has been studied at $SL = 2.0 \ \mu\text{m}$ in intact cells which were skinned afterwards. Force developed in intact cells never attained more than 70% of force in directly activated skinned cells (solid symbols). Curve A has been described at a longer sarcomere length ($2.30 \ \mu\text{m}$).

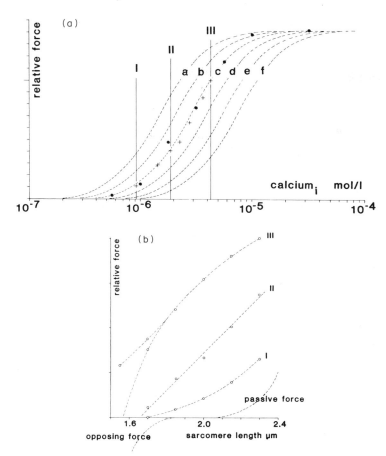

Curves B, D, E, F were interpolated assuming that the affinity change is proportional to sarcomere length (curve B, 2.15 μm; curve D, 1.84 μm; curve E, 1.70 μm; curve F, 1.55 μm). Force development (crosses) in intact trabeculae at SL = 2.00 μm at varied external calcium concentration fits curve C if $[Ca^{++}]_i = 0.0035[Ca^{++}]_o/(1 + 400[Ca^{++}]_o)$ and if F_{Max} is assumed to be 70% of the maximal force of directly stimulated myofilaments. Calcium concentration that is reached during the transient rise of Ca_i following calcium release is assumed to be independent of sarcomere length (vertical lines: I at an external calcium concentration of 0.25 mM; II at $[Ca^{++}]_o = 0.5$ mM; III at $[Ca^{++}]_o = 2.5$ mM. Intersection of lines I, II, and III with curves A through F yield force–sarcomere length relations in (b) at the corresponding $[Ca^{++}]_o$. Opposing force (panel (b)) has been assumed to increase exponentially with decreasing sarcomere length. The magnitude of opposing force corresponds to experimental estimates. Opposing force has been subtracted from active force (shown in curve III). The resultant force sarcomere–length relation should be compared with Figure 4.5

The excitation coupling apparatus is reduced to two compartments. Both compartments bind calcium. The uptake compartment exchanges calcium with the extracellular fluid and receives calcium that is recycled from the previous contraction. During steady state contractions the concentration of calcium that is bound to this compartment is a function of the extracellular calcium concentration ($[Ca^{++}]_o$). The release compartment contains sites (RS) that each bind a calcium ion from the uptake compartment. Hill's equation describes the relation between the concentration of 'release sites' in the cell to which calcium is bound and $[Ca^{++}]_o$. Complete release of calcium from the release sites is triggered by the action potential such that the free calcium concentration $[Ca^{++}]_i$ in the cell following release rises to equal [RSCa]. It is not possible to specify the properties of either compartment in detail. I therefore assumed that the simplest binding reaction between one binding site and one calcium ion occurs in both compartments. Furthermore, one of the compartments can saturate with calcium ions. I assumed that the relation between Ca_i following calcium release and Ca_o in rat trabecula at 25 °C and a low stimulus rate is given by

$$[Ca^{++}]_i = 0.0035[Ca^{++}]_o/(1 + 400[Ca^{++}]_o).$$

(The capacity of the uptake sites in rat myocardium may exceed that of the release sites a few (two to four) times. The uptake compartment thus is only half saturated during regular contractions at $[Ca^{++}]_o = 2.5$ mmol l^{-1} and at the optimum rate of 12 min^{-1}. The resultant effective K_1 for binding of Ca_o by the uptake compartment then is 400. If maximal $[Ca]_i = [CaRS]_i RC = 4.35$ μmol l^{-1}, it follows that $K_2 = 8.7 \times 10^{-6}$ as

$$[Ca]_i = \frac{K_1 \cdot K_2[Ca^{++}]_o}{1 + K_1[Ca^{++}]_o},$$

where K_2 is the affinity constant of the release sites (RS) and K_1 is affected by stimulus rate only.)

If we now calculate $[Ca]_i$ at various $[Ca^{++}]_o$ at a contraction rate of 12 min^{-1}, the resultant force–$[Ca]_i$ relation of rat trabeculae at a sarcomere length of 2.00 μm and 25 °C in our laboratory can be compared to the relation that has been found by Fabiato under similar circumstances (see Figure 4.10).

Binding two calcium ions to the myofilaments leads to activation of the force generators. The affinity of the filaments for calcium depends on sarcomere length. The exponential increase of affinity with increasing sarcomere length is manifest as a shift to the left of the Hill relations that relate force development to the free intracellular calcium concentration. Figure 4.10 shows that the relation between force and $\log[Ca^{++}]_i$ is compatible with the hypothesis that two calcium ions are bound to each force generator. An exponential increase of the affinity of the myofilaments for calcium with increasing sarcomere length is assumed. The increased affinity manifests itself (Figure 4.10) as a shift to the left of the force–calcium concentration curves with increasing sarcomere length. Two of these curves have been established experimentally (Hibberd and Jewell, 1979), the position of the other curves was assumed as indicated above. As length does not influence the amount of calcium that is released (cf. Figures 4.4, 4.10), force at any sarcomere length depends only on the intersection of the Ca_i (length-independent) lines (Figure 4.10) with the F–$[Ca^{++}]_i$ curves for various sarcomere lengths. The force–sarcomere length relations, at three external calcium concentrations (0.3, 0.5, and 2.5 mM) are depicted in Figure 4.10(b). The force at low sarcomere length has been corrected for the presence of opposing forces (see Figure 4.10(b)). It is clear from Figure 4.10(b) that qualitatively good agreement is obtained with the experimental data presented in Figure 4.5 (ter Keurs *et al.*, 1980a,b; cf. also Gordon and Pollack, 1980). Quantitative differences between the force–length relation depicted in Figure 4.10 and the experimental data of Figure 4.5 can be accounted for if it is also assumed that some length dependence of calcium release is present (Fabiato, 1980). We opted, though, not to incorporate this feature as insufficient data are available at present.

Three other observations can be accounted for by this working hypothesis. First, peak force of contraction will not depend on shortening early during contraction, as rapid exchange of calcium between myofilaments and the sarcoplasm is possible when myofilament sliding occurs while the calcium in the sarcoplasm is still elevated. Secondly, during isometric contractions relaxation rate should reflect the dissociation rate of calcium from the filaments. It is reasonable to assume that the dissociation rate is inversely proportional to the affinity of the filaments. Slow relaxation at long sarcomere length vs rapid relaxation at short sarcomere length is compatible with this aspect of the hypothesis. Relaxation will be enhanced by rapid sliding of the filaments as described in the previous paragraphs. Alternatively, if a significant amount of calcium is still present in the sarcoplasm during relaxation, enhanced relaxation will not occur, as can be seen in frog or mammalian ventricle in hypoxia or in the presence of caffeine.

The mechanism of the shift of the force–calcium concentration curves is not well understood. It may be that double overlap of actin filaments, that occurs below 2.2 μm (Robinson and Winegrad, 1977), interferes with binding of calcium to the actomyosin sites. Such a mechanism has been proposed in a theory of sarcomere dynamics as described by Iwazumi (Noble, 1979). In this theory, the cross projections of myosin are supposed to interact with the tips of thin filaments by electrostatic forces.

The field generated by the cross projections depends on the local concentration of calcium ions. The local concentration of calcium ions depends itself on calcium bound to troponin and on the distance between troponin and the cross projection. As the repeat distance of cross projections (42.9 nm) and of troponin (40.0 nm) differs, the local concentration of calcium falls with distance from the tip to a minimum at approximately 320 nm away from the tip. This would imply that in double overlap tips of the actin filaments are always screened off from the calcium-recipient cross projection by the distal shaft of another actin filament that carries suboptimal calcium to the projection. Thus the effective calcium concentration in the neighbourhood of the cross projections decreases to a sarcomere length of 1.6–1.7 μm and then rises again such that force in its turn falls with SL to a minimum at around 1.60 μm.

CLINICAL IMPLICATIONS

Through geometrical transformation, the relation between force and length is equivalent to the relation originally described by Frank (1895). Early shortening during contraction does not alter the instantaneous relation between force and sarcomere length, as we have seen. This was recognized by Suga (1969) and Suga and Sagawa (1974) in isolated canine ventricle and led to the concept that the relation between pressure and volume at the end of systole is largely independent of the history of contraction (see Figure 4.11). Application of this concept of the relation between end-diastolic volume and stroke volume or stroke work at constant load yields directly the relation that has been described by Starling (1965) (see Figure 4.11).

It is certainly important to study the end-systolic pressure-volume relation in the diseased heart, as one can expect that in case of abnormal loading conditions such as in valvular disease (e.g. mitral valve prolapse or obstructive cardiomyopathy) the relation may be sensitive to the abnormal shortening pattern during systole. This also holds for pathological motion in a ventricle with ischaemic regions or a large aneurysm.

A study of the effects of catecholamines on the relation between pressure and volume at the end of systole would be intriguing, as it is conceivable that there may be cancellation of their effects on calcium release and on the affinity of the myofilaments.

This brings back the question that must have stuck in the mind of the reader since noting the heading of this chapter on calcium and contractility.

Figure 4.11 *Cardiac pump function:* diagrammatic illustration of various pump function aspects of the heart. During diastole ventricular volume increases; during systole blood is expelled from the heart under pressure. The left panel relates end-diastolic and end-systolic properties of the left ventricle and shows the influence of end-diastolic volume (V_{ed}) and end-systolic volume (V_{es}) on left ventricular pressure at the end of diastole (P_{lved}) or systole (P_{lves}) and on cardiac output. The volume (V_{ed}) and pressure (P_{ed}) in the heart at the end of diastole are related through its passive

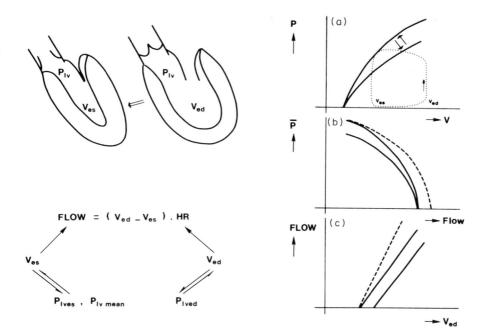

elastic properties. During systole blood is compressed and ejected by the ventricle, which shortens mainly along its short axis, as shown.

(a) The relation between P_{lves} and V_{es}. This relation is derived from end-systolic pressure and volume points of different contractions. The volume–pressure loop during a single cardiac contraction is indicated by the dotted line. Pressure (P_{lves}) and volume (V_{es}) at the end of systole are related in a constant fashion. The P_{es}–V_{es} relationship is allegedly not sensitive to end-diastolic volume. The effect of inotropic interventions consists of an increase of P_{es} at all V_{es} without a change in intercept. In (a), (b), and (c) the drawn lines refer to different inotropic states of the ventricle. The interrupted lines in the graphs refer to effects of heart rate or a change of V_{ed} (b) or to changes of aortic pressure or heart rate (c)

(b) describes the relation between mean developed intraventricular pump pressure ($\bar{P}$) and mean flow that is used to describe pump function of, for example, industrial pumps. This relation is affected both by changes in heart rate and V_{ed}, which modify $\bar{P}$ and flow. Inotropic interventions increase developed $\bar{P}$ without change of intercept.

(c) The modified Starling's relation. The original Starling curve of cardiac pump function depicted the relation between P_{ed} and flow. Starling suggested that: 'The law of the heart is therefore the same as that of skeletal muscle, namely that the energy set free on passage from the resting state to the contracted state depends on the area of "chemically active surfaces", i.e. on the length of the muscle fibres'. We used the relation between V_{ed} and flow, which can be derived from the relation between P_{ed} and V_{ed}. This relation is sensitive to blood pressure and inotropic interventions, which cause parallel shift of the curves, and to heart rate, which changes the slope of the curve (part (c))

Until we know the process in full detail, the definition of contractility can be given only provisionally: the transient interrelation between force, length, and velocity of shortening which is modulated by shortening and load.

REFERENCES

Abbott, B. C., and Mommaerts, W. F. H. M. (1959). A study of inotropic mechanisms in the papillary muscle preparation. *J. Gen. Physiol.*, **42**, 533–551.

Allen, D. G., and Kurihara, S. (1979). Calcium transients at different muscle lengths in rat ventricular muscle. *J. Physiol. (Lond.)*, **292**, 68–69P.

Allen, D. G., and Kurihara, S. (1980). Calcium transients in mammalian ventricular muscle. *Europ. Heart J.*, **1**, Suppl. A, 5–15.

Allen D. G., Blinks, J. R., and Prendergast, F. G. (1977). Aequorin luminescence: relation of light emission to calcium concentration – a calcium-independent component. *Science* **195**, 996–998.

Barany, M. (1967). ATPase activity of myosin correlated with speed of muscle shortening. *J. Gen. Physiol.*, **50**, 197.

Bodem, R., Skelton, C. L., and Sonnenblick, E. H. (1976). Inactivation of contraction as a determinant of the length–active tension relation in heart muscle of the cat. *Res. Exp. Med.* **168**, 1–13.

Brutsaert, D. L., and Sonnenblick, E. H. (1971). Nature of the force–velocity relation in heart muscle. *Cardiovasc. Res.*, Suppl. I, 18–33.

Brutsaert, D. L., Clerck, N. M. de, Goethals, M. A., and Housmans, P. R. (1978). Relaxation of ventricular cardiac muscle. *J. Physiol. (Lond.)*, **283**, 469.

Caroni, P. and Carafoli, E. (1980). An ATP-dependent Ca^{2+}-pumping system in dog heart sarcolemma. *Nature*, **283**, 765–767.

Caroni, P., Reinlib, L. and Carafoli, E. (1980). Charge movements during the $Na^+–Ca^{2+}$ exchange in heart sarcolemmal vesicles. *Proc. Natl. Acad. Sci.*, **77**, 6354–6358.

Clerck, N. M. de, Claes, V. A., and Brutsaert, D. L. (1977). Force velocity relations of single cardiac muscle cells calcium dependency. *J. Gen. Physiol.*, **69**, 221–241.

Couttenye, M. M., Clerck, N. M. de, Goethals, M. A., and Brutsaert, D. L. (1981). Relaxation properties of mammalian atrial muscle. *Circulation Res.*, **48**, 352–356.

Daniëls, M., Donselaar, W. van, Keurs, H. E. D. J. ter, Noble, M. I. M., and Wohlfart, B. (1982). Sarcomere force–velocity relations in rat myocardium. *J. Physiol. (Lond.)*, **324**, 23P.

Delay, M. J., Vassallo, D. V., Iwazumi, T., and Pollack, G. H. (1979). Fast response of cardiac muscle to quick length changes. In *Cross-bridge Mechanism in Muscle Contraction* (H. Sugi and G. H. Pollack, eds), Baltimore, University Park Press, pp. 71–102.

Donaldson, S. K. B., Best, Ph. M., and Kerrick, W. G. L. (1978). Characterization of the effects of Mg^{2+} on Ca^{2+}- and Sr^{2+}-activated tension; generation of skinned rat cardiac fibers. *J. Gen. Physiol.*, **71**, 645–655.

Ebashi, E. (1980). The Croonian Lecture 1979. Regulation of muscle contraction. *Proc. Roy. Soc. Lond.*, **207**, 259–286.

Edman, K. A. P. (1980). The role of non-uniform sarcomere behaviour during relaxation of striated muscle. *Europ. Heart J.*, 1, Suppl. A, 49–57.

Elzinga, G., and Westerhof, N. (1978). The effect of an increase in inotropic state and end-diastolic volume on the pumping ability of the feline left heart. *Circulation Res.*, **42**, 620–628.

Endo, M. (1973). Length dependence of activation of skinned muscle fibers by calcium. *Cold Spring Harbor Symp. Quant. Biol.*, **37**, 505–510.

Endo, M. (1977). Calcium release from the sarcoplasmic reticulum. *Physiol. Rev.*, **57**, 71–108.

Fabiato, A. (1980). Sarcomere length dependence of calcium release from the sarcoplasmic reticulum of skinned cardiac cells demonstrated by differential microspectrophotometry with arsenazo III. *J. Gen. Physiol.*, **76**, 15a.

Fabiato, A. (1981). Myoplasmic free calcium concentration reached during the twitch of an intact isolated cardiac cell and during calcium-induced release of calcium from the sarcoplasmic reticulum of a skinned cardiac cell from the adult rat or rabbit ventricle. *J. Gen. Physiol.*, **78**, 457–497.

Fabiato, A., and Fabiato, F. (1975a). Dependence of the contractile activation of skinned cardiac cells on the sarcomere length. *Nature*, **256**, 54–56.

Fabiato, A., and Fabiato, F. (1975b). Contractions induced by a calcium-triggered release of calcium from the sarcoplasmic reticulum of single skinned cardiac cells. *J. Physiol. (Lond.)*, **249**, 469–495.

Fabiato, A., and Fabiato, F. (1978a). Effects of pH on the myofilaments and the sarcoplasmic reticulum of skinned cells from cardiac and skeletal muscles. *J. Physiol. (Lond.)*, **276**, 233–255.

Fabiato, A., and Fabiato, F. (1978c). Myofilament-generated tension oscillations during partial calcium activation and activation dependence of the sarcomere length tension relation of skinned cardiac cells. *J. Gen. Physiol.*, **72**, 667–669.

Ford, L. E., Huxley, A. F., and Simmons, R. M. (1977). Tension responses to sudden length change in stimulated frog muscle fibers near slack length. *J. Physiol. (Lond.)*, **269**, 441–515.

Frank, O. (1895). Zur Dynamik des Herzmuskels. *A. Biol.*, **32**, 370–447.

Goethals, M. A., Housmans, P. R., and Brutsaert, D. L. (1980). Load-dependence of physiologically relaxing cardiac muscle. *Europ. Heart. J.*, **1**, Suppl. A, 81–87.

Gordon, A. M., and Pollack, G. H. (1980). Effects of calcium on the sarcomere length–tension relation in rat cardiac muscle, implications for the Frank–Starling mechanism. *Circulation Res.*, **47**, 610–619.

Gordon, A. M., and Ridgway, E. B. (1977). Calcium transients and relaxation in single muscle fibres. *Europ. J. Cardiol.*, **7**, Suppl., 27–35.

Gordon, A. M., Huxley, A. F., and Julian, F. J. (1966). The variation in isometric tension with sarcomere length in vertebrate muscle fibres. *J. Physiol. (Lond.)*, **184**, 170–192.

Grimm, A. F., and Wohlfart, B. (1974). Sarcomere lengths at the peak of the length–tension curve in living and fixed rat papillary muscle. *Acta Physiol. Scand.*, **92**, 575–577.

Heuningen, R. van, Rijnsburger, W. H., and Keurs, H. E. D. J. ter (1982). Sarcomere length control in striated muscle. *Amer. J. Physiol.*, **242**, H411.

Hibberd, M. G., and Jewell, B. R. (1979). Length dependence of the sensitivity of the contractile system to calcium in rat ventricular muscle. *J. Physiol. (Lond.)*, **290**, 30P.

Hill, A. V. (1973). The heat of shortening and the dynamic constants of muscle. *Physiol. Rev.*, **126**, 612–745.

Huntsman, L. L., and Stewart, D. K. (1977). Length dependent calcium inotropism in cat papillary muscle. *Circulation Res.*, **40**, 366–371.

Huxley, H. E., and Hanson, J. (1954). Changes in the cross-striation of muscle during contraction and stretch and their structural interpretation. *Nature*, **173**, 973–976.

Jewell, B. R. (1977). A reexamination of the influence of muscle length on myocardial performance. *Circulation Res.*, **40**, 221–230.

Julian, F. J., Sollins, M. R., and Moss, R. L. (1976). Absence of a plateau in length–tension relationship of rabbit papillary muscle when internal shortening is prevented. *Nature*, **260**, 340–342.

Katz, A. M. (1977). *Physiology of the Heart*, Raven Press, New York.

Keurs, H. E. D. J. ter, and Wohlfart, B. (1982). Influence of calcium concentration on maximal velocity of sarcomere shortening in rat trabeculae. *J. Physiol. (Lond.)*, **330,** 41P.

Keurs, H. E. D. J. ter, Rijnsburger, W. H., Heuningen, R. van, and Nagelsmit, M. J. (1980a). Tension development and sarcomere length in rat cardiac trabeculae; evidence of length-dependent activation. *Circulation Res.*, **46,** 703–714.

Keurs, H. E. D. J. ter, Rijnsburger, W. H., and Heuningen, R. van (1980b). Restoring forces and relaxation of rat cardiac muscle. *Europ. Heart. J.*, **1,** Suppl. A, 67–80.

Krueger, J. W., and Farber, S. (1980). Sarcomere length 'orders' relaxation in cardiac muscle. *Europ. Heart. J.*, **1,** Suppl. A, 37–47.

Krueger, J. W., and Pollack, G. H. (1975). Myocardial sarcomere dynamics during isometric contraction. *J. Physiol. (Lond.)*, **251,** 627–643.

Lakatta, E. G., and Jewell, B. R. (1977). Length-dependent activation. Its effect on the length-tension relation in cat ventricular muscle. *Circulation Res.*, **40,** 251–257.

McClellan, G. B., and Winegard, S. The regulation of calcium sensitivity of the contraction system in mammalian cardiac muscle. *J. Gen. Physiol.*, **72,** 737–764.

Marban, E., Rink, T. J., Tsien, R. W., and Tsien, R. Y. (1980). Free calcium in heart muscle at rest and during contraction measured with Ca^{2+}-sensitive microelectrodes. *Nature*, **286,** 845–850.

Moisescu, D. G. (1976). Kinetics of reaction in calcium-activated skinned muscle fibres. *Nature*, **262,** 610–613.

Moisescu, D. G., and Thieleczek, (1978). Length effects on the Ca^{++} and Sr^{++} activation curves in skinned frog muscle fibres. *J. Physiol. (Lond.)*, **275,** 241–262.

Nassar, R., Manring, A., and Johnson, E. A. (1974). Light diffraction of cardiac muscle: sarcomere motion during contraction. In *The Physiological Basis of Starling's Law of the Heart*, Elsevier/Excerpta Medica/North Holland, Amsterdam, pp. 57–91.

Noble, M. I. M. (1974). Force–velocity relation at different muscle lengths. In *The Physiological Basis of Starling's Law of the Heart*, Elsevier/Excerpta Medica/North Holland, Amsterdam, pp. 134–154.

Noble, M. I. M. (1979). *The Cardiac Cycle*. Blackwell Scientific Publications, Oxford.

Pollack, G. H., and Krueger, J. W. (1976). Sarcomere dynamics in intact cardiac muscle. *Europ. J. Cardiol.*, **4,** Suppl., 53–65.

Reuben, J. P., and Wood, D. S. (1979). Are cardiac muscle cells skinned by EGTA or EDTA? *Nature*, **280,** 700–701.

Reuter, H. (1974). Exchange of calcium ions in the mammalian myocardium. *Circulation Res.*, **34,** 599.

Robinson, T. F., and Winegrad, S. (1977). Variation of thin filament length in heart muscle. *Nature*, **267,** 74–75.

Sonnenblick, E. H. (1968). Correlation of myocardial ultrastructure and function. *Circulation*, **38,** 29–44.

Starling, E. H. (1965). Lecture on the circulatory changes associated with exercise. Given at the Royal Army Medical College 27-10-1919. In *Starling on the Heart* (C. B. Chapman and J. H. Mitchell, eds), Dawsons of Pall Mall, London.

Stephenson, D. G. S. and Julian, F. J. (1982). Ca^{++} effects on the unloaded speed of shortening (V_{max}) of mammalian skeletal muscle fibers. *Biophys. J.*, **37**, 358a.

Suga, H. (1969). Analysis of left ventricular pumping by its pressure–volume coefficient. *Jpn. J. Med. Elect. Biol. Eng.*, **7**, 406. [In Japanese with English abstract.]

Suga, H., and Sagawa, K. (1974). Instantaneous pressure–volume relationships and their ratio in the excised, supported canine left ventricle. *Circulation Res.*, **35**, 117.

Winegrad, S. (1979). Electromechanical coupling in heart muscle. In *Handbook of Physiology I: The Cardiovascular System* (R. M. Berne, N. Sperilakis, and S. R. Geiger, eds), American Physiological Society, Bethesda, Md, pp. 393–428.

Winegrad, S., McClellan, G., Robinson, T., and Lai, N.-P. (1976). Variable diastolic compliance and variable Ca-sensitivity of the contractile system in cardiac muscle. *Europ. J. Cardiol.*, **4**, Suppl., 41–46.

Winegrad, S., Weisberg, A., and McClellan, G. (1980). Are restoring forces important to relaxation? *Europ. Heart. J.*, **1**, Suppl. A, 59–65.

Cardiac Metabolism
Edited by A. J. Drake-Holland and M. I. M. Noble
© 1983 John Wiley & Sons Ltd

CHAPTER 5

Calcium Exchange

Bohdan Lewartowski

Medical Centre of Postgraduate Education, Marymoncka 99, 01-813 Warsaw, Poland

INTRODUCTION

Intracellular calcium exchanges with calcium contained in the extracellular space in resting cardiac muscle and this exchange is increased by the active state. I shall concentrate on calcium fluxes in the activated myocardium which will be referred to as the excitation-dependent exchange or excitation-dependent fluxes.

Contraction is triggered by an increase in free sarcoplasmic Ca^{++} concentration over the threshold value of several times 10^{-7} M (Bassingthwaighte and Reuter, 1972; Marban *et al.*, 1980). Velocity and maximal force of contraction depend on the amount of free Ca^{++} available in the sarcoplasm, although the relation is not simple and Ca^{++} might be not the sole factor (Ray and England, 1976; Marban *et al.*, 1980; Rezink *et al.*, 1981). As calculated by Solaro *et al.* (1974), an increment in free sarcoplasmic Ca^{++} content of about 0.08 mM is necessary for full activation of the contractile proteins. The crucial question on which the concept of the mechanism of excitation–contraction coupling depends is the source from which this free Ca^{++} is supplied to the sarcoplasm of the excited cell. The answer to this question may be provided by measurements of excitation-dependent Ca^{++} influx matched by excitation-dependent efflux on a beat-to-beat basis. If this influx is large enough to supply the amount of Ca^{++} sufficient for significant activation of contractile proteins, the mechanism of excitation–contraction coupling may be relatively simple. If this amount is too small, an intracellular source of activator Ca must be postulated, (Noble, Chapter 3 in this volume).

Calcium fluxes associated with contraction can be measured by isotopic methods, calculated as the charge transferred by slow inward Ca current or estimated by an indirect approach.

EXCITATION-DEPENDENT Ca^{++} EXCHANGE MEASURED BY ISOTOPIC METHODS

Amphibian Myocardium

The most careful studies on ^{45}Ca fluxes in the ventricle of the frog heart were performed by Niedergerke (1963). Excitation-dependent uptake was estimated from efflux curves. Stimulation applied during washout greatly accelerated ^{45}Ca efflux, the exchange kinetics being approximately exponential. This gave rise to the assumption that during activity the tracer enters and leaves some cellular compartment in which it mixes readily with unlabelled calcium. Therefore the uptake and release were calculated from equations describing the kinetics of such a single compartment whose capacity was assumed to be much larger than Ca^{++} influx per beat. These calculations yielded the value of influx of 1.67×10^{-6} M Ca per litre of cells (0.001 67 mM) per beat, matched by similar efflux. The studies on ^{45}Ca fluxes in the frog ventricle were repeated by the same author and his collaborators (Niedergerke et al., 1969) with a different experimental approach and an improved technique of investigating ^{45}Ca exchange between the tissue and perfusing solution (Niedergerke and Page, 1969). Calcium-45 uptake was investigated first in the resting ventricle and then the effects of activity were studied in ventricles which were stimulated after 40–60 min of tracer loading. The magnitude of extra ^{45}Ca influx was 1.3×10^{-6} M per litre of cells (0.0013 mM) per beat. Since ^{45}Ca efflux simultaneous with ^{45}Ca influx was not considered, this result may be treated as the uptake per beat and not as the absolute value of ^{45}Ca exchange per beat. The authors noticed that there was an absolute increase in Ca^{++} content due to activity.

Calculations described in the earlier paper (Niedergerke, 1963) were based on assuming only one compartment exchanging Ca^{++} with the extracellular space. Since the least number of excitations applied during loading with isotope was 50, Ca^{++} fluxes depending on some other compartment of low capacity and hence high rate of exchange could have been left unnoticed. For such a compartment, the bidirectional ^{45}Ca flux could reach a steady state equilibrium after the second beat and not affect the ^{45}Ca uptake later on. The initial slope of the uptake curves shown in both papers (Niedergerke, 1963; Niedergerke et al., 1969) did not suggest a large net extra influx during the first beat; however, the tissue was exposed to the tracer for up to 60 min prior to stimulation. Therefore, if the compartment of small capacity existed, it could exchange the extra influx of ^{45}Ca for the isotope already taken up at rest. (Lewartowski et al., 1982, and manuscript in preparation). The excitation-dependent efflux was studied (Niedergerke, 1963) after the initial 19 min of rest, during which some more readily exchanging compartment could have been already washed out.

Thus, close examination of the above mentioned papers leaves the impression that the measurements of ^{45}Ca fluxes performed by their authors could pertain to excitation-dependent accumulation of this tracer in, or loss from, some cellular compartment, which could be only a fraction of the total Ca^{++} fluxes per beat.

This concept has been further developed by Chapman and Niedergerke (1970a, b), who found that tension build-up or decline in isolated fragments of the frog ventricle in response to an increase or reduction in external Ca^{++} concentration occurred in two phases: rapid phase ($t_{1/2}$ between 3 and 10 s) and slow phase ($t_{1/2}$ between 50 and 180 s). Similar phases of the changes in contractile force were noticed when the heart rate was altered (Chapman and Niedergerke, 1970b). The rapid phase was completed during the first beat following an increase in extracellular Ca^{++} (Ca_o) concentration. Its magnitude depended on the magnitude of this increase and on the contractile force prior to the change. This in turn depended on the degree of development of 'hypodynamic state' of the heart and/or duration of exposure to low Ca_o concentration. In the hypodynamic hearts and in the hearts exposed for a long time to low Ca_o concentration, the rapid phase was small or absent. The authors explain their results by assuming that:

'Initiation of contraction, e.g. of a twitch, is due to the formation of compound Ca_1 from calcium entering heart cells during the action potential; relaxation results when Ca_1 dissociates. Some of the calcium ions released from Ca_1 combine with cellular sites to form Ca_2; the remainder, we tentatively suppose, are rapidly extruded from the cell (pathway α), although it should be noted that the evidence for such rapid calcium release is still indirect. Compound Ca_2, a "primer" of contraction, dissociates more slowly than Ca_1 and a separate pathway (pathway γ) may exist for efflux of the calcium released' (Chapman and Niedergerke, 1970b).

Compound Ca_1 may trigger Ca release from the intracellular store or activate the contractile system directly (Chapman and Niedergerke, 1970a). The authors prefer the second hypothesis, since Ca_1 is immediately dependent on Ca_o concentration. Compound Ca_2 could 'prime' the force of contraction initiated by Ca_1 by activating a separate, Ca-dependent enzyme system, or reside on sites of contractile proteins which might combine with two or more Ca ions at different rates.

Since the authors propose that Ca_1 diffuses into the cells during the action potential and is rapidly extruded, possibly on a beat-to-beat basis, measurements of $^{45}Ca^{++}$ fluxes described in earlier papers (Niedergerke, 1963; Niedergerke et al., 1969) apparently concerned the exchange and intracellular accumulation of compound Ca_2 only. Rapid exchange on a beat-to-beat basis could not be evaluated by these methods.

Mammalian Myocardium

Efflux of ^{45}Ca from the previously loaded guinea-pig left atria was studied by Winegard and Shanes (1962) and found to have rapid and slow phases. Excitation-dependent influx to the slow phase was calculated and yielded the maximal value of 0.6×10^{-6} mM Ca per gram of the tissue (0.0006 mM kg^{-1}) per beat. A linear relationship between the increase in the slow phase content and influx per beat and contractile force at various rates of stimulation was noticed. No effect of stimulation on efflux was found.

The authors calculated excitation-dependent ^{45}Ca uptake related only to the slow phase. The rapid phase was neglected despite the fact that according to the authors' estimate it contained 0.38 mM Ca per kilogram of tissue in a space in series or in parallel with the extracellular space (i.e. intracellular). Moreover, they did not consider possible simultaneous extrusion of ^{45}Ca from the cells calculating ^{45}Ca uptake simply by dividing the slow phase by the number of beats. This experimental approach ignores the ^{45}Ca exchange on the beat-to-beat basis. The same reasoning applies to the study of Little and Sleator (1969).

Grossman and Furchgott (1964) compared ^{45}Ca uptake by the left atria of the guinea-pig heart stimulated at a rate of 60 min^{-1} for 5 min during exposure to isotope with the uptake by the quiescent atria. This procedure resulted in estimation of a fraction of Ca^{++} associated with contraction, constituting 20% of total muscle calcium (about 0.4 mM kg^{-1}). Calculated ^{45}Ca uptake per beat did not exceed 10^{-6} M per litre of plasma water.

Langer and Brady (1963) tried to measure ^{45}Ca fluxes associated with contraction in ventricular muscle. Experiments were performed on the isolated, arterially perfused dog papillary muscle, in an experimental set-up enabling continued monitoring of the loading with and washout of isotope. The muscles were stimulated throughout both loading and washout. The authors found that increase in the rate of stimulation during loading increased the rate of ^{45}Ca uptake, the maximum increase being achieved within 11.4 min. Within the next 10 min the rate of uptake returned to its initial value despite a maintained increase in the rate of stimulation. Increase in the rate of stimulation did not affect the rate of washout. The authors concluded that increase in the rate of stimulation initiated a process of augmented Ca^{++} turnover with the influx first exceeding efflux. Dividing maximal increase in ^{45}Ca uptake by the number of beats, they obtained a value of 0.92 pM cm^2 for the external surface of the cell per beat. The total fibre external surface in the papillary muscle was estimated at 97 cm^2. Assuming the external fibre area to be 2350 cm^2 g^{-1} (Bassingthwaighte and Reuter, 1972) it gives a value of 0.002 15 mM Ca per kilogram of tissue per beat.

These experiments were repeated by Langer (1965) with the use of a similar technique. Net maximal increase in ^{45}Ca uptake due to increase in the rate of stimulation was divided by the number of stimuli in order to obtain uptake per beat. This yielded a value of 0.0022 mM Ca per litre of tissue water per beat. The methods used in both papers allow, at best, an estimate of the mean increase in ^{45}Ca uptake per beat but not the absolute value of Ca^{++} uptake or exchange per beat.

The papers reviewed on the preceding pages of this chapter are, to the author's knowledge, the only works aimed at measuring excitation-dependent Ca^{++} fluxes during a single beat by isotopic methods. Their results are currently quoted as the evidence that the amount of Ca^{++} diffusing into the excited cell from the extracellular space is too small for significant activation of the contractile system. This evidence seems rather feeble, since in fact Ca^{++} influx per beat has never been measured, at least in the mammalian myocardium.

Having reached this conclusion we tried to measure ^{45}Ca fluxes at a single excitation using a direct experimental approach (Lewartowski *et al.*, 1982) and to monitor ^{45}Ca exchange under post-rest and under steady state stimulation conditions (Pytkowski and Lewartowski, manuscript in preparation).

Experiments were performed on the isolated, perfused ventricles of the guinea-pig heart, after ventricular automaticity had been suppressed by severing the upper part of the His bundle and elevating potassium concentration in the perfusing solution to 7.5 mM. These experiments provided the following information.

Perfusion of the quiescent preparation with the solution containing ^{45}Ca resulted in the uptake of labelled calcium which attained a steady state level of 0.418 ± 0.093 mM kg^{-1} wet weight within approximately 8 min. A single excitation applied after 4 min of rest, during which the muscle was perfused with radioactive solution, resulted in the increase of the tissue ^{45}Ca content to 0.647 ± 0.027 mM kg^{-1} wet weight. Thus excitation-dependent ^{45}Ca uptake was 0.23 mM kg^{-1} wet weight. The single excitation did not affect the volume of extracellular space as measured with extracellular marker $^{35}SO_4^{--}$, nor did it change radioactivity of the tissue when ^{63}Ni in very low concentration (which did not affect the force of contraction) was substituted for ^{45}Ca. Due to similar size, same charge, and similar affinity to the sarcolemmal binding sites (Kohlhardt *et al.*, 1979), Ni ions should simulate ^{45}Ca distribution within the extracellular space. As blockers of the slow Ca channel, they should not diffuse across the excited membrane. Excitation-dependent ^{45}Ca uptake was almost completely inhibited by Ni ions in 2 mM concentration sufficient to block the slow inward Ca^{++} current (Kohlhardt *et al.*, 1973). These control experiments showed that the increase in ^{45}Ca content in the stimulated ventricles probably did not depend on the effect of the twitch on the distribution of isotope within the extracellular space. Moreover, excitation-dependent ^{45}Ca was not displaced from the tissue by lanthanum (La) ions, which showed that it was not adsorbed on the outer surface of sarcolemma (Sanborn and Langer, 1970; Langer and Frank, 1972). Therefore we concluded that excitation-dependent ^{45}Ca uptake by our preparations most probably resulted from the diffusion of Ca^{++} into the cells from the extracellular space.

Continued post-rest stimulation at the rate of $60\ min^{-1}$ resulted in a further increase in the tissue $^{45}Ca^{++}$ content, most of it being completed during the initial three beats. The steady state ($1.327 \pm 0.054\ mM\ kg^{-1}$ wet weight) was reached within about 240 beats and was maintained during the following 360 beats. Thus in the steady state, the net post-rest, excitation-dependent uptake reached about $0.91\ mM\ kg^{-1}$ wet weight. This accumulation of ^{45}Ca paralleled post-rest recovery of contractile force. When the stimulation was stopped again, tissue ^{45}Ca content dropped again to the resting level despite the continued perfusion with the isotope-containing solution. This experiment showed that there is an absolute loss of Ca^{++} from the rested ventricles. This loss of Ca^{++} is accompanied by decrease of the contractile force.

We took advantage of the possibility to exchange nearly completely the capillary fluid for the ^{45}Ca containing perfusate within 18 s, and of the evidence provided by Frank and Langer (1974) and by Philipson and Langer (1979) that capillary-to-cell exchange shunts the interstitial space, to develop a method of measuring ^{45}Ca uptake at a single excitation also under the conditions of steady state stimulation at a slow rate. Excitation-dependent uptake per beat at the rate of $12\ min^{-1}$ was $0.22\ mM\ kg^{-1}$ wet weight. The content of ^{45}Ca was not further increased by an increase in the number of beats up to 48. Calcium uptake at a single excitation could not be measured directly at the higher rates of stimulation; however, we were also able to show that at the rate of $60\ min^{-1}$ and $120\ min^{-1}$ it did not depend on the number of beats (from 15 to 240). However, when the rate was increased during exposure to isotope, ^{45}Ca content rose above the value found at the lower rate. Thus, we concluded that under the steady state conditions, ^{45}Ca uptake after a number of beats was equal to the uptake at single excitation. This could result only from extrusion of labelled calcium taken at one excitation during or due to the next excitation without mixing with other Ca^{++} already present within the cell. The value of uptake decreased with increase in rate. At the rate of $60\ min^{-1}$ it was $0.105\ mM\ kg^{-1}$ wet weight and at the rate of $120\ min^{-1}$ it dropped to $0.075\ mM\ kg^{-1}$ wet weight. This lower amount of Ca^{++} is still sufficient for full activation of contractile proteins (Solaro *et al.*, 1974).

Comparison of the results obtained under the post-rest conditions with those obtained under the steady state conditions lead us to an hypothesis very similar to that of Chapman and Niedergerke (1970a,b). Three functionally defined intracellular Ca^{++} fractions (compartments) may be distinguished. Fraction Ca_1 continuously exchanges with the extracellular space in resting conditions (background exchange). The volume of this fraction is about 0.14 mM kg^{-1} wet weight. Fraction Ca_2 diffuses across the excited membrane and triggers contraction. The amount of Ca forming this fraction is between 0.075 and 0.220 mM kg^{-1} wet weight and it is roughly inversely dependent on the rate of stimulation. Under the steady state conditions Ca_2 diffusing into the excited cell at one excitation is completely extruded at the next excitation without mixing with other fractions. In post-rest conditions or when the rate is increased, some Ca_2 is trapped at each beat within some intracellular compartment forming fraction Ca_3. Under the steady state conditions Ca_3 is bound (fixed) and does not exchange with other fractions nor with the extracellular space. The capacity of Ca_3 increases with increase in rate and decreases with decrease in rate. Accordingly, Ca^{++} is bound or released. At rest Ca_3 is completely released and extruded from the cell. Under the conditions of our experiments (rates from 0 to 120 min^{-1}) gain and loss of Ca_3 was accompanied by increase and loss of contractile force.

Fraction Ca_3 seems to have two important functions: (i) it controls the amount of Ca_2 diffusing across the excited membrane; (ii) it controls the response of the contractile system to Ca_2. Due to this double control, the force of contraction depends on the amount of Ca^{++} within Ca_3 and not on amount within Ca_2. The latter is always sufficient for activation of the contractile system.

It is difficult to imagine how Ca_3 can control the amount of Ca diffusing across the excited membrane; however, it is apparent that Ca_2 is inversely dependent on the content of Ca_3.

The control of the response of the contracile system to the triggering action of Ca_2 may depend on the effect on some enzyme as postulated already by Chapman and Niedergerke (1970a,b), and discussed by England (Chapter 16 in this volume).

Studies on efflux of ^{45}Ca from the resting, previously loaded ventricles showed that washout curves were composed of four mono-exponential components similar to those described by Shine et al. (1971). They were labelled phases 0 through 3. Their rate constants were 2.832, 1.523, 0.245, and 0.008, respectively. It was tempting to link phases of washout with some functionally defined Ca^{++} cellular compartments. However, in all experimental conditions the ratios of the contents of these washout phases were similar. In other words, disregarding the way by which labelled Ca^{++} entered the cells, it was washed out according to the same four-component kinetics. This result shows that the described phases cannot be linked with the functionally defined fractions Ca_1, Ca_2, and Ca_3. For example, if any of these phases were linked to fraction Ca_3 it should disappear from the washout curves in the experiments in which steady state stimulation was applied during loading with isotope, since under these conditions Ca_3 did not accumulate. In control experiments in which the ventricles were quiescent at loading, phases linked with Ca_2 and with Ca_3 should not appear; this was not the case. Although we are not able to propose at present the model of Ca turnover, it seems that the phases of washout reflect the various ways and processes of Ca transport between the cells and extracellular space, rather than the intracellular Ca compartments.

Calcium Influx Calculated from the Slow Inward Calcium Current

The application of the voltage clamp to myocardial preparations provided evidence of the existence of a slow inward current carried mostly by Ca ions and responsible for the final part of 0 phase and the maintenance of the plateau of the cellular action potential of cardiac muscle (Rougier *et al.*, 1969; Beeler and Reuter, 1970a; Bassingthwaite and Reuter, 1972; New and Trautwein, 1972, for a review see Carmeliet and Vereecke, 1979). The area enclosed by the net current trace in units of charge may be determined. Provided that this charge is carried exclusively by Ca ions the total calcium inflow into the intracellular volume can be calculated. The author of this chapter is aware of only three original papers in which the results of such calculations are reported. Beeler and Reuter (1970b) stated:

> 'A net gain in intracellular calcium between 1×10^{-6} and 5×10^{-5} M has been calculated from the charge transfer during the initial calcium inward current, the variation being dependent upon the potential at which I_{Ca} was activated and upon Ca_o concentration. This amount of Ca, however, would be sufficient to activate the contractile system appreciably'.

Unfortunately, the conditions under which these marginal values have been obtained were not specified by the authors, nor did they report Ca^{++} flux under conditions close to physiological. Also it is not certain for which units of tissue volume or weight these fluxes were calculated. One of the authors (Reuter, 1974), quoting this paper in his review article, wrote that, 'With an extracellular Ca concentration of 2 mM the gain in intracellular Ca ions during each action potential is of the order of $1-5 \times 10^{-6}$ moles per liter cell volume'. This amount cannot be sufficient for significant activation of the contractile system. New and Trautwein (1972) calculated Ca^{++} influx between 5×10^{-7} and 5×10^{-6} M Ca per litre of fibre volume per beat. Extracellular Ca^{++} concentrations in the experiments in which current traces used for calculations were obtained was 1.8 mM. The value obtained by Vassort and Rougier (1972) in frog atrial muscle was 1×10^{-5} M.

These values are similar to those reported by the authors who used isotopic techniques to estimate Ca^{++} fluxes, and they are more than one order of magnitude lower than ours. One of the possible reasons for this discrepancy could be that, due to technical difficulties (Fozzard and Beeler, 1975), calculations based on the recording of slow inward current may be regarded as a rough estimate only. The other, more likely, reason is the possibility that slow inward Ca^{++} current may constitute only a fraction of Ca^{++} transferred across the sarcolemma into the excited cell, the rest being transferred by means of the Na^+–Ca^{++} exchange system (Langer, 1976). This hypothesis has recently obtained experimental support.

Working with isolated sarcolemmal vesicles, Pitts (1979) and Young and Pitts (1980) established that the stoicheiometry of Na^+–Ca^{++} exchange is different from that described previously (see Chapman *et al.*, Chapter 6 in this volume). They found that at least three Na^+ ions exchange for one Ca^{++} ion instead of two. Thus Na^+–Ca^{++} exchange should be electrogenic and, as such, affected by membrane voltage. This has been demonstrated by Bers *et al.* (1980) and Philipson and Nishimoto (1980), in isolated sarcolemmal vesicles.

Horackova and Vassort (1979) found that Na^+–Ca^{++} exchange may be sensitive to membrane potential during the course of excitation, suggesting that Na^+–Ca^{++} exchange contributes significantly to total Ca^{++} influx during excitation. A reversal potential of electrogenic Na^+–Ca^{++} exchange that is about midway between their resting membrane potential and the plateau level (Mullins 1979; Langer, 1982) implies that the direction of Na^+–Ca^{++} exchange should be reversed at the plateau of the cardiac cellular action potential, resulting in Ca^{++} influx independent of the slow Ca^{++} channel.

Excitation-dependent Ca^{++} Fluxes Estimated by Means of an Indirect Approach (Efflux Studies)

Evidence concerning the source and amount of Ca^{++} which activates contraction has also been provided by workers who investigated the kinetics of ^{45}Ca and/or Ca efflux from the myocardium under various conditions.

Four or five kinetically defined phases of ^{45}Ca efflux from the isolated, arterially perfused papillary muscle (Langer and Brady, 1963; Langer, 1965), isolated, perfused interventricular septum of the rabbit heart (Shelburne *et al.*, 1967; Shine *et al.*, 1971) and from the isolated, perfused ventricles of the guinea-pig heart (Lewartowski *et al.*, manuscript in preparation) have been described (Figure 5.1). These phases have been labelled 0 through 3 or 4. All these authors collected the effluent from the heart for at least 1 h.

Bailey and Dresel (1968) and Bailey *et al.* (1972) studied the isolated cat heart perfused alternately with solution and gas. When these hearts were subjected to Ca^{++}-free perfusion, washout of calcium revealed three phases labelled I through III. Contractile force fell with Ca^{++}–free perfusion along a single exponential whose rate constant corresponded to that of phase II.

Saari and Johnson (1971) found that the rate constant of decay of contractile force of isolated, perfused rabbit heart occurring with Ca^{++}-free perfusion did not differ significantly from the rate constant of the rapid

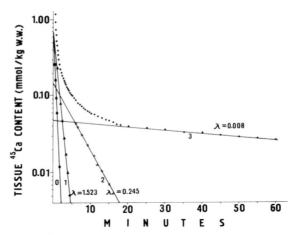

Figure 5.1 Efflux of $^{45}Ca^{++}$ from the isolated perfused ventricles of the guinea-pig heart. The ventricles were stimulated 240 times at the rate of $60\,min^{-1}$ during loading with isotope and quiescent throughout the washout. Mono-exponential components resolved by graphical analysis

phase of Ca tissue content decay. The kinetics of this phase were compara-ble with those of the interstitial space. A similar conclusion was reached by Teiger and Farah (1967) with respect to the isolated rabbit atria and by Ma and Bailey (1979a) with respect to the hamster ventricular muscle. The latter authors found that Ca content in the rapidly exchanging (extracellular) phase is much larger than the amount of Ca^{++} in the volume of interstitial fluid. This finding led to a conclusion that much of the extracellular Ca^{++} is adsorbed on the external surface of the sarcolemma and on other extracellu-lar structures.

More recently Philipson and Langer (1979) found that the kinetics of recovery of contractile force of isolated, perfused interventricular septum of the rabbit heart correlate best with the kinetics of exchange of the vascular space. Considering the morphological data provided by Frank and Langer (1974) they supposed that a large fraction of cellular–capillary exchange shunts the interstitial space. This supposition has recently been confirmed in our laboratory (Lewartowski *et al.*, manuscript in preparation). We found that excitation-dependent uptake of ^{45}Ca, when only the vascular space is equilibrated with $^{45}Ca^{++}$-containing solution, is as large as that obtained upon full equilibration of total extracellular space with radioactive perfusate. This could not be so if there were no direct cellular–capillary exchange.

Such findings led to the concept of specific sarcolemmal Ca^{++} receptors which are rapidly accessible to and remain in equilibrium with Ca^{++} in the extracellular space and which control contractility. This membrane-bound calcium either controls the release of Ca^{++} from intracellular stores or is itself a source of activator Ca^{++} supplied to the contractile system.

Two classes of membrane binding sites were distinguished (Philipson and Langer, 1979): a high affinity, low capacity class with association constant, $K_A = 46\,060$ M, and number of sites per milligram of protein $n = 54$ nM, and low affinity, high capacity class with $K_A = 830$ M and $n = 216$ nM per milligram of protein. The low affinity sites would be half-saturated at 1.2 mM Ca^{++}, which is similar to the Ca^{++} concentration at which rabbit ventricular myocardium reaches half-maximum contractility (Bers and Langer, 1979). The isolated membrane vesicles are able to bind 0.7 mM Ca per kilogram wet weight of the tissue (Bers and Langer, 1979) which, if delivered to the contractile proteins, is sufficient for activation of contraction (Solaro *et al.*, 1974). A similar amount is displaced from isolated membrane vesicles and from a cell culture by trivalent cations (e.g. lanthanum, Sanborn and Langer, 1970), the percentage of release being parallel to their uncoupling effectiveness (Bers and Langer, 1979).

Evidence has been provided by several authors that the external sarcolemmal surface coat, 'glycocalyx', rich in polysaccharides and associated primarily with membrane glycoproteins, plays an important role in Ca^{++} binding and cellular Ca^{++} exchange. Both these functions are impaired upon removal of sialic acid and Ca^{++} (Crevey *et al.*, 1978; Frank *et al.*, 1977; Langer *et al.*, 1976). Working with isolated fragments of cardiac cell membranes, Ma and Bailey (1979c) distinguished two classes of Ca^{++} binding sites; the low affinity sites with a capacity of 134.8 nM per milligram of protein and dissociation constant (K_D) of 2.17 mM 1^{-1} and the high affinity sites with a capacity of 5.2 nM per milligram of protein and K_D of 0.04 mM 1^{-1}. Neuraminidase treatment of the sarcolemmal fragments reduced the sialic acid content and low affinity binding capacity, but increased high affinity binding.

This hypothesis concerning the essential role of the glycocalyx in Ca^{++} binding and excitation–contraction coupling has been challenged by some recently published results. Philipson *et al.* (1980) found that vesicles built of phospholipids extracted from isolated fragments of cardiac sarcolemma bind 80% of the Ca^{++} adsorbable by intact sarcolemmal vesicles. Binding was inhibited by La and EGTA. Vesicles built of phospholipids previously treated with phospholipase-C lost up to 80% of their Ca^{++} binding capacity. Experiments in which the intact vesicles were treated with this enzyme provided less consistent results; however, their binding capacity was always decreased. On the other hand, treatment of these vesicles with neuraminidase, which results in removal of most of the sialic acid, did not appreciably affect their Ca^{++} binding. The authors concluded that phospholipids but not the glycocalyx may be the most important factor for sarcolemmal Ca^{++}

binding and for excitation–contraction coupling. This conclusion is similar to the view of Lüllmann *et al.* (see Chapter 1 in this volume).

Isenberg and Klöckner (1980) showed that the slow inward Ca^{++} current in the isolated rat myocyte is larger by up to one order of magnitude than in multicellular preparations. The procedure of isolation deprived these myocytes of all their glycocalyx. This result suggests that the glycocalyx is not essential for at least one of the possible ways of transfer of activator Ca^{++} into the excited cells. Harding and Halliday (1980) did not see any effect of removal of 75% of sialic acid from the isolated guinea-pig atria on their contractility or response to changes in external Ca^{++} concentration.

Regardless of the nature of the process of Ca^{++} binding to the external surface of the sarcolemma and its importance for excitation–contraction coupling, the papers reviewed in this section have provided evidence that Ca^{++} which activates contraction is derived directly from the extracellular space. This would mean that either the amount of Ca^{++} transferred across the excited membrane is sufficient for activation of the contractile system (i.e. it is of the order of 10^{-5}–10^{-4} M kg^{-1} wet weight per beat) or that it activates contraction by releasing more Ca from the intracellular stores, as proposed by Fabiato and Fabiato (1979a,b). Our own results (Lewartowski *et al.*, 1982), if confirmed, would support the former hypothesis.

Excitation-dependent Calcium Extrusion

Excitation-dependent Ca^{++} influx into the cells should be matched by Ca^{++} efflux, otherwise Ca^{++} accumulation within the cells would occur. Extrusion of extra Ca^{++} could be accomplished between beats by means of an Na^+–Ca^{++} exchange system (Chapman *et al.*, Chapter 6 in this volume) and by active transport (St Louis and Sulakhe, 1979). However, if a large influx takes place upon excitation, an equally large excitation-dependent efflux may be expected.

Niedergerke (1963) found that stimulation increased $^{45}Ca^{++}$ efflux from previously loaded frog ventricles. Calculated efflux per beat was very low (about 0.0017 mM per litre of the cells) and matched ^{45}Ca influx per beat. These measurements suffered from some shortcomings. No effect of stimulation on ^{45}Ca efflux from isolated guinea-pig atria was noticed (Winegrad and Shanes, 1962), or from the isolated dog papillary muscle (Langer and Brady, 1963) and isolated rabbit atria (Teiger and Farah, 1967).

We have recently found (Lewartowski *et al.*, 1982, manuscript in preparation) that a single excitation considerably increased ^{45}Ca efflux from the ventricles of guinea-pig hearts which were stimulated during loading and rested during washout. This rapid increase in efflux brought the washout curve to the level found in the control ventricles which were not stimulated during loading. Only early excitations, applied not later than 90 s after the beginning of washout (and rest) were effective. Moreover, increase in the number of excitations during washout did not increase the efflux any more, as if the single excitation extruded all the excitation-dependent Ca^{++} which entered the cells at the preceding excitations. These findings may explain discrepances between our results and the results of other workers quoted in this section. Excitation-dependent efflux per beat was of the order of $0.1 \, mM \, kg^{-1}$ wet weight, i.e. it could match excitation-dependent influx found in our experiments. However, it should be stressed that the isotopic technique does not allow one to differentiate the part of the cardiac cycle at which this extrusion associated with contraction occurred. It is possible that an increase in the rate of $Na^+–Ca^{++}$ exchange could occur during depolarization. Such a possibility is suggested by increased activity of the Na^+, K^+ pump (Boyett and Fedida, 1982) upon depolarization of Purkinje fibres. This could lead to an increased $Na^+–Ca^{++}$ exchange immediately after depolarization.

SUMMARY

Review of the literature shows that the apparently simple problem of the amount of Ca^{++} transferred across the excited cardiac sarcolemma has not been yet successfully solved. Calcium influx at a single excitation has never been measured by isotopic methods, at least in the mammalian myocardium. Our own results shed some light on this question; however, experiments have so far been performed on just one preparation obtained from one animal species only. Moreover, we have so far failed to provide direct evidence that the increase in ^{45}Ca content in stimulated preparations resulted from influx of Ca into the excited cells from extracellular space.

Calculations based on measurements of slow inward calcium current provide only a rather rough estimate. Moreover, this method can overlook large amounts of Ca^{++} transferred across the sarcolemma by means of a mechanism other than the slow inward Ca^{++} current.

This review leads to a rather challenging conclusion that reasoning based on the data concerning quantitative aspects of excitation-dependent Ca^{++} exchange (i.e. many models of excitation–contraction coupling) still lacks sound experimental background.

REFERENCES

Bailey, L. E., and Dresel, P. E. (1968). Correlation of contractile force with a calcium pool in the isolated cat heart. *J. Gen. Physiol.*, **52**, 969–982.

Bailey, L. E., Seok Doo Ong, and Queen, G. M. (1972). Calcium movement during contraction of the cat heart. *J. Mol. Cell. Cardiol.*, **4**, 121–138.

Bassingthwaighte, J. B., and Reuter, H. (1972). Calcium movements and excitation–contraction coupling in cardiac cells. In *Electrical Phenomena in the Heart* (W. C. DeMello, ed.), Academic Press, New York and London.

Beeler, G. W., and Reuter, H. (1970a). Membrane calcium current in ventricular myocardial fibres. *J. Physiol. (Lond.)* **207**, 191–209.

Beeler, G. W., and Reuter, H. (1970b). The relation between membrane potential, membrane currents and activation of contraction in ventricular myocardial fibres. *J. Physiol. (Lond.)*, **207**, 211–229.

Bers, D. M., and Langer, G. A. (1979). Uncoupling cation effects on cardiac contractility and sarcolemmal Ca^{2+} binding. *Amer. J. Physiol.*, **237**, H332–H341.

Bers, D. M., Philipson, K. D., and Nishimoto, A. Y. (1980). Sodium–calcium exchange and sidedness of isolated cardiac sarcolemmal vesicles. *Biochim. Biophys. Acta*, **601**, 358–371.

Boyett, M. R., and Fedida, D. (1982). Evidence for activation of the electrogenic Na-K pump at high rates of stimulation in cardiac Purkinje fibres. *J. Physiol.* **324**, 24P.

Carmeliet, E., and Vereecke, J. (1979). Electrogenesis of the action potential and automaticity. In *Handbook of Physiology, Section 2: The Cardiovascular System*, Vol. I, *The Heart*, American Physiological Society, Bethesda, Md, pp. 269–334.

Chapman, R. A., and Niedergerke, R. (1970a). Effects of calcium on the contraction of the hypodynamic frog heart. *J. Physiol. (Lond.)*, **211**, 389–421.

Chapman, R. A., and Niedergerke, R. (1970b). Interaction between heart rate and calcium concentration in the control of contractile strength of the frog heart. *J. Physiol. (Lond.)*, **211**, 423–443.

Crevey, B. J., Langer, G. A., and Frank, J. S. (1978). Role of Ca^{2+} in the maintenance of rabbit cell membrane structural and functional integrity, *J. Mol. Cell. Cardiol.*, **10**, 1081–1100.

Fabiato, A., and Fabiato, F. (1979a). Calcium and cardiac excitation–contraction coupling. *Annu. Rev. Physiol.*, **41**, 473–484.

Fabiato, A., and Fabiato, F. (1979b). Use of chlortetraegaline fluorescence to demonstrate Ca^{2+}-induced release of Ca^{2+} from the sarcoplasmic reticulum of skinned cardiac cells. *Nature*, **281**, 146–148.

Fozzard, H. A., and Beeler, G. W. (1975). The voltage clamp and cardiac electrophysiology. *Circulation Res.*, **37**, 403–413.

Frank, J. S., and Langer, G. A. (1974). The myocardial interstitium: its structure and its role in ionic exchange. *J. Cell Biol.*, **60**, 586–601.

Frank, J. S., Langer, G. A., Nudd, L. M., and Seraydarian, K. (1977). The myocardial cell surface, its histochemistry and the effect of sialic acid and calcium removal on its structure and cellular ionic exchange. *Circulation Res.*, **41**, 702–714.

Grossman, A., and Furchgott, R. F. (1964). The effects of frequency of stimulation on ^{45}Ca exchange and contractility of the isolated guinea-pig auricle. *J. Pharmacol. Exp. Ther.*, **143**, 120–130.

Harding, S. E., and Halliday, J. (1980). Removal of sialic acid from cardiac sarcolemma does not affect contractile function in electrically stimulated guinea pig left atria. *Nature*, **286**, 819–821.

Horackova, M., and Vassort, G. (1979). Sodium–calcium exchange in regulation of cardiac contractility. Evidence for an electrogenic, voltage dependent mechanism. *J. Gen. Physiol.*, **73**, 403–424.

Isenberg, G., and Klöckner, U. (1980). Glycocalix is not required for slow inward calcium current in isolated rat heart myocytes. *Nature*, **284**, 358–360.

Kohlhardt, M., Bauer, B., Krause, H., and Fleckenstein, A. (1973). Selective inhibition of the transmembrane conductivity of mammalian myocardial fibres by Ni, Co and Mn ions. *Pflügers Arch. Europ. J. Physiol.*, **338**, 115–123.

Kohlhardt, M., Mnich, Z., and Haap, K. (1979). Analysis of the inhibitory effect of Ni ions on slow inward current in mammalian ventricular myocardium. *J. Mol. Cell. cardiol.* **11**, 1227–1243.

Langer, G. (1965). Calcium exchange in dog ventricular muscle: relation to frequency of contraction and maintenance of contractility. *Circulation Res.*, **17**, 78–89.

Langer, G. A. (1976). Events at the cardiac sarcolemma: localization and movement of contractile-dependent calcium. *Fed. Proc.*, **35**, 1274–1278.

Langer, G. A. (1982). Sodium–calcium exchange in the heart. *Annu. Rev. Physiol.*, **44**, 435–449.

Langer, G. A., and Brady, A. J. (1963). Calcium flux in the mammalian ventricular myocardium. *J. Gen. Physiol.*, **46**, 703–719.

Langer, G. A., and Frank, J. S. (1972). Lanthanum in heart cell culture. *J. Cell Biol.*, **54**, 441–455.

Langer, G. A., Frank, J. S., Nudd, L. M., and Seraydarian, K. (1976). Sialic acid: effect of removal on calcium exchangeability in cultured heart cells. *Science*, **193**, 1013–1015.

Lewartowski, B., Pytkowski, B., Prokopczuk, A., Wasilewska, E., and Otwinowski, W. (1982). Amount and turnover of ^{45}Ca entering the cells of ventricular muscle of guinea pig heart at single excitation. *Advanc. Myocardiol.*, **3**, in press.

Little, G. R., and Sleator, W. W. (1969). Calcium exchange and contraction strength of guinea pig atrium in normal and hypertonic media. *J. Gen. Physiol.*, **54**, 494–511.

Ma, T. S., and Bailey, L. E. (1979a). Excitation–contraction coupling in normal and myopathic hamster hearts: I. Identification of a calcium pool involved in contraction. *Cardiovasc. Res.*, **13**, 487–498.

Ma, T. S., and Bailey, L. E. (1979b). Excitation–contraction coupling in normal and myopathic hamster hearts: II. Changes in contractility and Ca pools associated with development of cardiomyopathy. *Cardiovasc. Res.*, **13**, 499–505.

Ma, T. S., Baker, J. C., and Bailey, L. E. (1979c). Excitation–contraction coupling in normal and myopathic hamster hearts: III. Functional deficiences in interstitial glycoproteins. *Cardiovasc. Res.*, **13**, 568–577.

Marban, E., Rink, T. J., Tsien, R. W., and Tsien, R. Y. (1980). Free calcium in heart muscle at rest and during contraction measured with Ca^{2+}-sensitive microelectrodes. *Nature*, **286**, 845–850.

Mullins, L. I. (1979). The generation of electric currents in cardiac fibres by Na/Ca exchange. *Amer. J. Physiol.*, **236**, C103–C110.

New, W., and Trautwein, W. (1972). The ionic nature of slow inward current and its relation to contraction. *Pflügers Arch. Europ. J. Physiol.*, **334**, 24–38.

Niedergerke, R. (1963). Movements of Ca in beating ventricles of the frog heart. *J. Physiol. (Lond.)*, **167**, 551–580.

Niedergerke, R., and Page, S. (1969). A new method for the determination of calcium fluxes in the frog heart by means of high precision measurement of ^{45}Ca concentration. *Pflügers Arch. Europ. J. Physiol.*, **306**, 354–356.

Niedergerke, R., Page, S., and Talbot, M. S. (1969). Calcium fluxes in frog heart ventricles. *Pflügers Arch. Europ. J. Physiol.*, **306**, 357–360.

Philipson, K. D., and Nishimoto, A. Y. (1980). Na^+-Ca^{2+} exchange is affected by membrane potential in cardiac sarcolemmal vesicles. *J. Biol. Chem.*, **255**, 6880–6882.

Philipson, K. D., Bers, D. M., and Nishimoto, A. Y. (1980). The role of phospholipids in the Ca^{2+} binding of isolated cardiac sarcolemma. *J. Mol. Cell. Cardiol.*, **12**, 1159–1173.

Pits, B. J. R. (1979). Stoichiometry of sodium–calcium exchange in cardiac sarcolemmal vesicles. Coupling to the sodium pump. *J. Biol. Chem.*, **254**, 6232–6235.

Ray, K. P., and England, P. J. (1976). Phosphorylation of the inhibitory subunit of troponin and its effect on the calcium dependence of cardiac myofibril adenosine triphosphatase. *FEBS Lett.*, **70**, 11–16.

Reuter, H. (1974). Exchange of calcium ions in the mammalian myocardium. Mechanism and physiological significance. *Circulation Res.*, **34**, 599–605.

Rougier, O. G., Vassort, D., Gardiner, Y. M., Gargouil, Y. M., and Corabaeuf, E. (1969). Existence and role of a slow inward current during the frog atrial action potential. *Pflügers Arch. Europ. J. Physiol.*, **308**, 91–110.

Saari, J. T., and Johnson, J. A. (1971). Decay of calcium content and contractile force in the rabbit heart. *Amer. J. Physiol.*, **221**, 1572–1575.

St Louis, P. J., and Sulakhe, P. V. (1976). Adenosine triphosphate-dependent calcium binding and accumulation by guinea pig cardiac sarcolemma. *Canad. J. Biochem.*, **54**, 946–956.

Shelburne, J. C., Serena, S. D., and Langer, G. A. (1967). Rate–tension staircase in rabbit ventricular muscle: relation to ionic exchange. *Amer. J. Physiol.*, **213**, 1115–1124.

Shine, K. I., Serena, S. D., and Langer, G. A. (1971). Kinetic localization of contractile calcium in rabbit myocardium. *Amer. J. Physiol.*, **221**, 1408–1417.

Solaro, J. R., Wise, R. M., Shiner, J. S., and Briggs, F. N. (1974). Calcium requirements for cardiac myofibrillar activation. *Circulation Res.*, **34**, 525–530.

Teiger, G., and Farah, A. (1967). Calcium movements in resting and stimulated isolated rabbit atria. *J. Pharmacol. Exp. Therap.*, **157**, 8–18.

Vassort, G., and Rougier, O. (1972). Membrane potential and slow inward current dependence of frog cardiac mechanical activity. *Pflügers Arch. Europ. J. Physiol.*, **331**, 191–203.

Winegrad, S., and Shanes, A. M. (1962). Calcium flux and contractility in guinea pig atria. *J. Gen. Physiol.*, **45**, 371–394.

Young, C. O., and Pitts, B. J. R. (1980). Electrogenic Na, Ca exchange in cardiac sarcolemmal vesicles. *Proc. VIII Europ. Congr. Cardiol.*, Paris, 164, abstr. no. 1978.

Cardiac Metabolism
Edited by A. J. Drake-Holland and M. I. M. Noble
© 1983 John Wiley & Sons Ltd

CHAPTER 6

Sodium–Calcium Exchange in Mammalian Heart: the Maintenance of low Intracellular Calcium Concentration

R. A. Chapman, A. Coray, and John A. S. McGuigan

Department of Physiology, University of Berne, Bühlplatz 5, 3012 Berne, Switzerland

INTRODUCTION

The Na^+–Ca^{++} exchange mechanism and the factors controlling intracellular calcium concentrations $[Ca]_i$, have been adequately covered in several recent reviews, viz. Chapman (1979), Requena and Mullins (1979), Sulakhe and St Louis (1980), Borle (1981), Mullins (1981), and Reuter (1982). In this article we try to put the Na^+–Ca^{++} exchange system into perspective with regard to other calcium controlling systems of the heart.

Anatomy

The data in Figure 6.1 are taken from the review by Page (1978) and are for rat left ventricle. A striking feature (Figure 6.1(a)) is the relatively large volume occupied by membrane-bound structures, so that they occupy roughly 40% of the total. The cytoplasm of the cell fills the remaining 60% of the volume. This value must be even further reduced because this includes the myofibrils. Although the myofibrils are shown to occupy 47% in the diagram, the cytoplasmic value is not reduced by this amount since water will be present within the myofibrils.

For ionic movements across cell membranes (plasma, mitrochondria, or sarcoplasmic reticulum (SR)) it is not the volume but rather the surface area that is important, for transport at a given driving force is defined to be the amount per unit time per unit area. The relative surface areas of the three structures is shown in Figure 6.1(b), and it is seen that the ratio of the areas of plasma membrane : SR : mitochondria is $1:4:67$. (In this calculation the surface area of the T-system was not included in that of the plasma membrane.) What Figure 6.1(b) means is that even if the transport rate for an ion by the mitochondria was 17 times less than that for the same ion by

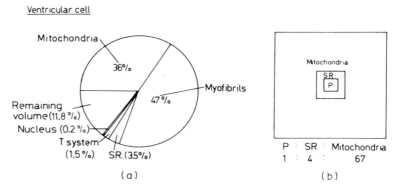

Figure 6.1 (a) Pie diagram of the relative volume of the various cell organelles. (b) Relative area of the plasma membrane (P), the sarcoplasmic reticulum (SR), and the mitochondria. Each square represents the surface area of the individual organelle

the SR, both structures would transport the same amount per unit time. This aspect of transport has recently been emphasized by Borle (1981) and Carafoli (1982).

General Predictions from Na^+–Ca^{++} Exchange

If $[Ca]_i$ is maintained at a low concentration by Na ions moving down their electrochemical gradient, by a tightly coupled exchange, then $[Ca]_i$ should be predicted by the following equation:

$$[Ca]_i = \left\{\frac{[Na]_i}{[Na]_o}\right\}^n [Ca]_o \exp\left\{\frac{(n-2)EF}{RT}\right\}. \tag{6.1}$$

If n is other than 2, then the exchange becomes electrogenic and a function of the membrane potential.

One of the predictions from this type of formalism is that Na^+ removal from the bathing solution should lead to Ca^{++} accumulation inside the cell and to a contracture. What actually happens in a bundle of cow ventricular fibres 0.8 mm in diameter is shown in Figure 6.2(a). Twitch tension is shown at the beginning of the recording. Stimulation was then switched off; between the arrows the bundle was exposed to sodium-free solution. Despite this there is little or no increase in tension. Similar findings have been reported previously by Scholz (1969), Bassingthwaighte *et al.* (1976), and Marban *et al.*, (1980).

In an attempt to explain such findings we calculated the time necessary for the diffusion of Na^+ and of Ca^{++} in the extracellular space and in the cell (Figure 6.2(b)).

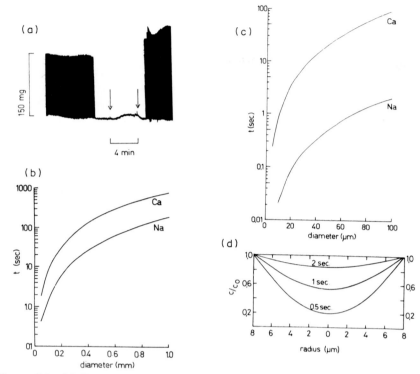

Figure 6.2 (a) Pen recording of twitch tension from a cow trabecula 0.8 mm in diameter. Between the arrows, the trabecula was perfused with Na-free Tyrode. (b) Diffusion times for Ca and Na to reach a mean of concentration of 97% of the original value in the extracellular space for trabeculae of various diameters. Diffusion coefficients for Na and Ca in extracellular space were 7.1×10^{-6} and 1.65×10^{-6} cm^2 s^{-1} respectively. (c) Diffusion times for Ca^{++} and Na$^+$ to reach a mean concentration of 97% inside the cell on a sudden change outside the cell for cells of various diameters. (d) Diffusion profile of Ca across a 16 μm cell (calculated from Figure 5.3 in Crank, 1967). c/c_0 is the ratio of the internal concentration to the surface concentration. Intracellular diffusion coefficients for Na and Ca were 6.02×10^{-6} and 1.4×10^{-7} cm^2 s^{-1} respectively

Diffusion in the Extracellular Space

For Na$^+$ we have used an apparent diffusion coefficient of 7.1×10^{-6} cm^2 s^{-1} (Page and Bernstein, 1964) and for Ca 1.65×10^{-6} cm^2 s^{-1} (Safford and Bassingthwaighte, 1977), and have calculated (using data from Hill, 1928) the time necessary to change the mean [Na]$_o$ in the bundle from 155 to 5 mM and the mean [Ca]$_o$ from 5.4 to 0.17 mM (the concentrations in our Tyrode); this time would be 2 min for Na$^+$ but 8 min for Ca^{++} (0.8 mm diameter muscle).

In our study of contractures we have used bundles of either guinea-pig or ferret ventricle under $300 \mu m$ in diameter and a rapid flow system (Chapman *et al.*, 1981a,b). The disappearance of the twitch on switching to a Ca-free solution had a $T_{1/2}$ of around 10 s. This provides only a rough estimate of the extracellular exchange time. If the diffusion coefficients for Na^{++} and Ca^{++} are different, and if their concentrations are simultaneously changed, transient effects are to be expected because of the differing rates at which these ions will be cleared from the extracellular space (cf. Horackova and Vassort, 1979).

Diffusion in the Cell

It is sometimes tacitly assumed that the diffusion of Na^+ and Ca^{++} inside heart and muscle cells is 'instantaneous', i.e. can for practical purposes be neglected. This is not necessarily so for skeletal muscle cells (Stephenson and Williams, 1981; Stephenson, 1981) and squid axon (Blaustein and Hodgkin, 1969). In Figure 6.2(c) we present results plotted in a similar way to those in Figure 6.2(b). We have, however, used the coefficient for intracellular diffusion found by Kushmerick and Podolsky (1969) for Na^+ and Ca^{++}. Figure 6.2(d) shows the theoretical distribution of Ca^{++} for a cell $16 \mu m$ in diameter at 0.5, 1, and 2 s.

Such theoretical considerations imply that during contractures lasting several minutes there should be a more or less even distribution across the cell (unless binding takes place at the inner surface of the membrane). However, events lasting less than 1 s could, at least temporarily, lead to diffusional Ca^{++} gradients across cardiac cells. If, as part of an experimental manoeuvre, the movement of Na^+ and Ca^{++} across the cell membrane is altered simultaneously, then, because the diffusion of Na^+ is 40 times faster than that of Ca^{++}, intracellular organelles may be confronted by changes in the $[Ca]_i : [Na]_i$ ratio which may last several seconds.

SODIUM WITHDRAWAL CONTRACTURES IN GUINEA-PIG AND FERRET TRABECULAE

Despite using a rapid flow system and thin bundles, Na^+ withdrawal contractures did not reach maximum tension, as is shown in Figure 6.3(a). That maximum tension was not reached is shown by the fact that the addition of 10 mM caffeine caused developed tension to more than double. Furthermore, as is shown in Figure 6.3(b), these sodium-free contractures relax over a period of minutes. This failure to develop maximal tension coupled with the fact that the contractures relax spontaneously at a rate similar to that of diffusion in a thick bundle, explains the previous failures to record increases in tension in ventricular muscle on Na^+ removal.

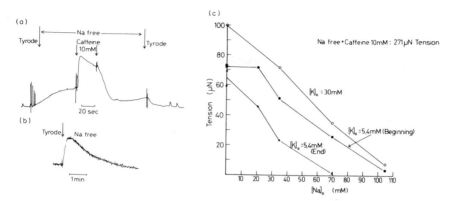

Figure 6.3 (a) Guinea-pig trabecula 100 μm in diameter. Between upper arrows it was perfused with Na-free Tyrode. During this perfusion the addition of 10 mM caffeine caused tension to increase to a maximal value of 0.9 mN, Na⁺ was replaced by tris(hydroxymethyl)aminomethane. (b) Ferret trabecula, 150 μm in diameter. At the arrow the trabecula was perfused with Na-free Tyrode and in this solution the contracture relaxes spontaneously. Maximum tension reached during this contracture was 0.45 mN. Na⁺ replaced by tetramethylammonium chloride. Note the different time scales in parts (a) and (b) of the figure. (c) Guinea-pig trabecula 125 μm in diameter. Measurement of Na⁺ withdrawal contractures at two different [K]ₒ. Room temperature

Na⁺–Ca⁺⁺ Exchange and [Ca]ᵢ

The various measurements of resting $[Ca]_i$ in ventricular muscle using Ca^{++} microelectrodes that have been carried out are tabulated in Table 6.1. These figures are given in units of concentration and the binding constant given by Schwarzenbach *et al.* (1957). From the values of Table 6.1, it is seen that the values lie between 200 and 360 nM. This is some 10 times higher than the value assumed by Mullins (1981), which will have important consequences when considering the stoicheiometry of the Na–Ca exchange.

Since measurements of $[Ca]_i$ in cardiac cells is difficult (see Blinks *et al.*, 1982), changes in tension are taken as indicating changes in $[Ca]_i$. To be able to convert tension into $[Ca]_i$ some relationship between $[Ca]_i$ and tension has to be assumed. An S-shaped relationship is regularly found for isolated myofibrils and skinned fibres (see Figure 1 in Chapman, 1979).

Three basic forms of equation have been described in the literature and a brief description of the derivation is given in Appendix 1 at the end of this chapter. The steepest form is given by the simultaneous reaction and a Hill plot (see Appendix 1) gives the minimum number of reacting sites (n) in the equation

$$T = \frac{K[Ca]_i^n}{1 + K[Ca]_i^n}. \tag{6.2}$$

Table 6.1 Resting $[Ca]_i$, $[Na]_o$, and $[Ca]_o$ in ventricular muscle

Tissue	Temperature (°C)	$[Ca]_i$ (nM)	$[Na]_o$ (mM)	$[Ca]_o$ (mM)	Reference
Ferret ventricle	24	260	150	1.8	Marban *et al.* (1980)
Rabbit ventricle	35–36	202	153	1.8	Lee *et al.* (1980)
Sheep ventricle	22–24	360	150	1.8	Coray *et al.* (1980)
Guinea-pig ventricle	22–24	270	150	1.8	Coray and McGuigan (1981)

All values except those of Lee *et al.* (1980) were calibrated using the EGTA binding constant of Schwarzenbach *et al.* (1957). The values of Lee *et al.* (1980) have been recalculated for a temperature of 36 °C. Values for $[Ca]_i$ are in concentrations. Sheu and Fozzard (1981) give a value of 310 nM for $[Ca]_i$ but do not quote a binding constant.

pCa–tension Curve in Cardiac Muscle

Chapman (1979) collected the various published values for tension and calcium concentration. He fitted this curve assuming two binding sites for Ca^{++} and the sequential type of reaction (Appendix 1), i.e.

$$T = \left\{ \frac{K[Ca]_i}{1 + K[Ca]_i} \right\}^2. \tag{6.3}$$

In a recent paper Fabiato [1981] has studied the pCa–tension curve in cardiac muscle. The measured points, especially at calcium concentrations less than a pCa of 5.6, would suggest a much steeper curve than that assumed by Chapman (1979); in fact a simultaneous reaction with $n = 2$ would fit the data much better. However, we have reservations about accepting the measured points at a pCa of less than 5.6, because of inadequate buffering with EGTA (Stephenson, 1981).

The steepness of the pCa–tension curve is important as it can give information about the number of calcium binding sites for muscle activation. However, the actual slope in cardiac muscle still awaits adequate determination.

Holroyde *et al.*, 1980; and Johnson *et al.*, 1980 find that cardiac troponin-C, binds only 1 mol of Ca per mole of troponin-C over the pCa range that leads to tension development, so the steepness of the pCa versus tension curve may be due to co-operativity elsewhere in the reaction sequence generating tension.

Relationship between [Na]$_o$ and [Ca]$_i$

It is usual to use a two-stage procedure (see Chapman and Tunstall, 1980). The [Ca]$_i$ is predicted from the level of [Na]$_o$ according to the following equation:

$$[Ca]_i = \left\{\frac{[Na]_i}{[Na]_o}\right\}^n \exp\left\{(n-2)\frac{EF}{RT}\right\}. \qquad (6.4)$$

This calculated [Ca]$_i$ is then used to predict the tension levels obtained under the experimental conditions from the pCa–tension relationship (equation (6.3)).

Such an analysis assumes that [Na]$_i$ remains constant, that the sensitivity of the myofibrils does not change during the contracture, and that the equation assumed for the pCa–tension relationship is an adequate description of this curve. As we will show later, [Na]$_i$ decreases during a contracture; the sensitivity of the myofibrils may change because of a decrease in [H]$_i$. Whether the equation of the form of (6.3) adequately describes the pCa–tension relationship in intact heart muscle is still undecided.

Figure 6.3(c) shows an experiment from guinea-pig ventricular trabeculae in which Na$^+$ withdrawal contractures have been measured at a [K]$_o$ of 5.4 and 30 mM K. The figure demonstrates two common difficulties in trying to evaluate these experiments along the same lines as that of Chapman and Tunstall (1980). First, maximum tension was not reached since addition of 10 mM caffeine causes a large additional contracture in Na$^+$-free fluid. Secondly, there was a drift down of the strength of the Na$^+$ withdrawal contractures during the course of the experiment. Due to these complications, curve fitting of the sort used for data from frog atrial trabeculae to these experiments was not possible.

However, in a qualitative way, it could be shown that increasing [Ca]$_o$ moves the tension–[Na]$_o$ curve upwards. This was also found for substances that increased [Na]$_i$, e.g. cardiac glycosides and monensin. Zero potassium had a similar effect but it also caused a depolarization of the cells.

RECENT EXPERIMENTAL RESULTS ON THE Na–Ca EXCHANGE SYSTEM WITH ION-SELECTIVE ELECTRODES AND A RAPID FLOW SYSTEM

To overcome the difficulties found with tension measuring experiments and because we thought that changes in [Na]$_i$ might be affecting the results, we adapted the rapid flow system to measure changes in [Na]$_i$ and [H]$_i$ during the development of contractures at 22–26 °C, with ion-sensitive microelectrodes using the following ligands: Na$^+$: Steiner *et al.*, (1979); H$^+$: Ammann *et al.*, (1981). Part of this work has been published in abstract form (Chapman *et al.*, 1981b, 1982).

[Na]$_i$ and Na–Ca Exchange

The average [Na]$_i$ under our conditions of perfusion (room temperature, 5.4 mM [Ca]$_o$, 155 mM [Na]$_o$) was 15.0 ± 5.6 mM (mean ±S.D.) expressed as a concentration (somewhat higher than at 37 °C, see review by Lee, 1981).

During a Na withdrawal contracture there is, as shown in Figure 6.4(a), a rapid decrease in [Na]$_i$. That a fall in [Na]$_i$ occurred on Na$^+$ withdrawal was shown as long ago as 1963 by Niedergerke in his experiments on frog ventricle (see his Figures 7 and 8). More recent experiments by Ellis (1977) using a Thomas Na$^+$ electrode have also shown a decrease in [Na]$_i$ in Purkinje fibres. The time course of the decrease was much slower, presumably related to the slower perfusion rate in these experiments and the larger size of the Purkinje fibres.

This decrease in [Na]$_i$ during perfusion with nominally Na-free perfusate or low Na (<2.5 mM) was not influenced by strophanthidin (5×10^{-5} M), suggesting that the Na pump does not play a role in this fall. A possible Na$^+$–H$^+$ exchange was excluded by changing pH$_o$ to 9.5, where the driving force for H$^+$ is outward. Even at this alkaline pH$_o$ the decrease in [Na]$_i$ during Na-free contractures was still present, thus excluding a Na$^+$–H$^+$ exchange. Furthermore, during a Na$^+$ withdrawal contracture the [H]$_i$ decreases (see later). Finally a passive loss of Na$^+$ in the experiment in Figure 6.4(a) can be excluded. The [Na]$_o$ was 2.5 mM and, with 17 mM [Na]$_i$, E_{Na} was equal to -41 mV, i.e. at an E_m of -80 mV the driving force on Na ions was inward.

The [Na]$_i$ can be altered by changing either [Ca]$_o$ or [Na]$_o$ and one such experiment is shown in Figure 6.4(b). An increase in [Ca]$_o$ from 5.4 to 15 mM caused a decrease in [Na]$_i$ from 18.5 to 12 mM. A reduction of the [Na]$_o$ from 155 to 100 mM at this calcium concentration caused a further reduction in [Na]$_i$ to 8.5 mM. On the reapplication of normal Tyrode (155 mM [Na]$_o$; 5.4 mM [Ca]$_o$) the [Na]$_i$ returned slowly to its original level.

From the experiments quoted above we conclude that Na$^+$ leaves the cell in exchange for Ca^{++}. We have only measured a change in [Na]$_i$ and it could be argued that the decrease was due to internal movement of the Na ions, e.g. between mitochondria and cytoplasm. This explanation is made unlikely in view of Na efflux experiments and the experiments which demonstrated that, in a variety of tissues, Na-free solutions (or sodium-poor solutions) lead to millimolar gains of cellular Ca (frog ventricle: Niedergerke, 1963; mammalian heart: Langer, 1964; Reuter and Seitz, 1968; Wendt and Langer, 1977; chick embryo cells: Murphy *et al.*, 1981).

To calculate the efflux of Na$^+$ from the cell during the Na$^+$ withdrawal contracture, we replotted the [Na]$_i$ during the contracture on a linear scale. The Na$^+$ efflux (J) at each [Na]$_i$ is then given by

$$J = \frac{\Delta[\text{Na}]_i}{\Delta t} \frac{V}{A}, \tag{6.5}$$

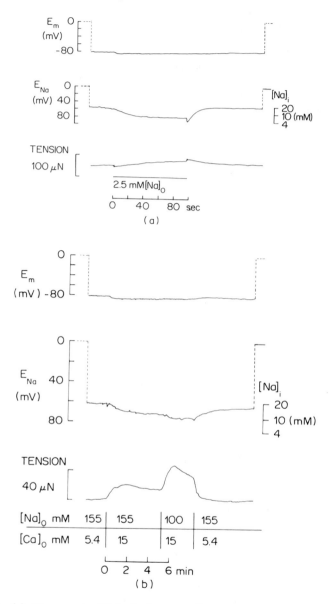

Figure 6.4 (a) Changes in [Na]$_i$ during a sodium withdrawal contracture ([Na]$_o$, 2.5 mM). The curves are, from above downwards: membrane potential, [Na]$_i$, tension. The sudden change on returning to normal Tyrode is a switching artefact. The contracture was 8% of the twitch amplitude. (b) Changes in [Na]$_i$ on altering either [Na]$_o$ or [Ca]$_o$. The curves are, from above downwards: membrane potential, [Na]$_i$, resting tension. The sequence of solution change is shown at the bottom. The maximum change in resting tension was 5% of twitch tension

where $\Delta[\mathrm{Na}]_i$ is the change in internal Na^+ concentration over the time interval Δt. V/A is the volume:surface area ratio; the value of 2.17×10^{-7} cm per litre cell volume was used (Page, 1978). Steps of either 10 or 30 s were taken. The average $[\mathrm{Na}]_i$ was then plotted against the efflux for each experiment and a smooth curve was drawn through the points. In order to combine all our results the effluxes at each $[\mathrm{Na}]_i$ were averaged.

The combined results from 30 experiments are shown in Figure 6.5(a), and suggest that the efflux is tending to a plateau at around

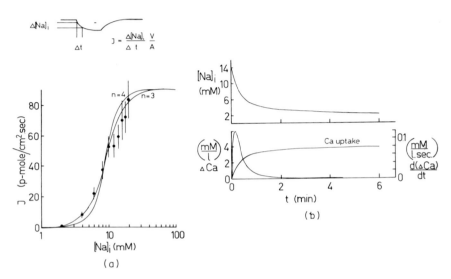

Figure 6.5   (a) Plot of Na^+ efflux (pmol cm^{-2} s^{-1}) against $[\mathrm{Na}]_i$ (mM). Each point is $\pm$S.E. The method of calculating the efflux in each experiment is shown in upper half of the figure. The S-shaped curves have been drawn according to the equation

$$J = J_{max} \frac{[\mathrm{Na}]_i^n}{(K_m)^n + [\mathrm{Na}]_i^n}$$

with n equal to 3 or 4, $J_{max} = 90$ pmol cm^{-2} s^{-1}, and a K_m of 9 mM. (b) Calculation of the decrease in $[\mathrm{Na}]_i$, Ca^{++} uptake (i.e. the total amount of calcium entering the cell via Na^+–Ca^{++} exchange), and $d(\Delta\mathrm{Ca})/dt$ during a Na-free contracture. A stoicheiometry of three Na^+ for one Ca^{++} was taken and it is assumed that Na efflux J is given by

$$J = J_{max} \frac{[\mathrm{Na}]_i^3}{(K_m)^3 + [\mathrm{Na}]_i^3},$$

where J_{max} is 90 pmol cm^{-2} s^{-1} and K_m 9 mM. In the lower curves the scale for calcium uptake is on the left; the scale for the rate of change of calcium is on the right

$90 \, \text{pmol cm}^{-2} \text{s}^{-1}$. The relationship between efflux and $[\text{Na}]_i$ appears S-shaped and has been fitted by an equation of the form

$$J = J_{max} \frac{[\text{Na}]_i^n}{(K_m)^n + [\text{Na}]_i^n}, \tag{6.6}$$

where J_{max} is taken as $90 \, \text{pmol cm}^{-2} \text{sec}^{-1}$ and K_m as $9 \, \text{mM} \, [\text{Na}]_i$. The curves are for n equal to 3 or 4.

In drawing these curves it has been assumed that only Na^+ binds to the carrier. If calcium binding to the carrier is allowed for, the above equation becomes

$$J = J_{max} \frac{[\text{Na}]_i^n}{(K_m)^n \left(1 + \dfrac{[\text{Ca}]}{K_{Ca}}\right) + [\text{Na}]_i^n}. \tag{6.7}$$

If resting calcium is $2 \times 10^{-7} \, \text{M}$ and K_{Ca} around $25 \times 10^{-6} \, \text{M}$, the factor $(1 + [\text{Ca}]/K_{Ca})$ becomes 0.008, which for practical purposes can be neglected.

Further assumptions are that the Na^+–Ca^{++} exchange system is at equilibrium and that intracellular ionic calcium is maintained at levels which will not interfere with the Na binding. While n equal to 3 would be the better fit to the data, due to the inaccuracies in calculation of the fluxes and the nature of the assumptions, other values for n cannot be entirely excluded.

However, this type of relationship explains the initial rapid decrease in $[\text{Na}]_i$, followed by a much slower decrease. Initially, at $[\text{Na}]_i \geqslant 15 \, \text{mM}$, the efflux is large, but at values of $3 \, \text{mM}$ or less the net efflux of Na^+ via the Na^+–Ca^{++} exchange system would seem for all practical purposes to have fallen to a low value.

A finding of such a high Na^+ efflux was surprising but there are reports of Na^+ effluxes of this magnitude. In comparing flux studies with one another it is essential to take into account the value used for V/A. The fluxes could, for instance, be misleadingly high if it is assumed that the cells are cylindrical and no account is taken of the folding of the surface membrane. The figures quoted below are for the V/A ratio per litre cell volume. Keenan and Niedergerke (1967) measured an unidirectional Na^+ efflux in frog ventricle of between 50 and $100 \, \text{pmol cm}^2 \text{s}^{-1}$. These fluxes were calculated on the basis of a V/A ratio of $8.77 \times 10^{-8} \, \text{cm}$, a figure obtained from planimeter measurements of electron microscope photographs. Recently, Lieberman and colleagues, using their growth-orientated chicken heart cell preparation (Horres *et al.*, 1977), quoted unidirectional Na efflux values of $98 \, \text{pmol cm}^{-2} \text{s}^{-1}$ (Wheeler *et al.*, 1980, 1981; Murphy *et al.*, 1981). These fluxes were calculated from a V/A ratio of 1.06×10^{-7} obtained by morphometric measurements of these cells (Horres *et al.*, 1977). These authors argue that 85% of this Na efflux is via a Na^+–Ca^{++} exchange since only 15%

is blocked by ouabain. If these fluxes are through the Na^+-Ca^{++} exchange system, it must mean that a form of exchange–diffusion is occurring through the carrier, i.e. the carrier is in a state of dynamic equilibrium.

Stoicheiometry of the Na^+-Ca^{++} Exchange System

Reuter and coworkers have argued that if the Na^+-Ca^{++} exchange was to control $[Ca]_i$ at a low value, the exchange would have to be greater than two Na^+ for one Ca^{++} (see Reuter, 1970, 1982). However, experiments on guinea-pig atria failed to show any effect of membrane potential on the Na-activated efflux (Jundt *et al.*, 1975). Recently, a number of separate studies have provided evidence in favour of the Na^+-Ca^{++} exchange system being dependent on the membrane potential and exchanging more than two Na^+ for each Ca^{++} (frog atrial trabeculae: Horackova and Vassort, 1979; Chapman and Tunstall, 1980; isolated sarcolemma vesicles: Pitts, 1979; Reeves and Sutko, 1980; Philipson and Nishimoto, 1980; Caroni *et al.*, 1980; ^{45}Ca fluxes in intact cardiac muscle: Busselen, 1981; Chapman *et al.*, 1981c; using ion-sensitive electrodes: Sheu and Fozzard, 1981). Although Mullins (1981) argues for a ratio of 4:1, this is based on $[Ca]_i$ 10 times lower than has ever been measured. (Furthermore, in his calculation he also assumed an $[Na]_i$ of 20 mM, about 30% higher than that actually found in our ferret preparations at rest.)

In our experiments the simultaneous measurement of the calcium uptake as well as the Na^+ loss would enable a direct calculation of this ratio to be made. However, since $[Ca]_i$ in the sarcoplasm is buffered, even if we measured sarcoplasmic Ca activity with a calcium electrode, we could still not calculate the exchange ratio directly because of the difference between the total cell calcium and the ionized calcium in the sarcoplasm.

It might be thought that from steady state measurements of $[Na]_i$, $[Ca]_i$, and E_m, as well as a knowledge of $[Na]_o$ and $[Ca]_o$, it would be possible to calculate n from equation (6.1). However, this equation is derived from equilibrium conditions when influx and efflux via the Na^+-Ca^{++} exchange are equal, but in heart muscle (even neglecting the calcium pump) we have the following situation:

$$\text{Efflux } (Na^+-Ca) = \text{Influx } (Na^+-Ca^{++}) + \text{Influx (leak)},$$

i.e. the internal ionized calcium will rise until the efflux via the Na^+-Ca^{++} exchange equals the set influx. (If $[Ca]_i$ is held constant, then $[Na]_i$ will change.) This is no longer an equilibrium state and if the measured values of $[Na]_i$, $[Na]_o$, $[Ca]_i$, $[Ca]_o$, and E_m are used and n calculated for equilibrium conditions a minimal value of n will be found. This value will not necessarily be a whole number and how far the calculated n deviates from the true value of n depends on the extent that $[Ca]_i$ deviates from the equilibrium value for Na–Ca exchange. This will depend on the extent of the calcium leak and the extent to which this is compensated by the calcium pump. The leak is of the order of 40 fmol cm^{-2} s^{-1} (Table 9 in Borle, 1981) and the maximum estimated efflux via the pump at 10^{-7} M is roughly 50 fmol cm^{-2} s^{-1}, suggesting that the Na$^+$–Ca^{++} exchange is not very far from equilibrium conditions. As a consequence, estimates of the coupling ratio made from measurements of $[Na]_i$, $[Ca]_i$, and E_m at different $[Na]_o$ and $[Ca]_o$ values may be close to the true value of n (e.g. Sheu and Fozzard, 1981; Bers and Ellis, 1982). Furthermore, current models of the Na$^+$–Ca^{++} exchange which require large passive Ca leaks would seem inappropriate.

Ca^{++} Uptake due to Na$^+$–Ca^{++} Exchange

From the data shown in Figure 6.5(a) and using the equation

$$J = J_{max} \frac{[Na]_i^3}{(K_m)^3 + [Na]_i^3} \tag{6.8}$$

it is possible to calculate the expected fall in $[Na]_i$, the increase in total cell Ca^{++} and the rate of change of $[Ca]_i$, assuming that all of the calcium flows into the cytoplasm during a Na-free contracture.

The equation, which assumes three Na$^+$ for one Ca^{++}, is a good fit to the data below 15 mM; it can be used to predict the changes in total calcium, even if the Na$^+$–Ca^{++} exchange is not at equilibrium. If the exchange is greater than three Na$^+$ for one Ca^{++} this would decrease the amount of calcium entering the cell. Such calculations are shown in Figure 6.5(b).

The decrease in $[Na]_i$ from the average value of 15.0 mM shows a rapid phase followed by a slow phase. This decrease is not mono-exponential and on a semi-log plot it gives the impression of consisting of two components. The calcium uptake is shown in the lower part of the figure. Initially, the Ca^{++} uptake is rapid, reaching a value of around 4 mM per litre cell volume after 2 min. The uptake thereafter falls steeply to a low value because the decrease in $[Na]_i$ has reduced the Na$^+$–Ca^{++} exchange (cf. Figure 6.5(a)). While the exchange is reduced, it would, in Na$^+$-free solution, eventually lead to Na depletion of the cells.

The rate of change of calcium (dΔCa/dt) is also given in this figure. The maximum rate is around 0.12 mM per litre cell volume per second. Due to the decrease in $[Na]_i$ this declines almost to zero after 2 min. The calcium uptake would correspond to a change from a resting value of 1 mM per litre cell volume to 5 mM per litre cell volume. An uptake of Ca^{++} in heart in Na-poor solutions has been reported (see above), but the most detailed study is that by Niedergerke (1963) for frog ventricle. He found that the Ca^{++} uptake in Na-free solution ranged from 2 to around 4 mM per litre cell volume associated with a decrease in $[Na]_i$ with a slower time course than those found for Ca^{++} in the present experiments. Murphy *et al.* (1981) find that under Na-free conditions the total Ca^{++} increases from 10 to 50 nM per milligram cell protein with a $T_{1/2}$ of 30 s, i.e. 90% uptake in 100 s, (also see Figure 6.5(b)). This figure does not take account of the resting Ca^{++} influx. However measured influxes are in the order of femtomoles per square centemetre per second (see Table 9 in Borle, 1981). Taking the largest value of 40 fmol $cm^{-2} s^{-1}$, this would correspond to an additional gain in calcium of 0.7 mM per litre cell volume over a 1 h period.

If the heart is also electrically stimulated in Na-free solutions at $0.1 s^{-1}$ (6 min^{-1}) and an average figure of 1 pmol cm^{-2} per beat is assumed for the extra Ca influx (see Table 4 in Chapman, 1979) this would correspond to an uptake of 1.7 mM per litre cell volume over 1 h of stimulation. Thus, even in Na-free solution, stimulated at $0.1 s^{-1}$ and allowing for passive leak, influx per beat and influx via the Na^+–Ca^{++} exchange systems, the total gain of calcium would be 6.4 mM $l^{-1} h^{-1}$. Whether or not there was a marked increase in $[Ca]_i$ in the cytoplasm and an increase in resting tension depends on the calcium buffering capacity of the cell.

Hyperpolarization due to the Na^+–Ca^{++} Exchange System

When more than two Na^+ ions move outward in exchange for one Ca^{++} ion during a Na^+ withdrawal contracture, there is a net outward movement of charge which should cause a hyperpolarization of the membrane. The extent of this hyperpolarization can be calculated, since the current is the flux multiplied by the Faraday constant. At an average $[Na]_i$ of 15 mM, the Na efflux is 74 pmol $cm^{-2} s^{-1}$. The λ of ferret ventricle is 0.67 mM (H. Hofmann, unpublished result) and assuming an R_i value of 470 Ω cm (Weidmann, 1970) yields a membrane resistance of 5200 Ω cm^2. The calculated hyperpolarizations from this value are 12 mV (3 Na:1 Ca), 7 mV (5 Na:2 Ca), and 18 mV (4 Na:1 Ca), values near to those measured experimentally.

In K-free Tyrode, when the Purkinje fibres are depolarized, Coraboeuf *et al.* (1981) found hyperpolarizations of 32 mV. Moreover, this hyperpolarization declined with time on exposure to Na-free fluid (see their Figure 2). On the basis of the data presented in Figure 6.5(a) this might be expected because as $[Na]_i$ declines so too does the net efflux of Na.

Changes in $[H]_i$ During Na Withdrawal Contractures

With the H ion resin we have measured $[H]_i$ at rest and during Na-free contractures. The average resting H^+ activity ($[Na]_o$, 155 mM; $[Ca]_o$, 5.4 mM; $[H]_o$, 39.8 nM (pH 7.4; room temperature)) in 13 experiments (47 impalements) was 51.1 ± 16 nM, mean $\pm$ S.D. which corresponds to a pH_i of 7.29 (pH range from 7.17 to 7.45).

During the Na-free contracture, the $[H]_i$ decreases to around half within

30 s, i.e. the cell becomes alkaline. This finding makes a Na^+–H^+ exchange for the decrease of the $[Na]_i$ unlikely, for if H ions moving inward were coupled with the efflux of Na^+, the cell would become acid, not alkaline. If Ca^{++} ions arriving in the sarcoplasm liberate H^+ ions, then, similarly, an increase in $[H]^+$ would be expected. A large fall in pH has been reported by Deitmer and Ellis (1980) in Purkinje fibres on lowering the $[Na]_o$ when $[Na]_i$ is high.

In summary, Na-free contractures are coupled with decreases in $[Na]_i$ and $[H]_i$, and with measured increases in total cell calcium. Despite these measurements we found little increase in tension, and Marban *et al.* (1980) found almost no change in $[Ca]_i$ during Na^+ withdrawal. These findings suggest to us that the Ca^{++} is removed from the cytoplasm and is in this sense buffered. Similar effects are seen in squid axons and in nerve endings (see Sulakhe and St Louis, 1980, for references).

SUBCELLULAR SYSTEMS CONCERNED WITH THE REGULATION OF $[Ca]_i$

It must be pointed out that in the regulation of $[Ca]_i$ the Na^+–Ca^{++} system is only one system among many. These various systems include the mitochondria, the sarcoplasmic reticulum, and the sarcolemmal Ca pump, as well as the Na^+–Ca^{++} exchange system. Other possible sites for Ca^{++} binding are the inner surface of the membrane, the myofibrils, and calmodulin. Other chapters in this book deal with these in more detail. The cytoplasmic calcium concentration, $[Ca]_i$, is in dynamic, not static equilibrium:

$$[Ca]_i = \frac{\text{Amount entering}}{\text{Unit time}} \quad \frac{\text{Amount removed}}{\text{Unit time}}, \tag{6.9}$$

where entry could be via Na^+–Ca^{++} exchange, passive leak, or through the slow inward current. Removal includes uptake into subcellular structures, binding to the inner side of the cell membrane, or transport out of the cell via the Na^+–Ca^{++} exchange system or by the calcium pump.

Methodological Problems

EGTA and calcium buffering

In studies of Ca^{++} uptake or binding, EGTA is often used to buffer the calcium. There are various values for the binding constant of EGTA in the literature but, as pointed out by Tsien and Rink (1980), the differences are more apparent than real, for they arose because of failure to take account correctly of the H^+ activity at various ionic strengths. If this is correctly carried out, the absolute values of the binding constant for EGTA calculated from the data in the literature are equal to the absolute constant determined by Schwarzenbach *et al.* (1957). For a discussion of this point see Fabiato (1981) and Blinks *et al.* (1982).

The binding constant of EGTA depends on ionic strength, pH, and temperature. (A method for correcting for temperature is given in Appendix 2, since the tables of Martel and Smith (1974) contain a misprint.) EGTA will only adequately buffer over a range ± 1 pCa unit from the log of the apparent binding constant. We correct the EGTA binding constant for temperature, ionic strength, and pH, using the value of the absolute constant obtained by Schwarzenbach *et al.* (1977). We have ignored the small amount of Ca^{++} binding to other ligands (e.g. ATP) and the effects of Mg^{++}.

Correction factors

The conversion from amount per gram wet weight (or amount per gram wet weight per second) was based on a tissue density of 1.063 (Yipintsoi *et al.*, 1977) and an extracellular space of 19% (Polimeni, 1974). From these figures a conversion factor of 1.31×10^3 can be calculated. The conversion for membrane surface area from mg protein used by Venosa and Horowicz (1981) was used.

Calcium Binding to Myofibrils and Calmodulin

The myofibrils bind calcium and, at any given $[Ca]_i$, a certain amount of calcium is bound to the contractile proteins. Solaro *et al.* (1974) measured the amount of calcium bound at different calcium concentrations. An increase of $[Ca]_i$ from a pCa of 7 to a pCa of 6 would only bind around 30 μM per litre cell volume, which is small considering that heart cells can take up millimolar amounts of calcium.

The calmodulin concentration is 0.09 g per litre cell volume (Grand *et al.*, 1979), which corresponds to a concentration of around 6×10^{-6} M. Even with all four sites binding Ca^{++} it would only bind 24 μM per litre cell volume. This means that the total binding of calcium from the myofibrils and calmodulin would be 54 μM per litre cell volume. This figure is in good agreement with that of Robertson *et al.* (1981) who estimate a total of between 50 and 100 μM Ca per litre cell volume when account is taken of the fact that they assume a resting $[Ca]_i$ of 10^{-8} M.

Sarcoplasmic Reticulum (SR)

A summary of the calcium uptake by the SR (from 1967 onwards) as measured by various authors is given in Table 6.2. These values are for 'calcium binding', i.e. uptake with no precipitating anion present. Where the data are given, we have converted uptake into nanomolarity per gram wet weight and millimolarity per litre cell volume at 25 °C. For this conversion

Table 6.2 Values for calcium binding by sarcoplasmic reticulum

Species	Temperature (°C)	pH	Uptake			$K_{0.5}$(M)	[Ca](M)	Millimolarity per litre (25°C)§	References
			Nanomolarity per milligram of protein	Milligrams of protein per gram wet weight	Nanomolarity per gram wet weight				
Dog	25	7	29	1.71	50	8.7×10^{-6}	5×10^{-5}	0.07	Katz and Repke (1967)
Rabbit	37	6.8	5	10	50	—	20×10^{-6}	0.04	Palmer and Posey (1967)
Dog	31	6.8	51	—	—	—	30×10^{-6}	—	Entman et al., (1972)
Rabbit	25	6.8	40	1–1.5	40–60	2.3×10^{-7}	4.5×10^{-6}	0.05–0.08	Harigara and Schwartz
Dog	25	6.8	75	1–1.5	75–1125	—	4.5×10^{-6}	0.1–0.15	(1969)
Dog	25	6.8	60–90	0.75	45–67.5	—	1.5×10^{-6}–2.4×10^{-6}	0.06–0.09	McCollum et al., (1972)
Dog	RT†	6.8	8–9	—	—	2.3×10^{-7}	1.2×10^{-6}	—	Repke and Katz (1972)
Dog	25	7	45	6.8	306	1.6×10^{-7}	4×10^{-6}	0.4	Solaro and Briggs (1974)
Guinea-pig	37	7	48	0.76	37	—	5×10^{-5}	0.04	Nayler et al. (1975)
Rat	37	7	28	0.78	22	—	5×10^{-5}	0.02	
Rat	37	6.8	42	0.78	33	—	3×10^{-5}	0.03	Nayler et al. (1976)
Rabbit	37	6.8	44	0.76	33	—	3×10^{-5}	0.03	
Guinea-pig	37	6.8	45	0.76	34	—	3×10^{-5}	0.03	
Chicken	29	6.8	50–60	3.5‡	175–210	2×10^{-7}	1×10^{-4}	0.21–0.25	Kitazawa (1976)
Rabbit	22	6.8	20	—	—	—	4×10^{-7}	—	Will et al. (1976)
Dog	25	6.8	63	0.6	38	—	1×10^{-4}	0.05	Dhalla et al. (1980)
Pigeon	37	6.8	72	3.2	230	—	7.5×10^{-6}	0.22	Levitsky et al. (1981)
Guinea-pig	37	6.8	71	2.1	150	—	7.5×10^{-6}	0.14	
Rat	25	6.8	70	—	—	—	2×10^{-6}	—	Malhotra et al. (1981)

† RT, room temperature.
‡ Estimated value.
§ To convert to millimolarity per litre (25 °C) a Q_{10} value of 1.3 was taken.

a Q_{10} of 1.3 was used, measured from Figure 4 of Entman *et al.* (1972). Taking the whole range of values the capacity of the SR would be between 0.2 and 0.5 mM per litre cell volume, a figure much too small to suggest that the SR accumulates the millimolar amounts of calcium obtained from the flux and ion-sensitive electrode studies.

The values for the rate of uptake of calcium (in nanomolarities per milligram protein per second) are summarized in Table 6.3. Like the capacity measurements, the rates of uptake are less than the calculated maximal uptake rate of 0.12 mM $l^{-1} s^{-1}$ of Ca removal from the sarcoplasm (see Figure 6.5(b)).

In summary, both in terms of capacity and rate of uptake, the SR is unable to accommodate the amount of calcium entering the cell during Na depletion. This could mean that either the published figures for capacity and rate are too low or structures other than the SR are taking part in calcium buffering.

That structures other than the SR are capable of taking up calcium in intact mammalian cardiac muscle is supported by experiments with the drug antazoline (5 mM), which is known to block calcium uptake into the SR (see Chapman, 1979). Application of this drug to ferret ventricular trabeculae increased the strength of the Na-free contracture, but even after prolonged exposure the contracture did not reach maximum tension, suggesting that the SR was not the only structure able to remove calcium from the sarcoplasm.

Mitochondria

As is shown in Figure 6.1, the mitochondria occupy some 36% of the cell volume. They also show, in the presence of ATP and inorganic phosphate, a very large calcium capacity of 2–3 μM per milligram of protein. With 100 mg mitochondria per gram wet weight, this corresponds to a net calcium uptake of 250–400 mM l^{-1} (see Carafoli and Crompton, 1976). While such large uptakes could well be non-physiological, they do indicate the very large Ca-buffering capacity of the mitochondria.

The mitochondria are capable not only of taking up calcium, but possess two additional antiporter systems (Carafoli, 1982). For a full discussion of mitochondrial transport see Chapter 7 (Williams, in this volume). With reduced $[Na]_0$, the ionised Ca^{++} in the sarcoplasm will increase and the $[Na]_i$ fall steeply, leading to an increased accumulation of Ca^{++} within the mitochondria, which provide the necessary Ca-buffering in our experiments.

Sarcolemma

Na–Ca exchange

It has recently become possible to isolate sarcolemmal vesicles from heart muscle and, using this preparation, an electrogenic Na–Ca mechanism

Table 6.3 Values for rate of uptake of calcium by sarcoplasmic reticulum

Species	Temperature (°C)	pH	Rate of uptake					References
			Nanomolarity per milligram of protein per second	Milligrams of protein per gram wet weight per second†	Nanomolarity per gram wet weight per second	[Ca](M)	Millimolarity per litre per second (25 °C)	
Rabbit	23	6.8	4.3	1–1.5	4–5	3×10^{-5}–4×10^{-5}	0.006–0.009	Harigara and Schwartz (1969)
Dog	31	6.8	0.3	—	—	3×10^{-5}	—	Entman et al. (1972)
Dog†	25	6.8	0.13	0.75	0.097	3×10^{-5}	0.0001	McCollum et al. (1972)
Dog	26	6.8	3–5	3	9–15	10×10^{-5}	0.011–0.019	Scarpa and Williamson (1974)
Guinea-pig	26	6.8	2.5–4.5	3	7.5–13.5	10×10^{-5}	0.009–0.017	
Rat	37	6.8	59	0.78	46	3×10^{-5}	0.04	Nayler et al. (1976)
Rabbit	37	6.8	8	0.76	6	3×10^{-5}	0.005	
Guinea-pig	37	6.8	11	0.76	8	3×10^{-5}	0.007	
Chicken	29	6.8	0.5	3.5†	2	1.4×10^{-7}	0.002	Kitazawa (1976)
Rabbit	22	6.8	20–30	—	70–105	1×10^{-4}	0.08–0.12	Will et al. (1976)
			3.8	—	—	10^{-7}	—	
			9			10^{-6}	—	
Guinea-pig	37	7.2	4.6	2.1	10	10^{-7}	0.008	Levitsky et al. (1981)
			11.5		24	10^{-6}	0.021	
		6.8	0		0	10^{-7}	—	
			9.5		20	10^{-6}	0.017	

† Estimated.

The values of Nayler et al. (1976) are the rates obtained over a 250 ms interval. To obtain the values at 10^{-7} and 10^{-6} M the uptake rates were plotted against the [Ca]$_o$ and the values read from the graph. In the paper by Levitsky et al. (1981) Figure 4 was redrawn for the corrected calcium concentrations. The listed values were obtained from this graph.

Table 6.4 Values for Na/Ca exchange in sarcolemma

Species	Ca uptake		K_m Ca (μM)	$[Na]_o$ (influx) (mM)	$K_m[Na]_o$ (efflux) (mM)	Reference
	Nanomolarity per milligram	Nanomolarity per milligram per second (V_{max})				
Rabbit	7–8	—	18	16	—	Reeves and Sutko (1980)
Dog	22	—	—	—	—	Pitts (1979)
Dog	90	—	—	—	—	Reeves and Sutko (1980)
Dog	80	15†	2‡			Caroni et al. (1980)
Dog	8	—	25§			Philipson and Nishimoto (1980)
Rabbit	25–35	—	30			Bers et al. (1980)
Dog	31				12.5	Philipson and Nishimoto (1981)
Dog	60–100	—	28‖			Philipson et al. (1982)

All measurement at 37°C and pH of 7.4.
† Reinlib et al. (1981) quote 20 nM mg s^{-1} as maximum value.
‡ Valinomycin present in solution.
§ Estimated from their Figure 1.
‖ Ca concentration between 6 and 40 μM.

probably exchanging more than two Na^+ for one Ca^{++} has been described by various authors. A summary of these recent experiments in Table 6.4 gives the maximum uptake values, as well as kinetic parameters when these have been measured. The uptake values of the more recent experiments are around 90 nM mg^{-1}, which are much larger than those found initially, presumably due to improvements in the methodology. These uptake values were, however, measured in the absence of ATP, and Reinlib *et al.* (1981) find that the addition of more than 2 μM ATP roughly doubles the calcium uptake (see their Figure 1). The mechanism of this increase is still unclear (cf. also Jundt and Reuter, 1976). This Ca uptake mechanism is also pH dependent, increasing as the pH becomes alkaline (Philipson *et al.*, 1982).

Kinetic descriptions are currently not very detailed. The K_m for external calcium for calcium uptake has been estimated in five studies. Four of these values lie between 18 and 30 μM. These values are for total calcium (a Ca buffer did not appear to be used) and are, therefore, probably too high. The value of Caroni *et al.* (1980) was estimated using an EGTA buffer. P. Caroni (personal communication) measured the binding constant for EGTA by a method similar to that of Bers (1981) and used a value of 3.16×10^7. This is slightly different from the value of 2.11×10^7 obtained by calculation from Schwarzenbach *et al.* (1957) and we have recalculated their results to make their K_m 2 μM, i.e. much less than the other reported values. Since it is important to have a good estimate of the K_m it would seem worthwhile for it to be determined in adequately buffered solutions.

Two sets of data show that the calcium uptake is half inhibited at a [Na] of 16 mM and that the calcium efflux is half maximally activated at a [Na] of 12.5 mM. While Caroni *et al.* (1980) give the maximal Ca uptake rate associated with the Na^+–Ca^{++} exchange as 15 nM $mg^{-1} s^{-1}$, in a later paper from Professor Carafoli's laboratory Reinlib *et al.* (1981) quote a value of 20 nM $mg^{-1} s^{-1}$. Assuming that 1 mg protein corresponds to an area of cell membrane of 1.9×10^3 cm^2, this converts to a maximal calcium exchange of 10.5 pmol $cm^{-2} s^{-1}$. This is less than the 30 pmol $cm^{-2} s^{-1}$ calculated from Figure 6.5(a). However, there are a number of reasons for believing that the Ca flux will be larger in intact cardiac cells; ATP can double the uptake rate and the figure of 10.5 pmol $cm^{-2} s^{-1}$ was obtained in the absence of ATP; in intact cells there is intracellular Ca buffering; the calcium uptake mechanism is potential dependent and the actual potential across the vesicular membrane under uptake conditions is not known, and the estimation of membrane area can only be regarded as an approximation. If we assume that ATP doubles the flux, the maximal uptake rate becomes 21 pmol $cm^{-2} s^{-1}$ at 37 °C. At 25 °C (assuming a Q_{10} for Na^+–Ca^{++} exchange of 1.35; Reuter and Seitz, 1968) this figure becomes 15 pmol $cm^{-2} s^{-1}$. While this is only half that measured from the decrease in $[Na]_i$, considering the assumptions involved in making the calculation, the agreement can be regarded as reasonable. This is especially true because a problem with the current preparations of vesicles is that they are composed of a mixture of right-side out, inside-out, and leaky vesicles (see Caroni *et al.*, 1980; Bers *et al.*, 1980; Trumble *et al.*, 1980). Whether the vesicular membrane is symmetrical in its reactions to Na^+ and Ca^{++} is at present an open question, but recently attempts have been made to separate the vesicles into right-side out and inside-out fractions (Mas-Oliva, *et al.*, 1980; Reinlib *et al.*, 1981).

With vesicles, no study has attempted to characterize Ca^{++} uptake as a function of $[Na]_i$. However, Reuter (1982) replotted the data obtained by Glitsch *et al.* (1970) using guinea-pig atria and found a K_m for total measured Na of 60 mM. Using neonatal mouse cells in which they could alter the internal Na^+, Wakabayashi and Goshima (1981) found a K_m for total Na^+ of 25 mM. It is difficult to compare these figures with the ionic activities measured with Na^+-sensitive microelectrodes, but if an apparent Na^+ activity coefficient of 0.175 (Lee and Fozzard, 1975) is assumed then these values correspond to a $[Na]_i$ of 10.5 and 4.4 mM respectively. We have expressed our results as sodium concentrations in our calibrating solutions. This being so, these activities correspond to sodium concentrations of 14 and 6 mM, values not all that different from the K_m of 9 mM obtained from our data.

Calcium pump

Previous attempts to establish the existence of an ATP-driven calcium pump in cardiac sarcolemma were equivocal due to possible contamination of the preparations with either SR or mitochondria (see review by Dhalla *et al.*, 1977). Recently, using more purified sarcolemmal vesicle preparations, it has been possible to demonstrate the existence of such a pump. This is discussed in more detail in Chapter 1 (Lullmann, Peters and Preuner, this volume).

Both the Na^+–Ca^{++} system and the calcium pump can remove calcium from the cell. In order to get some idea of the relative contributions of these systems, the efflux from the pump and via the Na^+–Ca^{++} exchange system, we used the following equations:

$$J_{pump} = V_{max} \frac{[Ca]_i}{K_{mCa} + [Ca]_i} ; \qquad (6.10)$$

$$J_{Na-Ca} = V_{max} \frac{[Ca]_i}{K_{mCa}(1 + [Na]_i^3 / K_{mNa}^3) + [Ca]_i} . \qquad (6.11)$$

The choice of constants has to be somewhat arbitrary. We have assumed a maximum efflux via Na^+–Ca^{++} exchange of 30 pmol cm^{-2} s^{-1} and a coupling ratio of three Na^+ for one Ca^{++}. The maximal flux through the pump has been taken as 100 times less than that of the Na^+–Ca^{++} exchange (0.3 pmol $cm^{-2} s^{-1}$).

The calcium flux through each system at any given calcium concentration depends, as would be expected, not only on the V_{max} of the system, but also on the K_m. If the K_{mCa} of the Na^+–Ca^{++} exchange system is 25 μM, then both pump and Na^+–Ca^{++} exchange would contribute to calcium efflux at the resting value in intact heart cells of 250 nM (pCa 6.6). If the K_{mCa} is 2 μM then the relative contribution of the Na^+–Ca^{++} exchange would be much increased.

Inner side of the membrane and other systems

Ca binding to sarcolemmal vesicles has been shown (see Pang, 1980; also Lullman and Peters, 1981) but since these vesicles are a mixture of inside-out and right-side out vesicles the exact site and magnitude of the binding must remain unclear. High affinity, non-energy-dependent Ca^{++} binding sites may be present such as those in giant axons (Baker and Schlaepfer, 1978). The role of Ca^{++} binding by the inner surface of the cell membrane is discussed elsewhere (Chapter 1 in this volume); we think this cannot be established without vesicles having a single membrane polarity.

Binding at the membrane's inner surface coupled with the slow diffusion will aggravate the calcium gradients with the sarcoplasm (see also Figure 6.2(c)).

While it has been useful to think of the Na^+–Ca^{++} exchange as a control mechanism for calcium in the cell, a distinction must be made between *total cell calcium* and *ionized calcium* in the sarcoplasm. From our experiments it is clear that the Na^+–Ca^{++} exchange does not directly control the ionized cell calcium in mammalian ventricular cells. This would seem to be set by the various cellular Ca buffers. This means that an additional constraint has been placed on the Na^+–Ca^{++} exchange; if the ionized calcium in the cell remains more or less constant, an alteration of either $[Na]_o$ or $[Ca]_o$ will cause increases or decreases in total cell calcium which will alter $[Na]_i$ and possibly the intracellular pH (see Figure 6.4(b)). Thus it is possible to load internal calcium stores while the ionized calcium in the cytoplasm is only marginally elevated.

CONCLUSIONS

For the study of Na^+–Ca^{++} exchange three possible environments now exist: (a) vesicles, (b) cultured or isolated cells, and (c) thin trabeculae. Each method has its advantages and disadvantages. It is especially important when dealing with intact cardiac muscle that the influence of diffusion delays in the extracellular spaces are borne in mind, for if interpretable results are to be obtained trabeculae of less than 300 μm must be used, in combination with a rapid perfusion system. Moreover, since Na^+ and Ca^{++} have different diffusion coefficients, a simultaneous alteration of both $[Na]_o$ and $[Ca]_o$ must be avoided.

As shown in this study (see Figure 6.4(b)) changes in either $[Ca]_o$ or $[Na]_o$ can cause concomitant changes in the internal ionic concentrations. This is also true for changes in pH (unpublished results). Such changes in the composition of the sarcoplasm induced by ionic substitutions in the perfusing fluid could have far-reaching consequences upon earlier results, particularly in interpretation of voltage clamp data.

We have tried to show in this chapter that the Na^+–Ca^{++} exchange is one of *several* systems involved in controlling cell calcium. In mammalian ventricular muscle it would seem not directly to control the ionized calcium in the sarcoplasm, but rather the total cell calcium. Thus increasing or decreasing external [Na] or [Ca] in the perfusing fluid will, within limits, not alter the ionized calcium in the sarcoplasm (cf. Marban *et al.*, 1980) but rather the amount of calcium in intracellular stores and the free Na^+.

Alterations of either $[Na]_o$ or $[Ca]_o$ will cause changes in stored calcium and $[Na]_i$, so in terms of the beating heart there would be little or no alteration in resting tension, but an increase or decrease in the amount of calcium released during contraction.

ACKNOWLEDGEMENTS

The work in this paper was supported by the Swiss National Science Foundation, grant no. 3.565.0.79. Dr R. A. Chapman was a Hoffmann-La Roche Visiting Investigator. We also wish to thank Miss M. Herrenschwand and Miss I. Schonberg for their patience and excellent technical help. Professor S. Weidmann made valuable comments on the manuscript.

APPENDIX 1

In this appendix we give a brief description of the derivations of the equations used to describe the pCa–tension curves. For each equation we (1) describe the reaction, (2) give the mathematical formulation, (3) show the sum of various forms of the carrier, and (4) describe the relationship between tension and $[Ca]_i$. Maximum tension is taken as 1; total carrier concentration is taken as 1.

K_1, K_2, and K_n are equilibrium constants. The equations have been derived for two binding sites but can be expanded for any number of sites. For further details and descriptions of these equations see Mahler and Cordes (1971, Chap. 6), Ashley and Moisescu (1972), Moisescu (1976), Miller and Moisescu (1976), and Stephenson and Williams (1981).

While the curves have been described for tension–pCa they can be used to describe such S-shaped relationships as Figure 6.5(a). The description is not meant as an accurate mathematical formulation, rather as an aid to the general reader to show how such equations can be derived. Furthermore, these equations describe an equilibrium situation.

Simultaneous

(1) This is the simplest form of these equations. In this reaction it is assumed that two molecules react simultaneously with the binding site. Tension is proportional to $[Ca_2X]$.

(2)
$$2\,Ca + X \overset{K_1}{\rightleftharpoons} Ca_2X,$$

$$K_1 = \frac{[Ca_2X]}{[Ca]^2[X]}.$$

(3)
$$[X] + [Ca_2X] = 1.$$

(4) Tension,
$$T = [Ca_2X] = \frac{K[Ca]^2}{1 + K[Ca]^2}.$$

The more general solution is

$$T = \frac{K[Ca]^n}{1 + K[Ca]^n}.$$

This is the Hill equation (Hill, 1910, 1913) and if $\log[T/(1-T)]$ is plotted against $\log K_{Ca}$, the result is a straight line with slope n and intercept at K on the y axis.

In this equation, if K is set equal to $1/(K_m)^n$, where K_m is the Ca value at which tension is half-maximal, it becomes

$$T = \frac{[Ca]^n}{(K_m)^n + [Ca]^n}.$$

Independent

(1) In this scheme Ca^{++} ions react independently with two different binding sites. If the fraction of sites at site 1 is θ_1, and that at site 2 θ_2, then since both sites have to be simultaneously occupied for tension to occur, tension is proportional to $\theta_1\theta_2$. This is best understood by considering probabilities when throwing two dice. The probability of getting one 6 with

one dice is 1/6; with the second dice it is also 1/6. The probability of achieving two 6s is $1/6 \times 1/6$ or 1/36.

(2)
$$Ca + X_1 \xrightleftharpoons{K_1} CaX_1,$$

$$Ca + X_2 \xrightleftharpoons{K_2} CaX_2,$$

$$K_1 = \frac{[CaX_1]}{[Ca][X_1]},$$

$$K_2 = \frac{[CaX_2]}{[Ca][X_2]}.$$

(3)
$$[CaX_1] + [X_1] = 1, \qquad [CaX_2] + [X_2] = 1.$$

(4) Since $[CaX] + [X]$ is defined as 1, $\theta = [CaX_1]$:

$$T = \theta_1 \theta_2$$

$$= \left\{ \frac{K_1[Ca]}{1 + K_1[Ca]} \right\} \left\{ \frac{K_2[Ca]}{1 + K_2[Ca]} \right\}.$$

If $K_1 = K_2$, then

$$T = \left\{ \frac{K_1[Ca]}{1 + K_1[Ca]} \right\}^2$$

Sequential

In this type of reaction the binding of one Ca^{++} ion is followed by the binding of the second (and third and so on). There are two forms of this type of reaction: (a) consecutive and (b) consecutive with spatial independent binding sites.

Consecutive

(1) In this form the binding follows a linear scheme. Tension is proportional to Ca_2X.

(2)
$$Ca + X \xrightleftharpoons{K_1} CaX + Ca \xrightleftharpoons{K_2} Ca_2X,$$

$$K_1 = \frac{[CaX]}{[Ca][X]}, \qquad K_2 = \frac{[Ca_2X]}{[CaX][Ca]}.$$

(3)
$$[X] + [CaX] + [Ca_2X] = 1.$$

(4)
$$T = [Ca_2X] = \frac{K_1 K_2[Ca]^2}{1 + K_1[Ca] + K_1 K_2[Ca]^2}.$$

Consecutive: independent and spatially separate sites

(1) In this kinetic scheme there are two sites for binding calcium. CaX and XCa represent different forms of the carrier. Tension is proportional to [Ca×Ca].

(2)

$$\frac{[XCa]}{[Ca][X]} = K_1, \qquad \frac{[CaX]}{[Ca][X]} = K_1,$$

$$\frac{[Ca \times Ca]}{[XCa][Ca]} = K_2, \qquad \frac{[Ca \times Ca]}{[CaX][Ca]} = K_2.$$

(3)
$$[X] + [CaX] + [XCa] + [Ca \times Ca] = 1.$$

(4)
$$T = [Ca \times Ca] = \frac{K_1 K_2 [Ca]^2}{1 + 2K_1[Ca] + K_1 K_2 [Ca]^2}.$$

If $K_1 = K_2$,

$$T = \left\{ \frac{K_1[Ca]}{1 + K_1[Ca]} \right\}^2.$$

APPENDIX 2

This appendix deals with the temperature for absolute binding constants. From Moore (1974, page 295, equation 8:30)

$$\log K_{T_2} = \log K_{T_1} + f(X),$$

$$f(X) = \frac{\Delta H}{2.303R} \left(\frac{1}{T_1} - \frac{1}{T_2} \right).$$

In this equation K_{T_2} and K_{T_1} are absolute binding constants at temperatures T_2 and T_1; T_1, T_2, and are absolute temperatures (in kelvins); R is the gas constant (in calories per mole per kelvin) ($= 1.987$); ΔH is the enthalpy (in calories per mole).

$f(X)$ simplifies to

$$0.218\,52\,\Delta H \left(\frac{1}{T_1} - \frac{1}{T_2} \right).$$

Since in the tables of Martel and Smith (1974), ΔH is given in kilocalories per mole, $f(X)$ becomes

$$218.52\,\Delta H\left(\frac{1}{T_1}-\frac{1}{T_2}\right).$$

ΔH is tabulated in Martel and Smith (1974). For an *increase* in temperature, if the tabulated ΔH is *negative* then $f(X)$ must be *subtracted* from $\log K_{T_1}$. If ΔH is *positive* for an *increase* in temperature then $f(X)$ has to be *added* to $\log K_{T_1}$.

The formula in Martel and Smith (1974, p. xii) should read

$$\log K_{T_2} = \log K_{T_1} + \Delta H(T_2 - T_1) \times 0.002\,46.$$

This is derived as follows:

$$\log K_{T_2} = \log K_{T_1} + \frac{\Delta H}{2.303R}\,\frac{(T_2 - T_1)}{T_1 T_2}.$$

Since $T_1 \simeq T_2$ at 25 °C, then

$$T_1 T_2 \simeq (T_1)^2 = (298)^2.$$

The above equation thus simplifies to

$$\log K_{T_1} = \log K_{T_2} + \Delta H(T_2 - T_1) \times 0.002\,46.$$

REFERENCES

Ammann, D., Lanter, F., Steiner, R. A., Schulthess, P., Shijo, Y., and Simon, W. (1981). Neutral carrier based hydrogen ion-selective microelectrode for extra- and intracellular studies. *Analyt. Chem.*, **53**, 2267–2269.

Ashley, C. C., and Moisescu, D. G. (1972). Model for the action of calcium in muscle. *Nature New Biol.* **237**, 208–211.

Baker, P. F., and Schlaepfer, W. W. (1978). Uptake and binding of calcium by axoplasm isolated from giant axons of *Loligo* and *Myxicola*. *J. Physiol. (Lond.)*, **276**, 103–125.

Bassingthwaighte, J. B., Fry, C. H., and McGuigan, J. A. S. (1976). Relationship between internal calcium and outward current in mammalian ventricular muscle; a mechanism for the control of the action potential duration? *J. Physiol. (Lond.)*, **262**, 15–37.

Bers, D. M. (1981). A simple method for the calculations of free [Ca] in EGTA buffered Ca solutions. *J. Physiol. (Lond.)*, **312**, 2–3P.

Bers, D. M., and Ellis, D. (1982). Intracellular calcium and sodium activity in sheep heart Purkinje fibres: effect of changes of external sodium and intracellular pH. *Pflügers Arch. Europ. J. Physiol.* **393**, 171–178.

Bers, D. M., Philipson, K. D., and Nishimoto, A. Y. (1980). Sodium–calcium exchange and sidedness of isolated cardiac sarcolemmal vesicles. *Biochim. Biophys. Acta*, **601**, 358–371.

Blaustein, M. P., and Hodgkin, A. L. (1969). The effect of cyanide on the efflux of calcium from squid axons. *J. Physiol. (Lond.)*, **200**, 497–527.

Blinks, J. R., Wier, W. G., Hess, P., and Prendergast, F. G. (1982). Measurement of Ca^{2+} concentrations in living cells. *Prog. Biophys. Molec. Biol.*, **40**, 1–114.

Borle, A. B. (1981). Control, modulation, and regulation of cell calcium. *Rev. Physiol. Biochem. Pharmacol.*, **90**, 13–153.

Busselen, P. (1981). The effect of high external K on the Na-activated fractions of Ca efflux in goldfish ventricles. *Arch. Int. Pharmacodyn. Ther.*, **249**, 309–311.

Carafoli, E. (1982). The transport of calcium across the inner membrane of mitochondria. In *Membrane Transport of Calcium* (E. Carafoli, ed.), Academic Press, London, pp. 109–139.

Caroni, P., and Carafoli, E. (1980). An ATP-dependent Ca^{2+}-pumping system in dog heart sarcolemma. *Nature*, **283**, 765–767.

Chapman, R. A. (1979). Excitation–contraction coupling in cardiac muscle. *Prog. Biophys. Molec. Biol.*, **35**, 1–52.

Chapman, R. A., and Tunstall, J. (1980). The interaction of sodium and calcium ions at the cell membrane and the control of contractile strength in frog atrial muscle. *J. Physiol. (Lond.)*, **305**, 109–123.

Chapman, R. A., Cigada, C., Coray, A., and McGuigan, J. A. S. (1981a). Sodium withdrawal contractures in mammalian ventricular muscle. *J. Physiol. (Lond.)*, **318**, 4P.

Chapman, R. A., Coray, A., and McGuigan, J. A. S. (1981b). Sodium/calcium exchange in mammalian ventricular muscle. *J. Physiol. (Lond.)*, **318**, 13–14P.

Chapman, R. A., Tunstall, J., and Yates, R. J. (1981c). The effect of K^+ upon the sodium activated efflux of calcium from atria of the frog *Rana pipiens*. *J. Physiol. (Lond.)* **316**, 31–32P.

Chapman, R. A., Coray, A., and McGuigan, J. A. S. (1982). $[Na]_i$ measurements at rest and during Na withdrawal contractures in mammalian ventricular muscle. *J. Physiol. (Lond.)*, **328**, 19–20P.

Coraboeuf, E., Gautier, P., and Guiraudou, P. (1981). Potential and tension changes induced by sodium removal in dog Purkinje fibres: role of an electrogenic sodium–calcium exchange. *J. Physiol. (Lond.)*, **311**, 605–622.

Coray, A., and McGuigan, J. A. S. (1981). Measurement of intracellular ionic calcium concentration in guinea pig papillary muscle. In *Ion Selective Microelectrodes and Their Use in Excitable Tissues* (E. Sykova, P. Hnik, and L. Vyklicky, eds), Plenum, New York, pp. 299–301.

Coray, A., Fry, C. H., Hess, P., McGuigan, J. A. S., and Weingart, R. (1980). Resting calcium in sheep cardiac tissues and in frog skeletal muscle measured with ion-selective microelectrodes. *J. Physiol. (Lond.)*, **305**, 60–61P.

Crank, J. (1967). *The Mathematics of Diffusion*, Clarendon Press, Oxford.

Deitmer, J. W., and Ellis, D. (1980). Interactions between the regulation of the intracellular pH and sodium activity of sheep cardiac Purkinje fibres. *J. Physiol. (Lond.)*, **304**, 471–488.

Dhalla, N. S., Ziegelhoffer, A., and Harrow, J. A. C. (1977). Regulatory role of membrane systems in heart functions. *Canad. J. Physiol. Pharmacol.*, **55**, 1211–1234.

Dhalla, N. S., Sulakhe, P. V., Lee, S. L., Singal, P. K., Varley, K. G., and Yates, J. C. (1980). Subcellular Ca^{2+} transport in different areas of dog heart. *Canad. J. Physiol. Pharmacol.*, **58**, 260–367.

Ellis, D. (1977). The effects of external cations and ouabain on the intracellular sodium activity of sheep heart Purkinje fibres. *J. Physiol. (Lond.)*, **273**, 211–240.

Entman, M. L., Bornet, E. P., and Schwartz, A. (1972). Phasic components of calcium binding and release by canine cardiac relaxing system (sarcoplasmic reticulum fragments). *J. Mol. Cell. Cardiol.*, **4**, 155–169.

Fabiato, A. (1981). Myoplasmic free calcium concentrations reached during the twitch of an intact isolated cardiac cell and during calcium-induced release of calcium from the sarcoplasmic reticulum of a skinned cardiac cell from the adult rat or rabbit ventricle. *J. Gen. Physiol.*, **78**, 457–497.

Glitsch, H. G., Reuter, H., and Scholz, H. (1970). The effect of the internal sodium concentration on calcium fluxes in isolated guinea-pig auricles. *J. Physiol. (Lond.)*, **209**, 25–43.

Grand, R. J. A., Perry, S. V., and Weeks, R. A. (1979). Troponin C-like proteins (calmodulins) from mammalian smooth muscle and other tissues. *Biochem. J.*, **177**, 521–529.

Harigara, S., and Schwartz, A. (1969). Rate of calcium binding and uptake in normal animal and failing human cardiac muscle. Membrane vesicles (relaxing system) and mitochondria. *Circulation Res.*, **25**, 781–794.

Hill, A. V. (1910). The possible effects of the aggregation of the molecules of haemoglobin on its dissociated curves. *J. Physiol. (Lond.)*, **40**, 4–7P.

Hill, A. V. (1913). The combinations of haemoglobin with oxygen and with carbon monoxide. *Biochem. J.*, **7**, 471–480.

Hill, A. V. (1928). The diffusion of oxygen and lactic acid through tissue. *Proc. Roy. Soc. Lond. B*, **104**, 39–96.

Holroyde, M. J., Robertson, S. P., Johnson, J. D., Solaro, R. J., and Potter, J. D. (1980). The calcium and magnesium binding sites on cardiac troponin and their role in the regulation of myofibrillar adenosine triphosphatase. *J. Biol. Chem.*, **255**, 11688–11693.

Horackova, M., and Vassort, G. (1979). Sodium–calcium exchange in regulation of cardiac contractility. Evidence for an electrogenic voltage dependent mechanism. *J. Gen. Physiol.*, **73**, 403–424.

Horres, C. R., Lieberman, M. and Purdy, J. E. (1977). Growth orientation of heart cells on nylon monofilament: determinations of the volume-to-surface area ratio and intracellular potassium concentration *J. Membr. Biol.*, **34**, 313–329.

Johnson, J. D., Collins, J. H., Robertson, S. P., and Potter, J. D. (1980). A fluorescence probe study of Ca^{2+} binding to the Ca^{2+} specific sites of cardiac troponin and troponin C. *J. Biol. Chem.*, **255**, 9635–9640.

Jundt, H., and Reuter, H. (1976). Is sodium-activated calcium efflux from mammalian cardiac muscle dependent on metabolic energy? *J. Physiol. (Lond.)*, **266**, 78–79P.

Jundt, H., Porzig, H., Reuter, H., and Stucki, J. W. (1975). The effect of substances releasing intracellular calcium ions on sodium dependent calcium efflux from guinea-pig auricles. *J. Physiol. (Lond.)*, **246**, 229–253.

Katz, A. M., and Repke, D. I. (1967). Quantitative aspects of dog cardiac microsomal calcium binding and calcium uptake. *Circulation Res.*, **21**, 153–162.

Kennan, M. J., and Niedergerke, R. (1967). Intracellular sodium concentration and resting sodium fluxes of the frog heart ventricle. *J. Physiol. (Lond.)*, **188**, 235–260.

Kitazawa, T. (1976). Physiological significance of Ca uptake by mitochondria in the heart in comparision with that by cardiac sarcoplasmic reticulum. *J. Biochem.*, **80**, 1129–1147.

Kushmerick, M. J., and Podolsky, R. J. (1969). Ionic mobility in muscle cells. *Science*, **166**, 1297–1298.

Langer, G. A. (1964). Kinetic studies of calcium distribution in ventricular muscle of the dog. *Circulation Res.*, **15**, 393–405.

Lee, C. O. (1981). Ionic activities in cardiac muscle cells and application of ion-selective microelectrodes. *Amer. J. Physiol.*, **241**, H459–H478.

Lee, C. O., and Fozzard, H. A. (1975). Activities of potassium and sodium ions in rabbit heart muscle. *J. Gen. Physiol.*, **65**, 695–708.

Lee, C. O., Uhm, D. Y., and Dresdner, K. (1980). Sodium–calcium exchange in rabbit heart muscle cells: direct measurement of sarcoplasmic Ca^{2+} activity. *Science*, **209**, 699–701.

Levitsky, D. O., Benevolensky, D. S., Levchenko, T. S., Smirnov, V. N., and Chazoc, E. I. (1981). Calcium-binding rate and capacity of cardiac sarcoplasmic reticulum. *J. Mol. Cell. Cardiol.*, **13**, 785–796.

Lullmann, H., and Peters, Th. (1981). Influence of cardiac glycosides on cell membrane. In *Handbook of Experimental Pharmacology*, Vol. 56/I, *Cardiac Glycosides* (K. Greef, ed.), Springer Verlag, Berlin, pp. 395–406.

McCollum, W. B., Besch, H. R., Entman, M. L., and Schwartz, A. (1972). Apparent initial binding rate of calcium by canine cardiac-relaxing system. *Amer. J. Physiol.*, **223**, 608–614.

Mahler, H. R., and Cordes, E. H. (1971). *Biological Chemistry*, 2nd edn, Harper and Row, New York.

Malhotra, A., Penpargkul, S., Schaible, T., and Scheuer, J. (1981). Contractile proteins and sarcoplasmic reticulum in physiologic cardiac hypertrophy. *Amer. J. Physiol.*, **241**, H263–H267.

Marban, E., Rink, T. J., Tsien, R. W., and Tsien, R. Y. (1980). Free calcium in heart muscle at rest and during contraction measured with Ca^{2+}-sensitive microelectrodes. *Nature*, **286**, 845–850.

Martel, A. E. and Smith, R. M. (1974). *Critical Stability Constants*, Vol. 1: *Amino Acids*, Plenum, New York.

Mas-Oliva, J., Williams, A. J., and Naylor, W. G. (1980). Two orientations of isolated cardiac sarcolemmal vesicles separated by affinity chromatography. *Analyt. Biochem.*, **103**, 222–226.

Miller, D. J., and Moisescu, D. G. (1976). The effects of very low external calcium and sodium concentrations on cardiac contractile strength and calcium–sodium antagonism. *J. Physiol. (Lond.)* **259**, 283–308.

Moore, W. J. (1974). *Physical Chemistry*, 5th edn, Longman, London.

Moisescu, D. G. (1976). Kinetics of reaction in calcium-activated skinned muscle fibres. *Nature*, **262**, 610–613.

Mullins, L. J. (1981). *Ion Transport in Heart*, Raven Press, New York.

Murphy, E., Wheeler, D. M., Anderson, L., Horres, C. R., and Lieberman, M. (1981). Sodium calcium exchange in cultured chick heart cells. *J. Gen. Physiol.*, **78**, 24a.

Nayler, W. G. Dunnett, J., and Berry, D. (1975). The calcium accumulating activity of subcellular fractions isolated from rat and guinea pig heart muscle. *J. Mol. Cell. Cardiol.*, **7**, 275–288.

Nayler, W. G., Dunnett, J., and Burian, W. (1976). Further observations on species determined differences in the calcium accumulating activity of cardiac microsomal fractions. *J. Mol. Cell. Cardiol.*, **7**, 663–675.

Niedergerke, R. (1963). Movements of Ca in frog heart ventricles at rest and during contractures. *J. Physiol. (Lond.)* **167**, 515–550.

Page, E. (1978). Quantitative ultrastructural analysis in cardiac membrane physiology. *Amer. J. Physiol.*, **235**, C147–C158.

Page, E., and Bernstein, R. S. (1964). Cat heart muscle *in vitro*. V. diffusion through a sheet of right ventricle. *J. Gen. Physiol.*, **47**, 1129–1140.

Palmer, R. F., and Posey, V. A. (1967). Ion effects on calcium accumulation by cardiac sarcoplasmic reticulum. *J. Gen. Physiol.*, **50**, 2085–2095.

Pang, D. C. (1980). Effect of inotropic agents on the calcium binding to isolated cardiac sarcolemma. *Biochem. Biophys. Acta*, **598**, 528–542.

Philipson, K. D., and Nishimoto, A. Y. (1980). Na$^+$–Ca^{2+} exchange is affected by membrane potential in cardiac sarcolemmal vesicles. *J. Biol. Chem.*, **255**, 6880–6882.

Philipson, K. D., and Nishimoto, A. Y. (1981). Efflux of Ca^{2+} from cardiac sarcolemmal vesicles. *J. Biol. Chem.*, **256**, 3698–3702.

Philipson, K. D., Bersohn, M. M., and Nishimoto, A. Y. (1982). Effects of pH on Na$^+$–Ca^{2+} exchange in canine cardiac sarcolemmal vesicles. *Circulation Res.*, **50**, 287–293.

Pitts, B. J. R. (1979). Stoichiometry of sodium–calcium exchange in cardiac sarcolemmal vesicles. Coupling to the sodium pump. *J. Biol. Chem.*, **254**, 6232–6235.

Polimeni, P. I. (1974). Extracellular space and ionic distribution in rat ventricle. *Amer. J. Physiol.*, **227**, 676–683.

Reeves, J. P., and Sutko, J. L. (1980). Sodium–calcium exchange activity generates a current in cardiac membrane vesicles. *Science*, **208**, 1461–1464.

Repke, D. I., and Katz, A. M. (1972). Calcium-binding and calcium uptake by cardiac microsomes: a kinetic analysis. *J. Mol. Cell. Cardiol.*, **4**, 401–416.

Reinlib, L., Caroni, P., and Carafoli, E. (1981). Studies on heart sarcolemma: vesicles of opposite orientation and the effect of ATP on the Na$^+$/Ca^{2+} exchange. *FEBS Lett.*, **126**, 74–76.

Requena, J., and Mullins, L. J. (1979). Calcium movement in nerve fibres. *Quart. Rev. Biophys.*, **12**, 371–460.

Reuter, H. (1970). Calcium transport in cardiac muscle. In *Permeability and Function of Biological Membranes* (L. Bolis, ed.), North Holland, Amsterdam, pp. 342–347.

Reuter, H. (1982). Na–Ca counter transport in cardiac muscle. In *Membranes and Transport*, Vol. 1. (A. Martonosi, ed.), Plenum, New York, in press.

Reuter, H., and Seitz, N. (1968). The dependence of calcium efflux from cardiac muscle on temperature and external ion composition. *J. Physiol. (Lond.)*, **195**, 451–470.

Scarpa, A., and Williamson, J. R. (1974). Calcium binding and calcium transport by subcellular fractions of the heart. In *Calcium Binding Proteins* (W. Drabikowki, H. Stzelecka-Gohazewska, and E. Carafoli, eds), Elsevier, Holland, pp. 547–585.

Scholz, H. (1969). Uber Unterschiede im Kontrakturverhalten bei Ventrikel- und Vorhofsproparaten aus Wärmbluter Herzen. *Pflügers Arch. Ges. Physiol.*, **312**, 63–81.

Schwarzenbach, G., Senn, H., and Auderegg, G. (1957). Komplexone XXIX. Ein grasser Chelateffeckt besondereer Art. *Helv. Chim. Acta*, **40**, 1886–1900.

Sheu, S. S. and Fozzard, H. (1981). The stoichiometry of the Na/Ca exchange in the mammalian myocardium. *Biophys. J.*, **33**, 11a.

Solaro, R. J., and Briggs, F. N. (1974). Estimating the functional capabilities of sarcoplasmic reticulum in cardiac muscle. Calcium binding. *Circulation Res.*, **34**, 531–540.

Solaro, R. J., Wise, R. M., Shiner, J. S., and Briggs, F. N. (1974). Calcium requirements for cardiac myofibrillar activation. *Circulation Res.*, **34**, 525–530.

Steiner, R. A., Oehme, M., Ammann, D., and Simon, W. (1979). Neutral carrier sodium ion-selective microelectrode for intracellular studies. *Analyt. Chem.*, **51**, 351–353.

Stephenson, D. G., and Williams, D. A. (1981). Calcium-activated force responses in fast and slow twitch skinned muscle fibres of rat at different temperatures. *J. Physiol. (Lond.)*, **317**, 281–302.

Stephenson, E. (1981). Activation of fast skeletal muscle: contributions of studies on skinned fibres. *Amer. J. Physiol.*, **240**, C1–C19.

Sulakhe, P. V., and St Louis, P. J. (1980). Passive and active calcium fluxes across plasma membranes. *Prog. Biophys. Mol. Biol.*, **35,** 135–195.

Tsien, R. Y., and Rink, T. J. (1980). Neutral carrier ion-selective microelectrodes for measurement of intracellular free calcium. *Biochim. Biophys. Acta*, **599,** 623–638.

Venosa, R. A., and Horowicz, P. (1981). Density and apparent location of the sodium pump in frog sartorius muscle. *J. Membr. Biol.*, **59,** 225–232.

Wakabayashi, S., and Goshima, K. (1981). Kinetic studies on sodium-dependent calcium uptake by myocardial cells and neuroblastoma cells in culture. *Biochim. Biophys. Acta*, **642,** 158–172.

Weidmann, S. (1970). Electrical constants of trabecular muscle from mammalian heart. *J. Physiol. (Lond.)*, **210,** 1041–1054.

Wendt, I. R., and Langer, G. A. (1977). The sodium–calcium relationship in mammalian myocardium: effect of sodium deficient perfusion on calcium fluxes. *J. Mol. Cell. Cardiol.*, **9,** 551–564.

Wheeler, D. M., Horres, C. R., and Lieberman, M. (1980). Sodium tracer kinetics in tissue-cultured chick heart cells. *Fed. Proc.*, **39,** 1841.

Wheeler, D. M., Horres, C. R., and Lieberman, M. (1981). Trans-membrane sodium fluxes in tissue cultured heart cells. *Fed. Proc.*, **40,** 617.

Will, H., Blanck, H. Smettan, G., and Wollenberger, A. (1976). A quench-flow kinetic investigation of calcium ion accumulation by isolated cardiac sarcoplasmic reticulum. Dependence of initial velocity on free calcuim ion concentration and influence of preincubation with a protein kinase, Mg ATP, and cyclic AMP. *Biochim. Biophys. Acta*, **449,** 295–303.

Yipintsoi, T., Scanlon, P. D., and Bassingthwaighte, J. B. (1977). Density and water content of dog ventricular myocardium. *Proc. Soc. Exp. Biol. Med.*, **141,** 1032–1035.

CHAPTER 7

Mitochondria

A. Williams

Cardiothoracic Institute, 2 Beaumont Street, London W1N 2DX, UK

INTRODUCTION

Mitochondria were identified using light microscopy around the turn of the century, but they were not isolated and characterized until the late 1950s with the introduction of cell fractionation techniques (de Dure, 1964). The fact that mitochondria occupy approximately 30% of the volume of the myocardial cell gives some indication of their importance in the normal functioning of cardiac muscle.

One of the most intensively investigated and probably the most important of their functions is the synthesis of adenosine triphosphate (ATP), the so-called 'energy-rich' compound which is used to power contraction. It is also becoming increasingly clear that mitochondria are capable of providing a superbly sensitive calcium buffering system within the cell. The energy supply required by both of these processes is provided by mitochondrial respiration, in which substrates, originally derived from lipids, carbohydrates, or proteins, are sequentially oxidized; the final electron acceptor being molecular oxygen.

Acetyl-CoA, the substrate for the tricarboxylic acid cycle is derived from pyruvate (from glucose or lactate) and free fatty acids (see Chapters 9, 10, and 13 in this volume). The process of free fatty acid oxidation occurs within the mitochondrial matrix. Free fatty acids cannot cross the inner mitochondrial membrane and require 'activation' to acyl-CoA. This process takes place in the cytosol in an ATP-consuming reaction. The acyl group is then transported across the mitochondrial inner membrane complexed with carnitine before re-associating with CoA in the mitochondrial matrix space (Pande, 1975). Acyl-CoA enters the beta-oxidation pathway yielding acetyl-CoA, the substrate for the tricarboxylic acid cycle. Pyruvate crosses the inner mitochondrial membrane and is oxidized to acetyl-CoA in a reaction mediated by the multi-enzyme complex pyruvate dehydrogenase.

Thus it can be seen that both fatty acid and carbohydrate metabolism produce a common intermediate, acetyl-CoA, which in turn enters the

151

tricarboxylic acid cycle. The tricarboxylic acid cycle, citric acid cycle, and Krebs cycle are names given to the series of reactions, catalysed by eight mitochondrial matrix enzymes, in which one molecule of acetyl-CoA is sequentially oxidized to yield two molecules of carbon dioxide and reduced coenzymes: namely, three molecules of nicotinamide adenine dinucleotide (NADH) and one molecule of flavin adenine dinucleotide ($FADH_2$). The reduced coenzymes are then reoxidized by donation of electrons to acceptors which are constituents of the respiratory or electron transport chain located in the mitochondrial inner membrane, which consists of a series of electron transferring components of increasing positive redox potential (Figure 7.1).

The transfer of a pair of electrons from NADH to the final acceptor, molecular oxygen, involves a redox potential change of 1.14 V (Figure 7.1), which is equivalent to a free energy drop of approximately 220 kJ. The question of how this available energy is stored and then used to generate

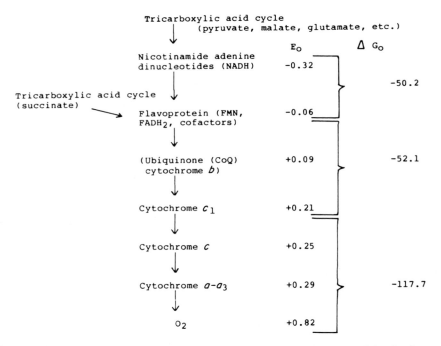

Figure 7.1 The components of the electron transport chain, located in the inner mitochondrial membrane, responsible for the sequential oxidation of cofactors, produced in the tricarboxylic acid cycle, and the liberation of free energy stored in the form of a proton gradient across the membrane. E_0 refers to the redox potential between the various components in volts and ΔG refers to the free energy change in kilojoules per molecule of NADH. Both values are determined at pH 7.0 and 25 °C

ATP and/or transport ions, such as calcium, across the mitochondrial inner membrane, has been the subject of intense investigation and debate.

It is now generally accepted that the free energy made available, as electrons flow along the respiratory chain, is stored in the form of an electrochemical proton gradient across the inner mitochondrial membrane. According to the chemiosmotic hypothesis, proposed in the early 1960s by Peter Mitchell (1966, 1968) the electron transfer components of the respiratory chain are arranged spatially and in sequence so that alternate electron and hydrogen atom (i.e. electron plus proton) transfers occur. The consequence of such an arrangement is that protons are transferred from the mitochondrial matrix space out across the inner membrane.

There is a considerable amount of experimental evidence supporting this hypothesis. A number of the components of the respiratory chain are arranged asymmetrically in the inner membrane (Racker, 1970, 1977), and some of the steps in electron transfer involve dehydrogenation reactions which are suitable candidates for electron plus proton transfers. However, not all regions of the system have obviously suitable components and the possibility that direct proton pumping is involved in the establishment of the proton gradient, for example by cytochrome oxidase, has also been suggested (Wikström and Krab, 1979).

Whatever the mechanism involved, it is now clear that electron transfer from NADH or $FADH_2$ to oxygen results in the establishment of an electrochemical proton gradient across the mitochondrial inner membrane (also known as the proton motive force, p.m.f., or $\Delta\bar{\mu}_{H^+}$) made up of a proton concentration gradient (Δ pH) and a charge separation or membrane potential ($\Delta\psi$). In respiring mitochondria the total $\Delta\bar{\mu}_{H^+}$ can reach approximately 220 mV (the matrix being negative with respect to the surroundings) with the major contribution (approximately 90%) coming from $\Delta\psi$ in the absence of other ion movements:

$$\Delta\bar{\mu}_{H^+} = \Delta\psi - \frac{2.3\,RT}{ZF}\,\Delta\,pH, \tag{7.1}$$

where R is the universal gas constant, T is the temperature in kelvins, F is the Faraday constant, and Z is the valency of the proton, i.e. 1.

Having established the electrochemical gradient it may then be used to drive the energy-consuming reactions of the mitochondron.

ATP SYNTHESIS

Coupling of $\Delta\bar{\mu}_{H^+}$ to the synthesis of ATP from ADP and inorganic phosphate (P_i) occurs via a protein complex located in and on the inner mitochondrial membrane; the elucidation of the site and components involved in the coupling of electron transport to the synthesis of ATP is described in detail in an enjoyable book by Efraim Racker (1976). In this section I will give only a brief outline of the findings.

The early experiments aimed at the elucidation of the mechanism of ATP synthesis were based on an assumption, which proved to be correct, that the ATPase activity seen in disrupted mitochondria represented the reversal of the usual ATP synthesis procedure. ATPase activity has proved considerably easier to monitor and a more reliable indicator of the coupling activity than ATP synthesis. Both reactions may be measured in submitochondrial particles (vesicles of inner mitochondrial membrane with an inside-out orientation produced by sonication or digitonin treatment of mitochondria (Loyter *et al.*, 1976)) under suitable conditions. Both activities are inhibited by oligomycin. These vesicles have a characteristic appearance when examined by electron microscopy following negative staining with phosphotungstic acid, being covered with 8 nm spheres which appear to be attached to the vesicle by small stalks. Treatment of submitochondrial particles with the proteolytic enzyme trypsin brought about an increase in the ATPase activity of the preparation; it has been established that this stimulation results from the proteolytic degradation of a protein inhibitor which associates with the ATPase in the absence of $\Delta\bar{\mu}_{H^+}$, so preventing ATP hydrolysis. If the particles were then treated with 2 M urea, the membrane component collected by centrifugation, and characterized both in terms of structure and enzyme activity, it was found that the membrane was devoid of 8 nm spheres and no longer displayed ATPase activity. However, the electron transport chain located in the membrane was still fully functional. The ATPase activity was discovered in the soluble phase associated with the small protein spheres released from the membrane by the urea treatment, but this activity was not inhibited by oligomycin.

These experiments suggested that the coupling factor between electron transport and ATP synthesis was the ATPase molecule, which could be seen lining the inner face of the inner mitochondrial membrane. The fact that the ATPase could be re-associated with the membrane and that following re-association ATPase activity returned to the membrane in an oligomycin-inhibitable form also suggested a role for a membrane-associated factor in ATP synthesis. It is now recognized that in addition to the ATPase or F_1 molecule, the complete ATP synthase contains a hydrophobic region (F_0) associated with the membrane and that this region contains a protein which binds oligomycin (oligomycin sensitivity conferring protein, OSCP). Other coupling factors, e.g. F_6, which is thought to be involved in the binding of F_1 with the membrane, have also been identified (Racker, 1976, 1977).

F_1 is actually a complex molecule composed of a number of subunits, the exact functions of which are still under investigation. The hydrophobic region (F_0) spans the membrane and during ATP synthesis specifically channels protons into the F_1 molecule. The highly endergonic process of

ATP synthesis is then driven by the free energy made available as protons flow down their electrochemical gradient back into the matrix space through F_1. The mechanisms involved in the reaction are still controversial with both direct coupling and proton-induced conformational changes suggested as possibilities (Boyer *et al.*, 1977).

The role of ATP synthase as the coupling factor is, however, well established. It has been possible to demonstrate ATP synthesis using mito-chondrial ATP synthase and a proton electrochemical gradient established by a system other than the electron transport chain. In these experiments purified ATP synthase from beef heart mitochondria was incorporated into liposomes in which a proton gradient was created by the bacteriorhodopsin proton pump which had been reconstituted into the same membrane (Racker and Stoeckenuis, 1974). These experiments provide strong support for the chemiosmotic coupling of electron transport and ATP synthesis.

ATP synthesis may be inhibited by a number of agents which fall into three major categories. The first of these are inhibitors of electron transport, e.g. rotenone, antimycin, and cyanide, which by blocking electron transport prevent the establishment of $\Delta\tilde{\mu}_{H^+}$, so removing the driving force for ATP synthesis. The second group of inhibitors are the uncouplers, examples of this group being carbonyl cyanide *p*-trifluoromethoxyphenylhydrazone (FCCP) and 2,4-dinitrophenol (DNP). These agents uncouple electron flow from ATP synthesis. They apparently act as proton ionophores, collapsing $\Delta\tilde{\mu}_{H^+}$ and hence accelerating electron flow along the respiratory chain. The final group are the energy transfer inhibitors, e.g. oligomycin and rutamycin, which, as we have already mentioned, have a direct blocking effect on ATP synthase, inhibiting both its forward and back reactions.

ATP synthesis occurs at the inner face of the mitochondrial inner mem-brane. Therefore, for ATP to be used as a fuel for cytosolic reactions it must first be transported out of the mitochondrion. This is achieved by another membrane-bound enzyme, the adenine nucleotide translocase (ANT) (Klingenberg *et al.*, 1975), which exchanges matrix ATP for extramito-chondrial ADP, so ensuring both a regular supply of cytosolic ATP and ADP for ATP synthesis. The translocase is driven by the respiration-generated membrane potential. At physiological pH values, ATP possesses four negative charges whilst ADP has three. The membrane potential (the matrix being approximately 200 mV negative to the cytosol) can therefore be used to drive ATP out of and ADP into the matrix.

The translocase is inhibited by a number of agents. Atractylate binds at the outer surface of the mitochondrial inner membrane and competes with ADP and ATP for binding to the translocase. Consequently atractylate is termed a non-penetrant inhibitor (Klingenberg *et al.*, 1975; Klingenberg, 1979). On the other hand, bongkrekic acid, in its protonated form, pene-trates the membrane and inhibits by increasing the binding of ADP and ATP to the translocase only on the matrix side of the inner membrane. Interestingly, it has been demonstrated that the translocase may also be inhibited by long chain acyl-CoA esters and that these act by binding to the translocase at either the outer or inner surface of the membrane (Chua and Shrago, 1977).

ATP transported from the matrix is not free to diffuse into the cytosol. An apparently close structural and functional relationship exists between the ANT and a creatine phosphokinase molecule (CPK) (Saks *et al.*, 1980; Moreadith and Jacobus, 1982). This enzyme converts the newly synthesized and exported ATP to creatine phosphate, liberating ADP which can be shuttled back into the matrix. Creatine phosphate travels into the cytosol and is converted to ATP by CPK at or near sites of ATP hydrolysis, for example the contractile proteins and the sarcolemma.

The other substrate for ATP synthesis, inorganic phosphate, is transported into the matrix in response to the ΔpH component of $\Delta\bar{\mu}_{H^+}$, either as a co-transport with protons or as an antiport with hydroxyl ions (Chapell and Crofts, 1965). This transporter may be inhibited by SH reagents such as N-ethyl maleimide (Meijer *et al.*, 1970).

This then is a brief description of the probable mechanisms involved in the synthesis of ATP from fatty acids and carbohydrate. Before proceeding to the other roles of myocardial mitochondria it may be useful to summarize and compare the quantities of ATP made available by the processes outlined above.

The complete oxidation of one molecule of a fatty acid such as palmitic acid ($C_{16}H_{32}O_2$) produces a total yield of 129 molecules of ATP. The complete oxidation of one molecule of glucose, including glycolysis, yields 38 molecules of ATP. Obviously, the oxidative synthesis of ATP described in the preceding section is completely dependent on a constant supply of the terminal electron acceptor, molecular oxygen. Should this supply cease to be available, for example in the case of total ischaemia, electron transport along the respiratory chain is blocked, $\Delta\bar{\mu}_{H^+}$ collapses, and the production of ATP by oxidative phosphorylation is stopped. In such a situation beta-oxidation would be completely inhibited and no energy could be obtained from fatty acids. The only possible source of ATP would be from the anaerobic component of carbohydrate metabolism, glycolysis; that is, two molecules of ATP per molecule of glucose. This represents a dramatic decline in the availability of ATP to the cell. Glycolysis is, to a great degree, regulated by the levels of ATP present in the cytosol. A major regulatory enzyme of the sequence, phosphofructokinase, is stimulated by ADP, AMP, and P_i and inhibited by ATP. In the absence of oxygen, with electron transport and oxidative phosphorylation blocked and the cytosolic ATP concentration declining, glycolysis is stimulated (Kübler and Spieckermann, 1970). However, this stimulation is really of limited usefulness; even working at maximal efficiency it has been estimated that glycolysis could supply only approximately 20% of the ATP necessary for normal cell function (Opie, 1968) and under ischaemic conditions glycolytic ATP production is inhibited due to the accumulation of lactic acid and protons and their action on phosphofructokinase (Neely *et al.*, 1975).

CALCIUM TRANSPORT

The other major function of mitochondria, and one which is of particular interest in cardiac metabolism, is calcium regulation. It is well known that the cytosolic calcium concentration is the factor which regulates the state of the contractile apparatus of the myocardial cell via its interaction with the regulatory troponin molecule. The intracellular calcium concentration varies between approximately 10^{-7} and 10^{-5} M during relaxation and contraction respectively. There is now a considerable body of evidence that the mitochondria of the myocardial cell may have an important long term buffering effect on the intracellular calcium concentration.

Mitochondria isolated from a variety of tissues are capable of accumulating large quantities of calcium, against a concentration gradient, in a respiration-dependent manner. The mechanism of calcium entry appears to be the same in all mitochondria so far investigated, occurring via a so-called uniport located in the inner membrane (Nicholls and Crompton, 1980). The driving force for calcium entry is provided by the membrane potential component of the respiration-generated $\Delta\bar{\mu}_{H^+}$. Strong evidence for such a mechanism was provided by experiments which demonstrated that calcium entry may also be driven by a K^+ diffusion potential set up in the presence of valinomycin (Scarpa and Azzone, 1970). Under these conditions a stoicheiometry of one calcium ion entering the matrix in exchange for two potassium ions leaving the matrix via valinomycin was observed.

Direct measurements of calcium–proton stoicheiometry during respiration-supported calcium transport also suggest that, in the absence of phosphate transport, calcium enters the mitochondrial matrix carrying two positive charges (Crompton and Heid, 1978; Reynafarje and Lehninger, 1977; Williams and Fry, 1979).

A hyperbolic relationship exists between the rate of the calcium entry via the uniport and the extra mitochondrial calcium concentration, with a Michaelis constant (K_m) in the range 10–15 μM calcium. This relationship becomes sigmoidal in the presence of the competitive inhibitor magnesium (Crompton *et al.* 1976b) or when uptake is measured at low temperatures (e.g. 10 °C) (Williams and Barrie, 1978). The uniport is also inhibited by the lanthanides and by the carbohydrate stain ruthenium red (Bygrave, 1977).

The presence of a permeant anion such as phosphate or acetate increases the total calcium storing capacities of isolated cardiac mitochondria. In addition, phosphate has been shown to increase the initial rate of calcium accumulation when succinate is used as the respiratory substrate. This effect is apparently due to an increased rate of succinate oxidation in the presence of phosphate (Crompton *et al.*, 1978).

Under the experimental conditions usually used to investigate calcium transport by isolated mitochondria the rate of calcium entry is limited, not by the uniport, but by the rate of proton ejection via the respiratory chain. Factors which increase the rate of respiration will also tend to increase rates of calcium transport via the uniport. Such a situation may be achieved by simply raising the extramitochondrial pH. At high external pH the proton gradient between the mitochondrial matrix and the surrounding medium is increased, leading to an enhanced rate of electron transport and proton ejection resulting in an increased rate of calcium entry into the mitochondria.

At high external pH the rapid phase of calcium entry is quickly superceded by a net release of calcium back into the medium (Figure 7.2). These experiments were carried out in the absence of any added permeant anion, such as phosphate, and they highlight the role that these anions play in the

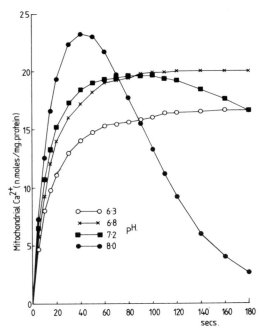

Figure 7.2   Time course of calcium transport into mitochondria isolated from rabbit myocardium at a range of extramitochondrial pH values. Ca^{2+} transport was monitored with a calcium-selective electrode (Williams and Fry, 1979), in a medium containing an initial free calcium concentration of 47 μM, 40 nmol N-ethylmaleimide (NEM) per milligram of protein, and no added phosphate

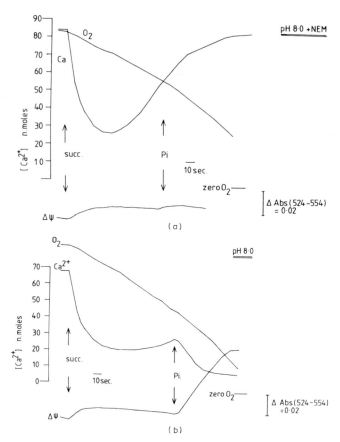

Figure 7.3 (a) Simultaneous measurement of calcium transport, oxygen consumption and $\Delta\psi$ of isolated rabbit cardiac mitochondria at pH 8.0. The medium contained 40 nmol NEM per milligram of protein and no added phosphate. A qualitative indication of $\Delta\psi$ was obtained using safranin as described in Åkerman and Wikström (1976) and Åkerman (1978). Phosphate was added to a final concentration of 3 mM as indicated by the arrow. (b) Calcium transport at pH 8.0 in the absence of added NEM. Conditions were identical to those in part (a) except that NEM was excluded from the medium. The arrow indicates the addition of phosphate to give a final concentration of 3 mM. Under these conditions this stimulates the generation of an appreciable $\Delta\psi$ and the reaccumulation of calcium

stabilization of calcium ions in the mitochondrial matrix by maintaining $\Delta\psi$ during calcium accumulation. A specific example is given in Figure 7.3(a). In this experiment calcium transport was monitored at pH 8.0 using a calcium-sensitive electrode (Fry and Williams, 1979) with no added permeant anion and in the presence of sufficient N-ethyl maleimide to prevent the transport of any endogenous phosphate. A qualitative estimate of the $\Delta\psi$ component of $\Delta\bar{\mu}_{H^+}$ has been obtained in a matched experiment using the fluorescent dye safranin (Åkerman and Wilkström, 1976; Åkerman, 1978), and this is included in the same figure. Adding succinate to initiate respiration stimulates the rapid accumulation of calcium with little or no generation of $\Delta\psi$. Following a phase of rapid calcium accumulation the matrix calcium reaches a level at which the electrochemical driving force reverses and calcium re-equilibrates via the uniport, producing a net calcium release. Under these conditions, in the presence of N-ethyl maleimide, adding phosphate to the system has no effect.

If the experiment is now repeated in the absence of N-ethyl maleimide (Figure 7.3(b)), we see an initially similar series of events, rapid calcium accumulation, and the onset of release. However, under these conditions the addition of phosphate stimulates the re-accumulation of calcium. This, in turn, is associated with the establishment of a significant membrane potential, the matrix becoming negative with respect to the surrounding medium.

As described above, calcium ions entering the matrix in response to a respiration-generated $\Delta\bar{\mu}_{H^+}$ carry with them two positive charges. As a consequence $\Delta\bar{\mu}_{H^+}$ will be expressed almost entirely as ΔpH under these conditions, the $\Delta\psi$ being dissipated by calcium ions. When phosphate is added to the system (Figure 7.3(b)) the anion enters the matrix in response to the pH gradient. Once in the more alkaline matrix space phosphate ions dissociate, donating protons to the medium, leaving negatively charged anions which convert the pH gradient established during calcium uptake into a potential gradient. As a result calcium ions re-enter the mitochondria down the newly established electrochemical gradient. Therefore permeant anions, such as phosphate and acetate, do not merely stabilize calcium in the mitochondrial matrix by precipitation, although this may play some role, they are also directly involved in the maintenance of the membrane potential component of $\Delta\bar{\mu}_{H^+}$ under calcium loading conditions.

The experiments described above represent a specific example of a more general phenomenon, that is calcium release from mitochondria induced by collapsing the membrane potential. Generally this occurs along with structural damage, loss of NADH, and other adenine nucleotides, requires very high levels of calcium, and may be enhanced by a range of components including atractylate (Asimakis and Sordahl, 1977), phosphoenol pyruvate (Roos *et al.*, 1978), and the oxidation of matrix NADH induced by acetoacetate (Nicholls and Brand, 1980). ATP and ADP have both been found to give some degree of protection against this form of damage, although the mechanism of this protection is unclear.

The release of mitochondrial calcium resulting from a lowering of the respiration-generated membrane potential, although of some pathological interest, as it might be predicted to occur under conditions of complete oxygen deprivation, has little relevance in terms of the role played by this organelle in the physiological buffering of calcium within the myocardial cell. Such a system would be required to function in the presence of the approximately 200 mV $\Delta\bar{\mu}_{H^+}$ needed to maintain normal ATP:ADP ratios.

The existence of a physiologically important release mechanism has been implied for a number of years. A simple calculation based on the observed membrane potential and the Nernst equation predicts that, at equilibrium, a 10^6-fold calcium concentration gradient should be established between the matrix and the cytosol, lowering the cytosolic free calcium concentration to 10^{-9} M. Clearly this is not what is observed *in vivo*. In addition to the calcium uniporter the cardiac mitochondrial inner membrane also contains an independent calcium release mechanism which is stimulated by sodium (Crompton *et al.*, 1976a,b; 1977).

If cardiac mitochondria are allowed to accumulate calcium in a respiration-dependent manner and the uniport is then blocked by the addition of ruthenium red, a slow leak of calcium (approximately 1 nmol min^{-1} mg^{-1}) into the surrounding medium is observed (Nicholls and Crompton, 1980). Calcium release is dramatically increased by the addition of sodium to the system, reaching a maximum of approximately 15 nmol min^{-1} mg^{-1} (Crompton *et al.*, 1977). Half-maximal release is seen with sodium concentrations of approximately 8 mm (Crompton *et al.*, 1977). A sigmoidal relationship exists between the initial rate of sodium-dependent calcium efflux and the extramitochondrial sodium concentration, with a Hill coefficient of approximately two (Nicholls and Crompton, 1980). These findings have been interpreted as suggesting that the exchanger operates electroneutrally, two sodium ions entering the matrix in exchange for each calcium ion. Recently it has been demonstrated that during sodium–calcium exchange the mitochondrial membrane potential remains unchanged, again implying a two sodium–one calcium exchange (Affolter and Carafoli, 1980).

The carrier will also exchange matrix calcium for extramitochondrial calcium with a one to one stoicheiometry (Crompton *et al.*, 1977). Some activity is also seen with lithium ions (Crompton *et al.*, 1977). Potassium is not carried by the exchanger but recently it has been demonstrated that potassium may have some stimulatory effect on the exchanger (Crompton *et al.*, 1980). The lanthanides are efficient inhibitors of the exchanger, acting equally on sodium–calcium and calcium–calcium exchange (Crompton *et al.*, 1978b).

A mechanism for the exchanger has been proposed in which the sodium–calcium antiporter is functionally linked to a sodium–proton antiporter known to be present in the mitochondrial inner membrane. In the suggested scheme (Figure 7.4) two sodium ions enter the mitochondrial matrix in exchange for one calcium ion; sodium ions are then recycled across the inner membrane in a one to one exchange with protons (Crompton, 1980). In this way calcium efflux is driven initially by the sodium gradient across the

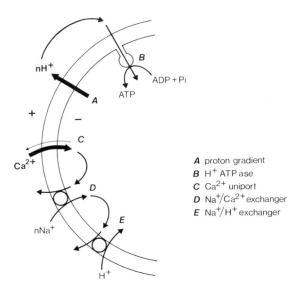

Figure 7.4 Diagram of the proposed mechanisms of calcium regulation carried out by cardiac mitochondria. Calcium ions enter the mitochondrial matrix in response to the proton gradient generated by respiration via a uniport system (C). Dissipation of the proton gradient may lead to an efflux of calcium by a reversal of the uniport. Calcium may also leave in exchange for sodium ions (D). It is now generally agreed that the system is electroneutral with $u = 2$. Sodium ions are then recycled out of the matrix on a sodium proton exchanger (E)

membrane and the sodium gradient is maintained by the respiration-generated proton gradient. This mechanism explains both the observed overall one calcium to two proton exchange measured during sodium-stimulated calcium release, and the electroneutrality of the system.

Sodium-stimulated calcium release is seen in mitochondria isolated from heart, skeletal muscle, brain, adrenal cortex, parotid gland, and brown adipose tissue (Crompton *et al.*, 1978c). Mitochondria from liver, smooth muscle, lung, and kidney have a ruthenium red-insensitive release system that is not stimulated by sodium but appears to involve a direct calcium–proton exchange (Nicholls and Crompton, 1980).

In all mitochondria the existence of independent calcium influx and efflux systems convey on them a superb ability to act as calcium buffers, The buffering capacity of cardiac mitochondria may be altered by interventions that affect either the independent influx or efflux systems. It is well known that the rate of uptake via the uniport is extremely dependent upon the extramitochondrial calcium concentration. In contrast the efflux pathway has been shown to work at a more or less constant rate once an internal calcium concentration of 10 nmol per milligram of protein has been achieved and is not significantly altered by changing extramitochondrial calcium (Nicholls,

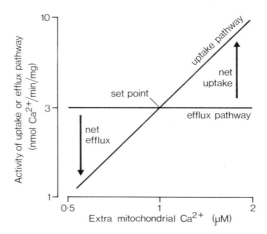

Figure 7.5 The buffering of the cytosolic calcium concentration by mitochondria (adapted from Nicholls, 1981). As the efflux system operates at a virtually constant rate and the uptake system responds to alterations in the extramitochondrial calcium concentration a cytosolic calcium concentration below the set point will induce net release from the mitochondria. A cytosolic calcium concentration above the set point will in turn induce net uptake. Reproduced with permission from Nicholls, *Trends Biochem. Sci.*, February 1981, pp. 36–38

1981). With a constant efflux rate the overall net movement of calcium will depend on the activity of the influx pathway.

If the extramitochondrial calcium concentration is relatively high the uptake system will be activated in an attempt to lower the extramitochondrial concentration; this in turn will lower the activity of the uniporter and a situation will be reached in which the rate of uptake is exactly balanced by the rate of efflux, the extramitochondrial calcium concentration reaching a so-called set point (Figure 7.5; Nicholls, 1981).

If for some reason the extramitochondrial calcium concentration is decreased to a level below the set point, the rate of uptake will decline and net efflux will occur, raising the extramitochondrial concentration towards the set point. The level of the set point can be altered by agents which affect the rate of the efflux mechanism; for example the addition of sodium to cardiac mitochondria will stimulate efflux and hence raise the set point. It can also be altered by factors which lower the rate of the uptake process at a given free calcium concentration, for example magnesium. A demonstration of this point is given in Figure 7.6, taken from Nicholls (1981). In this experiment, carried out with isolated brain mitochondria, an extramitochondrial free calcium concentration of approximately 0.35 μm is maintained in the absence of sodium. Following sodium addition and the activation of the sodium–calcium exchanger, a net efflux of calcium is seen

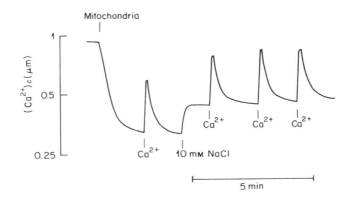

Figure 7.6 Alteration of the set point by stimulation of the efflux pathway. In this experiment net calcium transport is monitored with a calcium-sensitive electrode. The addition of 10 mM NaCl activates the Na^+–Ca^{++} exchanger, stimulating efflux and raising the set point. The new set point is maintained in the presence of additional extramitochondrial calcium (taken from Nicholls and Scott, 1980)

and a new, higher, set point is attained. The independent calcium influx and efflux mechanisms of mitochondria provide an efficient, sensitive calcium buffering system in the cardiac muscle cell. It should be emphasized that the rates of calcium movements carried out by mitochondria are relatively slow and consequently would probably not fluctuate on a beat to beat basis. The role played by mitochondria in buffering the calcium content of cells with elevated, or continuously rising, cytosolic calcium concentrations is likely to be extremely important and will be discussed further at the end of this chapter.

In addition to providing a system whereby mitochondria can buffer the cytosolic calcium concentration, independent influx and efflux pathways provide mitochondria with a system to buffer their own matrix calcium concentration. Recent studies by Denton and colleagues have demonstrated that intramitochondrial calcium may have important regulatory effects on a number of enzymes of the tricarboxylic acid cycle (Denton and McCormack, 1980). This mechanism may represent a method of extrinsic control of mitochondrial oxidative metabolism by hormones or neutrotransmitters.

MITOCHONDRIA IN THE ISCHAEMIC AND REPERFUSED MYOCARDIUM

Mitochondrial function, or to be more precise, mitochondrial dysfunction, is thought to play an important role in myocardial cell damage and death induced by ischaemia and reperfusion.

The severe reduction or abolition of flow to the isolated rabbit heart reduces cellular oxygen uptake, i.e., the terminal acceptor of the electron transport chain, leading to a dramatic inhibition of mitochondrial respiration and hence an inhibition of the oxidative production of ATP. Metabolites accumulate in the cell. These include NADH, acyl-CoA, lactate and protons (Jennings, 1969). Intracellular acidosis brings about a rapid cessation of the normal contractile behaviour of the myocardial cell (Figure 7.7, Cobbe and Poole-Wilson, 1979), because an elevated proton concentration decreases the affinity of the contractile apparatus for calcium (Katz and Hecht, 1969; Kentish and Nayler 1978 and inhibits the sarcolemma Ca^{++} channel (Sperelakis and Schneider, 1976).

Contraction utilizes approximately 75% of the total ATP production of the myocardial cell so that its cessation removes an enormous energy drain on the cell, allowing the remaining ATP to be used to drive pumps, which are vital for the maintenance of cell volume and cytosolic ionic composition. During this early period of ischaemia the initiation of flow will bring about a virtual complete recovery of normal cell function (Jennings, 1969). If the ischaemic period is extended the decline in the cytosolic ATP level continues (Figure 7.7) (Jennings *et al.*, 1978). The initial stimulation of anaerobic glycolysis, produced by ischaemia, is soon over-ridden by the inhibition of phosphofructokinase by lactate and protons (Neely *et al.*, 1975). Any residual oxidative phosphorylation is nullified as the adenine nucleotide translocase becomes increasingly inhibited by accumulating acyl-CoA, so preventing the export of ATP into the cytosol.

After approximately 45 min of no-flow ischaemia, resting tension begins to increase (Figure 7.7). Mitochondria isolated from hearts in this condition apparently have a slightly elevated calcium content (Figure 7.7), suggesting that they are capable of maintaining a membrane potential (thus preventing the re-equilibration of calcium via the uniport), and that the cytosolic calcium concentration is somewhat elevated. This is probably related to the breakdown of ATP-dependent calcium efflux systems such as the sarcolemmal calcium ATPase and the sodium–calcium exchange, which is ultimately driven by the sodium–potassium ATPase, and the storage of calcium in the sarcoplasmic reticulum. At this stage there is no alteration in the total tissue calcium concentration. Mitochondria isolated from such tissue function reasonably well, generating ATP at only slightly reduced rates (Nayler *et al.*, 1980).

Continuation of the ischaemic period to 90 min produces a steady increase in resting tension, no gain in tissue calcium, a slight increase in mitochondrial calcium content and a very small decline in the ATP-synthesizing capabilities of mitochondria isolated from the tissue (Figure 7.7). Reperfusion of the ischaemic myocardium at this stage does not lead to the re-establishment of normal function; it produces a marked increase in

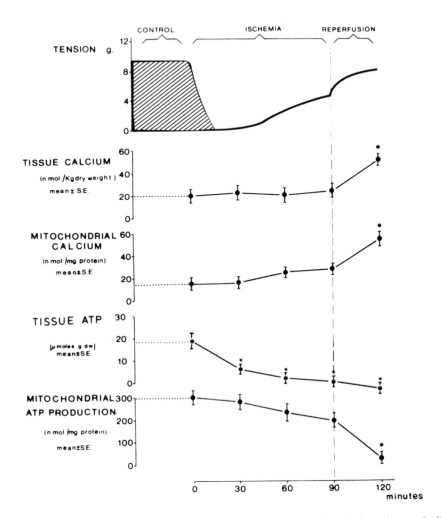

Figure 7.7 Effect of ischaemia and reperfusion on mechanical and metabolic function of isolated Langendorff-perfused hearts. Under control and reperfusion conditions the hearts were perfused with Krebs–Henseleit buffer, equilibrated with 95% O_2–5% CO_2 at a coronary flow of 25 ml min^{-1}. Ischaemia was induced by abolishing coronary flow. The hearts were paced at 180 beats min^{-1} and the wall temperature was maintained at 36 °C irrespective of coronary flow. The tension trace is representative of a typical experiment. The other parameters are mean values ±S.E. of at least five experiments. Tissue calcium, mitochondrial calcium, tissue ATP, and mitochondrial ATP production were determined as previously described (Nayler *et al.*, 1980). Asterisks indicate $p > 0.01$, referring to the difference between the experimental and control values

resting tension, no re-establishment of developed tension, a massive influx of calcium into the cell, and severe mitochondrial damage (Hearse, 1977).

It seems likely that the primary lesion occurs at the cell membrane, leading to a breakdown of the permeability barrier to ions such as calcium. The mechanism for this breakdown is unclear, but may be related to a detergent action of acyl-CoA and free fatty acids accummulated during ischaemia or free radical action initiated by the sudden reintroduction of oxygen to the cell. Whatever the mechanism there is no doubt that the intracellular calcium concentration rises significantly, the ATP content of the cell falls still further, and the mitochondria become severely damaged. Isolation of mitochondria from reperfused hearts has provided the following information (Ferrari *et al.*, 1982): (i) the yield of mitochondria isolated by methods designed to extract 'good' mitochondria falls, suggesting that a significant proportion of these organelles are structurally altered – this conclusion is supported by ultrastructural examination of the tissue; (ii) the isolated mitochondria contain large quantities of calcium; (iii) the oxidative phosphorylation capability of these organelles is severely disrupted.

A number of mechanisms have been suggested to explain these findings. It has been proposed that when faced with the possibility of producing ATP via oxidative phosphorylation or accumulating calcium, cardiac mitochondria will preferentially perform the latter task (Vercesi *et al.*, 1978). It is then argued that on reperfusion the mitochondria are exposed to high concentrations of calcium and ADP and the reintroduction of oxygen promotes calcium accumulation rather than the re-establishment of cellular ATP levels (Hearse, 1977). We have recently re-examined the basic premise, that calcium accumulation takes precedence over ATP synthesis, and have concluded that the two processes compete for respiratory energy. Furthermore, the interrelationship of these two processes is influenced by a number of factors such as respiratory substrate and intracellular effectors such as magnesium (Williams *et al.*, 1982).

In the presence of 1 mM free magnesium, a physiological concentration, the initial rate of ATP production seen in the absence of calcium is maintained at free calcium concentrations of up to 100 μM (Figure 7.8); above this concentration there is some inhibition. In the absence of magnesium all the concentrations of calcium which were tested decreased the initial rate of ATP production, the degree of inhibition increasing with calcium concentration. These findings presumably reflect the action of a physiological modulator of mitochondrial calcium transport, magnesium, in shifting the equilibrium between mitochondrial calcium transport and ATP synthesis towards ATP synthesis. These results may be interpreted as suggesting that at least in the presence of magnesium the rate of ATP synthesis would be maintained at free calcium concentrations in excess of those found in the normal myocardial cell.

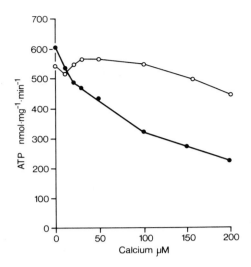

Figure 7.8 Effect of magnesium on the inhibition of ATP synthesis induced by calcium.

Initial rates of ATP production were determined enzymatically (Williams *et al.*, 1982). ATP synthesis was initiated by the addition of either ADP (475 nmol) or ADP plus varying amounts of calcium. When present, 1 mM magnesium was included in the reaction medium prior to the addition of mitochondria. ●—●, ATP production in the absence of magnesium; ○—○, ATP production in the presence of 1 mM magnesium

Turning to the situation pertaining to the reperfusion of the ischaemic myocardium we would envisage that the re-introduction of oxygen either causes damage to the cell membrane or finds the membrane already damaged, due to the factors outlined above. In addition to supplying oxygen, reperfusion also conveys large quantities of calcium to the cell, a cell that by this time is freely permeable to this ion. Calcium enters the cell causing a very significant elevation of the cytosolic concentration. We would predict that provided with oxygen and an enormous increase in the cytosolic calcium concentration, mitochondria would begin to accumulate calcium at maximal rates in an attempt to maintain the normal set point. With a continuous influx of calcium from the extracellular fluid this would inevitably lead to a massive accumulation of calcium and the associated mitochondrial damage.

Under these conditions ATP production would not be able to compete effectively for respiratory energy and the situation would be made worse by the fact that intracellular magnesium levels drop significantly during ischaemia and reperfusion (Shen and Jennings, 1972), so favouring the accumulation of calcium.

ACKNOWLEDGEMENTS

I am extremely grateful to Dr Roberto Ferrari for many useful discussions on ischaemia and reperfusion and for allowing me to present his unpublished data (Figure 7.7). This work was supported by the Medical Research Council.

REFERENCES

Affolter, H., and Carafoli, E. (1980). The Ca^{2+}–Na^{2+} antiporter of heart mitochondria operates electroneutrally. *Biochem. Biophys. Res. Commun.*, **95**, 193–196.

Åkerman, K. E. O. (1978). Changes in membrane potential during calcium influx and efflux across the mitochondrial membrane. *Biochim. Biophys. Acta*, **502**, 359–366.

Åkerman, K. E. O., and Wikström, M. K. F. (1976). Safranine as a probe of the mitochondrial membrane potential. *FEBS Lett.*, **68**, 191–197.

Asimakis, G. K., and Sordahl, L. A. (1977). Effects of atractyloside and palmitoyl coenzyme A on calcium transport in cardiac mitochondria. *Arch. Biochem. Biophys.*, **179**, 200–210.

Boyer, P., Chance, B., Ernster, L., Mitchell, P., Racker, E., and Slater, E. C. (1977). Oxidative phosphorylation and photophosphorylation. *Annu. Rev. Biochem.*, **46**, 955–1026.

Bygrave, F. L. (1977). Mitochondrial calcium transport. *Curr. Topics Bioenerget.*, **6**, 259–318.

Chappell, J. B., and Crofts, A. R. (1965). Gramicidin and ion transport in isolated liver mitochondria. *Biochem. J.*, **95**, 393–402.

Chua, B. H., and Shrago, E. (1977). Reversible inhibition of adenine nucleotide translocation by long chain acyl-CoA esters in bovine heart mitochondria and inverted submitochondrial particles. *J. Biol. Chem.*, **252**, 6711–6714.

Cobbe, S. M., and Poole-Wilson, P. A. (1979). Tissue acidosis in myocardial hypoxia. *J. Mol. Cell. Cardiol.*, **12**, 745–760.

Crompton, M. (1980). The sodium ion/calcium ion cycle of cardiac mitochondria. *Biochem. Soc. Trans.*, **8**, 261–262.

Crompton, M., and Heid, I. (1978). The cycling of calcium, sodium and protons across the inner membrane of cardiac mitochondria. *Europ. J. Biochem.*, **91**, 599–608.

Crompton, M., Capano, M., and Carafoli, E. (1976a). The sodium-induced efflux of calcium from heart mitochondria. A possible mechanism for the regulation of mitochondrial calcium. *Europ. J. Biochem.*, **69**, 453–462.

Crompton, M., Sigel, E., Salzmann, M., and Carafoli, E. (1976b). A kinetic study of the energy linked influx of Ca^{2+} into heart mitochondria. *Europ. J. Biochem.*, **69**, 429–434.

Crompton, M., Kunzi, M., and Carafoli, E. (1977). The calcium-induced and sodium-induced effluxes of calcium from heart mitochondria. *Europ. J. Biochem.*, **79**, 549–558.

Crompton, M., Hediger, M., and Carafoli, E. (1978a). The effect of inorganic phosphate on calcium influx into rat heart mitochondria. *Biochem. Biophys. Res. Commun.*, **80**, 540–546.

Crompton, M., Heid, I., Baschera, C., and Carafoli, E. (1978b). The resolution of calcium fluxes in heart and liver mitochondria using the lanthanide series. *FEBS Lett.*, **104**, 352–354.

Crompton, M., Moser, R., Lüdi, H., and Carafoli, E. (1978c). The interrelations between the transport of sodium and calcium in mitochondria of various mammalian tissues. *Europ. J. Biochem.*, **82**, 25–31.

Crompton, M., Heid, I., and Carafoli, E. (1980). The activation by potassium of the sodium–calcium carrier of cardiac mitochondria. *FEBS Lett.*, **115**, 257–259.

de Duve, C. J. (1964). Principles of tissue fractionation. *J. Theoret. Biol.*, **6**, 33–59.

Denton, R. M., and McCormack, J. G. (1980). The role of calcium in the regulation of mitochondrial metabolism. *Biochem. Soc. Trans.*, **8**, 266–269.

Ferrari, R., Williams, A. J., and Dilisa, F. (1982). The role of mitochondrial function in the ischemic and reperfused myocardium. *J. Molec. & Cell. Cardiol.*, **13**, Suppl 1, 25–26.

Fry, C. H., and Williams, A. J. (1979). Measurement of ionic exchange in organelle suspensions with ion selective electrodes. *J. Physiol. (Lond.)*, **289**, 2–3P.

Hearse, D. (1977). Reperfusion of the ischemic myocardium. *J. Mol. Cell. Cardiol.*, **9**, 605–616.

Jennings, R. B. (1969). Early phase of myocardial ischemic injury and infarction. *Amer. J. Cardiol.*, **24**, 753–765.

Jennings, R. B., Hawkins, H. K., Lowe, J. E., Hill, M. L., Klotman, S., and Reimer, K. A. (1978). Relation between high energy phosphate and lethal injury in myocardial ischemia in the dog. *Amer. J. Pathol.*, **92**, 187–207.

Katz, A. M., and Hecht, H. H. (1969). The early 'pump' failure of the ischemic heart. *Amer. J. Med.*, **47**, 497–502.

Kentish, J. C., and Nayler, W. G. (1978). Ca^{2+}-dependent tension generation in chemically 'skinned' cardiac trabeculae: effect of pH. *J. Physiol. (Lond.)*, **284**, 90–91.

Klingenberg, M. (1979). The ADP, ATP shuttle of the mitochondria. *Trends Biochem. Sci.*, November, 249–252.

Klingenberg, M., Grebe, K., and Schever, B. (1975). The binding of atractylate and carboxy-atractylate to mitochondria. *Europ. J. Biochem.*, **52**, 351–363.

Kübler, W., and Spieckermann, P. G. (1970). Regulation of glycolysis in the ischemic and anoxic myocardium. *J. Mol. Cell. Cardiol.*, **1**, 351–377.

Loyter, A., Christiansen, R. O., Steensland, H., Saltzgaber, J. and Ralcker, E. (1969). Energy-linked ion transduction in submitochondrial particles, *J. Biol. Chem.*, **244**, 4422–4427.

Meijer, A. J., Groot, G. S. P., and Tager, J. M. (1970). Effect of sulphydryl-blocking reagents on mitochondrial anion exchange reactions involving phosphate. *FEBS Lett.*, **8**, 41–44.

Mitchell, P. (1966). *Chemiosmotic Coupling in Oxidative and Photosynthetic Phosphorylation*, Glynn Research, Bodmin, UK.

Mitchell, P. (1968). *Chemiosmotic Coupling and Energy Transduction*, Glynn Research, Bodmin, UK.

Moreadith, R. W., and Jacobus, W. E. (1982). Creatine kinase of heart mitochondria. *J. Biol. Chem.*, **257**, 899–905.

Nayler, W. G., Ferrari, R., and Williams, A. J. (1980). Protective effect of pretreatment with verapamil, nifedipine and propranolol on mitochondrial function in the ischemic and reperfused myocardium. *Amer. J. Cardiol.*, **46**, 242–248.

Neely, J. R., and Morgan, H. E. (1974). Relationship between carbohydrate and lipid metabolism and the energy balance of heart muscle. *Annu. Rev. Physiol.*, **36**, 413–459.

Neely, J. R., Whitmer, J. T., and Rovetto, M. J. (1975). Effect of coronary blood flow on glycolytic flux and intracellular pH in isolated rat hearts. *Circulation Res.*, **37**, 733–741.

Nicholls, D. G. (1981). Some recent advances in mitochondrial calcium transport. *Trends Biochem. Sci.*, February, 36–38.

Nicholls, D. G., and Brand, M. D. (1980). The nature of the calcium ion efflux induced in rat liver mitochondria by the oxidation of endogenous nicotinamide nucleotides. *Biochem. J.*, **188**, 113–118.

Nicholls, D. G., and Crompton, M. (1980). Mitochondrial calcium transport, *FEBS Lett.*, **111**, 261–268.

Nicholls, D. G., and Scott, I. D. (1980). The regulation of brain mitochondrial calcium-ion transport. *Biochem. J.*, **186**, 833–839.

Opie, L. H. (1968). Metabolism of heart in health and disease, part I, *Amer. Heart J.*, **76**, 685–698.

Opie, L. H. (1969). Metabolism of the heart in health and disease, part II. *Amer. Heart J.*, **77**, 100–122.

Pande, S. V. (1975). A mitochondrial carnitine acylcarnitine translocase system. *Proc. Natl Acad. Sci.*, **72**, 883–887.

Racker, E. (1970). The two faces of the inner mitochondrial membrane. *Essays Biochem.*, **6**, 1–22.

Racker, E. (1976). *A New Look at Mechanisms in Bioenergetics*, Academic Press, New York.

Racker, E. (1977). Mechanisms of energy transformations. *Annu. Rev. Biochem.*, **46**, 1006–1014.

Racker, E., and Stoeckenius, W. (1974). Reconstitution of purple membrane vesicles catalysing light-driven proton uptake and adenosine triphosphate formation. *J. Biol. Chem.*, **249**, 662–663.

Reynafarje, B., and Lehninger, A. L. (1977). Electric charge stoichiometry of calcium translocation in mitochondria. *Biochem. Biophys. Res. Commun.*, **77**, 1273–1279.

Roos, I., Crompton, M., and Carafoli, E. (1978). The effect of phosphoenol pyruvate on the retention of calcium by liver mitochondria. *FEBS Lett.*, **94**, 418–421.

Saks, V. A., Kupriyanov, V. V., Elizarova, G. V., and Jacobus, W. E. (1980). Studies of energy transport in heart cells. The importance of creatine kinase localization for the coupling of mitochondrial phosphoryl creatine production to oxidative phosphorylation. *J. Biol. Chem.*, **255**, 755–763.

Scarpa, A., and Azzone, G. F. (1970). The mechanism of ion translocation in mitochondria. *Europ. J. Biochem.*, **12**, 328–335.

Shen, A. C., and Jennings, R. B. (1972). Myocardial calcium and magnesium in acute ischemic injury. *Amer. J. Pathol.*, **67**, 417–440.

Sperelakis, N., and Schneider, J. A. (1976). A metabolic control mechanism for calcium ion influx that may protect the ventricular myocardial cell. *Amer. J. Cardiol.*, **37**, 1079–1085.

Vercesi, A., Reynafarje, B., and Lehninger, A. L. (1978). Stoichiometry of H^+ ejection and Ca^{2+} uptake coupled to electron transport in rat heart mitochondria. *J. Biol. Chem.*, **253**, 6379–6385.

Wikström, M., and Krab, K. (1979). Proton-pumping cytochrome *c* oxidase. *Biochim. Biophys. Acta.* **549**, 177–222.

Williams, A. J., and Barrie, S. E. (1978). Temperature effects on the kinetics of calcium transport by cardiac mitochondria, *Biochem. Biophys. Res. Commun.*, **84**, 89–94.

Williams, A. J., Crie, J. S., and Ferrari, R. (1982). Factors influencing cardiac mitochondrial calcium transport and oxidative phosphorylation. *J. Molec. & Cell. Cardiol.* **13**, Suppl. 98.

Williams, A. J., and Fry, C. H. (1979). Calcium–proton exchange in cardiac and liver mitochondria, *FEBS Lett.*, **97**, 288–292.

Cardiac Metabolism
Edited by A. J. Drake-Holland and M. I. M. Noble
© 1983 John Wiley & Sons Ltd

CHAPTER 8

Cardiac Oxygen Consumption and the Production of Heat and Work

G. Elzinga

Department of Physiology, Free University, Amsterdam, The Netherlands

INTRODUCTION

The energy needed for cardiac contraction comes from the breakdown of chemical substances, substrates. In the heart this process occurs mainly aerobically, i.e. substrates are combined with oxygen to form water, carbon dioxide, and energy. The amount of oxygen consumed is often used as a measure of the total energy available. This could in principle hold equally true for the amount of water or carbon dioxide produced, but those are, for practical reasons, much less frequently used. The ultimate fate of the liberated energy is to take the form of heat. However, before this happens completely, part of the energy is used for contraction, a process during which the heart may perform external work, as is usually the case in the intact body. Then part of the liberated energy leaves the heart as work and becomes heat in the vascular system.

This chapter deals with whole heart energetics. Measurement and determinants of the work done, the heat produced, and the oxygen consumed will be discussed and comments will be made on some interrelationships.

Oxygen consumption has different dimensions and cannot therefore, be directly compared with heat and work, which are energy quantities, given in the same units, preferably joules. This has been known since the work of Joule (1818–89). Cardiac oxygen consumption is not a direct measure of the energy turnover by the myocardium. Nevertheless it is often used as such because it is regarded as a direct measure of the energy liberated with the oxidation of substrates. If one wants to compare the amount of oxygen consumed with the heat produced and the work done, one needs to know the ratio of the energy liberated over the oxygen used. This ratio is called the calorific value of oxygen or the energy equivalent of oxygen and is usually given in joules per millilitre of oxygen. The energy equivalent depends on the substrate burned by the heart (Table 8.1). The values given in Table 8.1 have been calculated from the heat of combustion given in the

Table 8.1 Energy equivalents for oxygen used for the combustion of three different substrates

Substrate	Reaction	Energy equivalent $J(ml\ O_2^{-1})$
Lactate	$C_3H_6O_3 + 3O_2 \rightarrow 3H_2O + 3CO_2 + 326.8\ kcal\ g^{-1}$	20.33
Glucose	$C_6H_{12}O_6 + 6O_2 \rightarrow 6H_2O + 6CO_2 + 669.94\ kcal\ g^{-1}$	20.84
Palmitate	$C_{16}H_{32}O_2 + 23O_2 \rightarrow 16H_2O + 16CO_2 + 2384.76\ kcal\ g^{-1}$	19.36

CRC Handbook of Chemistry and Physics (1977/78) for lactate, glucose, and palmitate at 25 °C. The volume of oxygen holds for standard conditions (STPD). No corrections have been made for the heat of solution. However, for these substrates this correction factor is rather small ($<1\%$) and also dependent on the concentration present in the solution (Moore, 1972).

The precise value of the energy equivalent the substrates burnt by the heart needs to be known. This requirement is not easily met because it does not suffice to measure concentration differences in the arterial and venous coronary blood and the coronary blood flow. From those three measurements one can calculate substrate uptake by the heart but they do not give information whether these substrates are burnt or stored (see Drake-Holland, Chapter 9, and Van der Vusse and Reneman, Chapter 10, in this volume). Therefore in most studies it remains unclear what substrates are used by the heart to liberate energy. Fortunately, the energy equivalents are, for substrates most commonly used by the heart, i.e. carbohydrates, fat, and lactate, rather close. It is therefore possible to assume an average value for the energy equivalent. Often 20 J per millilitre of oxygen is used. The maximal possible error made in the conversion is then reasonably small. It arises, according to Table 8.1, when the heart uses glucose only, and equals

$$\frac{20.84 - 20}{20.84} \times 100 = 4\%. \tag{8.1}$$

Elegant experimental proof that an average value for the energy equivalent of 20 J per millilitre of oxygen holds well for the heart has been given by Coulson (1976) using a calorimetric method in isolated Langendorff-perfused rabbit hearts (Figure 8.1). Note that rates have been plotted on both axes instead of amounts. However, this does not influence the value of the slope of the relationship. The slope indicates how much oxygen is converted into heat. Because Langendorff hearts do not perform external work, all the energy liberated becomes heat in the heart itself. The slope is therefore equal to the energy equivalent. Depending on how he did the regression analysis (x versus y, or y versus x) Coulson found for his data, shown in Figure 8.1, 19.75 or 20.48 J per millilitre of oxygen.

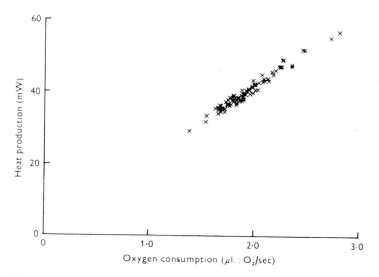

Figure 8.1 Relationship between the rate of heat production and oxygen consumption of isolated Langendorff-perfused rabbit hearts (Coulson, 1976). The slope of the relationship (19.75 or 20.48 J per millilitre of oxygen) equals the energy equivalent. [Reproduced with permission from R. L. Coulson, *J. Physiol.* (*Lond.*), **260**, 45–53 (1976).]

THE WORK DONE

By ejecting blood into the aorta at a given pressure the left ventricle performs work. The adjective 'external' is used here to indicate that energy in the form of work leaves the system under study, i.e. the left ventricle. It is also meant to indicate that the heart performs internal work. This internal fraction of the work may be defined as the work which degrades into heat inside the heart. A system which performs internal work needs to contain at least two components. The (internal) work can then be done during contraction by one component on the other and be returned during relaxation to become heat.

For some time it has been assumed, in parallel with previous studies on skeletal muscle, that at least two elements are present in isolated cardiac muscle, (Britman and Levine, 1964; Sonnenblick *et al.*, 1968) a contractile component and an elastic element in series with it. During contraction, work is done by the contractile element on the series elastic element when the latter is stretched. During relaxation the work stored in the elastic element is then used to stretch the contractile element where it degrades into heat. To calculate the absolute amount of internal work done, one requires the force and extent of shortening of the contractile component obtained from the stress–strain relationship of the series elastic element. Lengthening of the passive, series elastic element is then taken as a measure of the shortening of the active contractile component. Assuming the same stress–strain relationship of the series elastic element for isolated cardiac muscle and the intact heart, and calculating wall stress from pressure and dimensions, the internal work can be calculated for the whole heart. Unfortunately the mechanical properties of the series elastic element used in these calculations have been shown to be due mainly to the dead muscle ends in these isolated preparations (Krueger and Pollack, 1975; Donald *et al.*, 1980; ter Keurs *et al.*, 1980). It is therefore not justified to extrapolate those values to the intact heart. Even if the true, much smaller, series elasticity in isolated heart muscle were known, extrapolation to the intact heart would be hazardous. The presence of valves and asynchronicity of activation at the onset of contraction are severely limiting factors for such a calculation.

A small fraction of the work performed is used to compress the blood in the ventricular cavity. This portion of the work has been measured and put forward as a measure of ventricular performance (Stein and Sabbah, 1975). Since blood is virtually incompressible, the amount of work needed is negligible with respect to total energy turnover ($<0.001\%$). The time dependency of this minute fraction of the work is, at a given volume, directly related to the pressure in the ventricle, because compressibility of blood is constant over that range. Therefore it contains no more information than pressure.

In contrast to the internal work, external work can be calculated without assumptions on how the heart or arterial system functions. This is due to the fact that we can measure directly the amount of blood ejected by the ventricle and the pressure at which this occurs. The only requirement is to make a sharply defined separation between the system under study and its environment: in the case of the left ventricle, for example, we distinguish between the left ventricular wall (system) and the blood and arterial system (environment).

External work done by the heart is most often determined per unit time and then called power. Comparable to ordinary mechanics, two fractions of the external power performed by the left ventricle are distinguished: kinetic and potential power. Instantaneous potential power is found through the instantaneous multiplication of pressure (aortic or left ventricular) and flow (Milnor *et al.*, 1966):

$$\dot{w}_p = PF, \qquad (8.2)$$

where $\dot{w}_p$ is potential power, P is pressure, and F is volume flow. Power is zero when either pressure or flow is zero. Thus during an isovolumic contraction no external power is generated and no external work done. Integration of the product of equation (8.2) with respect to cycle time yields

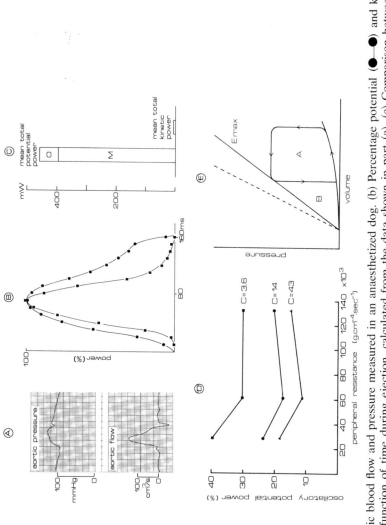

Figure 8.2 (a) Aortic blood flow and pressure measured in an anaesthetized dog. (b) Percentage potential (●—●) and kinetic power (■—■) as a function of time during ejection, calculated from the data shown in part (a). (c) Comparison between the magnitudes of mean total potential and mean total kinetic power. Mean total potential power is subdivided into mean potential power (M) and oscillatory potential power (O). (d) Percentage oscillatory potential power as a function of the peripheral resistance for three values of arterial compliance (C). Measurements were taken from Elzinga and Westerhof (1973). (e) End-diastolic and end-systolic (E_{max}) pressure–volume relationships of the left ventricle. The loop represents a contraction with ejection. The area A is equal to the external stroke work (cf. equation (8.3)). The whole pressure volume area (A + B) is used as an index of myocardial oxygen consumption. The dashed line indicates the change of E_{max} with an increase in contractility

potential stroke work. This value can also be determined from the area enclosed by the ventricular pressure volume loop (A in Figure 8.2(e)). This loop is found when instantaneous ventricular pressure is plotted against instantaneous ventricular volume. It then holds that

$$\oint P \, dV = \int_{t_1}^{t_1+T} P \frac{dV}{dt} \, dt = \int_{t_1}^{t_1+T} PF \, dt, \tag{8.3}$$

where P in this case is left ventricular pressure, V is left ventricular volume, and T the time of the cardiac cycle.

Kinetic power is the energy needed to give the blood a certain velocity during ejection. It can be calculated (McDonald, 1974) from

$$\dot{w}_k = \tfrac{1}{2}\rho(F^3/A^2), \tag{8.4}$$

where $\dot{w}_k$ is kinetic power, ρ is the density of blood, and A is the internal cross-sectional area of the aorta. As can be learned from equation (8.4), kinetic energy does not depend on the pressure generated by the ventricle, it depends mainly on blood flow. Its highest value, when arterial load is varied, is therefore found at the lowest pressure where potential power approaches zero.

The external power output of the ventricle is an oscillatory phenomenon because pressure and flow are oscillatory. Figure 8.2(a) shows aortic blood flow and pressure during a cardiac cycle, measured in an anaesthetized dog. From these two variables potential and kinetic power have been calculated according to equations (8.2) and (8.4). Time courses of the two power curves, normalized for their maximal values, have been plotted in Figure 8.2(b). Kinetic power rises much more sharply to its maximum value than potential power because, to obtain kinetic power, blood flow is raised to the third power, whereas potential power is proportional to flow. The shape of the potential power curve resembles the flow curve rather closely because pressure is fairly constant while the valve is open.

The average height of the two power curves plotted in Figure 8.2(b) may be called mean total potential power and mean total kinetic power. To obtain the power outputs per stroke, these values have to be divided by the period of the cardiac cycle. The absolute amounts of mean total potential and kinetic power have been compared in Figure 8.2(c). From this comparison it may be concluded that for practical purposes mean total kinetic power generated by the left ventricle is negligibly small (4.8 mW in Figure 8.2(c)). It therefore suffices to use only equation (8.2) to determine the power output of the ventricle.

There exists a fundamental difference between the calculation of the mean total potential power, obtained from the instantaneous power curve as discussed above, and the mean potential power value, which is obtained from the product of mean aortic pressure and mean aortic blood flow.

Mathematically speaking, the product of the means (mean potential power) differs from the mean of the product (the mean of total potential power); the difference is called oscillatory power (13% of total in the example in Figure 8.2(c)). However, the magnitude of this percentage depends on the nature of the arterial system. An artificial arterial system, frequently used for experimental work, causing large pressure oscillations during the cardiac cycle, can cause a considerable increase in oscillatory power.

The effects of the load on the percentage value of oscillatory potential power are shown in Figure 8.2(d). This graph uses cat data taken from Elzinga and Westerhof (1973). The resistance and compliance of the arterial system were physiological and could be changed selectively; a stiffer arterial system produced larger pressure oscillations. For the stiffest system oscillatory potential power was between 30 and 40% of total.

Power output of the heart depends not only on the setting of the arterial system but on the properties of the ventricle as a pump, can be changed by alterations in ventricular end-diastolic volume, inotropic state, or heart rate. However, when one wants to measure ventricular pump function at a given functional state such control mechanisms should be kept constant during the measuring process. This approach has been followed by Elzinga and Westerhof (1978, 1979, 1980) in studies on isolated ejecting cat hearts. They found an inverse relationship between mean ventricular pressure and output, the pump function curve (Figure 8.3(a) lower panel). Note that the scales on the ordinate for left and right ventricle are a factor of 5 different. The intercepts of the pump function graphs are found at the highest output, at zero pressure (abscissa), and with an isovolumic beat (ordinate). In any one situation external power must approach zero (cf. equation (8.2)) because one of the two variables of the product is zero. The graphs relating mean total power output to volume output are different in magnitude but similar in shape (Figure 8.3(a) top panel). Maximum power output is found at medium values of volume output, reflecting the parabolic shape of the relationship.

The differences in pump function between the two ventricles are related to the well known differences in wall thickness and geometry. A similar difference in pump function is also found when the inotropic state of the ventricle is changed at a fixed heart rate and ventricular end-diastolic pressure (Elzinga and Westerhof, 1978), but the position of the maximum power output is unchanged in such graphs.

On the other hand, changes in end-diastolic volume at a constant heart rate and inotropic state cause the pump function graph to move outwards and upwards. This effect is shown in the lower panel of Figure 8.3(b), where the effect of an increase in right ventricular filling is shown, as compared to the analagous situation in Figure 8.3(a). Right ventricular end-diastolic pressure rose from 1.9 mm Hg (Figure 8.3(a)) to 2.4 mm Hg (Figure 8.3(b)),

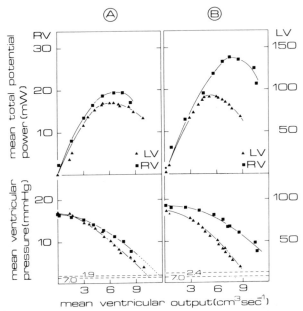

Figure 8.3 (a) Left and right ventricular pump function graphs are shown in the lower panel (note the scale differences). The dotted horizontal lines indicate left (7 mm Hg) and right (1.9 mm Hg) ventricular end-diastolic pressures. The upper panel shows mean total potential power as a function of output. (b) The same heart but now the end-diastolic pressure of the right ventricle has been increased (2.4 mm Hg), resulting in a different position of the right ventricular pump function graph and of the mean total potential power output graph

while end-diastolic pressure in the left ventricle was kept the same (7 mm Hg). A similar outward and upward shift was found for the left ventricle when filling was selectively increased (Elzinga and Westerhof, 1978). The change in pump function resulting from an increase in filling has a significant effect on position and height of the power curve (upper panels, Figure 8.3(a), (b)); the whole curve moves upwards and outwards.

When heart rate is changed at constant inotropic state and end-diastolic volume, the pump function graph shows an almost parallel outward shift (Elzinga and Westerhof, 1980). This implies that a selective change of this variable causes a similar shift of the power curve to that shown for an increase in end-diastolic volume, i.e. upwards and to the right.

THE HEAT PRODUCED

Heat produced by the intact working heart is difficult to measure. This is due to the fact that control of heat exchange between heart and environment in the intact body is almost impossible to realize. Therefore in most

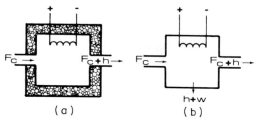

Figure 8.4 Schematic representation of the way in which energy leaves an intact Langendorff perfused heart in a Dewar flask (a) and an ejecting heart which has not been thermally isolated (b). F_c represents coronary blood flow, h and w stand for heat and work respectively
(for further explanation see text)

studies where an attempt has been made to measure the heat produced by the heart, a Langendorff-perfused heart in a Dewar flask was used as was done for the experiments of Coulson shown in Figure 8.1. Schematically this experimental situation is shown in Figure 8.4(a). A thermally isolated chamber in which energy is produced electrically represents the heat-producing myocardium. The flow through the chamber represents myocardial blood flow (F_c). Myocardial blood flow times the temperature difference between input and output (ΔT) times the specific heat of blood (c_h) equals the heat ($\dot{h}_m$) produced per unit time:

$$\dot{h}_m = F_c \Delta T c_h. \tag{8.5}$$

Such studies are unphysiological but useful to determine the energy equivalent in the intact heart (cf. Figure 8.1), provided that they operate under fully aerobic conditions. In the intact animal, the experimental situation resembles the model shown in Figure 8.4(b). External work is done and heat is lost to the surrounding tissues and the blood in the cavities. The work output can be measured quite accurately (see above), but this is not so for the heat lost through routes other than the coronary system, shown to be about 60% Neill *et al.* (1961).

Recently, an indirect method has been described to estimate the total amount of heat lost by *in situ* hearts (Ten Velden *et al.*, 1982). When a bolus of heat or cold is injected in the left atrium a transient change in temperature can be detected at the arterial and venous side of the coronary system. When no heat would be lost other than through the coronary system, the surface areas under the thermodilution curves which can be measured at entrance and exit would have to be the same. In reality this is not the case and the ratio, R, of the venous over the arterial thermodilution area is less than unity. Assuming that this injected bolus of heat (or cold) leaves the heart in the same way as the heat generated by metabolism, the ratio R represents the fraction of the total heat which leaves the heart via the coronary system. Total myocardial heat production should therefore be given by

$$\dot{h}_m = \frac{1}{R} F_c \Delta Tc_h. \tag{8.6}$$

Because some heat is lost per unit time to the endothermic biochemical reactions $(-\dot{h}_c)$ of haemoglobin deoxygenation and the reactions of carbon dioxide with blood, a correction term should be added:

$$\dot{h}_m = \frac{1}{R} F_c \Delta Tc_h - (-\dot{h}_c). \tag{8.7}$$

Measurement of the overall heat production of the whole heart may give no more information than can be obtained from the oxygen consumption and work measurements. However, if one wants to know more about local heat production at different locations in the myocardium, understanding of the way in which the heat generated by metabolism leaves the heart is a prerequisite.

Efforts have been made to measure local heat production in the myocardium by Kjekshus and Mjøs (1971). The method followed by these authors was based on the idea that when coronary blood flow was stopped suddenly, tissue temperature would rise for a few seconds because the metabolic processes would initially proceed undisturbed. The slope of the temperature rise would then be a measure of the metabolic activity. Tissue temperature was measured in this investigation with thermistors mounted on a needle introduced into the ventricular wall. Coronary blood flow to the left ventricle was stopped suddenly by occlusion of the main stem of the left coronary artery. Immediately following occlusion, temperature in the myocardium rose. However, different slopes were found at different locations.

It is unlikely that these differences in slope reflect local differences in metabolic rates because not all heat produced by the myocardium is transported by the coronary circulation. The temperature distribution over the left ventricular wall has a parabolic shape (Figure 8.5), with a maximum

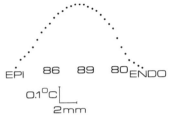

Figure 8.5 Temperature distribution over the left ventricular wall of a dog. Blood flows, as measured with microspheres, for epicardium, midwall, and endocardium are given by the numbers in the figure in millilitres per minute per 100 g

near the midwall. Blood flow, measured with microspheres in the study from which this graph was taken (Ten Velden, 1982), was the same in epicardial, mesocardial, and endocardial layers. The parabolic shape of the temperature profile results from diffusion of heat to epi- and endocardium. Assuming that heat taken up in the various myocardial layers by the coronary blood is proportional to the temperature present at that location, the slope of the rise in temperature following a coronary occlusion would then be proportional to that temperature. This suggests that the same distribution for temperature and rate of rise of temperature after coronary occlusion exist. This expectation implies that the latter variable cannot be a function of local metabolism alone; the way in which heat is transported just prior to the occlusion is also of great importance.

THE OXYGEN CONSUMED

Because the oxygen consumed by the heart can be measured with more ease than the heat produced, most studies on the energy requirements of the heart are based on the measurement of its oxygen consumption. The purpose of many of these studies has been to find a reliable oxygen consumption index for clinical use to avoid the more troublesome direct measurement of the oxygen consumption itself. The general lay-out of these studies is simple: oxygen consumption is varied over a wide range and related to a single variable and/or a combination of variables. The best linear fit is then selected and proposed as an index. Such a study is sometimes followed by another one to test the predictive value of the index by comparing prediction and measurement. In some studies different indices are compared (Kühn and Brachfeld, 1969; Baller *et al.*, 1979, 1981; Rooke and Feigl, 1982).

Many indices have been developed over the years and put forward as reliable measures of the oxygen consumption (Sarnoff *et al.*, 1958; Feinberg *et al.*, 1962; Sonnenblick *et al.*, 1965, 1968; Weber and Janicki, 1977; Baller *et al.*, 1979; Khalafbeigui *et al.*, 1979; Rooke and Feigl, 1982; see also Gibbs, 1978). The still increasing number of indices suggests that they can probably not be used reliably outside the range of experimental conditions tested. This situation has a negative effect on the clinical usefulness of these indices, for which they have often been developed. These analyses suffer in that they comprise only those variables measured in the study, which are often selected on the basis of their ease of measurement or on some more or less arbitrary basis. They may not be the ones most directly related to the energy required by the myocardium, and therefore not the ones giving the best prediction in other situations. Usually a number of variables are combined in some way or another to constitute the index. Following such an approach has a limited value for the improvement of our understanding of the energetic costs of the various processes responsible for the contraction of the heart.

I will not make a detailed analysis of the predictive power of the various indices proposed. This has recently been done by others (Kühn and Brachfeld, 1969; Baller *et al.*, 1979, 1981; Rooke and Feigl, 1982). The outcome almost inevitably depends to some extent on the experimental conditions chosen and the assumptions made. To demonstrate this I have compared in Figure 8.6 results obtained by three groups of investigators. All three found their index to correlate extremely well with myocardial oxygen consumption. Figure 8.6(a) has been obtained from Baller *et al.* (1979). They used the value E_t (see Table 8.2) to predict the oxygen consumed by the heart. Myocardial oxygen consumption was varied by the administration of catecholamines, isoproterenol, atropine, propranolol, and by hypo- and hypervolaemia. Data were obtained from 10 dogs; a correlation coefficient of 0.96 was found. Rooke and Feigl (1982) obtained the best results with their pressure–work index (Table 8.2; Figure 8.6(b)). This index was developed on basis of experiments (phase I) where changes in contractility were minimized by propranolol. Changes in myocardial oxygen consumption in phase I were obtained by combinations of two systolic blood pressures (120 and 180 mm Hg), two heart rates (80 and 120 beats min^{-1}) and two different stroke volumes. The index developed in phase I was subsequently tested in phase II where the protocol consisted of infusions of isoproterenol, noradrenaline, dobutamine, Nembutal, and propranolol. In phase II data were obtained from 11 dogs. They found for their index a correlation coefficient of 0.94.

The pressure–volume area as a measure of left ventricular oxygen consumption (Table 8.2) has been proposed by Suga *et al.* (1981). The pressure–volume area is the sum of the surface area of the left ventricular pressure–volume loop (E in Figure 8.2(e)) and the surface area enclosed by that loop, the E_{Max} line, and the diastolic pressure–volume relationship (A in Figure 8.2). Suga *et al.* (1981) obtained the pressure–volume area by varying stroke volume and end-diastolic volume. In each experiment heart rate was kept constant, but between dogs it ranged between 90 and 150 beats min^{-1} (Suga *et al.*, 1981). This means that their experimental interventions to vary oxygen consumption resemble those of phase I of Rooke and Feigl (1982) closely. For 10 experiments they found a mean correlation coefficient of 0.96. Comparing the three panels of Figure 8.6 and the correlation coefficients found for each of these relationships leads to the conclusion that all three indices are very powerful predictors of myocardial oxygen consumption. Comparison of the three completely different equations in Table 8.2, however, leads almost inevitably to the conclusion that we know little indeed about the fundamental determinants of myocardial oxygen consumption.

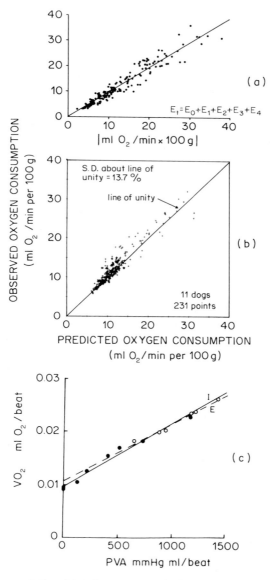

Figure 8.6 Three relationships between an index of oxygen consumption and measured oxygen consumption: (a) $r = 0.96$; (b) $r = 0.94$; (c) $r = 0.96$. [(a) reproduced with permission from D. Baller, H. J. Bretschneider, and G. Hellige, *Clin. Cardiol.*, **2,** 317–327 (1979); (b) reproduced by permission of the American Heart Association from G. A. Rooke and E. O. Feigl, *Circulation Res.*, **50,** 273–286 (1982); (c) reproduced with permission from H. Suga, T. Hayashi, and M. Shirahata, *Amer. J. Physiol.*, **240,** H39–H40 (1981).]

Although the pressure–work index is based on experiments of the type used by Suga *et al.* (1981) for the pressure–volume area, the indices seem to predict the effect of changes in contractile state on the amount of oxygen consumed differently. Changes in contractility have been shown to increase the slope of the E_{max} line (Suga *et al.*, 1976). This change is shown schematically in Figure 8.2(e) by the dashed line. The pressure–volume area for an isovolumic contraction of the same peak pressure would thus be less for higher levels of contractility. Therefore the pressure–volume area predicts a lower oxygen consumption under those conditions. It is unlikely that this would happen; at least, the prediction of the other two indices is different. One (Baller *et al.*, 1979) suggests that oxygen consumption would increase; the other (Rooke and Feigl, 1982) suggests that no change would occur. Such differences in prediction between indices which have been claimed to be very reliable measures of cardiac oxygen consumption shows that our ignorance in heart muscle is comparable to that for frog skeletal muscle, a preparation studied in more detail but in which a full biochemical explanation of the energy turnover during contraction has not yet been given (Curtis and Woledge, 1978).

The most important problem in studies on the determinants of oxygen consumption is probably that of the 'baseline' used to show an effect of some intervention. In his book *Trails and Trials in Physiology*, Hill (1965) has a separate chapter on this problem where he explains that it is often necessary in physiological experiments to assume a level, a baseline, from which some quantity or rate can be measured. This is of great importance in studies on cardiac oxygen consumption. An interesting example has been given in the study by Rooke and Feigl which has been discussed above (Rooke and Feigl, 1982) and concerns the oxygen wasting effect of catecholamines. This effect has been discussed by a number of investigators who showed that inotropic agents alter myocardial oxygen consumption more than predicted by indices such as mean pressure–rate product or the tension–time value (Sarnoff *et al.*, 1965; Sonnenblick *et al.*, 1965; Chandler *et al.*, 1968; Graham *et al.*, 1968; Boerth *et al.*, 1978). However, this oxygen wasting effect disappeared when the pressure–work index was used. One can probably not conclude from these studies whether such an oxygen wasting effect exists or not (see above). To do so, a precise definition and measurement of the chemical reactions involved is required. The example nevertheless shows clearly the dangers involved in such studies.

One of the baselines most often assumed in studies on cardiac oxygen consumption is that processes other than actin–myosin interaction consume a constant amount of energy independent of the total amount of energy liberated. What processes are important in this respect is usually not stated because they are not known in sufficient detail. All changes in oxygen consumption are then assumed to be related to changes in the energy requirements of the contractile apparatus. This procedure may not reflect the true situation, and the energy required by non-contractile processes may not be constant. If the energy required for the other processes changes in proportion to the total energy turnover, it would be hard to determine non-contractile energy requirements. However, when under specific conditions the latter would demand more energy without changes in the energy turnover of the contractile apparatus we might be able to detect them. Too little attention has been devoted to the energy required by such processes.

Without much doubt the Fenn effect is one of the most quoted phenomena in the energetics of muscle contraction. Fenn (1923a,b) showed for frog skeletal muscles at 0 °C that more heat was produced during contractions with shortening than during isometric contractions. The importance of the finding was that it contradicted the validity of simple viscoelastic models of muscle contraction, which were very much in vogue in those days. Viscoelastic models assumed that the contracting muscle can be represented

Table 8.2 Three indices of myocardial oxygen consumption

---

(1) $M\dot{V}O_2 = E_t$ (Baller *et al.*, 1979)

$E_t = E_0 + E_1 + E_2 + E_3 + E_4$

$E_0 = K_0$ $\qquad\qquad\qquad\qquad\qquad\qquad\qquad$ $K_0 = 7.0 \times 10^{-1}$

$E_1 = t_{syst} \times HR \times K_1$ $\qquad\qquad\qquad\qquad\quad$ $K_1 = 3.0 \times 10^{-2}$

$E_2 = SBP(ESV/100 \text{ g})^{1/2} \times sep \times HR \times K_2$ $\qquad$ $K_2 = 2.0 \times 10^{-4}$

$E_3 = (dP/dt_{max}) \times HR \times K_3$ $\qquad\qquad\qquad$ $K_3 = 1.2 \times 10^{-5}$

$E_4 = (d^2P/dt^2_{max}) \times HR \times K_4$ $\qquad\qquad\quad$ $K_4 = 1.0 \times 10^{-8}$

(2) *Pressure–work index* (Rooke and Feigl, 1982)

$$M\dot{V}O_2 = K_1(SBP \times HR) + K_2\left(\frac{(0.8SBP + 0.2DBP) \times HR \times SV}{BW}\right) + K_3$$

$\qquad\qquad\qquad\qquad\qquad\qquad\qquad\qquad\qquad$ $K_1 = 4.8 \times 10^{-4}$
$\qquad\qquad\qquad\qquad\qquad\qquad\qquad\qquad\qquad$ $K_2 = 3.25 \times 10^{-4}$
$\qquad\qquad\qquad\qquad\qquad\qquad\qquad\qquad\qquad$ $K_3 = 1.43$

(3) *Pressure–volume area* (Suga *et al.*, 1981)

$M\dot{V}O_2/HR = K_1 \times PVA + K_2$

$\qquad\qquad\qquad\qquad\qquad\qquad\qquad\qquad\qquad$ $K_1 = 1.64 \times 10^{-5}$
$\qquad\qquad\qquad\qquad\qquad\qquad\qquad\qquad\qquad$ $K_2 = 0.015$

$M\dot{V}O_2$, myocardial oxygen consumption (ml O_2 100 g^{-1} min^{-1}); t_{syst}, electrical duration of systole (s); *HR*, heart rate (beats min^{-1}); *SBP*, systolic blood pressure (mm Hg); *ESV*, end-systolic volume (ml); *sep*, systolic ejection period (s); dP/dt_{max}, maximal rate of rise of left ventricular pressure (mm Hg); *DBP*, diastolic blood pressure (mm Hg); *BW*, body weight (kg); *SV*, stroke volume (ml); *PVA*, pressure–volume area (mm Hg ml $beat^{-1}$).

by a spring and a dashpot in parallel arrangement. At the onset of contraction the spring changed in stiffness and acquired the ability to shorten. An inherent assumption is that the amount of energy needed to change the muscle properties was set at the onset of contraction as the change occurred. Fenn showed this not to be the case when he found that even more energy was released by a shortening muscle. Not all muscles show the Fenn effect and the presence of it depends also on the experimental circumstances. Frog sartorius muscles at 18 °C, for instance, do not produce more heat in contractions where shortening is allowed than in isometric ones (Homsher and Rall, 1973; Homsher *et al.*, 1973). The same holds true for isolated cardiac muscle (Gibbs and Gibson, 1970) and the intact heart (Elzinga and Westerhof, 1980).

The mechanical model of a spring and a dashpot in parallel has an electrical representation in the combination of a capacitor (spring) and a resistor (dashpot) in series. For the ventricle such models have become popular as a description of the mechanical properties of the heart (Sagawa, 1978). This is based on the existence of ventricular pressure–volume relationships such as shown in Figure 8.2(e). The index proposed by Suga *et al.* (1981) for the left ventricular oxygen consumption (Table 8.2; Figure 8.6(c)) implies that the energy required by the heart to contract is in accordance with a viscoelastic model of muscle contraction. One of the reasons that such a model may hold rather well for the left ventricle is that cardiac muscle does not show a Fenn effect. On the other hand, it would be very unlikely that heart muscle would differ fundamentally from skeletal muscle. Therefore, although the overall behaviour of the left ventricle seems to be similar to that of a time-varying compliance in combination with a resistor, it may not be based on fundamental myocardial properties.

RELATIONS BETWEEN THE OXYGEN CONSUMED, THE WORK DONE, AND THE HEAT PRODUCED BY THE HEART

The sum of heat produced ($\dot{h}$) and work done ($\dot{w}$) per unit time equals the oxygen consumption ($M\dot{V}O_2$) times its energy equivalent (EE). In the mathematical form:

$$\dot{h} + \dot{w} = M\dot{V}O_2 \times EE. \tag{8.8}$$

When no work is done, as was the case in Coulson's experiment (Figure 8.1), the heat produced equals the amount of oxygen consumed times the energy equivalent. Equation (8.8) has also been shown to hold, for the ejecting heart, which does perform external work, by Ten Velden *et al.* (1982) in open-thorax dogs. Assuming an energy equivalent of oxygen of 20.3 J ml^{-1} they found no difference between the sum of heat and power produced by the heart, and the oxygen consumed times 20.3.

Since there is ample evidence that equation (8.8) is valid for the heart, the amount of heat produced by the heart can be calculated in a reliable way by subtracting the external work from the oxygen consumption energy equivalent product. This has been done in Figure 8.7(a) for the left heart of a cat. In this experiment the end-diastolic pressure, heart rate, and inotropic state were kept constant and peripheral resistance varied (Elzinga and Westerhof, 1980). The result strongly resembles findings in isolated cardiac muscles where heat production is altered by varying the load at a given initial muscle

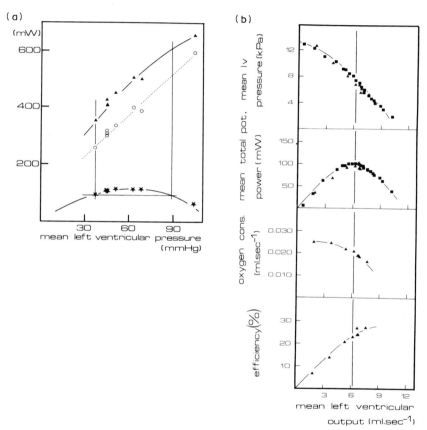

Figure 8.7 (a) Total energy liberated (▲), heart produced (○), and power generated (★) by an isolated ejecting cat heart related to mean left ventricular pressure. The two vertical lines are drawn at identical values of the power output. (b) As a function of mean left ventricular output have been plotted: mean left ventricular pressure, (the pump function graph), mean total potential power, oxygen consumption, and left ventricular efficiency. Measurements have been obtained from an isolated ejecting cat heart at constant end-diastolic volume, inotropic state, and heart rate. The vertical line goes through the optimum power output

length, stimulation frequency, and inotropic state (cf. Figure 3 of Gibbs, 1978). These findings show that the amount of work produced is only a weak determinant of the heat produced by the heart. Most of the heat is produced at the highest pressure, i.e. in isovolumic contractions.

Because the mean total potential power is parabolically related to the output of the ventricle at a fixed end-diastolic pressure, heart rate, and inotropic state, a given amount of work can be performed at two different levels of the cardiac oxygen consumption. This statement holds true only because oxygen consumption and work do not show the same dependence on ventricular output. The phenomenon is indicated in Figure 8.7(a) by the two vertical lines connecting the graphs. The two lines cross the mean power curve at the same value, but the heat and total energy curve at different values. Although the amount of work is equal, this is obtained by a low value for the pressure times a high value for the flow, and vice versa. As has been known for a long time (Evans and Matsuoka, 1914/15), 'pressure' work requires more energy than volume work. The finding that the same amount of external work can be found at two different pressure values only pertains to situations with a constant end-diastolic volume and inotropic state. If these two control mechanisms are allowed to vary also, the same amount of external work may be obtained by an infinite number of combinations of arterial pressure, filling, heart rate, and inotropic state.

Figure 8.7(a) also shows that the absolute amount of work produced in relation to the energy taken up by the heart is small. The ratio of these two quantities times 100 is called the efficiency:

$$Eff = \frac{\dot{w}}{\dot{h} + \dot{w}} \, 100 = \frac{\dot{w}}{M\dot{V}O_2 \times EE} \times 100. \qquad (8.9)$$

For a given ventricular pump function (cf. Figure 8.7(b)) efficiency is not constant but depends on the output (and therefore the arterial load) because both work and energy uptake depend on it. Thus, efficiency must be close to zero when the heart contracts isovolumetrically and when it does not generate any pressure (Figure 8.7(b)). An optimal value of the efficiency is not found at the same output at which the mean external power reaches its optimum value (vertical line; Figure 8.7(b)). This would have been the case if the energy required for the contraction had been independent of the arterial load. The highest value for the efficiency of the ventricle at a given heart rate, inotropic state, and end-diastolic volume is in reality found at higher outputs, and therefore lower pressures, than the highest mean external power (Figure 8.7(b)). In the example given the highest efficiency value equals almost 30%. In open thorax dogs Ten Velden *et al.* (1982) found values between 10 and 34%. These percentages do not reflect the efficiency of the contractile apparatus itself. That must be considerably higher because energy is also required to maintain the structure and change ionic concentration in different cellular compartments.

Wilcken *et al.* (1964) found in the conscious dog that the ventricle is controlled in such a manner that it operates near optimum mean power output, i.e. changes in arterial pressure, on a beat-to-beat basis, in either direction caused a decrease of mean power output of the beat following the intervention. This finding could suggest that the circulation is controlled to optimize maximum power transfer from the heart to the periphery. However, such a situation cannot be obtained at an optimum value for the efficiency (Figure 8.7(b)).

How can the circulation adapt itself in such a way that the heart operates at the top of the power parabola? Almost all mammals seem to have about the same blood pressure. This indicates that the body strongly demands the pump to be capable of generating that pressure. On the other hand the tissues in the body require a certain amount of blood flow to maintain their energy supply. Pressure and flow are not independent variables (Figures 8.3 and 8.7(b)). The best compromise to meet the double requirement of generation of pressure and flow is found at a given mean power value, but the control mechanisms (end-diastolic volume, heart rate, inotropic state,

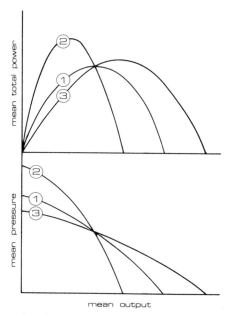

Figure 8.8 Schematic drawing of three pump function graphs with their respective mean total power curves (cf. Figure 8.3). They show that the same pressure and output can be generated in different ways

and hypertrophy) could provide the heart with many different pump characteristics suited to generate the same amount of pressure and flow for the periphery. Three such pump function graphs have been compared in Figure 8.8 in a schematic manner. Pump 1 works at the optimum of the mean power curve. Pump 2 generates the same pressure and flow at the working point but has a higher inotropic state and a smaller end-diastolic volume. Pump 3 has a higher end-diastolic volume but a somewhat lower inotropic state. All three pumps generate the same pressure, the same flow, and the same amount of mean external power. If in case 1 the heart would need the smallest amount of energy, we could understand why the heart evolved to operate at its power maximum. If it did not matter or if the energy required by cases 2 or 3 was less than in case 1, it is difficult to understand why the ventricle operates at the optimum mean power output. Unfortunately no experiments have been performed to explore this point specifically.

REFERENCES

Baller, D., Bretschneider, H. J., and Hellige, G. (1979). Validity of myocardial oxygen consumption parameters. *Clin. Cardiol.*, **2**, 317–327.

Baller, D., Bretschneider, H. J., and Hellige, G. (1981). A critical look at currently used indirect indices of myocardial oxygen consumption. *Basic Res. Cardiol.*, **76**, 163–181.

Boerth, R. C., Hammermeister, K. E., and Warbasse, J. R. (1978). Comparative influence of ouabain, norepinephrine and heart rate on myocardial oxygen consumption and inotropic state in dogs. *Amer. Heart J.*, **96**, 355–362.

Britman, N. A., and Levine, H. J. (1964). Contractile element work: a major determinant of myocardial oxygen consumption. *J. Clin. Invest.*, **43**, 1397–1408.

Chandler, B. M., Sonnenblick, E. H., and Pool, P. E. (1968). Mechanochemistry of cardiac muscle, III. Effects of norepinephrine on the utilization of high-energy phosphates. *Circulation Res.*, **22**, 729–735.

Coulson, R. L. (1976). Energetics of isovolumic contractions of the isolated rabbit heart. *J. Physiol. (Lond.)*, **260**, 45–53.

CRC Handbook of Chemistry and Physics, 58th edn (1977/78) (R. C. Weast, ed.), CRC Press, Palm Beach.

Curtis, N. A., and Woledge, R. C. (1978). Energy changes and muscular contraction. *Physiol. Rev.*, **58**, 690–761.

Donald, T. C., Reeves, R. N. S., Reeves, R. C., Walker, A. A., and Hefner, L. L. (1980). Effect of damaged ends in papillary muscle preparations. *Amer. J. Physiol.*, **238**, H14–H23.

Elzinga, G., and Westerhof, N. (1973). Pressures and flow generated by the left ventricle against different impedances. *Circulation Res.*, **32**, 178–186.

Elzinga, G., and Westerhof, N. (1978). The effect of an increase in inotropic state and end-diastolic volume on the pumping ability of the feline left heart. *Circulation Res.*, **42**, 620–628.

Elzinga, G., and Westerhof, N. (1979). How to quantify pump function of the heart. The value of variables derived from measurements on isolated muscle. *Circulation Res.*, **44**, 303–308.

Elzinga, G., and Westerhof, N. (1980). Pump function of the feline left heart;

changes with heart rate and its bearing to the energy balance. *Cardiovasc. Res.*, **14**, 81–92.

Elzinga, G., Piene, H., and de Jong, J. P. (1980). Left and right ventricular pump function and consequences of having two pumps in one heart. A study on the isolated cat heart. *Circulation Res.*, **46**, 564–574.

Evans, C. L., and Matsuoka, Y. (1914/15). The effect of various mechanical conditions on the gaseous metabolism and efficiency of the mammalian heart, *J. Physiol. (Lond.)*, **49**, 378–405.

Feinberg, H., Katz, L. N., and Boyd, E. (1962). Determinants of coronary flow and myocardial oxygen consumption. *Amer. J. Physiol.*, **202**, 45–52.

Fenn, W. O. (1923a). A quantitative comparison between the energy liberated and the work performed by the isolated sartorius muscle of the frog. *J. Physiol. (Lond.)*, **58**, 175–203.

Fenn, W. O. (1923b). The relation between the work performed and the energy liberated in muscular contraction. *J. Physiol. (Lond.)*, **58**, 373–395.

Gibbs, C. L. (1978). Cardiac energetics. *Physiol. Rev.*, **58**, 174–255.

Gibbs, C. L., and Gibson, W. R. (1970). Energy production in cardiac isotonic contractions. *J. Gen. Physiol.*, **56**, 732–750.

Graham, T. P., Covell, J. W., Sonnenblick, E. H., Ross, J., Jr, and Braunwald, E. (1968). Control of myocardial oxygen consumption. Relative influence of contractile state and tension development. *J. Clin. Invest.*, **47**, 375–385.

Hill, A. V. (1965). *Trails and Trials in Physiology*, Edward Arnold, London.

Homsher, E., and Rall, J. A. (1973). Energetics of shortening muscles in twitches and tetanic contractions. I. A reinvestigation of Hill's concept of the shortening heat. *J. Gen. Physiol.*, **62**, 663–676.

Homsher, E., Mommaerts, W. F. H. M., and Ricchiuti, N. V. (1973). Energetics of shortening muscles in twitches and tetanic contractions, *J. Gen. Physiol.*, **62**, 677–692.

ter Keurs, H. E. D. J., Rijnsburger, W. H., van Heuningen, R., and Nagelsmit, M. J. (1980). Tension development and sarcomere length in rat cardiac trabeculae. Evidence of length dependent activation. *Circulation Res.*, **46**, 703–714.

Khalafbeigui, F., Suga, H., and Sagawa, K. (1979). Left ventricular systolic pressure–volume area correlates with oxygen consumption. *Amer. J. Physiol.*, **237**, H566–H569.

Kjekshus, J. K., and Mjøs, O. D. (1971). Local metabolic rate and left ventricular oxygen consumption in the intact dog heart. *Scand. J. Clin. Lab. Invest.*, **28**, 379–388.

Krueger, J. W., and Pollack, G. H. (1975). Myocardial sarcomere dynamics during isometric contraction. *J. Physiol. (Lond.)*, **251**, 627–643.

Kühn, P., and Brachfeld, N. (1969). Zur Wertigkeit des Tension-Time-Index und der maximalen linksventrikulären Druckanstiegsgeschwindigkeit (dP/dt_{max}) in der Korrelation zum myokardialen Sauerstoffverbrauch. *Z. Kreislaufforsch.*, **58**, 244–251.

McDonald, D. A. (1974). *Blood Flow in Arteries*, 2nd edn, Edward Arnold, London.

Milnor, W. R., Bergel, D. H., and Bargainer, J. D. (1966). Hydraulic power association with pulmonary blood flow and its relation to heart rate. *Circulation Res.*, **19**, 467–480.

Moore, W. J. (1972). *Physical Chemistry*, 5th edn. Longman, London, and Prentice Hall, Englewood Cliffs, N.J.

Neill, W. A., Levine, H. H., Wagman, R. J., Messer, J. V., Krasnow, N., and Gorlin, R. (1961). Left ventricular heat production measured by coronary flow and temperature gradient. *J. Appl. Physiol.*, **16**, 883–890.

Rooke, G. A., and Feigl, E. O. (1982). Work as a correlate of canine left ventricular oxygen consumption, and the problem of catecholamine oxygen wasting. *Circulation Res.*, **50**, 273–286.

Sagawa, K. (1978). The ventricular pressure–volume diagram revisited. *Circulation Res.*, **43**, 677–687.

Sarnoff, S. J., Braunwald, E., Welch, G. H., Jr, Case, R. B., Stainsby, W. N., and Macruz, R. (1958). Hemodynamic determinants of oxygen consumption of the heart with special reference to the tension–time index. *Amer. J. Physiol.*, **192**, 148–156.

Sarnoff, S. J., Gilmore, J. P., Weisfeldt, M. L., Daggett, W. M., and Mansfield, P. B. (1965). Influence of norepinephrine on myocardial oxygen consumption under controlled hemodynamic conditions, *Amer. J. Cardiol.*, **16**, 217–226.

Sonnenblick, E. H., Ross, J., Jr, Covell, J. W., Kaiser, G. A., and Braunwald, E. (1965). Velocity of contraction as a determinant of myocardial oxygen consumption. *Amer. J. Physiol.*, **209**, 919–927.

Sonnenblick, E. H., Ross, J., Jr, and Braunwald, E. (1968). Oxygen consumption of the heart. Newer concepts of its multifactoral determination. *Amer. J. Cardiol.*, **22**, 328–336.

Stein, P. D., and Sabbah, H. N. (1975). Ventricular performance in patients based upon rate of change of power during isovolumic contraction. *Amer. J. Cardiol.*, **35**, 258–263.

Suga, H. Sagawa, K., and Kostiuk, D. P. (1976). Controls of ventricular contractility assessed by pressure–volume ratio, E_{max}. *Cardiovasc. Res.*, **10**, 582–592.

Suga, H., Hayashi, T., and Shirahata, M. (1981). Ventricular systolic pressure–volume area as predictor of cardiac oxygen consumption. *Amer. J. Physiol.*, **240**, H39–H44.

Ten Velden, G. H. M. (1982). Heat production of the canine left ventricle. PhD thesis, Free University, Amsterdam.

Ten Velden, G. H. M., Elzinga, G., and Westerhof, N. (1982). Left ventricular energetics. Heat loss and temperature distribution of canine myocardium. *Circulation Res.*, **50**, 63–73.

Weber, K. T., and Janicki, J. S. (1977). Myocardial oxygen consumption: the role of wall force and shortening. *Amer. J. Physiol.*, **233**, H421–H430.

Wilcken, D. E., Charlier, A. A., Hoffman, J. I. E., and Guz, A. (1964). Effects of alterations in aortic impedance on the performance of the ventricles. *Circulation Res.*, **14**, 283–293.

Cardiac Metabolism
Edited by A. J. Drake-Holland and M. I. M. Noble
© 1983 John Wiley & Sons Ltd

CHAPTER 9

Substrate Utilization

Angela J. Drake-Holland

Department of Medicine 1, St Georges Hospital Medical School, Cranmer Terrace, London SW17 0RE, UK

INTRODUCTION

Myocardial oxygen consumption ((MVO_2)) is affected by mechanical determinants such as heart rate, left ventricular pressure, and, to a lesser extent, by other haemodynamic and metabolic variables. These factors have been extensively studied (Weber and Janicki, 1977) and reviewed (Gibbs, 1979; Elzinga, Chapter 8 in this volume). If the metabolic rate is increased, there will be a concommitant increase in utilization of subtrates to meet the increased metabolic demand. In the normal myocardium the production of adenosine triphosphate (ATP) is strictly coupled to the MVO_2 (La Noue and Schoolwerth, 1979).

In order to produce ATP, the myocardium must extract its substrate from a source. Thus the process of substrate 'extraction' is the disappearance of a substance from arterial blood into the myocardium. Substrate 'oxidation' is the conversion of that substrate to carbon dioxide and water. These two processes may not necessarily be the same if some of the substrate, once into the myocardium, is utilized by being diverted into other pathways, e.g. glycogen or triglyceride synthesis.

Pathways of Substrate Utilization

Energy production occurs in all living cells as the result of catalysed reactions, i.e. enzyme systems. It is beyond the scope of this book to give a detailed account of all the phases of intermediary metabolism; the processes involved in substrate utilization will be briefly outlined.

The overall process of energy production involves the complete oxidation of substrates to carbon dioxide and water. Throughout the intermediary reactions, although energy is both absorbed and liberated, it is carried mainly in the form of adenosine triphosphate (ATP). In myocardium, the energy released from the breakdown of ATP is used to perform mechanical work. All the three major myocardial substrates, carbohydrates, fats, and proteins, can be used to produce ATP, though the amount of each substrate used is subject to variability.

Energy (as ATP) can be generated in the myocardium by two metabolic pathways, glycolysis (anaerobic) and oxidative phosphorylation (aerobic). The majority (90%) of ATP is produced by the latter pathway (Kobayashi and Neely, 1979). However, under conditions of limited oxygen supply (e.g. anoxia/ischaemia) the production of ATP by the anaerobic pathway is important in order to compensate, in part, for the decrease in ATP production from the aerobic pathways (see Opie, Chapter 13 in this volume). Before carbohydrate (in the form of glucose) can enter the tricarboxylic acid cycle (aerobic phase), it must be broken down via the glycolytic pathway (anaerobic phase). Lactate, the other major carbohydrate fuel, is dependent on the activity of lactate dehydrogenase (LDH) and the pyruvate dehydrogenase complex (see Figure 9.1). Non-esterified fatty acids (NEFA) can only be used for generation of energy by oxidative processes; the same is the case for proteins, via amino acids. However, proteins contribute very little of the substrate for normal cardiac function. Both the carbohydrates and fats are oxidized in the mitochondria. It is the regeneration of the oxidized form of nicotinamide adenine dinucleotide (NAD) from the reduced form (NADH) produced by these reactions, via the cytochrome chain, that leads to the majority of ATP formation.

Control of glycolysis is extremely complex (see Figure 9.1). Control can be exerted at several points. First at the entry of glucose into the pathway and also at three important enzyme steps. In the aerobic heart, the most important of these is phosphofructokinase (PFK) (reaction 1 in Figure 9.1). This complex enzyme is subject to many controlling factors, mainly those related to the energy requirements of the cell. The next most important enzyme in this pathway is glyceraldehyde-3-phosphate dehydrogenase (G3PDH) (reaction 2, Figure 9.1) which becomes important under anaerobic conditions as this enzyme responds to changes in the essential supply of cofactors for oxidation. The final step in aerobic glycolysis is the conversion of pyruvate to acetate (reaction 3, Figure 9.1), which then enters the tricarboxylic acid cycle. Similar two-carbon fragments, split off from the fatty acids during the steps of fatty acid oxidation (beta-oxidation), can also enter the tricarboxylic acid cycle at this point. Entry to the cycle is not as the free acetate, but in a complex bound with coenzyme A (acetyl-CoA, often abbreviated to CoASH). These reactions after pyruvate dehydrogenase take place in the mitochondria and form another major site for control of energy production.

The conversion of pyruvate to acetyl-CoA involves a series of interrelated reactions, catalysed by a multi-enzyme compound of large molecular weight,

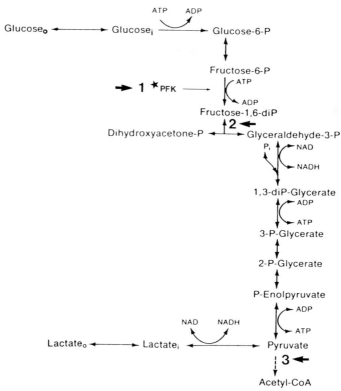

Figure 9.1 A diagrammatic representation of the inclusion of substrates into the tricarboxylic acid cycle via acetyl-CoA. Control points are at phosphofructokinase (PFK) (reaction 1), glycceraldehyde 3-phosphate dehydrogenase (G3PDH) (reaction 2), and pyruvate dehydrogenase (PDH) (reaction 3). For further explanations see text

the pyruvate dehydrogenase complex. This reaction is situated at the crossroads between aerobic and anaerobic metabolism, and its complexity gives rise to many means of exercising controls. The fact that there are multiple controls on glycolyis and its interaction with oxidative metabolism is in accord with the general rule, that the more critical the reaction the more it is subject to checks and balances.

Descriptive Indices of Substrate Extraction

In studies on cardiac metabolism it is desirable to measure both extraction and total utilization of substrates. This is no problem in isolated heart studies (Opie, Chapter 13 in this volume), but it is more difficult in intact animal studies around which this chapter is orientated and in which less adequate indices are often used. Substrate extraction is obtained by measuring the arterial–coronary sinus (AV) difference and multiplying by the coronary blood flow. This then is substrate consumption. Substrate utilization (be it oxidation or storage) is measured by the labelling of the substrates

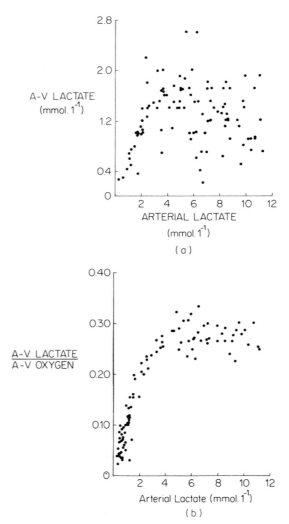

Figure 9.2 (a) AV (coronary sinus) lactate plotted against lactate concentration. Values obtained from 30 normal dogs. (b) The same data as in (a), now plotted as AV lactate/AV oxygen content against arterial lactate

with isotopes (stable or unstable) and measurement of the conversion of these labelled substrates into labelled end-products. However, in the majority of studies, because of the technical difficulties involved, it is not possible to make absolute measurements of substrate oxidation. Other indices of these processes are often used, and this can lead to considerable confusion. Therefore, the descriptive indices of substrate extraction, oxidation and utilization will be defined in this Chapter in the same way as in a recent review (Drake, 1982).

However it is important to re-emphasise that extraction ratios (AV substrate difference divided by arterial concentration) are of little value. They are given for lactate by the slope of the lines (not drawn in illustration) joining the points in Figure 9.2(a) to the origin. When the same data is converted to AV substrate difference divided by AV oxygen difference (Fig. 9.2(b)), a clear and expected dependence of substrate uptake upon arterial concentration is demonstrated.

The rate of tissue metabolism (uptake or release) can only be measured by multiplying the AV difference by the blood flow if the flow, the arterial concentration, and the rate of tissue metabolism are all constant. The effect of a non-steady state on simultaneous AV difference means that a solitary AV difference is uninterpretable. The immediate history of the system must be known (Zierler, 1961).

SUBSTRATE PREFERENCE

The regulatory mechanisms optimize the utilization of the substrates under the conditions which exist at any given moment. These mechanisms involve circulating hormones and membrane transport properties, as well as specific effects on the enzymes involved such as product inhibition, the supply of cofactors, and allosteric effects. Finally, substrate utilization is controlled by substrate availability. Thus the regulatory mechanisms in the aerobic heart ensure that the rate of production of ATP will always equal the consumption of ATP.

To produce the ATP required for contraction the heart must use a substrate, the major extracellular myocardial fuels being the carbohydrates glucose and lactate, as well as the non-esterified fatty acids (NEFA). Though it has been established for some time that the myocardium is able to utilize such fuels as pyruvate, acetate, ketone bodies, and proteins, the normal circulating levels are too low for them to be considered as major sources of energy. Even when the external supply is raised, the relative contribution of these fuels is too small for them to be the major myocardial sources of energy. The heart can also use its internal stores of energy, viz. glycogen and lipid, under certain circumstances (see van der Vusse and Reneman, Chapter 10 in this volume).

It is interesting to consider the amount of useful energy that the heart can 'capture' out of substrates. As the heart derives most of its energy from oxidative metabolism, enthalpy changes can be taken to be equivalent to the oxygen consumption. This holds true when considering the oxidation of the various substrates. For, though the amount of heat liberated per gram of fat oxidized (approximately 9 kcal) is more than twice that per gram of carbohydrate or protein (approximately 4 kcal), the enthalpies, when expressed per litre of oxygen consumed, are quite similar (fat 4.69 kcal; carbohydrate 5.05 kcal; protein 4.60 kcal). This is because more oxygen is required to oxidize a gram of fat than carbohydrate or protein. This means that the energy available to the myocardium per gram or carbohydrate or fat is roughly equivalent. Thus in terms of energy yield, carbohydrates would seem to be preferable to fats as they cost less, in terms of energy, to get into and to be broken down in the cell.

However, there is still some controversy about which is the preferred myocardial substrate. In spite of the fact that the role of lipid as the major myocardial fuel has been over-emphasized (Opie, 1969), it is often stated that lipid is the preferred myocardial substrate (Bing, 1965; Neely and Morgan, 1974; Zierler, 1976). This is so in spite of evidence in the past literature.

In 1933, McGinty showed that the mammalian heart would take up lactate, though he thought that this was independent of the arterial concentration. The usage of lactate in blood-perfused dog hearts was found to be dependent on several factors, mainly the blood lactate and glucose levels, the rate of work, and the oxygen supply (Evans *et al.*, 1933, 1935). When the extractions of glucose and lactate were compared it was found that an increase in the concentration of one in the blood led to an increased extraction of that substance, and a decreased extraction of the other (Evans *et al.*, 1935). It was also shown that the addition of glucose did not inhibit the lactate oxidation as much as the addition of lactate lowered the glucose oxidation. From these findings it was concluded that the heart prefers lactate to glucose (Evans, 1939). It was suggested that lactate was used by the myocardium to yield energy, and the glucose was used mainly to replace glycogen (Evans, 1939). The intermediates of glycolysis can be used for the synthesis of important cell constituents such as phospholipids, amino acids, purines, and pyrimidines (Randle, 1963), rather than just as a source of pyruvate.

The thought that other fuels beside glucose and lactate may be used by the myocardium arose from the fact that the sum of the glucose and lactate extractions could not account for all the oxygen extracted. The other source of fuel suggested was fats. The idea was supported by changes in respiratory quotient, although the difficulties in obtaining meaningful results from respiratory quotients was fully realized (Bogue *et al.*, 1935; Evans, 1939).

Using a Starling heart–lung aglycaemic preparation in dogs, Cruickshank and Startup (1933) showed that the heart would become depleted of glycogen, and that only when 50% of this store had been used would other endogenous fuels be mobilized, i.e. fat or protein. Later the endogenous fuel so used was measured, and it was found to be fat (Cruickshank and Kosterlitz, 1941). However, most studies on the myocardial utilization of unesterified fatty acids in humans have been undertaken in resting fasting subjects. In this state, the circulating NEFA levels are high (over $1000 \ \mu Eq \ l^{-1}$) (Bing *et al.*, 1953; Rothlin and Bing, 1961), and thus may provide up to three-fifths of the myocardial energy requirements (Bing, 1954). But, if the energy requirements are satisfied by the supply of carbohydrates, the NEFA extraction will be decreased (Ballard *et al.*, 1960).

Evidence for the Preference of Lactate

The use of radioactive, ^{14}C- or ^{3}H-labelled isotopes has facilitated the study of substrate utilization and extraction. Using these techniques and a constant flow perfusion system, it was shown that the primary fate of lactate in the myocardium is oxidation (Griggs *et al.*, 1966). These findings confirmed the postulate of the early physiologists Bogue *et al.* (1935) and Evans (1939), who were unable to make absolute measurements because of the limited methods available.

Using [^{14}C]palmitate and [^{3}H]oleate, Spitzer and Spitzer (1972) and Spitzer (1974) showed that in resting, fasting dogs, NEFA was utilized as the major substrate, with lactate supplying about one-third of the metabolic CO_2 production. In neither study was the lactate raised above $2.4 \ mmol \ l^{-1}$. Thus the utilization of lactate would not be at its maximum (see Figure 9.3(a)). However, Isekutz *et al.* (1965) had already shown that, in dogs, an elevated blood lactate (over $10 \ mmol \ l^{-1}$) caused a 30% reduction in the oxidation of NEFA, together with a 15% reduction in glucose oxidation. This effect, which was described by them as a 'glucose-sparing effect' could also be interpreted as a preference for lactate over glucose, if lactate levels are raised. This preference for lactate can be shown at the cellular level by isolated myocytes (Liu and Spitzer, 1978). In the elegant studies of Rose and Goresky (1977), the uptake of tritiated palmitate was inhibited by $5.5 \ mmol \ l^{-1}$ lactate, in intact dogs. This gives further support to the preference of lactate as a myocardial fuel, if it is available.

Thus resolution of the question of myocardial substrate preference is critically dependent on the availability of substrates in the circulation during the experiment. It is crucial that substrate utlization always be studied with defined substrate availability. Preference can only be studied when all substrates are available in adequate concentration. The major substrate utilized will depend not only on preference but also on availability. Normally the circulating levels of NEFA and glucose are fairly constant. NEFA

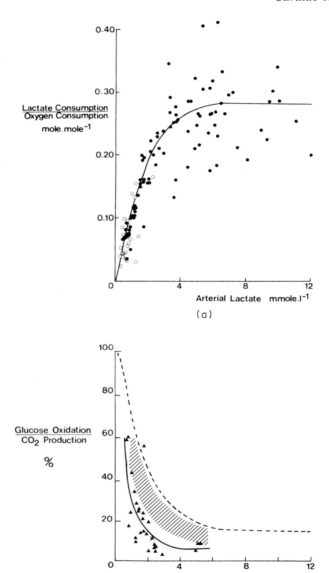

Figure 9.3 (a) AV lactate/AV oxygen plotted against arterial lactate: O, control dogs; ●, lactate infusion studies; $r_s = 0.892$ (Spearman rank test) for data up to an arterial lactate of 4.5 mmol l^{-1}. (b) Unpublished data for dogs in which glucose oxidation as a ratio of total CO_2 production is plotted against arterial lactate. The dashed line is the inverse of the lactate data in part (a)

levels will only be increased with prolonged fasting (Lassers *et al.*, 1972), whilst glucose levels are tightly controlled. Confusion as to the preferred myocardial substrate arises from studies in which the arterial lactate is uncontrolled, unknown, or in an unsteady state. The level of circulating lactate is normally very low at rest, about 1 mmol l^{-1}. At this low resting level, total extraction of lactate by the heart would not provide sufficient energy for contraction, and thus other substrates must be utilized. Lactate cannot be taken up when it is not available. In a human, resting, *fasting* subject, NEFA will be oxidized (Carlsten *et al.*, 1961). However, if there is a rise in the arterial lactate, it has been shown that there is an increase in the myocardial utilization of lactate (Bing *et al.*, 1953). During exercise the contribution of lactate to myocardial substrate metabolism is increased (Keul *et al.*, 1965). With moderate exercise, the arterial lactate rises to about 5.0 mmol l^{-1} (Margaria *et al.*, 1963), due to the lactate discharged from the working skeletal muscles. During severe exercise, lactate levels may rise to 12.0 mmol l^{-1} or more (Shepard *et al.*, 1968). The lactate so produced can be used for immediate energy production in the heart. In the situation where the normal dog heart has been given the choice of lactate, glucose, or fat as fuel, lactate has been shown to be the preferred substrate (Drake *et al.*, 1980).

In Figure 9.3(a) is shown a scheme of the ratio of lactate consumption to oxygen consumption (from Drake *et al.*, 1980). This ratio has a theoretical maximum at 0.33, where 100% of the fuel oxidized is lactate. There is a relationship between arterial-coronary sinus lactate difference and arterial-coronary sinus oxygen content difference, up to an arterial lactate of 4.5 mmol l^{-1}. The shape of the curve points towards a partially stereospecific system. A similar curve has been shown in the plasma membrane of the rat hepatocyte (Monson *et al.*, 1982). If the entry of lactate into the cell was merely by passive diffusion, then the amount entering should be the same no matter what the extracellular concentration. If there was a saturable system (suggesting a transport mediator, or a limitation in oxidation rate) then the uptake should fall to negligible levels at a constant extracellular concentration. This was no so (Monson *et al.*, 1982). Whether this behaviour also applies to myocardial cells is uncertain. Opie thinks that lactate entry into the cell may be governed by an enzyme – lactate permease (see Opie, Chapter 13 in this volume).

From the unpublished data in dogs shown in Figure 9.3(b), where the ratio of glucose oxidized to total CO_2 production is measured using $[^{14}C]$-D-glucose, it can be seen that the amount of glucose oxidized decreases with increasing arterial lactate (solid line). The dashed line is the inverse of the lactate data of Figure 9.3(a). The shaded area between the curves is the oxidation of substrates other than glucose and lactate. Figure 9.3 shows once again that lactate utilization is a function of lactate availability, and that above an adequate arterial concentration lactate is preferred. The latter conclusion is reinforced by the fact that the curve in Figure 9.3(a) is not shifted by changes in glucose and NEFA arterial concentrations.

Though it has been shown that the heart can burn fuels other than carbohydrates (such as ketone bodies and pyruvate), these studies have been undertaken in isolated, Krebs–Henseleit-perfused rat hearts. The question of resolving the problem of substrate preference in these studies is difficult. The isolated perfused rat heart frequently produces lactate under 'control' conditions, indicative of anoxia. Also, the substrates are given at abnormally high levels or when there are no other substrates available (e.g. Williamson and Krebs, 1961; Garland *et al.*, 1962; Olsson, 1962).

Thus, in normal heart, when lactate is available for energy production, it will be utilized. Lactate oxidation occurs because though the equilibrium constant (K_m) for lactate dehydrogenase is in the direction of lactate formation (Kaplan *et al.*, 1956), the lactate dehydrogenase isoenzyme found in heart has a low affinity for pyruvate. In addition the hydrogen ion, pyruvate, and nicotinamide adenine dinucleotide (NADH; reduced form) formed by the lactate dehydrogenase reaction are rapidly removed in the aerobic heart, forcing the reaction in the direction of the formation of pyruvate. Therefore, little or no pyruvate in the aerobic heart will be converted to lactate. Lactate will only be produced if the oxygen supply becomes limited and the pyruvate levels become very high. The NADH produced by the formation of pyruvate from lactate is rapidly transferred to the mitochondria for reoxygenation via the malate–aspartate shuttle. In the well oxygenated myocardium, the flux through the tricarboxylic acid cycle is geared towards oxidative phosphorylation, the rate being controlled by changes in both the high energy phosphate and NAD:NADH ratios. If such a substrate as lactate, which is easily incorporated into the tricarboxylic acid cycle, is available, it will tend to be used, thereby preserving the myocardial glycogen and triglyceride stores for use under circumstances of inadequate exogenous substrate supply.

Glucose versus Lipid

The problem of whether glucose is preferred to NEFA or vice versa in the normal heart is interesting. Unfortunately, actual measurement of glucose or NEFA oxidation is beset with methodological problems. The level of circulating glucose is high (about $4.5 \, \text{mmol} \, l^{-1}$) compared to the arterial-coronary sinus differences measured (of the micromole per litre order). This gives rise to large errors. These can be overcome to some extent by the use of [^{14}C]glucose in animals, but not in studies in man. The use of ^{13}C-labelled compounds in man is making measurement of substrate oxidation feasible. NEFAs are another problem in that the circulating NEFAs are normally a mixture of unesterified fatty acids, the ratios of which vary with the species and individual. If a specific labelled NEFA was used (e.g. [^{14}C]palmitate), would this be handled in the same way as the circulating mixture of NEFA? The turnover of the triglyceride pool in the myocardium is short: 10 min has been proposed (Opie, 1973). The duration of radioactive infusion experiments is usually of the order of 30 min, or longer, thus it would be very difficult to distinguish between the oxidation and/or turnover of triglyceride pools of the NEFA taken up. Also the ratios of the individual NEFAs change as they cross the myocardium (van der Vusse and Reneman, Chapter 10; this volume).

Experimentally, using [^{14}C]glucose it is possible to obtain information on the actual oxidation of glucose. In the dog the relative extraction of glucose and NEFA is shown in Figure 9.4 (Drake-Holland, 1982). The ratio of glucose oxidation to CO_2 production was $17.28 \pm 6.26\%$, which was reduced to $8.95 \pm 6.82\%$ by high NEFA. The NEFA levels reached (increased by the infusion of Intralipid and heparin) were over 2500 $\mu Eq\,l^{-1}$. The reduction in glucose oxidation suggests that the heart switched from glucose to NEFA as substrate.

The question of preference of glucose to NEFA remains unresolved in humans, once again because of variability in the availability of these substrates and the difficulties of making absolute measurements. It is well established that unesterified fatty acid is the blood lipid fraction primarily concerned with the supply of fats to tissues, including the myocardium, for oxidative metabolism (Gordon and Cherkes, 1956). This extraction of NEFA could be completely abolished by the administration of glucose and insulin. In subjects who have recently eaten, it has been known for some time that carbohydrate provides 90–100% of the fuel to the myocardium (Goodal *et al.*, 1950). In the resting, fasting state, or after a high fat meal, there will be

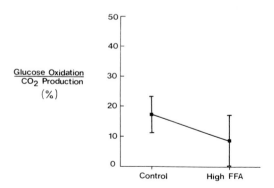

Figure 9.4 Unpaired study of glucose oxidation to total CO_2 production in dogs with normal arterial glucose and NEFA (= control) and high NEFA ($n = 6$). [Reproduced from *Basic Res. Cardiol.*, **77**, 1–11 (1982).]

a high NEFA extraction providing up to about 60% of the substrate for energy production (Bing *et al.*, 1953). However, there must also be some storage of fats, as the oxygen extraction ratios quoted for NEFAs are often over 100%. In the fasting state there may also be changes in the composition of the mixture of NEFAs as the blood crosses the myocardium (Rothlin and Bing, 1961), indicating a rapid turnover of the triglyceride and NEFA pool.

In summary it could be said that the myocardium in the resting state probably changes its relative utilization of glucose or NEFA according to the availability of NEFA and to the influence of hormonal factors such as insulin and glucagon.

The Effect of Substrates on Myocardial Oxygen Consumption (MVO$_2$)

The question of whether the substrate oxidized by the heart for energy production alters the MVO$_2$ has been a topic for a large amount of discussion. Many of the controversies about the effect of NEFAs on MVO$_2$ may well be due to differences in the experimental preparations and procedures used. It is very difficult to accept the fact that tissue that is perfused only with a solution of ions is comparable to the intact situation, where the tissue is perfused with red blood cells in a solution which has a high osmotic pressure. Other variations in the experimental techniques have been the variables measured, and the anaesthetics used. The use of barbiturate anaesthetics may lead to differing results as the heart is depressed by pentobarbitone. This anaesthetic is highly lipid soluble and is able to bind to both the cell and microsomal membranes. In addition the preparation described is often only offered one substrate, and that at unphysiologically high levels.

It has been proposed that elevated NEFA levels increase the oxygen consumption in the isolated rat heart (Challoner and Steinberg, 1966) and in the intact dog, i.e. in one Ringer-perfused and one blood-perfused preparation. An increase in myocardial oxygen consumption with NEFA stimulation has also been shown in man (Regan *et al.*, 1961). However, contrary evidence has been obtained in man (Rogers *et al.*, 1977) as well as in the isolated intact dog (Most *et al.*, 1973), the isolated cat heart (Drake-Holland *et al.*, 1983), and Ringer-perfused rat hearts (Gmeiner *et al.*, 1975). In isolated cat hearts perfused with red cells suspended in Krebs–Henseliet buffer, there are no changes in mechanical performance on changing from one substrate to another apart from a brief transient (Figure 9.5). This is important if artefactual (mechanics-dependent) increases in oxygen consumption are not to be attributed to the substrate change. In the intact dog studies of Most *et al.* (1973), the animals were studied in a closed-chest preparation having been previously implanted with the appropriate instrumentation. Thus at the

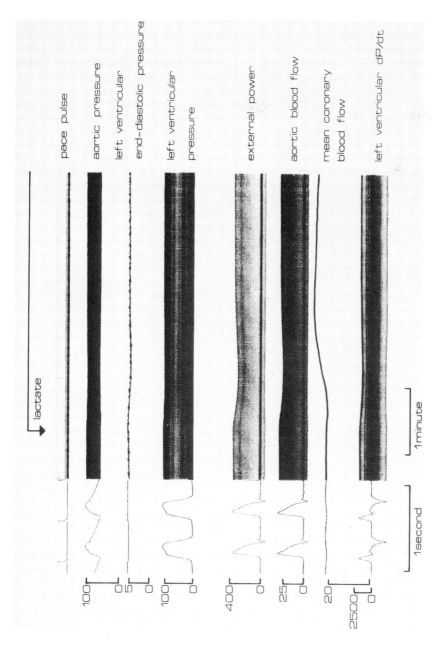

Figure 9.5 Chart recording of haemodynamic variables measured in the isolated ejecting cat heart. There were some transient changes at the beginning of the lactate period (see arrow), which did not persist

time of the study they were in a stable haemodynamic state. This may not always be the case in the open-chest preparation. Another problem in the intact animal is the effect of catecholamine release. Myocardial oxygen consumption could well be affected by catecholamine release (Hauge and Oye, 1966) promoted by substrate infusion or surgical stress. In the isolated preparation this would not be a problem as all sources of catecholamine supply have been removed. It may well be advisable to carry out intact animal experiments under a beta-adrenergic blocking agent. The absence of red cells in some preparations probably causes an inadequate oxygen supply (Gibbs *et al.*, 1980). Lactate production is indicative of such an inadequacy, and lactate production is frequently found in isolated rat heart studies (e.g. Willebrands and Van der Veen, 1967; Severied *et al.*, 1969). The normal, well oxygenated heart never produces lactate (Olsson, 1963; Liedtke *et al.*, 1978). Lactate is a normal myocardial substrate and is consistently taken up in normal human hearts (Bing *et al.*, 1953; Keul *et al.*, 1965) and in the normal dog heart (Drake *et al.*, 1980).

Substrate Withdrawal Studies

In the comparisons of myocardial substrates presented in previous sections, the hearts contained normal endogenous stores. In early experiments with the heart–lung preparation (Evans, 1939) aglycaemic perfusion was shown to deplete glycogen stores. Studies of substrate-free perfusion, which deplete both glycogen and triglyceride, enable exogenous substrates to be compared in a situation where oxidation is obligatory for ATP production, i.e. on their reintroduction after such depletion of endogenous stores. In the study of Drake and ter Keurs (1981), the isolated rat trabeculum was used for ease of substrate manipulation. The preparation was of such a size that diffusion of oxygen is not a problem. The isolated rat trabeculum is suitable because of the thin ribbon-like shape (80 μm thick × 150 μm wide × 2000 μm long). These muscle preparations are very stable. At a stimulation rate of 3 Hz (180 beats min^{-1}) the preparation is stable over a period of at least 90 min at 25 °C. Though it is not possible to measure actual substrate uptakes or oxidation in such small preparations, it is reasonable to assume that if a substrate is supplied and there is no deterioration in mechanical performance it is used for ATP production. In such muscles there was no change in the mechanical performance when each substrate was supplied in turn without prior substrate withdrawal. After a period of such withdrawal, there was no difference in recovery rate, for lactate (4 mmol l^{-1}), glucose (11.0 mmol l^{-1}), or palmitate (approximately 1 mmol l^{-1}, bound to albumin). There was also no difference between the long term effects of the lactate, glucose, or NEFAs on the mechanical performance. It would seem reasonable to conclude from these studies that each was good in terms of energy supply for ATP production.

A second withdrawal period was used to examine the effectiveness of endogenous store repletion in the period of substrate supply following the first withdrawal period. In this situation glucose and palmitate were equally effective in restoring endogenous stores. Lactate cannot be converted to glucose or glycogen in the heart (Opie and Newsholme, 1967) and was ineffective.

Changes in Substrate Extraction and Relevance to Ischaemia

The question arises as to whether the myocardium can change from one substrate to another and whether this is beneficial or deleterious. Inhibition of glucose oxidation by NEFAs is at the mitochondrial level (Shug *et al.*, 1975). The entry of carbohydrate fuels into the citrate cycle from glucose or lactate is via pyruvate and the pyruvate dehydrogenase complex (Figure 9.1). The pyruvate dehydrogenase complex and the link into the tricarboxylic acid cycle via acetyl CoA is independent of the acyl CoA–carnitine transferase mechanism, upon which the complete oxidation of NEFAs is dependent. Therefore high NEFA should not inhibit the oxidation of lactate and does not in the intact dog (Drake *et al.*, 1980).

As pointed out at the beginning of this chapter, one of the most important rate-limiting enzymes of glycolysis is phosphofructokinase (Mansour, 1972). Factors which tend to inhibit this enzyme, leading to a decrease in the relative contribution of pyruvate derived from glucose for entry into the citrate cycle, may thus have an indirect influence on myocardial substrate utilization. These factors may well push the heart away from glucose and towards the oxidation of NEFA. A high rate of oxidation of NEFA is said to inhibit the oxidation of glucose, presumably through the mediation of an intermediate metabolite, probably citrate (Katz, 1977), which inhibits the conversion of glucose to pyruvate at the rate limiting step, phosphofructokinase. The low oxidation rate of [^{14}C]glucose in dogs with high NEFA levels (A. J. Drake-Holland, unpublished) supports this contention.

Conversely a switch to glucose away from NEFA may be beneficial under some circumstances. Hypoxaemia is in itself a stimulus for greater relative oxidation of glucose (A. J. Drake-Holland, unpublished observations). Drugs which can stimulate glucose oxidation by the myocardium (Drake *et al.*, 1982) may enable the cells to oxidize even more glucose.

As the metabolic response of the heart to oxygen deprivation depends on the severity of the simultaneous reduction in coronary blood flow (Bing, 1954–55), anoxia (more correctly hypoxaemia) must be distinguished from ischaemia (Opie, Chapter 13, in this volume). Hypoxaemia is a reduction in oxygen supply but with no reduction in coronary blood flow, whereas in ischaemia the reduction in oxygen supply is due to the reduction or cessation of blood flow. The ischaemic condition is more complex in its response than hypoxaemia as there is not only a decrease in the delivery of substrates, but also a build up of the products of anaerobic glycolytic metabolism (e.g. protons, lactate) which in turn will inhibit glycolysis (Rovetto *et al.*, 1975; Gevers, 1977). Endogenous substrate stores will also be mobilised (see van der Vusse and Reneman, Chapter 10 in this volume).

The problem of an increase in myocardial oxygen consumption by increased utilization of NEFA has raised much interest because of the possible deleterious effects to the myocardium. The deleterious effect would be particularly marked under conditions of limited oxygen supply, be it ischaemia (Mjøs, 1971; Kjekshus and Mjøs, 1972) or anoxia (Opie, 1976). Other aspects of the deleterious consequences of NEFA oxidation and benefits of glycolysis are discussed by Opie (Chapter 13 in this volume).

Whether or not drugs which stimulate glucose oxidation are beneficial under ischaemic circumstances is a point worthy of definition. Ischaemia is further complicated by patterns of flow which are heterogenous; it is possible for oxygen to reach some myocardial cells by continued collateral flow. Thus the supply of 'oxygen-sparing' substrates such as glucose may be critical under these conditions. There may well be areas where the glucose oxidation stimulating effect of hypoxaemia prevails whereas in other areas with lower blood flow, inhibition of glucose oxidation predominates. The effect of drugs designed to switch the myocardium from NEFA to glucose oxidation would then be extremely difficult to predict or to measure.

REFERENCES

Ballard, F. B., Danforth, W. H., Naegles, S., and Bing, R. J. (1960). Myocardial metabolism of fatty acids. *J. Clin. Invest.*, **39**, 717–723.

Bing, R. J. (1954–55). The metabolism of the heart. In *Harvey Lecture Series*, Academic Press, New York, pp. 27–70.

Bing, R. J. (1965). Cardiac metabolism. *Physiol. Rev.*, **45**, 171–213.

Bing, R. J., Siegel, A., Vitale, A., Balboni, F., Sparks, E., Taeschler, M., Klapper, M., and Edwards, S. (1953). Metabolic studies on the human heart *in vivo*. I. Studies on carbohydrate metabolism of the human heart. *Amer. J. Med.*, **15**, 284–296.

Bogue, J., Evans, C. L., Grande, F., and Hsu, F. Y. (1935). Effects of adrenaline and of increased work on carbohydrate metabolism of mammalian heart. *Quart. J. Exp. Physiol.*, **25**, 213–228.

Carlsten, A., Hallgren, B., Jagenburg, R., Svanborg, A., and Werko, L. (1961). Myocardial metabolism of glucose, lactic acid, amino acids and fatty acids in healthy human individuals at rest and at different work loads. *Scand. J. Clin. Lab. Invest.*, **13**, 418–428.

Challoner, D. R., and Steinberg, D. (1966). Effect of free fatty acid on the oxygen consumption of the perfused rat heart. *Amer. J. Physiol.*, **210**, 280–286.

Cruickshank, E. W. H., and Kosterlitz, H. W. (1941). The utilization of fat by the aglycaemic mammalian heart. *J. Physiol. (Lond.)*, **99**, 208–223.

Cruickshank, E. W. H., and Startup, C. (1933). The respiratory quotient, oxygen consumption and glycogen content of the heart in aglycaemia. *J. Physiol. (Lond.)*, **80**, 179–192.

Drake, A. J. (1982). Substrate utilization in the myocardium. *Basic Res. Cardiol.* **77**, 1–11.

Drake, A. J., and ter Keurs, H. E. D. J. (1981). Myocardial mechanical performance is unaffected by added substrate unless endogenous stores are depleted. *J. Physiol. (Lond.)*, **300**, 46P.

Drake, A. J., Haines, J. R., and Noble, M. I. M. (1980). Preferential uptake of lactate by the normal myocardium in dogs. *Cardiovasc. Res.*, **14**, 65–72.

Drake, A. J., Passingham, J. E., and Noble, M. I. M. (1982). Factors influencing the proportion of glucose oxidized to total substrate oxidized *in vivo*. *Europ. J. Clin. Invest.*, **12**, part 11, 9.

Drake-Holland, A. J., Elzinga G, ter Keurs H. E. D. J., Nobel M. I. M., Wempe F. N. (1982). The effect of palmitate and lactate on mechanical performance and metabolism of cat and rat myocardium. *J. Physiol.* in press.

Evans, C. L. (1939). The metabolism of cardiac muscle. In *Recent Advances in Physiology*, 6th edn, London: Churchill, London, pp. 157–215.

Evans, C. L., de Graff, A. C., Kosaka, T., MacKenzie, K., Murphy, G. E., Vacek, T., Williams, D. H., and Young, F. G. (1933). The utilization of blood sugar and lactate by the heart–lung preparation. *J. Physiol. (Lond.)*, **80**, 21–40.

Evans, C. L., Grande, F., and Hsu, F. Y. (1935). The glucose and lactate consumption of the dog heart. *Quart. J. Exp. Physiol.*, **24**, 347–365.

Garland, P. B., Newsholme, E. A., and Randle, P. J. (1962). Effect of fatty acids, ketone bodies, diabetes and starvation on pyruvate metabolism in rat heart and diaphragm muscle. *Nature*, **195**, 381–383.

Gevers, W. (1977). Generation of protons by metabolic processes in heart cells. *J. Mol. Cell. Cardiol.*, **9**, 867–874.

Gibbs, C. L. (1979). Cardiac energetics. *Physiol. Rev.*, **58**, 174–254.

Gibbs, C. L., Papadoyannis, D. E., Drake, A. J., and Noble, M. I. M. (1980). Oxygen consumption of the non-working and KCl arrested dog heart. *Circulation Res.*, **47**, 408–417.

Gmeiner, R., Apstein, C. S., and Brachfeld, N. (1975). Effect of palmitate on hypoxic cardiac performance. *J. Mol. Cell. Cardiol.*, **7**, 227–235.

Goodal, W. T., Olsson, R. E., and Hackel, D. B. (1950). Myocardial glucose, lactate and pyruvate metabolism of normal and failing hearts studied by coronary sinus catheterization in man. *Fed. Proc.*, **9**, 49.

Gordon, R. S., and Cherkes, A. (1956). Unesterified fatty acid in human blood plasma. *J. Clin. Invest.*, **35**, 206–212.

Griggs, D. M., Nagano, S., Lipana, J. G., and Novack, P. (1966). Myocardial lactate oxidation *in situ*, and the effects thereon of reduced coronary flow. *Amer. J. Physiol.*, **211**, 335–340.

Hauge, A., and Oye, I. (1966). The action of adrenaline in cardiac muscle. *Acta Physiol. Scand.*, **68**, 295–303.

Isekutz, B., Miller, H. I., and Rodahl, K. (1965). Effect of lactic acid on free fatty acids and glucose oxidation in dogs. *Amer. J. Physiol.*, **209**, 1137–1144.

Kaplan, N. O., Ciotti, M. M., and Stolzenbach, F. E. (1956). Reaction of pyridine nucleotide analogues with dehydrogenases. *J. Biol. Chem.*, **221**, 833–844.

Katz, A. M. (1977). *Physiology of the Heart*, Raven Press, New York.

Keul, J., Doll, E., Steim, H., Fleer, U., and Reindell, H. (1965). Uber den Stoffweschel des menschlichen Herzens III. Der oxydative Stoffweschel des menschichen Herzens under vershiedenen Arbitsbedingungen. *Pflügers Arch. Ges. Physiol.*, **282**, 43–53.

Kjekshus, J. K., and Mjøs, O. D. (1972). Effect of free fatty acids on myocardial function and metabolism in the ischaemic dog heart. *J. Clin. Invest.*, **51**, 1767–1776.

Kobayashi, K., and Neely, J. R. (1979). Control of maximum rates of glycolysis in rat cardiac muscle. *Circulation Res.*, **44**, 166–175.

La Noue, K. F., and Schoolwerth, A. C. (1979). Metabolic transport in mitochondria. *Annu. Rev. Biochem.*, **48**, 871–922.

Lassers, W., Kaijser, L., and Carlson, L. A. (1972). Myocardial lipid and carbohydrate metabolism in healthy fasting mean at rest: studies during infusion of ^{3}H-palmitate. *Europ. J. Clin. Invest.*, **2**, 348–358.

Liedtke, A. J., Nellis, S., and Neely, J. R. (1978). Effect of excess free fatty acids on mechanical and metabolic function in normal and ischaemic myocardium in swine. *Circulation Res.*, **43**, 652–661.

Liu, M.-S., and Spitzer, J. J. (1978). Oxidation of palmitate and lactate by beating myocytes isolated from adult dog heart. *J. Mol. Cell. Cardiol.*, **10**, 415–426.

McGinty, A. (1933). Studies on the coronary circulation. I. Absorption of lactic acid by heart muscle. *Amer. J. Physiol.*, **98**, 244–254.

Mansour, T. E. (1972). Phosphofructokinase. *Curr. Topics Cell Regul.*, **5**, 2–46.

Margaria, R., Cerretelli, P., Aghemo, P., and Sassi, G. (1963). Energy cost of running. *J. Appl. Physiol.*, **18**, 367–370.

Mjøs, O. D. (1971). Effect of free fatty acids on myocardial function and oxygen consumption in intact dogs. *J. Clin. Invest.*, **50**, 1386–1389.

Monson, J. P., Smith, J. A., Cohen, R. D., and Iles, R. A. (1982). Evidence for a lactate transporter in the plasma membrane of the rat hepatocyte. *Clin. Sci.*, **62**, 411–420.

Most, A. S., Lipsky, M. H., Skydlik, P. A., and Bruno, C. (1973). Failure of FFA to influence myocardial oxygen consumption in the intact anaesthetized dog. *Cardiology*, **58**, 220–228.

Neely, J. R., and Morgan, H. E. (1974). Relationship between carbohydrate and lipid metabolism and the energy balance of heart muscle. *Annu. Rev. Physiol.*, **36**, 413–459.

Olsson, R. E. (1962). Effect of pyruvate and acetoacetate on the metabolism of fatty acids by the perfused rat heart. *Nature*, **195**, 597–599.

Olsson, R. E. (1963). 'Excess lactate' and anaerobiosis. *Ann. Intern. Med.*, **59**, 960–963.

Opie, L. H. (1969). Metabolism of the heart in health and disease II. *Am. J. Cardiol.*, **77**, 100–122.

Opie, L. H. (1973). Lipid metabolism of the heart and arteries in relation to ischaemic heart disease. *Lancet*, *i*, 192–195.

Opie, L. H. (1976). Effects of anoxia and regional ischaemia on metabolism of glucose and fatty acids. Relative rates of aerobic and anaerobic energy production during first six hours of experimental myocardial infarction. *Circulation Res.*, **38**, Suppl. 1, 52–68.

Opie, L. H., and Newsholme, E. A. (1967). The activities of fructose 1,6-diphosphatase, phosphofructokinase and phosphoenolpyruvate-kinase in white and red muscle. *Biochem. J.*, **103**, 391–399.

Opie, L. H., and Stubbs, W. A. (1976). Carbohydrate metabolism in cardiovascular disease. *Clin. Endocrinol.*, **5**, 703–729.

Randle, P. J. (1963). Endocrine control of metabolism. *Annu. Rev. Physiol.*, **25**, 291–321.

Regan, T. J., Binak, K., Gordon, S., Defazio, V., and Hellens, H. K. (1961). Myocardial oxygen consumption during post prandial lipema and heparin induced lipolysis. *Circulation*, **23**, 55–63.

Rogers, W. J., McDaniel, H. G., Moraski, R. E., Rackley, C. E., and Russel, R. O. (1977). Effect of heparin-induced free fatty acid elevation on myocaridal oxygen consumption in man. *Amer. J. Cardiol.*, **40**, 365–372.

Rose, C. P., and Goresky, C. A. (1977). Constraints on the uptake of labelled palmitate by the heart. *Circulation Res.*, **41**, 534–545.

Rothlin, M. E., and Bing, R. J. (1961). Extraction and release of individual free fatty acids by the heart and fat depots. *J. Clin. Invest.*, **40**, 1380–1386.

Rovetto, M. J., Lamberton, W. F., and Neely, J. R. (1973). Mechanisms of glycolytic inhibition in ischaemic rat hearts. *Circulation Res.*, **32**, 699–711.

Severeid, L., Connor, W. E., and Long, J. P. (1969). The depressant effect of fatty acids on the isolated rabbit heart. *Proc. Soc. Exp. Biol. Med.*, **131**, 1239–1243.

Shephard, R. J., Allen, C., Benade, A. J. A., Davies, C. T. M., di Prampero, P. E., Hedman, R., Merriman, J. E., Myhre, K., and Simmons, R. (1968). The maximum oxygen intake. An international reference standard in cardio-respiratory fitness. *Bull. WHO*, **38**, 757–764.

Shug, A. L., Shrago, E., Bittar, N., Folts, J. D. and Kokes, J. R. (1975). Long chain fatty acyl CoA inhibition of adenine nucleotide translocase in the ischaemic myocardium. *Amer. J. Physiol.*, **228**, 689–692.

Spitzer, J. J. (1974). Effect of lactate infusion on canine myocardial free fatty acid metabolism *in vivo*. *Amer. J. Physiol.*, **226**, 213–217.

Spitzer, J. J., and Spitzer, J. A. (1972). Myocardial metabolism in dogs during haemorrhagic shock. *Amer. J. Physiol.*, **222**, 101–105.

Weber, J. T., and Janicki, J. S. (1977). Myocardial oxygen consumption: the role of wall force and shortening. *Amer. J. Physiol.*, **233**, H421–H430.

Willebrands, A. F., and van der Veen, K. J. (1967). Influence of substrate on oxygen consumption of the isolated perfused rat heart. *Amer. J. Physiol.*, **212**, 1529–1535.

Williamson, J. R., and Krebs, H. A. (1961). Acetoacetate as a fuel of respiration in the perfused rat heart. *Biochem. J.*, **80**, 540–547.

Zierler, K. L. (1961). Theory of the use of arteriovenous concentration differences for measuring metabolism in steady and non-steady states. *J. Clin. Invest.*, **40**, 2111–2125.

Zierler, K. L. (1976). Fatty acids as substrates for heart and skeletal muscle. *Circulation Res.*, **38**, 459–463.

CHAPTER 10

Glycogen and Lipids (Endogenous Substrates)

Ger J. van der Vusse and Robert S. Reneman

*Department of Physiology, Biomedical Centre, University of Limburg, Maastricht,
The Netherlands*

INTRODUCTION

It is the purpose of this survey to consider the chemical nature, the cellular localization, the regulation of synthesis and breakdown, and the quantitative significance of the presence of lipids and glycogen as endogeneous substrates in myocardial tissue. Particular emphasis will be given to their importance in ischaemic heart disease and open-heart surgery.

CHEMICAL NATURE OF GLYCOGEN AND LIPIDS

Glycogen

Carbohydrates are stored in myocardial tissue as polysaccharides of high molecular weight. These polysaccharides consist of D-glucose and are called glycogen. D-Glucose molecules are coupled by $\alpha(1 \rightarrow 4)$ linkages; the glucose chains so formed are highly branched. The branch linkages are $\alpha(1 \rightarrow 6)$. Studies performed some three decades ago (Merrick and Meyer, 1954; Russell and Bloom, 1955) strongly suggest the presence of two different forms of glycogen in myocardial tissue, i.e. acid-extractable and non-acid-extractable glycogen. Whether these two forms of glycogen represent basically different chemical structures remains uncertain.

Lipids

In myocardial tissue, fatty acids are present in the unesterified and esterified forms. The fatty acids of the first group are called non-esterified fatty acids (NEFA) or free fatty acids (FFA). The use of the name NEFA is preferred to FFA since non-esterified fatty acids are not 'freely' present but are predominantly bound to proteins or other chemical structures. Esterified fatty acids are present in the myocardium as triacylglycerol, cholesteryl esters, and phosphoglycerides.

Esterification of the three hydroxyl groups of glycerol with fatty acids yields triacylglycerol. In heart tissue di- and mono-esterified glycerols are also found, but to a much lesser extent (Wheeldon *et al.*, 1965; Olsson and Hoeschen, 1967; Lochner *et al.*, 1978).

Phosphoglycerides generally consist of glycerol, of which the hydroxyl groups at the 1 and 2 positions are esterified to fatty acids and at the 3 position to phosphoric acid. The various types of phosphoglycerides present in myocardial tissue are characterized by the alcohol component esterified to the phosphoric acid moiety (Ansell *et al.*, 1973).

Fatty acids esterified to the 3β-hydroxyl group of cholesterol yield cholesteryl esters.

In normoxic dog myocardium, less than 0.1% of the fatty acids are present in the non-esterified form; 0.5% is incorporated in cholesteryl esters, whereas triacylglycerol contains about 14% of myocardial fatty acids. The majority of the fatty acids are incorporated in phosphoglycerides (van der Vusse *et al.*, 1980, 1982b). The relative fatty acid composition of each lipid class in normoxic dog myocardium has been summarized in these reports.

The function of the relatively small amount of cholesteryl esters in myocardial tissue is as yet not clarified. A possible role as endogenous substrate is not feasible. The main function of phosphoglycerides is as essential components of biological membranes. Although phosphoglycerides are subject to a continuous turnover process, the experiments of Crass and Shipp (1972) and Olsson and Hoeschen (1967) provided evidence that phosphoglycerides in heart tissue cannot be considered as a store of fatty acids available for mitochondrial energy production. In general, triacylglycerol is the most likely candidate for the endogenous lipid store.

CELLULAR AND SUBCELLULAR LOCALIZATION OF GLYCOGEN AND LIPIDS

Glycogen

Glycogen is generally present in myocardial tissue in the form of granules with a diameter of 10–40 nm. The granules are localized in abundance in the interstices surrounding the mitochondria, the interfibrillar sarcoplasm, the perinuclear areas, and the areas around subsarcolemmal cisternae. They are also visible in the I-band when the fibres are in the relaxed state. Entman *et al.* (1976) have reported that part of the glycogen is closely associated with the cardiac sarcoplasmic reticulum, together with enzymes linked to glycogenolysis, such as adenylate cyclase, cyclic AMP-dependent protein kinase, phosphorylase kinase, phosphorylase, and 'debrancher' enzyme.

Glycogen is not homogeneously distributed among the various cardiac cells. Jedeikin (1964) reported that the endocardial layers in the right and left ventricles of rabbit hearts contain almost twice the glycogen content of the epicardial layers. The conductive tissue, i.e. bundle of His and Purkinje fibres, contain great amounts of glycogen (Jedeikin, 1964; Crass and Sterrett, 1975).

Lipids

A sarcoplasmic localization of NEFA has to be considered since specific NEFA-binding proteins could be isolated from the cytosolic compartment of the heart (Mishkin *et al.*, 1972; Gloster and Harris, 1977). Attachment of part of the NEFA to other protein and lipid material in granules or membranes cannot be excluded (Wheeldon *et al.*, 1965; Masters and Glaviano, 1972).

Triacylglycerol is thought to be stored in lysosomes and as lipid droplets in the sarcoplasm (Hülsmann and Stam, 1979; Stam *et al.*, 1980). An

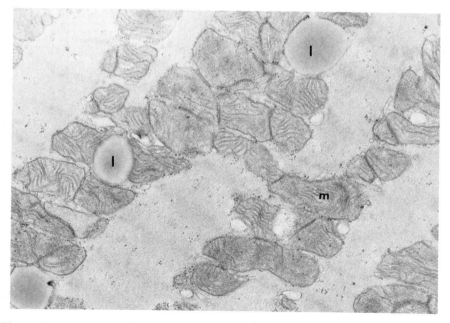

Figure 10.1 Human left ventricle (subepicardium). Lipid droplets (l) are found in between the mitochondria (m). Magnification ×21 450. [Reproduced by courtesy of Dr M. Borgers.]

interstitial localization of substantial amounts of lipid droplets has also been reported (Roy, 1975). Electron micrographs (Figure 10.1) show that the intracellular lipid aggregates are in the vicinity of mitochondria. The diameter of these droplets varies from 0.5 to 1.0 μm. The possibility that endogenous triacylglycerol is also stored in smaller aggregates, not directly discernible in electron micrographs, has to be considered (Masters and Glaviano, 1972).

Triacylglycerol is present in abundance in the left and right auricles of the dog heart, whereas the content tends to be higher in the right than in the left ventricle (Bruce and Myers, 1973). The content of triacylglycerol in the epicardial layers of the free wall of the left ventricle was reported to be about 2.5 times higher than that in the mesocardial and endocardial layers (Leunissen and Piatnek-Leunissen, 1975; Jesmok et al., 1978; Andrieu et al., 1979; van der Vusse et al., 1982b). Since fat is macroscopically visible in the perivascular epicardial regions, the observed transmural gradient of triacylglycerol does not necessarily imply a difference in content of fat between the myocytes of the various layers.

QUANTITATIVE ASPECTS OF GLYCOGEN AND LIPIDS AS ENDOGENOUS SUBSTRATE STORES

Glycogen

Table 10.1 shows that moderate differences in myocardial glycogen content exist within one species. Remarkable differences, however, are present between species. In goldfish and turtle hearts, high amounts of glycogen can be detected, whereas the hearts of mice contain small amounts of this substrate. Elective variations of the extraction technique of glycogen from heart tissue have revealed that these polysaccharides are present in two forms, i.e. free glycogen, which is readily extractable by dilute acids, and protein-bound glycogen. The latter form can be extracted completely by treatment with alkaline solution (Merrick and Meyer, 1954; Russell and Bloom, 1955). The percentage of acid-extractable glycogen appears to be species dependent. Merrick and Meyer (1954) found that the proportion of acid-extractable glycogen present was 100% in goldfish hearts, 87% in dog hearts, 55% in rat hearts, and 19% in mouse hearts.

Lipids

The variation in values of NEFA found by different investigators is noteworthy (Table 10.2). The effects of anesthetics used during the experiments, feeding conditions of the animals, and other unknown differences in

Table 10.1   Content of glycogen in myocardial tissue of various species (micromoles of glucose per gram wet weight)

Species	Area of the heart	Amount	References
Baboon	Left ventricle, epi	55	Opie *et al.* (1976)
	Left ventricle, endo	60	Opie *et al.* (1976)
Dog	Left ventricle, trans	22	Jedeikin (1964)
	Left ventricle, epi	33	Allison *et al.* (1977)
	Left ventricle, endo	43	Allison *et al.* (1977)
	Left ventricle, epi	55	Ichihara and Abiko (1975)
	Left ventricle, endo	69	Ichihara and Abiko (1975)
Goldfish	Total heart	135	Merrick and Meyer (1954)
Guinea-pig	Left ventricle, trans	32	Vincent and Ellis (1963)
Human	Left ventricle, trans	35	van der Vusse (unpublished)
	Left ventricle, trans	42	Lolley *et al.* (1979)
Mouse	Total heart	5	Merrick and Meyer (1954)
Pig	Left ventricle, trans	44	Liedtke *et al.* (1975)
	Left ventricle, trans	55	Salerno and Choing (1980)
Rabbit	Left ventricle, endo	28	Jedeikin (1964)
	Left ventricle, epi	11	Jedeikin (1964)
Rat	Total heart	12	Merrick and Meyer (1954)
	Total heart	19	Evans (1934)
	Left ventricle, trans	20	Jedeikin (1964)
	Total heart	35	Russell and Bloom (1965)
Turtle	Total heart	150	Brachfeld *et al.* (1972)

experimental circumstances are possible causes for the variation of myocardial NEFA content. However, we suggest that improper storage conditions of the biopsies and methods of lipid extraction and unspecific assay systems employed to determined NEFA readily result in an overestimation of NEFA in myocardial tissue (Christie, 1973; Kramer and Hulan, 1978; van der Vusse *et al.*, 1980, 1981).

In contrast with NEFA, no striking discrepancy exists between the values of triacylglycerol as published by different investigators. For rat tissue,

Table 10.2 Content of NEFA in the left ventricle of the dog and rat heart during normoxic circumstances (nanomoles per gram wet weight)

Species	Amount	Assay method	Reference
Dog	29	Gas–liquid chromatography	Van der Vusse *et al.* (1980)
	56	Gas–liquid chromatography	Hunneman *et al.* (1981)
	175	Gas–Liquid chromatography	Weglicki *et al.* (1973)
	900	Gas–liquid chromatography	Weishaar *et al.* (1979)
	1 240	Gas–liquid chromatography	Weishaar *et al.* (1977)
	10 800	Titrimetry	Haider *et al.* (1977)
	11 000	Colorimetry	Andrieu *et al.* (1979)
Rat	45	Colorimetry (after thin-layer chromatography	Garland and Randle (1964)
	90	Gas–liquid chromatography	van der Vusse (unpublished)
	140	Gas–liquid chromatography	Kramer and Hulan (1978)
	500	Gas–liquid-chromotography	Olsson and Hoeschen (1967)
	795	Gas–liquid chromatography	Lochner *et al.* (1978)
	7 000	Gas–liquid chromatography	Houtsmuller *et al.* (1970)
	12 680	Titrimetry	Shipp *et al.* (1964)

0.7–2.3 μmol triacylglycerol (glycerol) per gram of wet weight tissue have been reported (Crass, 1972; Lochner *et al.*, 1978; Kramer and Hulan, 1978). The contents of triacylglycerol in the endo-, meso-, and epicardial layers of dog left ventricle have been found to be 1.5–5.2, 1.0–1.7, and 4.2–9.1 μmol triacylglycerol (glycerol), respectively (Crass and Sterrett, 1975; Jesmok *et al.*, 1978; Andrieu *et al.*, 1979; van der Vusse *et al.*, 1982b).

In the dog, under normal circumstances, the energy requirement per minute is about 45 cal per 100 grams of left ventricle (Neill *et al.*, 1961). Under steady state conditions, uptake of exogenous substrates such as glucose, lactate, pyruvate, and lipids will be sufficient to meet this requirement. However, circumstances such as increased workload and impeded oxygen or substrate supply may give rise to utilization of the endogenous stores of glycogen and lipids. In the case of glycogen, a mean content of 40 μmol glycogen (glucose) per gram of dog left ventricle represents about 28.8 cal (Lehninger, 1970). Theoretically, this amount will be sufficiently high to meet the myocardial energy demands for 62 min.

Triacylglycerol has a high calorie value of about $9\,kcal\,g^{-1}$ (Lehninger, 1970). Assuming a mean triacylglycerol content of $2\,\mu mol$ per gram of myocardial tissue, this amount can meet the energy requirements for 38 min, when the heart has to depend on the oxidation of endogenous fat as sole source for energy delivery. If 30 nmol NEFA per gram approximates the real myocardial NEFA content, this amount represents $0.07\,cal$ per gram of tissue, or energy for less than 10 s of myocardial performance. It is therefore unlikely that NEFAs play a role of quantitative importance as an endogenous substrate store.

SYNTHESIS AND BREAKDOWN OF GLYCOGEN AND TRIACYLGLYCEROL IN MYOCARDIAL TISSUE

Glycogen

The starting point of synthesis of glycogen in heart tissue is the conversion of glucose-6-phosphate to glucose-1-phospate (equation (10.1)). This conversion is catalysed by phosphoglucomutase. Glucose-1-phosphate is metabolized to uridine diphosphoglucose (UDP-glucose), a reaction step controlled by UDP-glucose pyrophosphorylase (equation (10.2)). The glucose moiety of UDP-glucose is subsequently transferred to the glucose residue at the end of an amylose chain. In this reaction step, catalysed by glycogen synthetase, the 4-hydroxyl group of the terminal glucose residue of the polysaccharide chain is coupled to carbon atom 1 of the UDP-glucose molecule, forming the $\alpha(1 \rightarrow 4)$ linkage of glycogen (equation (10.3)). Amylo$(1, 4 \rightarrow 1, 6)$transglucosidase is required to create branching points in the glycogen network. After splitting an oligosaccharide of six or seven glucosyl residues from the end of a polysaccharide chain, an $\alpha(1 \rightarrow 6)$ linkage is made by coupling this terminal oligosaccharide to a 6-hydroxyl group of a glucose moiety of the same or another glucosyl chain.

$$\text{Glucose-6-phosphate} \leftrightharpoons \text{Glucose-1-phosphate} \qquad (10.1)$$

$$\text{Glucose-1-phosphate} + \text{UTP} \leftrightharpoons \text{UDP-glucose} + \text{PP}_i \qquad (10.2)$$

$$\text{UDP-glucose} + (\text{glucose})_n \rightarrow \text{UDP} + (\text{glucose})_{n+1} + \text{H}^+ \qquad (10.3)$$

The first step in the catabolism of glycogen is phosphorolysis of the terminal non-reducing $\alpha(1 \rightarrow 4)$ linkage. This reaction is controlled by glycogen phosphorylase (equation (10.4)). This enzyme does not have the ability to attack $\alpha(1 \rightarrow 6)$ glycoside linkages. When an $\alpha(1 \rightarrow 6)$ linkage has been reached after repetitive removal of glucose residues linked to each other with $\alpha(1 \rightarrow 4)$ bonds, $\alpha(1 \rightarrow 6)$ glucosidase is required for subsequent degradation of the glycogen strain. The enzymatic activity of $\alpha(1 \rightarrow 6)$ glucosidase, hydrolysing the $\alpha(1 \rightarrow 6)$ bonds at the branching points, gives freedom for further breakdown of glycogen by glycogen phosphorylase. After conversion of glucose-1-phosphate to glucose-6-phosphate by phosphoglucomutase (equation (10.5)), the latter substrate becomes available for the glycolytic pathway.

$$(\text{Glucose})_n + \text{HPO}_4^{--} \leftrightharpoons (\text{Glucose})_{n-1} + \text{glucose-1-phosphate}; \quad (10.4)$$

$$\text{Glucose-1-phosphate} \leftrightharpoons \text{Glucose-6-phosphate} \qquad\qquad (10.5)$$

Both the anabolic and catabolic pathways are irreversible in the myocardial cell (Larner, 1976). Reaction (10.4), catalysed by phosphorylase, is freely reversible *in vitro*. In the intracellular environment, the reaction is driven towards glycogen degradation due to the high cytoplasmic concentration of inorganic phosphate relative to that of glucose-1-phosphate. Reaction (10.3), catalysed by glycogen synthetase, has been found to be irreversible both *in vitro* and intracellularly. The reaction is shifted towards synthesis due to neutralization of the H^+ ion produced. Moreover, hydrolysis of the pyrophosphate (PP_i) produced in reaction (10.2) renders this reaction step essentially irreversible.

The key enzyme in the synthesis of glycogen is glycogen synthetase. This enzyme exists in two forms: an inactive phosphorylated D-form and an active dephosphorylated I-form (Figure 10.2). The conversion of the active to the inactive form is ATP dependent and catalysed by glocogen synthetase kinase. Glycogen synthetase kinase itself can be activated by cyclic AMP and hence is under hormonal control. Inactive phosphorylated glycogen synthetase can become enzymatically active in its phosporylated form in the presence of a high intracellular concentration of glucose-6-phosphate and is therefore called the D (dependent) form. Dephosphorylation of the phosphorylated glycogen synthetase is controlled by glycogen synthetase phosphatase.

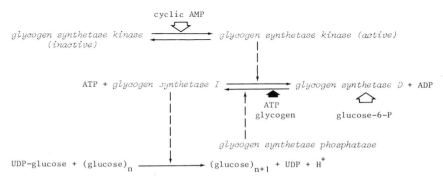

Figure 10.2 Cascade of the regulation of glycogen synthetase activity. Thin broken arrows, conversion controlled by enzyme; open big arrows, enzyme activated by chemical substance; solid big arrows, enzyme inhibited by chemical substance

Breakdown of glycogen is under control of glycogen phosphorlyase. This enzyme can be present in an activated form as phosphorylase *a* and an inactive form as phosphorylase *b*. The conversion of phosphorylase *a* into the *b* form is controlled by phosphorylase phosphatase. The conversion of the phosphorylase *b* into the *a* form is activated by phosphorylase kinase in an ATP-dependent reaction. The enzymatic activity of phosphorylase *b* kinase is controlled by another protein kinase, i.e. phosphorylase *b* kinase kinase, which is subjected to hormonal regulation via cyclic AMP. The cascade of the regulation of phosphorylase activity is depicted in Figure 10.3. The significance of these enzyme cascades in cellular metabolic processes and phosphorylation–dephosphorylation of enzymes has been surveyed in detail by Chock *et al.* (1980) and Krebs and Beavo (1979).

The activities of the enzymes involved in the regulation of the actual rate of glycogen synthesis or breakdown are controlled by hormonal as well as intracellular mechanisms. The advantages of this dual control mechanism have been discussed in detail by Newsholme (1965). Extracellular hormones transfer both glycogen synthetase and glycogen phosphorylase into a form which becomes less sensitive to intracellular, metabolically regulated control mechanisms. In the absence of hormonal stimuli, the rates of synthesis and degradation of glycogen are subject to the control exerted by the intracellular concentration of various metabolic intermediates.

Under normoxic conditions, about 90% of glycogen synthetase is present in the D-form (Opie, 1968). The activity of this form is strongly dependent on a high intracellular glucose-6-phosphate concentration. Intracellular factors such as high ATP and high glycogen contents seem to keep glycogen synthetase in its D-form. After administration of insulin, over 75% of the glycogen synthetase was found to be in the I-form. This form is enzymatically active, irrespective of the cytoplasmic glucose-6-phosphate concentration. The conversion of the active I-form to the inactive D-form is thought to be regulated by catecholamine activity via cyclic AMP-stimulated synthetase I kinase.

Although, in liver, glucagon stimulates the conversion of the I-form of glycogen synthetase into the D-form, there is no substantial evidence that myocardial glycogen formation is regulated by this pancreatic hormone. On the other hand, the inotropic properties of glucagon have been clearly established (Kruty *et al.*, 1978).

Besides conversion of phosphorylase *b* into the *a* form, phosphorylase *b* can be directly activated by intracellular AMP by increasing the affinity of phosphorylase *b* for its substrates P_i and glycogen (Opie, 1968). Phosphorylase *b* activity is inhibited by ATP, ADP, and glucose-6-phosphate at physiological concentrations in the normoxic cell. This glycogen-degrading enzyme can escape from inhibition by ATP and glucose-6-phosphate by conversion into phosphorylase *a*. This conversion is stimulated by thyroid

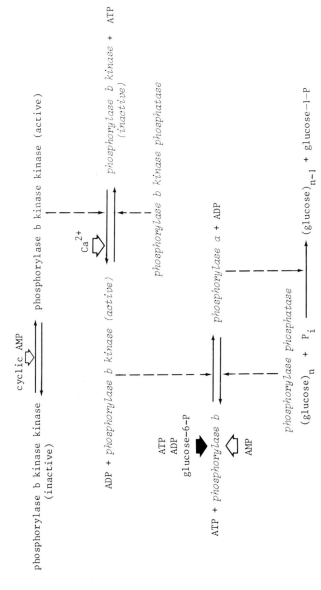

Figure 10.3   Cascade of the regulation of glycogen phosphorylase activity. See Figure 10.3 for key

hormones, glucagon, and catecholamines through increased intracellular cyclic AMP levels (Sutherland and Rall, 1968). In contrast with liver, intracellular calcium ions attached to calmodulin will stimulate the conversion of phosphorylase *b* into the *a* form in cardiac cells (Klee *et al.*, 1980; Walsh *et al.*, 1980). Moreover, Namm *et al.* (1968) and Dobson *et al.* (1976) have shown that the presence of Ca^{++} is also essential in the action of catecholamines on cardiac glycogen phosphorylase activity.

Triacylglycerol

Triacylglycerol is synthesized in heart muscle cells from glycerol 3-phosphate (or α-glycerol phosphate) and fatty acyl-CoA. The overall reaction is given in equation (10.6). In general, glycerol 3-phosphate is generated from dihydroxyacetone phosphate in an NADH-dependent reaction catalysed by cytoplasmic glycerol phosphate dehydrogenase (equation (10.7)). Dihydroxyacetone phosphate is an intermediate in the glycolytic pathway. Glycerol 3-phosphate can also be produced by direct phosphorylation of glycerol (equation (10.8)). The latter reaction is catalysed by glycerol kinase (Robinson and Newsholme, 1967).

Prior to esterification, NEFAs have to be coupled to coenzyme A by the action of fatty acid CoA synthetase (equation (10.9)). The free hydroxyl groups of glycerol-3-phosphate are acylated with fatty acyl-CoA by the action of glycerophosphate acyltransferase to form phosphatidic acid, an important intermediate in the synthesis of both triacylglycerol and phosphoglycerides (equation (10.10)). Subsequent hydrolysis of the phosphate group at the 3 position by phosphatidate phosphohydrolase yields diacyl glycerol (equation (10.11)).

The third free hydroxyl group of the glycerol residue is now attacked by fatty acyl-CoA to form triacylglycerol (equation (10.12)).

$$\text{L-Glycerol-3-phosphate} + 3\text{ acyl-CoA} \rightarrow \text{Triacylglycerol} + 3\text{ CoASH} + P_i; \tag{10.6}$$

$$\text{Dihydroxyacetone phosphate} + \text{NADH} + H^+ \leftrightharpoons \text{L-Glycerol-3-phosphate} + NAD^+; \tag{10.7}$$

$$\text{ATP} + \text{glycerol} \rightarrow \text{L-Glycerol-3-phosphate} + \text{ADP}; \tag{10.8}$$

$$\text{Fatty acid} + \text{CoASH} + \text{ATP} \rightarrow \text{Fatty acid CoA} + \text{AMP} + PP_i; \tag{10.9}$$

$$2\text{ Fatty acid CoA} + \text{L-glycerol-3-phosphate} \rightarrow \text{L-Phosphatidic acid} + 2\text{ CoASH}; \tag{10.10}$$

$$\text{L-Phosphatidic acid} + H_2O \rightarrow \text{Diacylglycerol} + P_i; \tag{10.11}$$

$$\text{Diacylglycerol} + \text{fatty acyl CoA} \rightarrow \text{Triacylglycerol} + \text{CoASH}. \tag{10.12}$$

Release of fatty acids stored in triacylglycerol is accelerated by the action of triacyglycerol lipase (equation (10.13)). Hydrolysis, of diacylglycerol to monoacylglycerol and subsequently glycerol, will yield two additional fatty acids (equations (10.14) and (10.15)). Reaction step (10.13) has been considered to be the rate-limiting step in overall lipolysis. A variety of lipolytic enzymes are involved in the stepwide degradation of myocardial triacylglycerol (Severson, 1979a,b).

$$\text{Triacylglycerol} + H_2O \rightarrow \text{Diacylglycerol} + \text{fatty acid;} \qquad (10.13)$$

$$\text{Diacylglycerol} + H_2O \rightarrow \text{Monoacylglycerol} + \text{fatty acid} \qquad (10.14)$$

$$\text{Monoacylglycerol} + H_2O \rightarrow \text{Glycerol} + \text{fatty acid.} \qquad (10.15)$$

The synthesis of triacylglycerol in the myocardium is likely to be regulated by the intracellular NEFA concentration. High concentrations of NEFA have been found to exert deleterious effects on, for instance, enzymes in the glycolytic pathway, Na^+,K^+-stimulated ATPase and adenine nucleotide translocase (see, for a review, Katz and Messineo, 1981; van der Vusse, 1983), This can be avoided by channelling these fatty acids to triacylglycerol. A direct hormonal effect on cardiac triacylglycerol formation has not been described.

Both exogenous and endogenous catecholamines and glucagon are proposed to stimulate myocardial lipolysis. (Severson, 1979a), mediated by adenylate cyclase, cyclic AMP, and protein kinase (Keely *et al.*, 1975) and simulated by dibutyryl cyclic AMP, (Gartner and Vahouny, 1972; Crass, 1973). Hron *et al.* (1977) found that hormone-stimulated lipolysis in the perfused rat heart is dependent on extracellular calcium ions. Under inotropic stimulation, triacylglycerol utilization may be enhanced indirectly due to an increased demand for oxidizable substrates. Hülsmann and Stam (1979) have recently proposed that enhanced activation and subsequent oxidation of NEFAs will prevent product inhibition of the lipolytic enzymes and give rise to accelerated degradation of triacylgycerol.

DYNAMIC CHARACTERISTICS OF THE SUBSTRATE STORES

Glycogen

No successful determinations of glycogen turnover rate in myocardial tissue have been described. A glycogen turnover rate of approximately 5 h can be calculated from studies of Crass *et al.* (1969) and Chain *et al.* (1969). This turnover rate, however, is a rough approximation. It remains uncertain whether all glucose moieties of myocardial glycogen are involved in the turnover process. Only the outer branches of the polysaccharide chains and the acid-extractable glycogen forms may be metabolically active (Russell and Bloom, 1955). Glycogen in isolated heart preparations depletes even in the presence of exogenous substrates (Crass and Pieper, 1975). Extrapolation to the heart *in situ* under more physiological conditions should therefore be carried out with caution.

Triacylglycerol

The half-life time of ^{14}C-labelled palmitate in the triacylglycerol pool of dog hearts *in situ* was found to be about 40 min (Crass, 1979). Assuming a homogeneous distribution of the labelled fatty acid over all triacylglycerol molecules in myocardial tissue, the turnover of the triacylglycerol pool will be of the same order of magnitude. However slower and faster metabolizing stores may be present.

The fate of labelled palmitate injected into the coronary artery of dog hearts *in situ* is rapid incorporation in the endogenous triacylglycerol stores (Crass, 1979; Klein *et al.*, 1979), suggesting that a considerable amount of [^{14}C]palmitate was found back in the esterified form instead of being oxidized. This result confirms the earlier findings of Scheuer and Brachfeld (1966) in isolated dog hearts. Kong and Friedberg (1971) suggested that about half of the fatty acids taken up by the heart *in situ* is promptly delivered to the site of oxidation. Results of experiments with isolated rat hearts perfused with labelled NEFA, however, are less indicative that the majority of NEFA has been chemically bound prior to oxidation (Stein and Stein, 1963; Whitmer *et al.*, 1978).

GLYCOGEN AND LIPIDS UNDER HYPOXIC AND ISCHAEMIC CONDITIONS

Reduction of oxygen supply to the heart *in vivo* as well as *in vitro* results in an impaired myocardial performance and in changes in carbohydrate and lipid metabolism in the myocardial cells. In general, the effect of oxygen restriction on myocardial substrate stores is considered as depletion of glycogen and accumulation of triacylglycerol. This generalized concept will be discussed in more detail.

In dog hearts *in situ*, acute reduction of myocardial blood flow by stenosis of a coronary artery almost immediately causes cessation of fibre shortening in the endocardial layers of the left ventricle (Prinzen, 1982). Approximately 20 s later, the fibre shortening in the epicardial layers is also affected. Reduction of endo- and epicardial glycogen content, however, could not be detected before 10 min of ischaemia. Reduction of the myocardial glycogen content continued during prolonged ischaemia. After 2 h, the epi- and endocardial levels were found to be 65 and 35% of their corresponding pre-ischaemic values respectively (Prinzen, 1982). Thus, impairment of myocardial performance during the shortage of oxygen cannot be due to depletion of the myocardial polycarbohydrate stores (Rovetto, 1979), at least in the first 2 h.

The trigger for enhanced glycogen breakdown under ischaemic conditions is not fully elucidated. Activation of the phosphorylase system can be achieved during ischaemia by activation of phosphorylase *b* due to changed intracellular concentration of regulating agents, and an accelerated conversion of phosphorylase *b* into the active *a* form. An increase in the activity of phosphorylase *b* can be caused by elevation of the sarcoplasmic concentration of inorganic phosphate and AMP, as well as reduced ATP and glucose 6-phosphate concentrations (Opie, 1968). Wollenberger and Krause (1968) have shown that in dog myocardium phosphorylase *b* activity increased within 1 min of the onset of ischaemia. The findings of Opie (1976) that, in dog myocardial tissue, the contents of inorganic phosphate and AMP were significantly raised and of ATP significantly decreased after 1 min of ischaemia, supports the observation of an early activation of phosphorylase *b*.

Conversion of phosphorylase *b* into the enzymatically active *a* form in ischaemic myocardial tissue has been reported by Wollenberger and Krause (1968), Kübler and Spieckermann (1970), Hough and Gevers (1975), and Sakai and Abiko (1981). As has been discussed earlier, this conversion is controlled by phosphorylase *b* kinase (Figure 10.3). The latter enzyme is activated by Ca^{++} (Drummond and Duncan, 1966) or indirectly by cyclic AMP. Drummond and Duncan (1966) were able to activate cardiac phosphorylase *b* kinase by Ca^{++} in a highly purified preparation, devoid of natural endogenous inhibitors of the calcium ion effect, but no conclusive evidence has been published that cytoplasmic Ca^{++} rises in the early ischaemic phase (Shen and Jennings, 1972).

The hypothesis that glycogenolysis is activated by elevated cytoplasmic cyclic AMP concentrations, due to release of endogenous catecholamines during ischaemia, is supported by a variety of experimental findings (Wollenberger and Shahab, 1965; De Leiris *et al.*, 1975). Podzuweit *et al.* (1978) have disputed the crucial role of intracellular cyclic AMP in the rapid transition from aerobic to anaeorbic metabolism with the onset of myocardial ischaemia. Since these authors were studying merely tissue samples of the epicardial layers in which no change in cyclic AMP content could be detected during 60 min of ischaemia, transmural gradients may have been overlooked.

Rovetto *et al.* (1973) have reported that the rate of glycogen utilization is much faster in anoxic rat hearts, perfused with oxygen-free fluid than in flow-restricted (ischaemic) hearts presumably because the latter are associated with accumulation of tissue lactate and with a decreased intracellular pH. Conn *et al.* (1959) have shown that the acid-extractable form of glycogen becomes depleted in isolated anoxic dog hearts, without any change in the content of the non-acid-extractable glycogen.

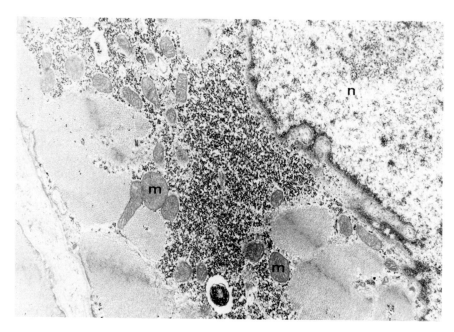

Figure 10.4 Human left ventricle (subendocardium). Glycogen is abundantly present near the nucleus (n) and around the mitochondria (m) of a cell derived from an akinetic wall. Magnification × 15 425. [Reproduced by courtesy of Dr M. Borgers.]

Hardly any data are available concerning the behaviour of myocardial glycogen under chronic ischaemic conditions. Electron microscopic examination of biopsies taken from hypo- and akinetic left ventricular walls of patients undergoing aorto-coronary bypass surgery revealed a large percentage of cells adapted to the oxygen-limited situation. These cells were characterized by a partial loss of sarcomeres, sarcoplasmic reticulum, and T-tubules, the presence of numerous small mitochondria, and an increased amount of glycogen-like material (Figure 10.4) (Flameng *et al.*, 1981a).

Accumulation of endogenous triacyglycerol seems to be a late phenomenon during myocardial ischaemia. Histochemical evaluation of experimentally infarcted dog myocardium demonstrated that no abnormal accumulation of fat occurred for as long as 1 h after ligation of a coronary artery (Wartman *et al.*, 1956). After 6 h of ischaemia, marked accumulation was observed which persisted as long as 2 weeks. On the basis of biochemical determination of endogenous fat, Jesmok *et al.* (1978) reported that in the ischaemic region subepicardial triacylglycerol decreased 30 min after the onset of ischaemia. However, ischaemia did not influence the triacylglycerol content of subepi-, meso-, and subendocardial layers between 1 and 2 h after ligation of a coronary artery (Jesmok *et al.*, 1978; van der Vusse *et al.*, 1982b). After 4 h, endogenous triacylglycerol was found to be increased in the ischaemic area (Bruce and Myers, 1973; Crass and Sterrett, 1975; Jesmok *et al.*, 1978). With respect to the transmural accumulation, the published results are at variance. Crass and Sterrett (1975) reported a greatly enhanced subendocardial accumulation. In contrast, Jesmok *et al.* (1978) found a marked increase in the subepicardial layers.

Experimental findings of Crass *et al.* (1976) and Crass (1976) support the idea of impaired lypolytic activity. This is not due to feedback inhibition by NEFA and acyl-CoA in the early phase of ischaemia because Prinzen (1982) has shown that in the ischaemic region NEFA does not accumulate until after 10 min of coronary artery stenosis. Tissue acyl-CoA increases rapidly after inducement of ischaemia (Whitmer *et al.*, 1978). Although the authors did not prove it, they claimed that the rise in acyl-CoA occurred mainly in the mitochondrial matrix. As a consequence, these fatty acids derivatives are not available for inhibition of sarcoplasmic and lysosomal lipase activity.

Previous studies of Scheuer and Brachfeld (1966) suggest an accelerated rate of intracellular esterification of the extracted NEFA in myocardial triacylglycerol under ischaemic circumstances. Opie *et al.* (1973) have reported that NEFA competed unfavourably with glucose for the residual oxygen in ischaemic dog hearts. As a consequence, the availability of intracellular NEFA or their derivatives for esterification will increase. The sarcoplasmic concentrations of α-glycerol phosphate, a key precursor for triacylglycerol formation, has been found to increase several-fold in the early ischaemic phase (Kübler and Spieckermann, 1970; Opie, 1976; Liedtke, 1981). The observation of a virtually unchanged net content of triacylglycerol during the first 2 h of ischaemia, despite rapidly increased key precursor products, is consonant with the concept that α-glycerol phosphate and acyl-CoA are localized in different compartments (Liedtke, 1981). Access of acyl-CoA, for instance, after loss of integrity of the mitochondrial inner membranes, to α-glycerol and the triacylglycerol synthesizing enzyme machinery will give rise to the readily observed lipid accumulation during prolonged oxygen deprivation of myocardial tissue.

GLYCOGEN AND MYOCARDIAL PROTECTION DURING OPEN-HEART SURGERY

Precise repair of intracardiac defects and performance of aorto-coronary artery bypass grafts require a quiet and practically bloodless operating field. To this purpose, cross-clamping of the ascending aorta is generally applied, resulting in an ischaemically arrested heart, whereas the systemic blood supply is sustained by extracorporeal circulation. Various biochemical, physical, and pharmacological manipulations have been proposed to minimize the possible hazards of ischaemia for the heart under these circumstances.

Lolley *et al.* (1979) have postulated the importance of pre-operative myocardial glycogen levels in cardiac preservation; this effect may be additive to potassium chloride cardioplegia (Lolley *et al.*, 1979). However functional recovery of the heart is good after complete anoxic arrest in combination with cold, high potassium-containing cardioplegic solutions, despite virtually unaffected myocardial glycogen content (Ellis *et al.*, 1977; Salerno and Choing, 1980; Roberts *et al.*, 1980; Grover *et al.*, 1981; van der Vusse *et al.*, 1982a).

The situation will be different during anoxic cardiac arrest at higher myocardial temperatures when electromechanical activity is still present and a considerable energy requirement will exist. Utilization of endogenous glycogen in ischaemically arrested hearts has been established in animals (Hewitt *et al.*, 1974; Ellis *et al.*, 1977; Levitsky *et al.*, 1977; Tyers *et al.*, 1977; Grover *et al.*, 1981) and humans (Flameng *et al.*, 1981b; van der Vusse *et al.*, 1982a) at temperatures ranging from 25 to 34 °C. At these temperatures, Hewitt *et al.* (1974) found a better functional recovery of dog hearts with high pre-ischaemic glycogen levels.

Biochemical, ultrastructural, and functional variables have been suggested and applied as indices to study the efficacy of myocardial protection during open-heart surgery (Hearse *et al.*, 1981). Indications from animal studies (Ellis *et al.*, 1977; Roberts *et al.*, 1980; Salerno and Choing, 1980; Grover *et al.*, 1981) that myocardial glycogen utilization is a sensitive marker for the ischaemic process during elective ischaemic arrest prompted us to employ this biochemical index in the clinical setting (Flameng *et al.*, 1981b; van der Vusee *et al.*, 1982a). We found that, in the human heart, the myocardial glycogen content decreases during the inevitable period of ischaemia. Therefore the glycogen content was used for evaluation of the efficacy of cardio-protective manipulations. Glycogen is readily detectable in small biopsies (about 2–3 mg dry weight) with a fluorometric technique for the determination of the glucose moieties in the polycarbohydrate chains. The drawback of the large intra-individual variation (ranging from 90 to 300 μmol glucose per gram dry weight of tissue) can be overcome by assessment of glycogen in both pre- and post-ischaemic biopsies, using the patient as his or her own control (G. J. van der Vusse *et al.*, manuscript in preparation). Determination of glycogen as well as 'high energy' phosphates in myocardial biopsies enables us to conclude that cold, high potassium cardioplegia is superior to intermittent aortic cross-clamping in myocardial preservation of patients undergoing extensive aorto-coronary bypass grafting (van der Vusse *et al.*, 1982a).

ACKNOWLEDGEMENTS

The authors are greatly indebted to Mrs Els Geurts for her help in preparing this manuscript.

REFERENCES

Allison, T. B., Ramey, C. A., and Holsinger, J. W. (1977). Transmural gradients of left ventricular tissue metabolites after circumflex artery ligation in dogs. *J. Mol. Cell. Cardiol.*, **9**, 837–852.

Andrieu, J. L., Vial, C., Font, B., Goldschmidt, D., Lievre, M., and Faucon, G. (1979). Myocardial biochemical modifications induced by theophylline with reference to its value as antianginal drug. *Arch. Internat. Pharmacodyn.*, **237**, 330–342.

Ansell, G. B., Hawthorne, J. N., and Dawson, R. M. C. (1973). *Form and Function of Phospholipids*, BBA Library, vol. 3, Elsevier, Amsterdam.

Brachfeld, N., Ohtaka, Y., Klein, I., and Kawada, M. (1972). Substrate preference and metabolic activity of the aerobic and the hypoxic turtle heart. *Circulation Res.*, **31**, 453–467.

Bruce, T. A., and Myers, J. T. (1973). Myocardial lipid metabolism in ischemia and infarction. *Recent Advanc. Stud. Cardiac Struct. Metab.*, **3**, 773–780.

Chain, E. B., Mansford, K. R. L., and Opie, L. H. (1969). Effects of insulin on the pattern of glucose metabolism in the perfused working and Langendorff heart of normal and insulin-deficient rats. *Biochem. J.*, **115**, 537–546.

Chock, P. B., Rhee, S. G., and Stadtman, E. R. (1980). Interconvertible enzyme cascades in cellular regulation. *Annu. Rev. Biochem.*, **49**, 813–843.

Christie, W. W. (1973). *Lipid Analysis*, Pergamon Press, Oxford.

Conn, H. L., Wood, J. C., and Morales, G. S. (1959). Rate of change in myocardial glycogen and lactic acid following arrest of coronary circulation. *Circulation Res.*, **7**, 721–727.

Crass, M. F., III (1972). Exogenous substrate effects on endogenous lipid metabolism in the working rat heart. *Biochim. Biophys. Acta* **280**, 71–81.

Crass, M. F., III (1973). Heart triglycerides and glycogen metabolism: effects of catecholamines, dibutyryl cyclic AMP, theophylline and fatty acids. *Recent Advanc. Stud. Cardiac Struct. Metab.*, **3**, 275–290.

Crass, M. F., III (1979). Myocardial triacylglycerol metabolism in ischemia. *Texas Rep. Biol. Med.*, **39**, 439–452.

Crass, M. F., III and Pieper, G. M. (1975). Lipid and glycogen metabolism in the hypoxic heart: effects of epinephrine. *Amer. J. Physiol.*, **299**, 885–889.

Crass, M. F., III, and Shipp, J. C. (1972). Metabolism of exogenous and endogenous fatty acids in heart muscle. *Recent Advanc. Stud. Cardiac Struct. Metab.*, **1**, 115–126.

Crass, M. F., III, and Sterrett, P. R. (1975). Distribution of glycogen and lipids in the ischemic canine left ventricle: biochemical and light and electron microscopic correlates. *Recent Advanc. Stud. Cardiac Struct. Metab.*, **10**, 251–263.

Crass, M. F., III, McCaskill, E. S., and Shipp, J. C. (1969). Effect of pressure development on glucose and palmitate metabolism in perfused heart. *Amer. J. Physiol.*, **216**, 1569–1576.

Crass, M. F., III, Shipp, J. C., and Pieper, G. M. (1976). Utilization of endogenous lipids and glycogen in the perfused rat heart: effects of hypoxia and epinephrine. *Recent Advanc. Stud. Cardiac Struct. Metabl.*, **7**, 219–224.

De Leiris, J., Begue, J. M., Gauduel, Y., and Feuvray, D. (1979). Lesions cellulaires précoces induites par l'hypoxie myocardique: rôle éventuel de l'AMP cyclique. *J. Physiol. (Paris)*, **76**, 813–819.

Dobson, J. G., Ross, J., and Mayer, S. E. (1976). The role of cyclic adenosine 3′,5′-monophosphate and calcium in the regulations of contractility and glycogen phosphorylase activity in guinea pig papillary muscle. *Circulation Res.*, **39**, 388–395.

Drummond, G. I., and Duncan, L. (1966). The action of calcium ion on cardiac phosphorylase *b* kinase. *J. Biol. Chem.*, **241**, 3097–3103.

Drummond, G. I., and Duncan, L. (1966). The action of calcium ion on cardiac phosphorylase *b* kinase. *J. Biol. Chem.*, **241**, 3097–3103.

Ellis, R. J., Pryor, W., and Ebert, P. A. (1977). Advantages of potassium cardioplegia and perfusion hypothermia in left ventricular hypertrophy. *Ann. Thorac. Surg.*, **24**, 299–306.

Entman, M. L., Kaniike, K., Goldstein, M. A., Nelson, T. E., Bornet, E. P., Futch, T. W., and Schwartz, A. (1976). Association of glycogenolysis with cardiac sarcoplasmic reticulum. *J. Biol. Chem.*, **251**, 3140–3146.

Evans, G. (1934). The glycogen content of the rat heart. *J. Physiol.*, **82**, 368–480.

Flameng, W., Suy, R., Schwarz, F., Borgers, M., Piessens, J., Thoné, F., Van Ermen, H., and De Geest, H. (1981a). Ultrastructural correlates of left ventricular contraction abnormalities in patients with chronic ischemic heart disease: determinants of reversible segmental asynergy postrevascularization surgery. *Amer. Heart J.*, **102**, 846–857.

Flameng, W., van der Vusse, G. J., Borgers, M., De Meyere, R., and Suy, R. (1981b). Intermittent aortic crossclamping at 32°C, a safe technique for multiple aortocoronary bypass grafting. *Thorac. Cardiovasc. Surg.*, **29**, 216–222.

Garland, P. B., and Randle, P. J. (1964). Regulation of glucose uptake by muscle. *Biochem. J.*, **93**, 678–687.

Gartner, S. L., and Vahouny, G. V. (1972). Effects of epinephrine and cyclic 3′,5′-AMP on perfused rat hearts. *Amer. J. Physiol.*, **222**, 1121–1124.

Gloster, J., and Harris, P. (1977). Fatty acid binding to cytoplasmic proteins of myocardium and red and white skeletal muscle in the rat. A possible new role for myoglobin. *Biochem. Biophys. Res. Commun.*, **74**, 506–513.

Grover, F. L., Fewel, J. G., Ghidoni, J. J., and Trinkle, J. K. (1981). Does lower systemic temperature enhance cardioplegic myocardial protection? *J. Thorac. Cardiovasc. Surg.*, **81**, 11–20.

Haider, B., Ahmed, S. S., Moschos, C. B., Oldewurtel, H. A., and Regan, T. R. (1977). Myocardial function and coronary blood flow response to acute ischemia in chronic canine diabetes. *Circulation Res.*, **40**, 577–584.

Hearse, D. J., Braimbridge, M. V., and Jynge, P. (1981). *Protection of the Ischemic Myocardium: Cardioplegia*, Raven Press, New York.

Hewitt, R. L., Lolley, D. M., Adrouny, G. A., and Drapanas, T. (1974). Protective effect of glycogen and glucose on the anoxic arrested heart. *Surgery*, **75**, 1–10.

Hough, F. S., and Gevers, W. (1975). Catecholamine release as mediator of intracellular activation in ischemic perfused rat hearts. *South Afr. Med. J.*, **49**, 538–543.

Houtsmuller, U. M. T., Struyk, C. B., and Van der Beek, A. (1970). Decrease in rate of ATP synthesis of isolated rat heart mitochondria induced by dietary erucic acid. *Biochim. Biophys. Acta*, **218**, 564–566.

Hron, W. T., Jesmok, G. J., Lombardo, J. B., Menahan, L. A., and Lech, J. J. (1977). Calcium dependency of hormone stimulated lipolysis in the perfused rat heart. *J. Mol. Cell. Cardiol.*, **9**, 733–748.

Hülsmann, W. C., and Stam, H. (1979). Lipolysis in heart and adipose tissue: effects of inhibition of glycogenolysis and uncoupling of oxidative phosphorylation. *Biochem. Biophys. Res. Commun.*, **88**, 867–872.

Hunneman, D. H., Schweickhardt, C., Gebhard, M. M., Preusse, C. J., and Bretschneider, H. J. (1981). Intramyocardial FFA concentration after treatment with verapamil. *Pflügers Arch. Europ. J. Physiol.*, Suppl., **391**, R12.

Ichihara, K. and Abiko, Y. (1975). Differences between endocardial and epicardial utilization of glycogen in the ischemic heart. *Amer. J. Physiol.*, **229**, 1585–1589.

Jedeikin, L. A. (1964). Regional distribution of glycogen and phosphorylase in the ventricles of the heart. *Circulation Res.*, **14**, 202–211.

Jesmok, G. J., Warltier, D. C., Gross, G. J., and Hardman, H. F. (1978). Transmural triglycerides in acute myocardial ischaemia. *Cardiovasc. Res.*, **12**, 659–665.

Katz, A. M., and Messineo, F. C. (1981). Lipid–membrane interactions and the pathogenesis of ischemic damage in the myocardium, *Circulation Res.*, **48**, 1–46.

Keely, S., Corbin, J. D., and Park, C. R. (1975). Regulation of adenosine 3′,5′-monophosphate-dependent protein kinase. Regulation of the heart enzyme by epinephrine, glucagon, insulin and 1-methyl-3-isobutylxanthine. *J. Biol. Chem.*, **250**, 4832–4840.

Klee, C. B., Crouch, T. H., and Richman, P. G. (1980). Calmodulin. *Annu. Rev. Biochem.*, **49**, 489–515.

Klein, M. S., Goldstein, R. A., Welch, M. J., and Sobel, B. E. (1979). External assessment of myocardial metabolism with ^{11}C-palmitate in rabbit hearts. *Amer. J. Physiol.*, **237**, H51–H57.

Kong, Y., and Friedberg, S. J. (1971). Rapid intracoronary radiopalmitate injection and myocardial fatty acid oxidation. *Metabolism*, **20**, 681–690.

Kramer, J. K. G., and Hulan, H. W. (1978). A comparison of procedures to determine free fatty acids in rat heart. *J. Lipid Res.*, **19**, 103–106.

Krebs, E. G., and Beavo, J. A. (1979). Phosphorylation–dephosphorylation of enzymes. *Annu. Rev. Biochem.*, **48**, 923–959.

Kruty, F., Gvozdjak, A., Bada, V., Niederland, T. R., Gvodzdjak, J., and Kaplan, M. (1978). The effect of glucagon on the heart muscle: relation between metabolic processes and contractility. *Biochem. Pharmacol.*, **27**, 2153–2155.

Kübler, W., and Spieckermann, P. G. (1970). Regulation of glycolysis in the ischaemic and anoxic myocardium. *J. Mol. Cell. Cardiol.*, **1**, 351–377.

Larner, J. (1976). Mechanism of regulation of glycogen synthesis and degradation. *Circulation Res.*, **38**, suppl. 1, 2–7.

Lehninger, A. L. (1970). *Biochemistry*, Worth, New York.

Leunissen, R. L. A., and Piatnek-Leunissen, D. A. (1975). Transmural metabolic gradients of the canine left ventricle in coronary constriction, systemic hypoxia, hemorrhagic shock and isoproterenol infusion. *Recent Advanc. Stud. Cardiac Struct. Metab.*, **6**, 145–150.

Levitsky, S., Wright, R. N., Rao, K. S., Holland, C., Roper, K., Engelman, R., and Feinberg, H. (1977). Does intermittent coronary perfusion offer greater myocardial protection than continuous aortic crossclamping? *Surgery*, **82**, 51–59.

Liedtke, A. J., Hughes, H. C., and Neely, J. R. (1975). Metabolic responses to varying restrictions of coronary blood flow in swine. *Amer. J. Physiol.*, **228**, 655–662.

Liedtke, A. J. (1981). Alterations of carbohydrate and lipid metabolism in the acutely ischemic heart. *Prog. Cardiovasc. Dis.*, **23**, 321–336.

Lochner, A., Kotze, J. C. N., Benade, A. J. S., and Gevers, W. (1978). Mitochondrial oxidative phosphorylation in low-flow hypoxia: role of free fatty acids. *J. Mol. Cell. Cardiol.*, **10**, 857–875.

Lolley, D. M., Ray, J. F., III, Myers, W. O., Sautter, R. D., and Tewksbury, D. A. (1979). Importance of preoperative myocardial glycogen levels in human cardiac preservation. *J. Thorac. Cardiovasc. Surg.*, **78**, 678–687.

Masters, T. N., and Glaviano, V. V. (1972). The effects of norepinephrine and propranolol on myocardial subcellular distribution of triglycerides and free fatty acids. *J. Pharmacol. Exp. Ther.*, **182**, 246–255.

Merrick, A. W., and Meyer, D. K. (1954). Glycogen fractions of cardiac muscle in the normal and anoxic heart. *Amer. J. Physiol.*, **177**, 441–443.

Mishkin, S., Stein, L., Gatmaitan, Z., and Artias, I. M. (1972). The binding of fatty acids to cytoplasmic proteins: binding to Z protein in liver and other tissue of the rat. *Biochem. Biophys. Res. Commun.*, **47**, 997–1003.

Namm, D. H., Mayer, S. E., and Maltbie, M. (1968). The role of potassium and calcium on the effect of epinephrine on cardiac cyclic adenosine 3',5'-monophosphate, phosphorylase kinase and phosphorylase. *J. Mol. Pharmacol.*, **4**, 522–530.

Neill, W. A., Levine, H. J., Wagman, R. J., Messer, J. V., Krasnow, N., and Gorlin, R. (1961). Left ventricular heat production measured by coronary flow and temperature gradient. *J. Appl. Physiol.*, **16**, 883–890.

Newsholme, E. A. (1965). Regulation of enzyme activity. *Sci. Prog.* **52**, 237–255.

Olsson, R. E., and Hoeschen, R. J. (1967). Utilization of endogenous lipid by the isolated perfused rat heart. *Biochem. J.*, **103**, 796–801.

Opie, L. H. (1968). Metabolism of the heart in health and disease. Part I. *Amer. Heart J.*, **76**, 685–698.

Opie, L. H. (1976). Effects of regional ischemia on metabolism of glucose and fatty acids. *Circulation Res.*, **38**, Suppl. 1, 52–74.

Opie, L. H., Owen, P., and Riemersma, R. S. (1973). Relative rates of oxidation of glucose and free fatty acids by ischaemic and non-ischaemic myocardium after coronary artery ligation in the dog. *Europ. J. Clin. Invest.*, **3**, 419–435.

Opie, L. H., Owen, P., and Lubbe, W. (1976). Estimated glycolytic flux in infarcting heart. *Recent Advanc. Stud. Cardiac Struct. Metab.*, **7**, 249–255.

Podzuweit, T., Dalby, A. J., Cherry, G. W., and Opie, L. H. (1978). Cyclic AMP levels in ischaemic and non-ischaemic myocardium following coronary artery ligation: relation to ventricular fibrillation. *J. Mol. Cell. Cardiol.*, **10**, 81–94.

Prinzen, F. W. (1982). Gradients in blood flow, mechanics and metabolism in the ischemic left ventricular wall of the dog. Thesis, University of Limburg, Maastricht, The Netherlands.

Roberts, A. J., Abel, R. M., Alonso, D. R., Subramanian, V. A., Paul, J. S., and Gay, W. A. (1980). Advantages of hypothermic potassium cardioplegia and superiority of continuous versus intermittent aortic crossclamping. *J. Thorac. Cardiovasc. Surg.*, **79**, 44–58.

Robinson, J., and Newsholme, E. A. (1967). Glycerol kinase activities in rat heart and adipose tissue. *Biochem. J.*, **104**, 2c–4c.

Rovetto, M. J., Whitmer, J. T., and Neely, J. R. (1973). Comparison of the effects of anoxia and whole heart ischemia on carbohydrate utilizaton in isolated working rat hearts. *Circulation Res.*, **32**, 699–710.

Rovetto, M. J. (1979). Energy metabolism in the ischemic heart. *Texas Report Biol. Med.*, **39**, 397–407.

Roy, P.-E. (1975). Lipid droplets in the heart interstitium: concentration and distribution. *Recent Advanc. Stud. Cardiac Struct. Metab.*, **10**, 17–27.

Russell, J. A., and Bloom, W. L. (1955). Extractable and residual glycogen in tissues of the rat. *Amer. J. Physiol.*, **183**, 345–355.

Sakai, K., and Abiko, Y. (1981). Acute changes of myocardial norepinephrine and glycogen phosphorylase in ischemic areas after coronary ligation in dogs. *Jpn. Circulation J.*, **45**, 1250–1255.

Salerno, T. A., and Choing, M. A. (1980). Cardioplegic arrest in pigs. Effects of glucose-containing solutions. *J. Thorac. Cardiovasc. Surg.*, **80**, 929–933.

Scheuer, J., and Brachfeld, N. (1966). Myocardial uptake and fractional distribution of palmitate-1-^{14}C by the ischaemic dog heart. *Metabolism*, **15**, 945–954.

Severson, D. L. (1979a). Regulation of lipid metabolism in adipose tissue and heart. *Canad. J. Physiol. Pharmacol.*, **57**, 923–937.

Severson, D. L. (1979b). Characterization of triglyceride lipase activities in rat heart. *J. Mol. Cell. Cardiol.*, **11**, 569–583.

Shen, A. C., and Jennings, R. B. (1972). Myocardial calcium and magnesium in acute ischemic injury. *Amer. J. Pathol.*, **67**, 417–440.

Shipp, J. C., Thomas, J. M., and Crevasse, L. (1964). Oxidation of carbon-14-labeled endogeneous lipids by isolated perfused rat heart. *Science*, **142**, 371–373.

Stam, H., Geelhoed-Mieras, M. M., and Hülsmann, W. C. (1980). Erucic acid-induced alteration of cardiac triglyceride hydrolysis. *Lipids*, **15**, 242–250.

Stein, O., and Stein, Y. (1963). Metabolism of fatty acids in the isolated perfused rat heart. *Biochim. Biophys. Acta*, **70**, 517–530.

Sutherland, E. W., and Rall, R. W. (1968). The relation of adenosine 3′,5′-phosphate and phosphorylase to the actions of catecholamines and other hormones. *Pharmacol. Rev.*, **12**, 265–299.

Tyers, G. F. O., Williams, E. H., Hughes, H. C., and Todd, G. J. (1977). Effect of perfusate temperature on myocardial protection from ischemia. *J. Thorac. Cardiovasc. Surg.*, **73**, 766–771.

van der Vusse, G. J. (1983). Myocardial free fatty acids under normoxic and ischemic circumstances. *J. Drug Res.*, in press.

van der Vusse, G. J., Roemen, T. H. M., and Reneman, R. S. (1980). Assessment of fatty acids in dog left ventricular myocardium. *Biochim. Biophys. Acta*, **617**, 347–352.

van der Vusse, G. J., Roemen, T. H. M., Prinzen, F. W., and Reneman, R. S. (1981). The concentration of non-esterified fatty acids in biopsies from normoxic dog myocardium. *Basic Res. Cardiol.*, **76**, 389–393.

van der Vusse, G. J., Flameng, W., Borgers, M., De Meyere, R., and Suy, R. (1982a). Myocardial protection in extensive myocardial revascularization. A preliminary report of a randomized study. In *Coronary Artery Disease Today. Diagnosis, Surgery and Prognosis* (A. V. G. Bruschke, G. van Herpen, and F. E. E. Vermeulen, eds), Excerpta Medica, Amsterdam, pp. 227–236.

van der Vusse, G. J., Roemen, T. H. M., Prinzen, F. W., Coumans, W. A., and Reneman R. S. (1982b). Uptake and content of fatty acids in dog myocardium under normoxic and ischemic conditions. *Circulation Res.*, **50**, 538–546.

Vincent, N. H., and Ellis, S. (1963). Inhibitory effect of actylcholine on glycogenolysis in the isolated guinea pig heart. *J. Pharmacol. Exp. Ther.*, **139**, 60–68.

Walsh, M. P., LePeuch, C. J., Vallet, B., Cavadore, J. C., and Demaille, J. G. (1980). Cardiac calmodulin and its role in the regulations of metabolism and contraction. *J. Mol. Cell. Cardiol.*, **12**, 1091–1101.

Wartman, W. B., Jennings, B., Yokoyama, H. O., and Clabough, G. F. (1956). Fatty change of the myocardium in early experimental infarction. *Arch. Pathol.*, **62**, 318–323.

Weglicki, W. B., Owens, K., Urschel, C. W., Serrur, J. R., and Sonenblick, E. H. (1973). Hydrolysis of myocardial lipids during acidosis and ischemia. *Recent Advanc. Stud. Cardiac Struct. Metab.*, **3**, 781–793.

Weishaar, R., Sarma, J. S. M., Maryama, Y., Fisher, R., and Bing, R. J. (1977). Regional blood flow, contractility and metabolism in early myocardial infarction. *Cardiology*, **62**, 2–20.

Weishaar, R., Ashikawa, K., and Bing, R. J. (1979). Effect of diltiazem, a calcium antagonist, on myocardial ischemia. *Amer. J. Cardiol*, **43**, 1137–1143.

Wheeldon, L. W., Schumert, Z., and Turner, D. A. (1956). Lipid composition of heart muscle homogenate. *J. Lipid Res.*, **6**, 481–489.

Whitmer, J. T., Idell-Wenger, J. A., Rovetto, M. J., and Neely, J. R. (1978). Control of fatty acid metabolism in ischaemic and hypoxic hearts. *J. Biol. Chem.*, **253**, 4305–4309.

Wollenberger, A., and Krause, E. G. (1968). Metabolic control characteristics of the acutely ischemic myocardium. *Amer. J. Cardiol.*, **22**, 349–359.

Wollenberger, A., and Shahab, L. (1965). Anoxia-induced release of noradrenaline from the isolated perfused heart. *Nature*, **207**, 88–89.

CHAPTER 11

Heat Production

J. Brian Chapman

Department of Physiology, Monash University, Clayton, Victoria 3168, Australia

INTRODUCTION

The myothermic technique for measuring the heat production of isolated muscle preparations dates back to 1848 when Helmholtz first detected the temperature rise in contracting leg muscles of the frog, using three thermocouples in series with a galvanometer. Although a great deal of descriptive information was gleaned from myothermic studies during the late nineteenth century, notably by Fick (1889) and his pupil Blix, it was not until 1913 that A. V. Hill published the first account relating the heat production of muscle in absolute units to the mechanical output by means of direct electrical calibration of the muscle–thermopile system. The subsequent half-century was dominated by Hill, his colleagues, and his pupils, and witnessed the introduction of numerical analysis of the time course of heat production (Hill and Hartree, 1920), ultra-thin thermopiles (Hill, 1937), and the progressive improvement of galvanometers from the moving magnet type to the moving coil type with photoelectric amplication, much of the technical innovation being due to the expertise of Hill's assistant, A. C. Downing.

In the 1960s two new types of thermopile were introduced. Wilkie (1963, 1968) used only two chromel–constantan junctions to detect the temperature changes in an insulated silver strip in contact with the muscle. The Ricchiuti thermopile (Ricchiuti and Mommaerts, 1965) is constructed by electroplating silver on a fine, continuous constantan wire and retains the low thermal capacity and rapid time resolution of the later Hill–Downing thermopiles. This has been modified to study right ventricular papillary muscles such as can be isolated from rabbits, cats, and guinea-pigs, or left ventricular papillary muscles of rats (Gibbs, 1978).

The latest development in thermopile technology has been introduced by Mulieri *et al.* (1977) wherein thermopiles of very low heat capacity are constructed by vacuum deposition of antimony and bismuth on thin mica sheets. These thermopiles allow even greater sensitivity and time resolution than is available from the Ricchiuti thermopiles. Their relative fragility is compensated for by the fact that they can be produced in a comparatively short time.

It should be emphasized that all measurements of heat production in isolated cardiac muscle preparations are necessarily made while the muscles are drained of their physiological bathing medium. This is because the high heat loss and low thermal capacity of these small preparations, together with the low temperature rise following contraction (of the order of 0.001 K), make recording in a temperature-stabilized gas mixture essential. It is not possible to measure the immediate effects on heat production of a change in the composition of the bathing medium and therefore only the steady state properties of myocardial heat production can be investigated with respect to the effects of drugs, metabolic inhibitors, substrates, and ionic composition.

The detailed experimental data obtained in the above ways from isolated papillary muscles are in general agreement with the more limited data obtained from calorimetric measurements on isolated perfused whole hearts (Neill and Huckabee, 1966; Coulson, 1976; McDonald, 1971) or from thermometric studies in the coronary sinus and ascending aorta of anaesthetized dogs (Afonso *et al.*, 1965).

SOURCES OF MYOCARDIAL HEAT PRODUCTION

Cardiac muscle is similar to other body tissues in depending for its immediate energy source on the free energy available from the splitting of ATP. The three main energy-transducing enzymes or ATPases concerned with the initiation and execution of myocardial contraction are as follows: (1) the Na,K-ATPase of the sarcolemmal electrogenic sodium pump (Schwartz, 1962) which not only maintains the ionic gradients necessary for electrical excitability but also contributes directly to the membrane current, thereby influencing the shape of the cardiac action potential (Chapman *et al.*, 1979; Johnson *et al.*, 1980); (2) the Ca-ATPase of the sarcoreticular calcium pump which influences relaxation of activated muscle (Weber *et al.*, 1966); (3) the myosin ATPase of the contractile mechanism which develops force, produces myofibrillar shortening, and transforms some of the chemical energy available from ATP into mechanical work (Weber *et al.*, 1963; Barany *et al.*, 1964).

The first two underwrite small amounts of electrochemical work and the last one underwrites the larger energy consumption of the contractile mechanism itself (Chapman *et al.*, 1970; Chapman, 1974). The free energy available from ATP for these ATPases is buffered throughout the cytoplasm by the creatine kinase reaction (Pool and Sonnenblick, 1967).

The long term restoration and maintenance of the free energy of ATP derives from the oxidation of glucose or glycogen, lactic acid and fatty acids (Opie, 1969), the major fraction of the ATP coming from reversal of the mitochondrial proton-motive ATPase (Mitchell, 1961, 1979) supplemented by substrate-level phosphorylations occurring in the cytoplasmic glycolytic pathway and the mitochondrial citric acid cycle (Jobsis, 1964).

According to the first law of thermodynamics all the summed enthalpy of chemical change will appear as heat evolved within the muscle, with or without a component of the enthalpy appearing as external work performed by the muscle on its surroundings, depending on the mechanical conditions under which the contraction occurs. In practically all of the studies to date on cardiac muscle preparations all the external work performed by the muscle, either in deforming levers during isometric contraction or in lifting loads during isotonic contraction, is returned to the muscle as heat during the relaxation process. Consequently, the final heat recorded is a direct measure of the total enthalpy of all the chemical reactions underwriting the initiation, execution, and recovery metabolism of the contractile event.

The thermal consequences of respiratory gas exchange between the muscle and its environment are so relatively negligible that it is possible to treat isolated cardiac muscle on a thermopile as a closed thermodynamic system exchanging energy but not matter with its surroundings (Gibbs and Chapman, 1979a). This being so, the heat production of muscles measured on thermopiles (including degraded work) is a complete reflection of the extent of chemical change occurring within the muscles. Any free energy of ATP splitting utilized for the electrochemical work of active transport within the muscle tissue is 'internal' work and does not diminish the total enthalpy of ATP splitting recorded by the thermopile (Chapman and Gibbs, 1972).

The enthalpy of ATP splitting in muscle is known to be $-48 \, \text{kJ mol}^{-1}$ (Homsher and Kean, 1978) while the enthalpy of substrate oxidation is -19.84 and $-21.14 \, \text{kJ l}^{-1}$ of oxygen for fat and carbohydrate, respectively (Ruch and Patton, 1965). When isolated cardiac muscle contracts, the total heat recorded above the baseline level from the moment of stimulation to the end of all heat production associated with restoration of all the ATP consumed by the contraction is simply the enthalpy of oxidation of substrate, provided that any external work performed by the muscle is degraded into the heat during relaxation. The ratio of the heat associated with the initial consumption of ATP to the total heat recorded following resynthesis of the ATP is 0.587 and 0.583 for fat and carbohydrate oxidation, respectively. As isolated cardiac muscle preparations supplied with glucose derive their energy from a mixed oxidation of glucose and endogenous lipid (Opie, 1969) it is convenient to assume a mean ratio of 0.585 (Chapman, 1974; Chapman and Gibbs, 1974).

RESTING HEAT PRODUCTION

Although 'rest' is an unphysiological state for the heart, the heat production of quiescent isolated cardiac muscle preparations yields the so-called resting heat baseline, above which active heat production associated with contraction is measured. In right ventricular papillary muscles isolated from rabbits at 20 °C, the resting heat rate is 1.8 mW per gram of muscle in the presence of glucose as exogenous metabolic substrate (Gibbs *et al.*, 1967). Four major factors have been found to influence the resting heat rate:

(1) Stretching the muscle by 20% beyond its normal length generally increases the resting heat rate by about 50% (Gibbs *et al.*, 1967).

(2) When pyruvate replaces glucose as the exogenous substrate the resting heat rate (at normal length) is increased by 68% while the active force development increased by 34%. Acetate and lactate also produce lesser increases (relative to pyruvate) in resting heat production and active mechanical output (Chapman and Gibbs, 1974). No significant alterations of the resting heat rate are produced by caffeine, adrenaline, ouabain, or altered calcium ion concentration (Gibbs and Gibson, 1969; Gibbs, 1967a,b; 1978; Gibbs and Vaughan, 1968).

(3) The resting heat production of isolated cardiac muscle preparations characteristically decreases with the duration of an experiment, declining by about 15% or more between the first and fourth hours following cardiectomy, while the active force development increases by about 8% (Chapman and Gibbs, 1974);

(4) The resting heat rate shows large variation among species, there being a negative correlation with animal size (Loiselle and Gibbs, 1979).

The metabolic basis of cardiac resting heat remains unresolved. Using a calorific equivalent for protein synthesis of 5.9 kJ per gram of protein (Millward *et al.*, 1976), a myocardial protein content of 15% of wet weight, and an average protein turnover rate of 10% per day, the possible contribution of protein synthesis to resting heat could be of the order of 1 mW g^{-1} (C. L. Gibbs, personal communication). However, the fact that the resting heat declines continuously in isolated preparations, together with the observation that the oxygen consumption of arrested hearts on cardio-pulmonary bypass is decreased when Krebs solution is substituted for blood perfusion (Gibbs *et al.*, 1980), raises doubts as to whether protein synthesis continues normally in isolated cardiac muscle.

Although it was suggested earlier that sarcolemmal Na–K transport would account for less than 10% of the resting heat production (Gibbs and Chapman, 1979a,b), more recent studies of ion fluxes in cultured rat heart cells at 37 °C have yielded Na^+ transport rates that would imply, assuming three Na^+ transported per ATP, a total contribution exceeding 4 mW g^{-1} for the equivalent enthalpy rate of substrate oxidation. This is the same order of magnitude as the total resting heat production of rat papillary muscle at 27 °C (Loiselle and Gibbs, 1979, Loiselle, 1981).

Thus it would appear that Na^+ transport might account for much, if not most, of the resting heat production of isolated preparations with the remainder possibly coming from protein synthesis. The latter process would be expected to be much greater in blood-perfused hearts which have a higher quiescent oxygen consumption. The effect of stretch remains unexplained although it may be speculated that stimulation of protein synthesis as would occur in hypertrophy could account for some of the increase in resting heat production in stretched muscles (Rabinowitz, 1971; Cooper *et al.*, 1973; Everett *et al.*, 1977).

INITIAL AND RECOVERY HEAT

The distinction between initial and recovery heat production was classically described by Hartree and Hill (1922) for amphibian skeletal muscle. They showed that the initial heat appears at 0 °C within a few seconds of a single contraction and is followed over the ensuing 20–30 min by the appearance of recovery heat, the two components being roughly equal in magnitude. In terms of the enzymatic sources of myocardial heat production (see above) one would identify initial heat as arising from the initial metabolism associated with the activity of the Na,K-ATPase, the Ca-ATPase, and the myosin ATPase, together with the buffering activity of the creatine kinase enzymes. The recovery heat would be identified with the recovery metabolism associated with the enzymes of intermediary metabolism and oxidative phosphorylation (Chapman, 1974).

However, the metabolic properties of cardiac muscle, either *in vivo* or isolated at room temperature, militate against any clear distinction between initial and recovery heat production. First, the myocardium is not adapted to sustain any significant oxygen debt; this means that the initial cost of a contraction, in terms of ATP molecules consumed, is rapidly repaid via intermediary metabolism and oxidative phosphorylation, the initial and recovery metabolism proceeding simultaneously in the continuously beating heart.

Secondly, even the enzymatic distinction between initial and recovery processes is blurred in cardiac muscle by the role of the creatine kinase enzyme which is distributed abundantly in both the cytoplasm and the mitochondria (Jacobus and Lehninger, 1973; Scholte, 1973; Saks *et al.*, 1975). It is now thought that this enzyme not only buffers the energy available to the various ATPases, but also regulates mitochondrial oxidative phosphorylation and transmits the energy of oxidative phosphorylation across the outer mitochondrial membrane as the cellular, high energy phosphate potential (Jacobus and Lehninger, 1973; Saks *et al.*, 1975).

Thirdly, myothermic records obtained from isolated papillary muscles at room temperature provide no clear temporal justification for the terms initial heat and recovery heat. Figure 11.1 shows original records of force

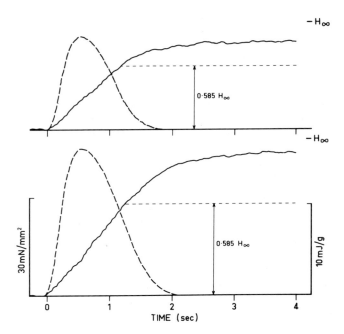

Figure 11.1 Records of heat production (solid) and mechanical stress development (dashed) for a papillary muscle equilibrated with glucose (upper diagram) and pyruvate (lower diagram) as substrate. Each record is averaged from the responses to 16 stimuli delivered at 1 min intervals. Final heat recorded for each contraction shown at extreme right (H_∞). Dashed horizontal lines show proportion of total heat attributable to initial ATPase activity (see text)

development and heat production elicited from a papillary muscle equilibrated at room temperature first with glucose as substrate (upper diagram) and then with pyruvate as substrate (lower diagram). The records are averaged from 16 single twitches evoked at 1 min intervals in each solution and show the time course of mechanical and myothermic response during the first 4 s following the stimulus together with the final heat values, H_∞ recorded after 30 s (pyruvate) or 40 s (glucose) had elapsed. By a line of reasoning converse to that used by Wilkie (1968) to calculate the number of phosphorylations arising from recovery metabolism in skeletal muscle, it is possible to draw certain limits on the time course of evolution of heat from the different enzymatic sources in these experiments (Chapman and Gibbs, 1974). The same reasoning also allows the derivation of the ratio of 0.585 for the initial enthalpy associated with the consumption of ATP to the total enthalpy following restoration of the original ATP levels (see above).

The horizontal lines drawn back to their intersection with the respective heat traces in Figure 11.1 represent 0.585 of the total heat recorded in each case. This is the maximum enthalpy of ATP breakdown that could have been recorded from these contractions: all heat production greater than this amount must be attributed to the recovery metabolic processes. More than 0.585 of the total heat was evolved even before the end of each mechanical event, suggesting that recovery metabolism had commenced within the first 2 s following the stimulus. If ATP is consumed by both the sarcoreticular Ca-ATPase and the myosin ATPase at least to the end of mechanical relaxation, the recovery processes and their associated heat production were well under way within the first second of each contraction.

This conclusion is supported by fluorometric monitoring of the level of reduction of mitochondrial pyridine nucleotides in the same preparation (Chapman, 1972). The fluorometric transient following a single twitch is fully developed in proportion to that following a train of contractions and the peak oxidation of pyridine nucleotide, signalled by a decrease in fluorescence and indicating the occurrence of oxidative phosphorylation, appears at the end of the mechanical event. Heat production occurs in an early fast phase followed by a later slower phase (see Figure 11.1), but it is not possible to correlate these phases with initial and recovery metabolism as can be done in amphibian skeletal muscle at low temperature.

The faster time resolution of the vacuum-deposited thermopiles has led their users to describe their recording of the early fast phase as 'initial heat' production (Alpert *et al.*, 1979; Alpert and Mulieri, 1982). However, in view of the foregoing arguments it would be erroneous to equate such early fast heat production solely with sarcolemmal, sarcoreticular, and myofibrillar ATPase activity as this early phase clearly derives in part from the oxidative recovery processes, while the commencement of the slow phase of heat production must necessarily derive in part from the Ca-ATPase and myosin ATPase during the final stages of relaxation (see Figure 11.1).

One can still detect differences in the intrinsic speed of recovery metabolism by examining the relative proportions of the fast and slow components and the time course of the late phase of heat production. Such a study established that the rate of late heat production proceeds most rapidly with pyruvate as substrate, followed by lactate, acetate, and glucose (Chapman and Gibbs, 1974). This finding confirmed indirectly the earlier finding that the kinetics of the fluorometric response proceeded more rapidly with pyruvate than with glucose (Chapman, 1972), indicating that the intrinsic rate of cardiac oxidative recovery metabolism depends on the dominant metabolic pathway underwriting the consumption of oxygen.

COMPONENTS OF MYOCARDIAL HEAT PRODUCTION

Mention has already been made of the distinct enzymatic sources of myocardial heat production and it would seem that these should form the sole biochemical basis for subdivision of the enthalpy cost of myocardial contraction into discrete components. We have also noted in the preceding section that, although one can ascribe 0.585 of the total enthalpy of contraction to the enthalpy of sarcolemmal, sarcoreticular, and myofibrillar ATPase activity, it is not possible to deduce a complete description of the time course of this enthalpy production as distinct from the enthalpy production of oxidative recovery metabolism.

This leaves the only reasonable subdivision of total enthalpy production as being the enthalpy of ATP consumption (including the associated oxidative recovery heat) apportioned among the three ATPases, i.e. the sarcolemmal Na,K-ATPase, the sarcoreticular Ca-ATPase, and the myofibrillar myosin ATPase. Enthalpy production associated with the myosin ATPase is directly involved with the development of force, myofibrillar shortening, and the performance of mechanical work. Enthalpy production associated with the other two ATPases has usually been described as force-independent heat, tension-independent heat, stress-independent heat, and activation heat (Gibbs and Chapman, 1979a,b; Loiselle and Gibbs, 1979). The term activation heat is analogous to the heat component of the same name in amphibian skeletal muscle, although in that case the heat derives almost entirely from the enthalpy of calcium transport (Chapman and Gibbs, 1972; Homsher *et al.*, 1972; Smith, 1972), whereas in cardiac muscle the enthalpy of sodium and potassium transport is likely to be significant (Chapman *et al.*, 1970).

Activation Heat

Myocardial activation heat is measured in isolated papillary muscles by pre-shortening the muscles to eliminate detectable force development. Consequently it is likely that, following stimulation, internal shortening without the development of force results in some contamination from residual myofibrillar ATPase activity. Moreover, the release of calcium within the muscle appears to be deactivated by shortening (Huntsman and Stewart, 1977; Jewell, 1977; Lakatta and Jewell, 1977). Hence the measurement of activation or force-independent heat in cardiac muscle is confounded to an unknown extent by two factors that, although working in opposite directions, cannot be assumed to cancel each other.

Na,K-ATPase

The enthalpy of ATP consumption for active transport of ions appears completely as heat during myothermic recording because all the useful work performed by the ATPase in conferring free energy on the transported ions is internal work as far as the muscle tissue is concerned, and because the enthalpy of ion translocation along electrochemical gradients is zero in the first approximation (Chapman *et al.*, 1970; Chapman and Gibbs, 1972; Gibbs and Chapman 1979a). Also Hodgkin (1951) has shown that any electrical work dissipated by local circuit currents during excitation in nerve is balanced by an absorption of heat making the overall excitatory event thermally neutral in the first approximation.

Langer (1967) estimated the sodium flux per excitation to be 66 nmol per gram of dog ventricle at 24 °C. Assuming a sodium pump stoicheiometry of three Na^+ per ATP (Baker, 1965; Harris, 1967) and $-48 \, kJ \, mol^{-1}$ for the enthalpy of ATP splitting *in vivo* (Homsher and Kean, 1978), this amount of sodium flux, if actively transported, would generate about 1 mJ per gram of ventricular muscle or $1.8 \, mJ \, g^{-1}$ if the oxidative recovery heat is included (Gibbs and Chapman, 1979a). This is probably an upper limit because unidirectional flux measurements tend to overestimate the true net extent of complex chemical reactions owing to contamination by reversible exchange processes in intermediate steps (Chapman, 1982).

Ca-ATPase

About 100 nmol of calcium ion per gram of tissue is required to achieve full activation of myocardial contraction (Solaro *et al.*, 1974). Assuming a calcium pump stoicheiometry of two Ca^{++} per ATP (Weber *et al.*, 1966), the corresponding heat of active calcium transport would be 2.4 or 4.1 mJ per gram of tissue if recovery heat is included. This estimate is the minimum enthalpy of total metabolism required to remove the calcium from maximally activated cardiac myofilaments.

Thus, the expected combined contribution of active transport to the total enthalpy of just maximally activated cardiac muscle is somewhat less than $6 \, mJ \, g^{-1}$. In papillary muscles stimulated in blocks of 10–20 contractions at 0.25 Hz at room temperature the activation heat is usually of the order of $2 \, mJ \, g^{-1}$ (see Figure 11.2). This low figure is presumably due to incomplete activation occurring at low stimulus frequency and pre-shortened length. However, the experimental value may be greatly altered by agents that alter myocardial contractility.

The activation heat is more than trebled under the combined influence of caffeine and catecholamines (Gibbs, 1967a,b; Chapman *et al.*, 1977). At room temperature an increase in stimulus rate from 0.1 to 0.67 Hz increases the activation heat by about 25% (Gibbs and Gibson, 1970a), as does a therapeutic dose of cardiac glycoside (Gibbs and Gibson, 1969) or a low dose of catecholamine (Gibbs, 1967a,b; Gibbs and Gibson, 1972). However, a change in activation heat does not always correlate with a change in contractility. In experiments where contractility was altered by varying the

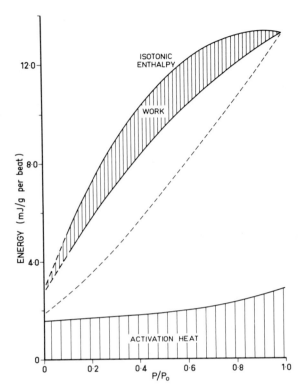

Figure 11.2 Isotonic enthalpy–load curve for papillary muscle at room temperaure. Loads (*P*) expressed as fraction of the maximum stress developed under isometric conditions, P_0. Data are usually not available for loads less than $0.1P_0$. Dashed line shows isometric heat production obtained at pre-shortened lengths (see text)

ratio of calcium ion concentration to the square of the sodium ion concentration in the bathing medium, it was found that the large inotropic effects did not correlate with the magnitude of the activation heat. These results were interpreted in terms of activation heat arising from both the Na,K-ATPase and the Ca-ATPase along with the associated recovery heat (Chapman *et al.*, 1970).

Contractile Element Heat and Work

The enthalpy production of cardiac muscle shares a feature in common with all other muscle types that have been studied in that, for a given level of activation, the energy consumption of a single contraction depends upon the mechanical conditions under which the contraction takes place; that is, the total ATP consumption by the myosin ATPase is intrinsically regulated according to the mechanical constraints. Figure 11.2 shows the variation in total enthalpy production of isometric contractions and afterloaded isotonic contractions, the loads being expressed as a fraction of the isometric stress P_0. (For an explanation of how these data are obtained see Gibbs *et al.*, 1967; Gibbs and Gibson, 1970b.) The activation heat is represented as a curvilinear function of load in Figure 11.2 to allow for the possible deactivation of calcium release during isotonic shortening (Blinks, 1970; Taylor and Rudel, 1970; Allen *et al.*, 1974; Jewell and Lakatta, 1976) and its intercept at zero load has been made slightly lower than the experimentally determined average value of 2 mJ g^{-1} to allow for internal myofibrillar shortening in preshortened muscles (see above).

The total isotonic enthalpy curve in Figure 11.2 shows more than a threefold variation down from the isometric value to that obtained with the lightest possible loads (usually about 0.1 P_0). This might be regarded as a manifestation of the Fenn effect in cardiac muscle, although the isotonic enthalpy does not exceed the isometric value over the load range as it does in amphibian skeletal muscle at low temperature (Fenn, 1924). Rather, in cardiac muscle the Fenn effect simply means that the total energy of a contraction is continuously variable over the isotonic load range, indicating an intrinsic regulatory property of the contractile mechanism dependent on the mechanical conditions.

Work and efficiency

The external mechanical work performed in lifting the isotonic loads is shown as a component of the enthalpy–load relation of Figure 11.2. Characteristically, the maximum work per contraction is performed against an isotonic load somewhat less than half the maximum isometric stress. The efficiency of myocardial contraction can be expressed in three ways:

(1) *Mechanical efficiency* This is defined as the magnitude of the external work divided by the total enthalpy of contraction and the corresponding efficiency–load relation is shown in Figure 11.3. Because the total enthalpy falls off so markedly at light isotonic loads (see Figure 11.2) the mechanical efficiency tends to peak at lower loads than does the external work.

(2) *Myosin ATPase mechanical efficiency* If the activation heat is subtracted from the enthalpy–load relation of Figure 11.2 and the remainder is multiplied by 0.585, then the result is the enthalpy of ATP breakdown directly attributable to the mechanical event. Dividing this quantity into the external work yields the direct mechanical efficiency of the contractile mechanism. This efficiency is, of course, considerably higher than its counterpart expressed relative to the total enthalpy of contraction including activation and recovery enthalpy (see Figure 11.3).

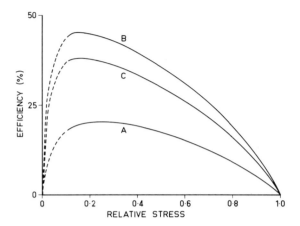

Figure 11.3 Efficiency–load curves computed from the data of Figure 11.2, the isotonic loads being expressed as fractions of the maximum isometric stress. Curve A, mechanical efficiency defined as external work per total enthalpy including activation and recovery heat; curve B, mechanical efficiency of the myosin ATPase defined as external work per enthalpy of ATP breakdown attributable to myosin; curve C, thermodynamic efficiency of the myosin ATPase defined as external work per free energy of ATP breakdown attributable to myosin

(3) *Myosin ATPase thermodynamic efficiency*   As the enthalpy of ATP breakdown is $-48 \, \text{kJ} \, \text{mol}^{-1}$ (Homsher and Kean, 1978) and the corresponding free energy change is $-57 \, \text{kJ} \, \text{mol}^{-1}$ in cardiac muscle (Hassinen and Hiltunen, 1975), it is possible to divide the external work by the calculated free energy change of the myosin ATPase and so obtain a direct estimate of the thermodynamic efficiency of the contractile mechanism in converting free energy into mechanical work under isotonic conditions. The resulting thermodynamic efficiency–load relation is also plotted in Figure 11.3. This curve falls below the corresponding mechanical efficiency curve for the myosin ATPase because the free energy of ATP splitting is larger than the enthalpy change. Nevertheless, the maximum thermodynamic efficiency of about 38% at $0.2P_0$ is quite high for chemomechanical transduction processes.

Further subdivivision of the enthalpy–load relation

There have been descriptions of 'shortening heat' and 'tension-dependent heat' but they are fraught with problems (Chapman and Gibbs, 1972; Gibbs and Chapman, 1979a). The dashed line in figure 11.2 shows the isometric enthalpy relation obtained by pre-shortening the muscle to different rest lengths and plotting the total enthalpy of contraction against the peak isometric stress developed. Following in the traditions stemming from A. V. Hill's classic studies (for a comprehensive review of this tradition see Mommaerts, 1969) it has been customary to refer to the isometric enthalpy less the activation heat as the 'tension-dependent' or 'stress-dependent' heat (Gibbs and Chapman, 1979a). It can be seen in Figure 11.2 that, if the external work were to be multiplied by 1.7 to include its counterpart in the enthalpy of recovery metabolism, it would account for almost all of the isotonic enthalpy in excess of the activation and 'tension-dependent' heat, thus leaving little or no room for any 'shortening heat'. While this might possible raise the question as to whether 'shortening heat' exists in cardiac muscle the following should be borne in mind:

(1) Isolated cardiac muscle preparations do not release energy at a higher rate during shortening than during isometric contraction (Gibbs and Gibson, 1970b). Thus, the classic manifestation of 'shortening heat' as originally defined by Hill (1938) in amphibian skeletal muscle is lacking in mammalian cardiac muscle.

(2) Because of the high compliance (Krueger and Pollack, 1975) and non-uniform force distribution (Pinto and Win, 1977) of papillary muscles there is much internal shortening, perhaps at quite high velocity (Manring *et al.*, 1977).

(3) The whole concept of 'shortening heat' is of doubtful significance and has tended to obscure, rather than enhance, thermodynamic insight into the essential properties of chemomechanical transduction in muscle (Chapman and Gibbs, 1972; Gibbs and Chapman, 1979a). Its continued propagation in present-day literature serves no obvious purpose and it would seem timely to abandon quantitative partitioning of muscle energy consumption into stress-dependent and shortening-dependent components, particularly as stress and shortening are phenomenologically inseparable in cardiac muscle. More understanding is likely to derive from thermodynamically constrained kinetic modelling of a stoicheiometrically defined mechanism such as that developed by Eisenberg and Hill (1978).

CARDIAC ENERGETICS *IN VIVO*

Enthalpy–load relations similar to that shown in Figure 11.2 have been obtained using chemical (Pool *et al.*, 1968), fluorometric (Chapman *et al.*, 1976), and polarographic (Coleman, 1968) techniques. The data usually obtained from isolated papillary muscle preparations are static, in that they only apply to a particular preload or prestimulus length and to a fixed set of physiological conditions. Similar findings are also obtained from studies of the influence of arterial load on the oxygen consumption, mean external power, and external efficiency of the isolated perfused cat heart (Elzinga and

Westerhof, 1980). However, it is important to emphasize that enthalpy–load relations are highly dynamic phenomena *in vivo*; both the maximum force or pressure developed and the maximum energy consumption per beat will vary according to the prevailing level of contractility and upon the length or end-diastolic volume from which the contraction commences (Gibbs and Chapman, 1979a,b).

The dependence of initial fibre length is a complex combination of the influence of myofilament overlap (Julian and Sollins, 1975) and the length dependence of activation (Jewell, 1977). The level of contractility *in vivo* will be influenced by the pattern and history of the rate of cardiac excitation, the neural discharge from the autonomic nervous system, and circulating hormones or drugs.

Recent myothermic studies of the effects of pressure overload and thyrotoxic hypertrophy have shown that the economy of tension development becomes chronically altered under these pathological conditions (Alpert *et al.*, 1979). The data were interpreted to suggest that pressure-overload hypertrophy causes a decrease in cross-bridge cycling rate with an increase in the proportion of time spent in the attached state by the individual cross-bridges, resulting in an increased economy of force or pressure development. The opposite effects were found in association with thyrotoxic hypertrophy.

ACKNOWLEDGEMENTS

Much of the work reviewed herein was supported by Grants-in-Aid from the National Heart Foundation of Australia and from the Australian Research Grants Council. I thank my colleagues Drs C. L. Gibbs and D. S. Loiselle for their reading and helpful criticism during the preparation of this chapter.

REFERENCES

Afonso, S., Rowe, G. G., Lugo, J. E., and Crumpton, C. W. (1965). Left ventricle heat production in intact anaesthetized dogs. *Amer. J. Physiol.*, **208**, 946–953.

Allen, D. G., Jewell, B. R., and Murray, J. W. (1974). The contribution of activation processes to the length-tension relation of cardiac muscle. *Nature*, **248**, 606–607.

Alpert, N. R., and Mulieri, L. A. (1982). Heat, mechanics, and myosin ATPase in normal and hypertrophied heart muscle. *Fed. Proc.*, **14**, 192–198.

Alpert, N. R., Mulieri, L. A., and Litten, R. Z. (1979). Functional significance of altered myosin adenosine triphosphatase activity in enlarged hearts. *Amer. J. Cardiol.*, **44**, 947–953.

Baker, P. F. (1965). Phosphorus metabolism of intact crab nerve and its relation to the active transport of ions. *J. Physiol. (Lond.)*, **180**, 383–423.

Barany, M., Gaetjens, E., Barany, K., and Karp, E. (1964). Comparative studies of cardiac and skeletal myosins. *Arch. Biochem. Biophys.*, **106**, 280–293.

Blinks, J. R. (1970). Factors influencing the prolongation of the active state by stretch in isolated mammalian heart muscle. *Fed. Proc.*, **29**, 611.

Chapman, J. B. (1972). Fluorometric studies of oxidative metabolism in isolated papillary muscle of the rabbit, *J. Gen. Physiol.*, **59**, 135–154.

Chapman, J. B. (1974). Energy sources of cardiac contraction. *Advanc. Cardiol.*, **12**, 128–138.

Chapman, J. B. (1982). A kinetic interpretation of 'variable' stoichiometry for an electrogen sodium pump obeying chemiosmotic principles. *J. Theoret. Biol.*, **95**, 665–678.

Chapman, J. B., and Gibbs, C. L. (1972). An energetic model of muscle contraction. *Biophys. J.*, **12**, 227–236.

Chapman, J. B., and Gibbs, C. L. (1974). The effect of metabolic substrate on mechanical activity and heat production in papillary muscle. *Cardiovasc. Res.*, **8**, 656–667.

Chapman, J. B., Gibbs, C. L., and Gibson, W. R. (1970). Effects of calcium and sodium on cardiac contractility and heat production in rabbit papillary muscle. *Circulation Res.*, **27**, 601–610.

Chapman, J. B., Gibbs, C. L., and Gibson, W. R. (1976). Heat and fluorescence changes in cardiac muscle: effects of substrate and calcium. *J. Mol. Cell. Cardiol.*, **8**, 545–558.

Chapman, J. B., Gibbs, C. L., and Loiselle, D. S. (1977). Simultaneous heat and fluorescence changes in cardiac muscle at high rates of energy expenditure. *J. Mol. Cell. Cardiol.*, **9**, 715–732.

Chapman, J. B., Johnson, E. A., and Kootsey, J. M. (1979). A kinetic model for determining the consequence of electrogenic active transport in cardiac muscle. *J. Theoret. Biol.*, **80**, 405–424.

Coleman, H. N. (1968). Effect of alterations in shortening and external work on oxygen consumption of cat papillary muscle. *Amer. J. Physiol.*, **214**, 100–106.

Cooper, G., Puga, F. J., Zujko, K. J., Harrison, C. E., and Coleman, H. N. (1973). Normal myocardial function and energetics in volume-overload hypertrophy in the cat. *Circulation Res.*, **32**, 140–148.

Coulson, R. L. (1976). Energetics of isovolumic contractions of the isolated rabbit heart. *J. Physiol. (Lond.)*, **260**, 45–53.

Eisenberg, E., and Hill, T. L. (1978). A cross-bridge model of muscle contraction. *Prog. Biophys. Mol. Biol.*, **33**, 55–82.

Elzinga, G., and Westerhof, N. (1980). Pump function of the feline left heart: changes with heart rate and its bearing on the energy balance. *Cardiovasc. Res.*, **14**, 81–92.

Everett, A. W., Taylor, R. R., and Sparrow, M. P. (1977). Protein synthesis during right ventricular hypertrophy after pulmonary-artery stenosis in the dog. *Biochem. J.*, **166**, 315–321.

Fenn, W. O. (1924). The relation between the work performed and the energy liberated in muscular contraction. *J. Physiol. (Lond.)*, **58**, 373–395.

Fick, A. (1889). *Myothermische Untersuchungen*, Bergmann, Wiesbaden.

Gibbs, C. L. (1967a). Changes in cardiac heat production with agents that alter contractility, *Austral. J. Exp. Biol. Med. Sci.*, **45**, 379–392.

Gibbs, C. L. (1967b). Role of catecholamines in heat production in the myocardium. *Circulation Res.*, **21**, Suppl. 3, 223–230.

Gibbs, C. L. (1978). Cardiac energetics. *Physiol. Rev.*, **58**, 174–254.

Gibbs, C. L., and Chapman, J. B. (1979a). Cardiac energetics. In *Handbook of Physiology – The Cardiovascular System I* R. M. Berne, N. Sperelakis, and S. R. Geiger, eds), American Physiological Society, Bethesda, Md, pp. 775–804.

Gibbs, C. L., and Chapman, J. B. (1979b). Cardiac heat production, *Annu. Rev. Physiol.*, **41**, 507–519.

Gibbs, C. L., and Gibson, W. R. (1969). Effect of ouabain on the energy output of rabbit cardiac muscle. *Circulation Res.*, **24**, 951–967.

Gibbs, C. L., and Gibson, W. R. (1970a). Effect of alterations in the stimulus rate upon energy output, tension development and tension–time integral of cardiac muscle in rabbits. *Circulation Res.*, **27**, 611–618.

Gibbs, C. L., and Gibson, W. R. (1970b). Energy production in cardiac isotonic contractions. *J. Gen. Physiol.*, **56**, 732–750.

Gibbs, C. L., and Gibson, W. R. (1972). Isoprenaline, propranolol and the energy output of rabbit cardiac muscle. *Cardiovascular Res.*, **6**, 508–515.

Gibbs, C. L., and Vaughan, P. C. (1968). The effect of calcium depletion upon the tension-independent component of cardiac heat production. *J. Gen. Physiol.*, **52**, 532–549.

Gibbs, C. L., Mommaerts, W. F. H. M., and Ricchiuti, N. V. (1967). Energetics of cardiac contractions. *J. Physiol. (Lond.)*, **191**, 25–46.

Gibbs, C. L., Papadoyannis, D. E., Drake, A. J., and Noble, M. I. M. (1980). Oxygen consumption of the nonworking and potassium chloride-arrested dog heart. *Circulation Res.*, **47**, 408–417.

Harris, E. J. (1967). The stoichiometry of sodium ion movements from frog muscle. *J. Physiol. (Lond.)*, **193**, 455–458.

Hartree, W., and Hill, A. V. (1922). The recovery heat production of muscle. *J. Physiol. (Lond.)*, **56**, 367–381.

Hassinen, I. E., and Hiltunen, K. (1975). Respiratory control in isolated perfused rat heart. Role of the equilibrium relations between the mitochondrial electron carriers and the adenylate system. *Biochim. Biophys. Acta*, **408**, 319–330.

Hill, A. V. (1913). The absolute mechanical efficiency of the contraction of an isolated muscle. *J. Physiol. (Lond.)*, **46**, 435–469.

Hill, A. V. (1937). Methods of analysing the heat production of muscle. *Proc. Roy. Soc. Lond. B*, **124**, 114–136.

Hill, A. V. (1938). The heat of shortening and the dynamic constants of muscle. *Proc. Roy. Soc. Lond. B*, **126**, 136–195.

Hill, A. V., and Hartree, W. (1920). The four phases of heat production of muscle. *J. Physiol. (Lond.)*, **54**, 84–128.

Hodgkin, A. L. (1951). The ionic basis of electrical activity in nerve and muscle. *Biol. Rev.*, **26**, 339–409.

Homsher, E., and Kean, C. J. (1978). Skeletal muscle energetics and metabolism. *Annu. Rev. Physiol.*, **40**, 93–131.

Homsher, E., Mommaerts, W. F. H. M., Ricchiuti, N. V., and Wallner, A. (1972). Activation heat, activation metabolism and tension-related heat in frog semitendinosus muscles. *J. Physiol. (Lond.)*, **220**, 601–625.

Huntsman, L. L., and Stewart, D. K. (1977). Length-dependent calcium inotropism in cat papillary muscle. *Circulation Res.*, **40**, 366–371.

Jacobus, W. E., and Lehninger, A. L. (1973). Creatine kinase of rat heart mitochondria. Coupling of creatine phosphorylation to electron transport. *J. Biol. Chem.*, **248**, 4803–4810.

Jewell, B. R. (1977). A reexamination of the influence of muscle length on myocardial performance. *Circulation*, **40**, 221–230.

Jewell, B. R., and Lakatta, E. G. (1976). Potentiation of cardiac muscle: dependence on resting muscle length. *J. Physiol. (Lond.)*, **258**, 79P.

Jobsis, F. F. (1964). Basic processes in cellular respiration. In *Handbook of Physiology. Respiration I* (W. O. Fenn and H. Rahn, eds), American Physiological Society, Washington, D.C., pp. 63–124.

Johnson, E. A., Chapman, J. B., and Kootsey, J. M. (1980). Some electrophysiological consequences of electrogenic sodium and potassium transport in cardiac muscle: a theoretical study. *J. Theoret. Biol.*, **87,** 737–756.

Julian, F. J., and Sollins, M. R. (1975). Sarcomere length–tension relations in living rat papillary muscle. *Circulation Res.*, **37,** 299–308.

Krueger, J. W., and Pollack, G. D., (1975). Myocardial sarcomere dynamics during isometric contraction. *J. Physiol. (Lond.)*, **251,** 627–643.

Lakatta, E. G., and Jewell, B. R. (1977). Length-dependent activation. Its effect on the length–tension relation in cat ventricular muscle. *Circulation Res.*, **40,** 251–257.

Langer, G. A. (1967). Sodium exchange in dog ventricular muscle. Relation to frequency of contraction and its possible role in the control of myocardial contractility. *J. Gen. Physiol.*, **50,** 1221–1239.

Loiselle, D. S. (1981). The effect of temperature on the resting metabolism of cardiac muscle. *J. Mol. Cell. Cardiol.*, **13,** Suppl 3, 5P.

Loiselle, D. S., and Gibbs, C. L. (1979). Species differences in cardiac energetics. *Amer. J. Physiol.*, **237,** H90–H98.

McDonald, R. H. (1971). Myocardial heat production: its relationship to tension development. *Amer. J. Physiol.*, **220,** 894–900.

Manring, A., Nassar, R., and Johnson, E. A. (1977). Light diffraction of cardiac muscle: an analysis of sarcomere shortening and muscle tension. *J. Mol. Cell. Cardiol.*, **9,** 441–459.

Millward, D. J., Garlick, P. J., James, W. P. T., Sender, P., and Waterlow, J. C. (1976). Protein turnover. In *Protein Metabolism and Nutrition* (D. J. A. Cole, K. N. Boorman, P. J. Buttery, D. Lewis, R. J. Neale, and H. Swan, eds), Butterworths, London, pp. 46–69.

Mitchell, P. (1961). Coupling of phosphorylation to electron and hydrogen transfer by a chemi-osmotic type of mechanism. *Nature*, **191,** 144–148.

Mitchell, P. (1979). Keilin's respiratory chain concept and its chemiosmotic consequences. *Science*, **206,** 1148–1159.

Mommaerts, W. F. H. M. (1969). Energetics of muscular contraction. *Physiol. Rev.*, **49,** 427–508.

Mulieri, L. A., Luhr, G., Trefry, J., and Alpert, N. R. (1977). Metal-film thermopiles for use with rabbit right ventricular papillary muscles. *Amer. J. Physiol.*, **233,** 146–156.

Neill, W. A., and Huckabee, N. W. (1966). Anaerobic heat production by the heart. *J. Clin. Invest.*, **45,** 1412–1420.

Opie, L. H. (1969). Metabolism of the heart in health and disease. II. *Amer. Heart. J.*, **77,** 100–122.

Pinto, J. G., and Win, R. (1977). Non-uniform strain distribution in papillary muscles. *Amer. J. Physiol.*, **233,** H410–H416.

Pool, P. E., and Sonnenblick, H. E. (1967). The mechanochemistry of cardiac muscle. I. The isometric contraction. *J. Gen. Physiol.*, **50,** 951–965.

Pool, P. E., Chandler, B. M., Seagren, S. C., and Sonnenblick, H. E. (1968). Mechanochemistry of cardiac muscle. II. The isotonic contraction. *Circulation Res.*, **22,** 465–472.

Rabinowitz, M. (1971). Control of metabolism and synthesis of macromolecules in normal and ischaemic heart. *J. Mol. Cell. Cardiol.*, **2,** 277–292.

Ricchiuti, N. V., and Mommaerts, W. F. H. M. (1965). Technique for myothermic measurements. *Physiologist*, **8**, 259.

Ruch, T. C., and Patton, H. D. (ed) (1965). *Physiology and Biophysics, 19th edn,* Saunders, Philadelphia.

Saks, V. A., Chernousova, G. B., Gukovsky, D. E., Smironov, V. N., and Chazov, E. I. (1975). Studies of energy transport in heart cells. Mitochondrial isoenzyme of creatine phosphokinase: kinetic properties and regulatory action of Mg^{2+} ions. *Europ. J. Biochem.*, **57**, 273–290.

Scholte, H. R. (1973). On the triple localization of creatine kinase in heart and skeletal muscle cells of the rat: evidence for the existence of myofibrillar and mitochondrial isoenzymes. *Biochim. Biophys. Acta*, **305**, 413–427.

Schwartz, A. (1962). A sodium and potassium stimulated adenosine triphosphatase from cardiac tissues. I. Preparation and properties. *Biochem. Biophys. Res. Commun.*, **9**, 301–312.

Smith, I. C. H. (1972). Energetics of activation in frog and toad muscle. *J. Physiol. (Lond.)*, **220**, 583–599.

Solaro, R. J., Wise, R. M., Shiner, J. S., and Briggs, F. N. (1974). Calcium requirements for cardiac myofibrillar activation. *Circulation Res.*, **34**, 525–530.

Taylor, S. R., and Rudel, R. (1970). Striated muscle fibres: inactivation of contraction induced by shortening. *Science*, **167**, 882–884.

Weber, A., Herz, R., and Reiss, I. (1963). On the mechanism of the relaxing effect of fragmented sarcoplasmic reticulum. *J. Gen. Physiol.*, **46**, 679–702.

Weber, A., Herz, R., and Reiss, I. (1966). Study of the kinetics of calcium transport by isolated fragmented sarcoplasmic reticulum. *Biochem. Z.*, **345**, 329–369.

Wilkie, D. R. (1963). The wafer thermopile: a new device for measuring the heat production of muscles. *J. Physiol. (Lond.)*, **167**, 39P.

Wilkie, D. R. (1968). Heat, work and phosphorylcreatine breakdown in muscle. *J. Physiol. (Lond.)*, **195**, 157–183.

CHAPTER 12

Cardiac Metabolism and the Control of Coronary Blood Flow

J. D. Laird

Department of Physiology and Physiological Physics, University of Leiden, Leiden, The Netherlands

INTRODUCTION

Since the early years of this century the control of coronary blood flow has intrigued an exponentially growing number of scientists. The variety of species, preparations, and interventions was already substantial (see Markwalder and Starling, 1913) and has only grown in the intervening decades. There have been several excellent reviews of this enormous body of literature encompassing many hundreds of research reports in the last few years and I would contribute little to our search for an understanding of this important problem by adding yet another compilation (Belloni, 1979; Berne and Rubio, 1979; Berne, 1980; Hoffman, 1980; Olsson, 1981; Sparks, 1981). The sad state of affairs is that despite the efforts of many, many researchers over the years, and notwithstanding the important improvements in experimental and analytical techniques, we are forced to conclude that we really do not understand what governs the vascular resistance of the coronary bed even in normal circumstances, let alone in the more complex situation characterized by ischaemic heart disease.

For both intellectual and practical reasons we will confine our discussion to the control of coronary flow under normal physiological conditions. There are three standard experiments which merit consideration: hypoxic vasodilation, autoregulation, and metabolic vasodilation. The search for THE FACTOR responsible for determining coronary flow is often confined to complex measurements applied to any one of these standard experimental situations. While I appreciate that I do a great injustice to all the very elegant and complex studies cited in the reviews mentioned above, it is striking that from the time of Starling up to the most recent research reports, two substances repeatedly crop up as controlling factors: oxygen and adenosine.

While there is a great body of evidence supporting a role for either of these substances in the control of coronary blood flow, there are also, for each, studies which can be cited which are inconsistent with a dominant role (see Belloni, 1979). There are several reasons for this state of affairs. Preparations used to elicit phenomena involve different species, different perfusion conditions, and a variable degree of control over other factors known to influence coronary blood flow. Moreover, the experiment which is relatively easy to do may be so complex that interpretation of the results and extrapolation to the normal basal state may be nearly impossible. I have come to the conclusion that reactive hyperaemia is just such an example. Further, if one comes to the conclusion that substance x is involved in, for example, autoregulation, then one is often forced to a different preparation, or study, to examine the role of x in metabolic vasodilation. There are very few reports in which both autoregulation and metabolic vasodilation have been studied in the same animal in the same study, under comparable conditions. To my knowledge there are none in which all three standard experiments can be compared.

It is, after all, one system, which responds to intervention by the experimenter, in differing ways: to an increase in oxygen consumption or a decrease in its availability with a vasodilation, but to an increase in perfusion pressure with a vasoconstriction. Perhaps if we are ever to unravel the puzzle of the control of coronary blood flow we should consider it as truly a control system disturbed in various ways by the researcher and by disease.

IS CORONARY FLOW REALLY CONTROLLED?

I presume that most readers would have no difficulty with the idea that coronary flow is controlled. We know that coronary flow does adjust to varying circumstances. The adjustment to an increased metabolic rate is usually called 'metabolic vasodilation'. The decrease in vascular resistance subsequent to a decreased arterial oxygen content is referred to as 'hypoxic vasodilation'. Finally, the increase in vascular resistance accompanying increased perfusion pressure in the isolated coronary bed preparation is termed 'autoregulation'.

A Brief Digression on Control Systems

This is all evidence for an active vascular bed but as such it does not constitute a proof that coronary flow is controlled by the system. A true control system has a number of quite specific characteristics. Let us consider first a control system with which we are all familiar, the central heating system of a home. If the fire has been turned off for the summer, or the fuel supply has been shut off, then the 'steady state response of the system' to changes in outside temperature is easy to predict, as is sketched in Figure 12.1(a). Of course, the inside temperature will be the same as the outside

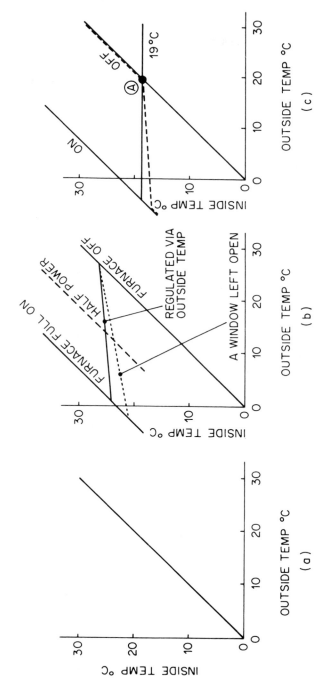

Figure 12.1 Inside-outside temperature characteristics for a centrally heated home. (a) Without heating; inside temperature equals outside temperature. (b) Limits of temperature with furnace full on, half on, and off. Full on maintains constant temperature difference with outside. By varying furnace power, it is possible to maintain inside temperature nearly constant, but disturbance of system (window open) not compensated when outside temperature used as control signal. (c) Using inside temperature as control signal, regulation (broken line) not so sensitive to disturbances, but cannot be perfect (solid line). Point A represents apparent set point (see text)

temperature. Now, let us consider what will happen when the furnace is fired up. Consider the simple case in which the fire runs at its maximum output, delivering a certain power (watts or calories per hour or even BTUs per hour). This power will be sufficient to keep the house a certain number of degrees higher than the outside air temperature. Note that we have assumed that the energy lost per hour from the house is linearly proportional to the temperature difference between the inside and the outside air. This case is shown in Figure 12.1(b), and constitutes a simple shift from the case without the heating system in operation. In neither of these extreme examples can we speak of a control system. Now if we wish to maintain a constant temperature in the house, it is clear that it is no use letting the boiler run full blast regardless of either the outside or the inside temperature. What is required is a more subtle approach in which we let the power development (on the average) depend on the circumstances. It is clear that running the furnace at half power will result in a relationship between inside and outside temperature lying between the two limits shown in Figure 12.1(b).

In this simple example, we have a choice with regard to which 'signal' we use to 'control' the heating system. 'Clearly', the colder it is outside the harder the furnace should run. Let us suppose that we have been very careful in determining such a relationship, such that the inside temperature can be kept constant by measuring the outside air temperature and 'the colder it gets outside, the more the furnace runs'. Is this now a true control system for the inside air temperature. No! To see that this is not the case, consider what will happen when someone leaves a window open. The colder it gets the more energy will be lost to the outside and it will get colder inside. In other words, our perfect balance between 'supply' and 'demand' has been lost. Even though the furnace is not at its maximum limit of power, the system, while still responding in a proportional way, is not really controlling the inside air temperature. It is important to note that a disturbance of the system has not been adequately compensated. You will agree, in this case, that one would not have expected anything else! If we really want to control the inside air temperature, we will have to measure it and base our corrective action on that temperature. You cannot control a variable if you don't measure it!

So, let us now consider the behaviour of our system when we use the inside air temperature as a basis for action. We shall have to decide what temperature we would like to have inside the house, let us say 19 °C (about 68 °F). This is, in technical systems, usually referred to as the set point of the system. In biological systems there is debate on the usefulness of the concept (Riggs, 1976; Verveen, 1978, 1979). Clearly, if the outside temperature is precisely 19 °C, we would still like to keep the furnace off. This gives us one measurement point labelled 'A', in Figure 12.1(c). As the outside temperature falls we will have to let the furnace run harder if we are to maintain the inside temperature close to the desired value of 19 °C.

Note that it is not possible to keep the inside temperature *exactly* equal to 19 °C, since then we wouldn't know whether the furnace should be turned off (because it's 19 °C outside) or continue to run (because it is 10 °C outside). It is only by allowing a small error that we can drive the system harder when it gets colder outside. This leads to the relationship shown in Figure 12.1(c), in which the actual inside temperature is not really constant, but shows a small slope. If we find the maximum error to be too great, we can make the heating system more sensitive to the small error signal. In control system terms, we increase the gain of the system. Once again, we can never remove the error completely.

Our trivial example of a proportional control system is characterized by a number of features, in the steady state:

(1) The information for driving the system, in this case the power output of the furnace, is proportional to an error signal.

(2) The error signal is derived from measuring the true value of the variable which is to be controlled, in this case, the actual inside air temperature, and subtracting it from the desired (set-point) value.

(3) The overall performance of the system will always be imperfect. The higher the gain of the system the less remaining static error.

(4) Nearly all physically realizable systems operate with true control, only over a limited range. Outside this range control is lost (see Figure 12.1(c)).

The purpose, of course, of this digression on some elementary aspects of control systems was not that of understanding how the central heating system in a home works. Rather, it is my hope that by reflecting on the characteristics of a control system we all 'understand', it may be possible to view, with fresh objectivity, our state of knowledge with respect to the so-called regulation of coronary blood flow.

There are other ways of approaching this problem: we could have used the mathematics of control systems theory (Riggs, 1976), but I fear the worst for those readers who have not suffered the pain and pleasure of a more mathematically orientated training (or education?) Thus, with all due apologies to the more formally trained of you, I have elected to 'analyse' the problem at hand through the use of analogy. I concede that such an approach is fraught with pitfalls, and both the writer and the reader should be cautious in accepting such an approach.

Does the Coronary Bed Behave Like a Control System?

If we consider the four points noted above, can we find an analogy in the experimentally determined characteristics of the coronary circulation. Consider point (4), the presence of regulation over a limited range. It would

seem reasonable to expect such a behaviour in the coronary bed since the
vascular resistance clearly has a minimum value, corresponding to the fully
dilated bed. Moreover, since the vascular resistance is determined by the
action of vascular smooth muscle, it seems likely that the resistance cannot
exceed a certain maximum, determined by the maximum value of tension
produced by the smooth muscle cell in the resistance vessel wall.

Autoregulation is an experiment in which one elicits a change in vascular
resistance by altering perfusion pressure. As one increases perfusion pressure in a preparation, flow remains quite constant. This can only happen if
the resistance increases, to 'counteract' the effects of the increased pressure.
Although the literature is rich in examples of this phenomenon, I take the
liberty of presenting some of our own results (Laird and Spaan, 1982a,b).

In Figure 12.2, one can see the measured relationship between coronary
blood flow and perfusion pressure over the range 40–180 mm Hg. As can be
seen, in this example, the flow is 'autoregulated' between approximately 80
and 130 mm Hg. On the low pressure side, we see the flow–pressure
relationship corresponding to the fully vasodilated bed. Every increase in

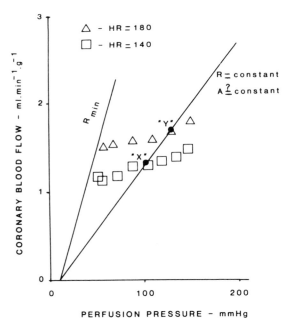

Figure 12.2 Coronary blood flow versus perfusion pressure with constant aortic
pressure. Data is presented at a heart rate of 140 (□) and 180 (△) beats min[-1]. The
maximal vasodilation line R_{min} is shown, as well as another arbitrary but constant
resistance line. If concentration of a vasodilator, A, is uniquely related to resistance,
points 'X' and 'Y' will have same concentration (see text)

pressure is accompanied by a corresponding increase in flow. This is in contrast to the autoregulated region, where a pressure increase is largely counteracted by a resistance increase to keep flow constant. At the high pressure end, I concede that imagination is required in order to see any evidence of the maximally constricted bed. I presume that the experimentalists among the readers will excuse our not having gone to such high and 'non-physiologic' perfusion pressures.

Thus, a limit of minimal resistance (furnace turned off) has been demonstrated, but what of the other limit? Is it possible to find the maximum resistance which the vascular bed is capable of reaching? In results from our laboratory obtained during long diastoles (Spaan and Laird, 1981; Laird and Spaan, 1982c) we have found that the resistance can rise to very high values indeed. In Figure 12.3, we see the time course of flow, under constant pressure perfusion conditions, during such a long diastole. The flow falls, with a time constant of approximately 4 s, to a flow value less than 20% of the control flow obtained with a constant perfusion pressure of 100 mm Hg. Since the flow can increase by approximately a factor of four with full dilatation, and can decrease by a factor of roughly five with active vasodilation, the full range of vascular resistance is roughly 20-fold.

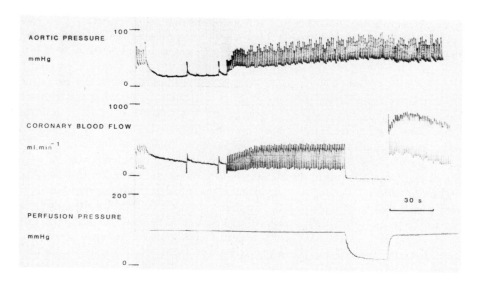

Figure 12.3 Aortic pressure, coronary flow, and perfusion pressure (filtered) versus time in an open-chest dog with AV block electrically paced. Shutting off pacer produces a long diastole and concomitant vasoconstriction. Compare with right half, where occlusion/release reactive hyperaemia demonstrates range of resistance of coronary bed

In summary, the active controller of coronary flow, the vascular resistance, is subject to real limits, both at the high end and at the low end. It is in between these limits that we must search for other measurable characteristics of a control system, if we are to be able to state whether or not coronary flow is truly controlled.

Isn't Auto-regulation Itself Proof of the Control of Flow?

The simple answer is, of course, yes. Flow changes only slightly (a small error?) while perfusion pressure changes over a wide range. Moreover, during autoregulation experiments, the limit of maximal vasodilation is easily demonstrated. So it's simple, flow is controlled; but the control itself has a maximum limit, just like the heating system in the home!

But . . .

If we now increase heart rate, and thereby oxygen consumption, at a constant perfusion pressure, the flow will, of course, increase. If we now, at this elevated oxygen consumption rate, vary the perfusion pressure, we obtain yet another example of autoregulation. It is very interesting, and probably significant, that this new autoregulation curve is apparently simply shifted to the new flow level. The slope, or perhaps better stated, the 'flatness' of the curve is the same. The effective gain of the system does not seem to change when the heart rate is increased. But, you will say, the 'thermostat' has simply been turned up. In technological terms, the set point has perhaps been altered. My question to you, then, is, by what mechanism was this achieved? Has the set point really been changed or is something else being regulated, other than the flow itself? Perhaps the regulated variable is a quantity which is only partially dependent on the flow.

A note of caution here is in order with regard to my somewhat incautious use of the word set point. In technical systems, such as the central heating system considered above, it is a perfectly useful idea, and can be identified with a physical component of the system – the thermostat. In physiological control systems it has been pointed out (Verveen, 1978, 1979) that the use of the term is 'inadvisable' and perhaps I should use the term 'reference state' instead. Part of this difficulty is related to an often futile attempt to search for the comparator, but there remain more fundamental objections to the use of the term. In the system under consideration here the comparator which is responsible for the 'error signal' may be nothing more mysterious than the law of conservation of mass, of the substance in question. Influx and outflux terms being 'compared' to each other.

IF IT'S NOT THE FLOW WHICH IS BEING CONTROLLED, WHAT IS IT THEN...?

The autoregulation experiment illustrates an important feature of a control system. A disturbance in the perfusion pressure is largely neutralized, leading to a minor change in flow. Taken by itself this suggests a true control of flow. Indeed, flow must be somewhere in the control loop. However, it is also known that a perturbation, or modest reduction in arterial oxygen content, leads to the well known phenomenon of hypoxic vasodilation. At constant perfusion pressure, lowering arterial oxygen tension leads to an increase in flow. In other words, this perturbation is not at all compensated for by keeping flow constant. The literature on hypoxic vasodilation does not permit a clear-cut interpretation. Some investigators (e.g. Stowe, 1980) find proportional increases in flow for every lowering of oxygen content in the perfusate at constant perfusion pressure. In the blood-perfused heart the matter is more complicated (Duvelleroy *et al.*, 1976, 1980) and many find an increase in flow only after arterial oxygen tension has been appreciably lowered (Berne *et al.*, 1957; Daugherty *et al.*, 1967). We shall return later to this important topic but I presume that all authors would agree that there exists a level of hypoxia where finally flow increases while the heart, itself, is not ischaemic. So, on the basis of this intervention alone, perhaps oxygen delivery, oxygen content multiplied by the flow, would be a good candidate for the parameter which is regulated.

However, if we perturb oxygen consumption by increasing heart rate, while keeping perfusion pressure and arterial oxygen content constant, the flow increases (see Figure 12.2). The increase in oxygen consumption is associated with a vasodilation. During the autoregulation experiment the increased perfusion pressure caused a 15–20% increase in oxygen consumption, but also led to a vasoconstriction! No wonder it is all a bit unclear.

A Single Mechanism? ... or a Combination of Effects?

At the beginning of this chapter attention was drawn to the recurrence of indications of an important role for both adenosine and oxygen. Let us now attempt to analyse these agents separately. Should that fail to explain the observed behaviour of the coronary system in the three standard experiments we will then consider briefly whether the two agents can act synergistically to save the day.

The adenosine hypothesis (Linder and Rigler, 1931; Berne, 1963; Gerlach *et al.*, 1963) is very attractive and would appear to offer the potential of 'explaining' the three standard experiments discussed above:

(1) Exogeneous adenosine is a potent vasodilator.

(2) The production rate of adenosine by the myocardial cell appears to parallel oxygen consumption (Berne, 1980; Knabb *et al.*, 1980).

(3) The dose–response relationship between vascular resistance and interstitial adenosine concentration should be appropriate and consistent with the changes induced by the standard interventions of the autoregulation, metabolic vasodilation, and hypoxic vasodilation experiments.

While much support can be found for the first two points, the relationship between interstitial concentration and vascular resistance raises questions. Moreover, it still remains to be demonstrated that the response of interstitial concentration is quantitatively consistent with observed changes in vascular conductance over the normal regulatory range.

The adenosine dose–response curve is a keystone of the hypothesis, and since the first study identifying its vasoactive properties (Drury and Szent Györgyi, 1929) has been a matter of continuous study and some debate (Breuls, 1981). The attempts to quantify the vasoactivity can be divided into two categories, dependent on whether or not an attempt was made to assay tissue adenosine concentration directly. The results have been quite variable, depending on the preparation and techniques used. The range in sensitivity is illustrated by noting that Schrader *et al.* (1977) found a 100-fold increase in concentration was required in order to decrease resistance by a factor of 3, whereas at the other extreme, Breuls (1981) found that a doubling in concentration was required to achieve the same effect.

Such studies are complicated by the recent evidence that no longer most of the adenosine content in a tissue sample can be regarded as being located in the extracellular space (see Chapter 23 by Olsson in this volume). Moreover, the assumption that plasma adenosine is equal to interstitial concentration fails to appreciate the contribution due to on-going release by the myocardial cell as well as the complexities of the washout problem (Breuls, 1981).

IS THE VASCULAR RESISTANCE SENSITIVE ENOUGH TO ADENOSINE?

This important question has received surprisingly little attention. Given the difficulties of determining the adenosine concentration at the site of action – the interstitium, we have in our laboratory attempted to make inferences based on compartmental models of a mass balance of adenosine. These range from the very simple (Laird *et al.*, 1981) to a rather more complex analysis (Breuls, 1981).

The Limiting Case

One of the more remarkable features of the family of autoregulation curves at different levels of oxygen consumption is, of course, the tight regulation of flow. The system shows a high sensitivity to small changes in flow. In control system terms, the gain is high: a 10–20% change ('error') in flow is associated with a three-fold change in resistance.

Let us consider a limiting case in which there is the tightest of coupling between flow and the interstitial concentration of adenosine. In order to do this, we have assumed (Laird *et al.*, 1981), that there is no diffusion barrier between the vascular and interstitial space. We regard the interstitial space as a 'well mixed' compartment into which adenosine is released by the myocardial cell. The steady state concentration is then determined by a balance between the rates of release and 'disappearance'. Adenosine released into the compartment can be (1) degraded or inactivated by endothelium and/or myocardial cells, (2) taken up again by myocardial cells, and (3) washed out of the interstitial space. (1) and (2) above are likely to be complex but it seems reasonable to presume that they are to be described as some function of the interstitial adenosine concentration, $Ch[A_i]$, the form of which is unknown but irrelevant. The rate of washout is, for this simple model, simply the plasma flow multiplied by the interstitial concentration. We can now set up the mass balance equation, in the steady state, for the interstitial compartment:

Production rate = (Degradation + uptake) rate + washout rate

or

$$Pr = Ch[A_i] + Q_p[A_i].\qquad(12.1)$$

If vascular resistance is determined by adenosine concentration, then we may draw a connection between two points at different heart rates in Figure 12.2, which have the same resistance and 'hence' the same adenosine concentration. Let us call such a pair of points 'X' and 'Y'. Since the adenosine concentration is the same, then it follows that the uptake/degradation rate will also be equal. If we then set up the mass balance equation (12.1) for two such points and subtract them from each other, we get, after re-arranging (Laird *et al.*, 1981)

$$\Delta Q = \frac{\Delta Pr}{[A_i]};\qquad(12.2)$$

that is, the amount by which the flow increases due to an increase in production rate of adenosine is proportional to the change in production rate, ΔPr, but inversely proportional to the adenosine concentration, along any line of constant adenosine concentration.

Recall and note that an increase in oxygen consumption is accompanied by a nearly parallel increase in flow, independent of perfusion pressure. Hence essentially independent of the adenosine concentration.

These two results can only be consistent with each other if the change in adenosine concentration required to cover the three-fold change in resistance is very small indeed. A range in adenosine concentration of 50% would already lead to a significant departure from a parallel shift. We conclude from this simple model that the known sensitivity of the vascular resistance to adenosine falls far short of that required to explain the observed changes in flow due to altered oxygen consumption and perfusion pressure. This simple model has been elegantly expanded by Breuls (1981), but the central conclusion remains unaltered. Adenosine is apparently not potent enough to explain autoregulation and metabolic vasodilation, or one is forced to make complex assumptions for which there is no experimental support.

There are some other results which are cause for concern in attempting to attribute an important role to adenosine in the regulation of coronary flow under normoxic conditions. It has recently been demonstrated (Hester *et al.*, 1982) that in the presence of massive infusions of adenosine, presumably overshadowing intrinsic adenosine production, after passage of some time the skeletal muscle flow returns to near control level and yet the exercise hyperaemia response remains intact.

The results obtained with various pharmacological and enzymatic agents intended to influence either the interstitial adenosine concentration or its action on vascular smooth muscle are not entirely consistent with each other.

The adenosine hypothesis is still attractive in its simplicity and plausibility even though, as Berne (1980) has pointed out, a number of questions remain unanswered. With all the respect due to those who have contributed so much to our understanding of the action of adenosine, some of the open questions really are quite crucial to the acceptance of a dominant role for adenosine in the regulation of coronary blood flow in the normal physiological range of conditions. The balance of rates responsible for determining the interstitial concentration of adenosine and the subsequent vasodilation form the main stumbling blocks.

WHAT ABOUT OXYGEN?

Since every student of physiology learns that a primary purpose of the circulation is to deliver oxygen and nutrients to hardworking tissues, it is no wonder that oxygen itself was an early candidate as the mediator of coronary blood flow. In 1982, while there remain cogent arguments against a role for oxygen, others keep coming to the conclusion that oxygen is somehow involved. The state of the debate concerning oxygen is even more bewildering than that concerning adenosine. This is, in my view, due in no small part to the fact that seldom is the 'oxygen hypothesis' stated in a form which is sufficiently well defined to permit a carefully designed experimental test to be made. When considering a potential role for oxygen in the regulation of coronary blood flow, it is important to be quite specific about the anatomical location of the presumed sensitivity.

The Mid-wall 'Oxygen Hypothesis'

In this version of the oxygen hypothesis, one takes note of the fact that the *lumen* of the resistance vessels are exposed to the oxygen tension of the *blood supply*, whereas the *outermost layer* is bathed in the oxygen tension of the *interstitial space*. This gradient in oxygen tension across the wall implies that the vascular smooth muscle 'sees' a p_{O_2} which is, in part, determined by the interstitial space. This would appear to offer the potential of coupling the vascular resistance to tissue oxygenation. In adition, of course, to others, this idea has been extensively examined over the years by Duling and his coworkers in a variety of preparations and has been extensively reviewed by Sparks (1981).

There are two major considerations which argue against a dominant role for vessel wall p_{O_2} in the regulation of flow. Firstly, the average vessel wall p_{O_2} would be expected to be proportionally sensitive to intraluminal oxygen, and in the normal regulation range every lowering of arterial oxygen content should be associated with a proportional vasodilation. This appears not to be the case (Berne *et al.*, 1957; Daugherty *et al.*, 1967), although these two crucial studies will be considered again later in this chapter. Duling and Berne (1970, 1971) have demonstrated that the transmural oxygen gradient leads to the transport of oxygen and to a subsequent fall in intraluminal oxygen content, decreasing the transmural gradient in the distal portions of an arteriole. Both model studies (Sparks, 1981) and experiments (Gorczynski and Duling, 1976) suggest that average wall p_{O_2} may not fall with metabolic vasodilation, and in fact may even rise at high levels of oxygen consumption.

The degree of oxygen sensitivity is also a matter of some debate. Many *in vitro* studies have used larger, relatively thick walled vessels and the question of contamination of the results by an anoxic core arises. However, Chang and Detar (1980) have recently shown an appropriate sensitivity in preparations which appear to be free of 'anoxic core' problems. Taken as a whole, the evidence that *vessel wall* p_{O_2} is directly responsible for the control of coronary blood flow is not very convincing.

Tissue Oxygen?

Ever since the pioneering studies early in this century (Markwalder and Starling, 1913; Hilton and Eichholtz, 1925) the idea that tissue oxygenation determines coronary blood flow persists. There is evidence both for and against, and Belloni (1979) concludes that oxygen is probably involved in hypoxic vasodilation and requires further evaluation in both autoregulation and metabolic vasodilation. An explanation for this confusing state of our knowledge is once again the fact that so many different preparations have been used to study each phenomenon (i.e. autoregulation, or metabolic vasodilation, or . . .). Rather than attempt to review the body of evidence for or against the role of tissue oxygen, I take the liberty of considering some of our recent work in this area (Laird and Spaan, 1982a,b,c).

While this work is, of course, also vulnerable to criticism, we have attempted to study both autoregulation and metabolic vasodilation in the same animal under comparable conditions. In five anaesthetised dogs the left main coronary artery was perfused under constant but adjustable pressure. The heart rate was also controlled by ventricular pacing after first inducing an AV block by intraseptal injection of 0.2 ml formaldehyde. Arterial-venous oxygen content difference was also measured continuously. Thus heart rate and coronary perfusion pressure were under control of the experimenter, while arterial pressure remained within narrow limits. From a given baseline condition an autoregulation curve was obtained by varying perfusion pressure while keeping heart rate constant. Then heart rate was increased while keeping perfusion pressure constant. A direct comparison was now possible and these results were also 'simulated' using a theoretical model in which interstitial oxygen tension was presumed to linearly determine vascular conductance.

The results of a typical experiment are shown in Figure 12.4 for the autoregulation intervention and in Figure 12.5 for the metabolic vasodilation experiment. As can be seen in Figure 12.4, the preparation showed the parallel shift of autoregulation curves as well as a decline in AV oxygen difference as perfusion pressure increased. Most intriguing is the fact that the oxygen model 'predicts' a similar response, even though no serious attempt was made to fit the model parameters to the experiment.

When perfusion pressure was kept constant and heart rate was increased, the standard metabolic vasodilation curve results (Figure 12.5). Oxygen extraction also increased with increasing heart rate. These results are also broadly consistent with the model simulations, although the AV difference would appear to be less sensitive to perfusion pressure than predicted by the model. It is important to realize that such experiments take time to do and there is always the risk that the baseline condition of the dog may have altered. If one is interested in the effect of perfusion pressure as variable, one should examine the autoregulation results of Figure 12.4. For heart rate effects, Figure 12.5 should serve as the reference.

The increased conductance resulting from increasing heart rate is the usual demonstration of the tight coupling between oxygen consumption and

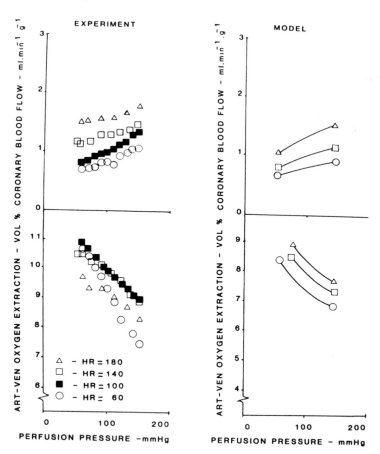

Figure 12.4 Coronary flow and arteriovenous oxygen extraction versus perfusion pressure at different heart rates. Left panel: experimental results in one dog. Right panel: model results assuming interstitial oxygen tension regulates conductance. Oxygen consumption ranges from lowest (open circles) to highest (open triangles). (See text)

flow. It is interesting to note that during autoregulation, flow increases slightly as perfusion pressure increases, while AV oxygen extraction declines. The product, however, does increase by 10–20%. This is then an experiment in which there is an inverse relationship between conductance and oxygen consumption, since at the higher perfusion pressure the resistance has increased to maintain flow close to constant. This illustrates the necessity of caution when interpreting such experiments.

The conductance as a function of venous oxygen content is shown in Figure 12.6. This result can be compared with the important and often

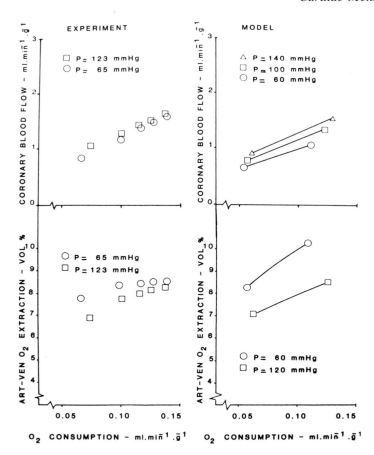

Figure 12.5 Coronary flow and arteriovenous oxygen extraction versus oxygen consumption with constant perfusion pressure for same dog as shown in Figure 12.4 (left panel). O_2 consumption was increased by increasing heart rate. Model results (right panel) assume interstitial oxygen tension to be controller of vascular conductance (see text)

quoted study by Berne *et al.* (1957), in which 'reduction of oxygen content of arterial blood produced increases in coronary blood flow only when coronary sinus oxygen levels fell below about 5.5 volumes percent'. Our own results partially confirm Berne's finding that at the lower oxygen levels (less than 3.5 vol%), the sensitivity is greatly enhanced. However, the sensitivity between 3 and 6 vol% is clearly non-zero. In this experiment the dilution was substantial and the haemoglobin concentration was 8 g per 100 ml, which is responsible for the low coronary venous oxygen content in control states. Since the study by Berne *et al.* (1957) is a key basis for

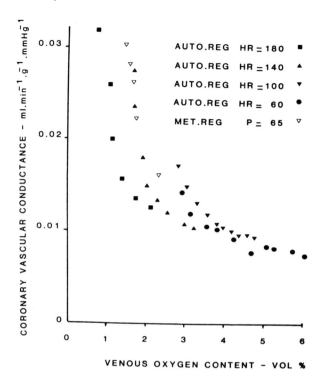

Figure 12.6 Vascular conductance versus coronary venous oxygen content for both autoregulation (solid symbols) and metabolic vasodilation (open symbols), for same dog as shown in Figures 12.4 and 12.5. No corrections made for changes in arterial O₂ content due to haemodilution (see text)

rejecting the oxygen hypothesis in the blood-perfused heart, this small but important difference deserves further attention.

So What?

The broad agreement between the predictions of the model and the experiment must be viewed with caution. While satisfying to the model builder, it means only that 'it *could* work that way'. The agreement with a model based on interstitial oxygen tension could be quite direct via some as yet unidentified receptor, or very indirect via one or more metabolic products acting as a signal reflecting tissue oxygen. Probably, the only way to unravel the direct versus the indirect hypothesis is via pharmacological studies in which actions are blocked. The results of such efforts in the adenosine story do not encourage an overly optimistic expectation in this.

WHAT ABOUT COMBINED EFFECTS?

As noted above, there are major difficulties in attributing *the role* of mediator of coronary flow regulation to any one of the long list of candidate substances. This has led many if not most authors to the belief that it is a combination of several effectors which somehow saves the day (Haddy and Scott, 1975). Given the difficulties of studying just one substance, it is not surprising that the combined hypothesis has received relatively little attention.

What should one have as a framework for thinking about combined effects? Consider, for a moment, the 'simple' case of the combined effects of oxygen and adenosine. If oxygen can be held responsible for 20% of a given response and adenosine for another 20%, is it correct to assume that the combination will be 40%? Using a variety of preparations and strategies, the facts are not clear and range (Lamerant and Becsei, 1972; Moir and Jones, 1973; Gellai *et al.*, 1973; Stowe, 1980) from simple addition to either impaired or enhanced interaction. These studies provide little encouragement for the combined hypothesis, although one is also forced to the conclusion that we just do not have the methods either to analyse combined systems or to design the right experiments. Attention needs to be devoted to the task of developing such tools.

PERHAPS WE'VE OVERSIMPLIFIED

The oxygen model discussed here (Laird, 1982b) is not really new (Grunewald, 1968; Middleman, 1972; Granger and Shepherd, 1973; Duvelleroy *et al.*, 1973, Grunewald and Sowa, 1977; Mild and Linderholm, 1981). For practical reasons we have all used a very simple geometry ranging from a well mixed compartment to an ordered array of Krogh cylinders uniformly perfused. The briefest of glances at the microvascular system of the heart (Brown, 1965; Bassingthwaighte *et al.*, 1974) is enough to put a cold chill through the spine of this model builder. It is hard to imagine that either a well mixed compartment or a uniformly perfused array of capillaries would give an accurate description of mass transport in such a complex system.

However, the experimentalist might also gain food for thought, since it is clear that tissue oxygen tension is not at all uniform in the myocardium (Whalen, 1971; Lösse *et al.*, 1975; Grunewald and Lübbers, 1975; Schubert *et al.*, 1978), and that the oxidative metabolic state shows substantial heterogeneity (Steenbergen and Williamson, 1980; Williamson *et al.*, 1982). This means that simple thinking, whether in a model or in the design, and interpretation of an experiment is an invitation to drawing incorrect and incomplete conclusions. We have made a first model step by trying 'simply' to calculate the flow distribution in the capillary network (Wieringa *et al.*,

1982), and it remains to be seen how far this can be extended to include mass transport aspects. The work of Schubert (1978), Honig and Odoroff (1981), Steinhausen *et al.* (1978), and Tillmanns *et al.*, (1981) may point in the right direction. The tools will just have to be developed to grapple with the complexity of reality. Until then, many of the statements (including ours) about the determinants of coronary flow will have to be taken with a 'grain of salt' (or perhaps adenosine).

It is difficult to write a chapter in which one must conclude that we just do not understand the regulation of coronary blood flow. I take heart in the fact that I would appear to be in very distinguished company (see references).

ACKNOWLEDGEMENTS

I am grateful to members of the staff and students in our laboratory who have permitted me to make liberal use of their results. In particular, my colleague Dr Ir Jos A. E. Spaan deserves special mention along with Dr P. N. W. M. Breuls, whose thesis work on adenosine has been most enlightening.

We are most grateful to Dr Mark Noble and Dr Angela Drake-Holland for the collaboration which has led to the autoregulation/metabolic flow experiments of Figures 12.4, 12.5, and 12.6. The technical assistance of Mr A. Boekee along with many students made the experiments possible and the figures readable. Our secretary, Mrs J. Bok-Krieger, did her best to compensate for my tardy production of this chapter.

REFERENCES

Bassingthwaighte, J. B., Yipintsoi, T., and Harvey, R. B. (1974). Microvasculature of the dog left ventricular myocardium. *Microvasc. Res.*, **7**, 229–249.
Belloni, F. L. (1979). Review: the local control of coronary blood flow. *Cardiovasc. Res.*, **13**, 63–85.
Berne, R. M. (1963). Cardiac nucleotides in hypoxia: possible role in regulation of coronary blood flow. *Amer. J. Physiol.* **204**, 317–322.
Berne, R. M. (1980). The role of adenosine in the regulation of coronary blood flow. *Circulation Res.*, **47**, 807–813.
Berne, R. M., and Rubio, R. (1979). Coronary circulation. In *Handbook of Physiology, The Cardiovascular System, The Heart* (R. M. Berne, ed.), Bethesda, Md, American Physiological Society, Sec. 2, Vol. 1, Chap. 25.
Berne, R. M., Blackmon, J. R., and Gardner, T. H. (1957). Hypoxemia and coronary blood flow. *J. Clin. Invest.*, **36**, 1101–1106.
Breuls, P. N. W. M. (1981). Adenosine and the control of coronary blood flow. Thesis, Leiden University, Leiden, the Netherlands.
Brown, R. E. (1965). The pattern of the microcirculatory bed in the ventricular myocardium of domestic mammals. *Amer. J. Anat.*, **116**, 355–374.
Chang, A. E., and Detar, R. (1980). Oxygen and vascular muscle contraction revisited. *Amer. J. Physiol.*, **238**, H716–H728.

Daugherty, R. M., Scott, J. B., Dabney, J. M., and Haddy, E. J. (1967). Local effects of O_2 and CO_2 on Limb, Renal, and Coronary Vascular Resistances. *Amer. J. Physiol.*, **213**, 1102–1110.

Drury, A. N., and Szent-Györgyi, A. (1929). The physiological activity of adenine compounds with special reference to their action upon the mammalian heart. *J. Physiol. (Lond.)*, **68**, 213–237.

Duling, B. R., and Berne, R. M. (1970). Longitudinal gradients in periarteriolar oxygen tension. *Circulation Res.*, **27**, 669–678.

Duling, B. R., and Berne, R. M. (1971). Oxygen and the local regulation of blood flow: possible significance of longitudinal gradients in arterial blood oxygen tension. *Circulation Res.*, **28**, Suppl. 1, 65–69.

Duvelleroy, M. A., Mehmel, H., and Laver, M. B. (1973). Hemoglobin–oxygen equilibrium and coronary blood flow: an analog model. *J. Appl. Physiol.*, **35**, 480–484.

Duvelleroy, M. A., Duruble, M., Martin, J. L., Teisseire, B., Droulez, J., and Cain, M. (1976). Blood perfused working isolated rat heart. *J. Appl. Physiol.*, **41**, 603–607.

Duvelleroy, M. A., Martin, J. L., Teisseire, B., Gauduel, Y., and Duruble, M. (1980). Abnormal hemoglobin oxygen affinity and the coronary circulation. *Bibl. Haemat.*, **46**, 70–77.

Duvelleroy, M. A., Martin, J. L., Teisseire, B., Duruble, M., and Laver, M. B. (1981). Graphical analysis of the effect of changes in hemoglobin oxygen affinity on myocardial oxygen supply. *Bull. Europ. Physiopath. Resp.*, **17**, 365–380.

Gellai, M., Norton, J. M., and Detar, R. (1973). Evidence for direct control of coronary vascular tone by oxygen. *Circulation Res.*, **32**, 279–289.

Gerlach, E., Deuticke, B., and Dreisbach, R. H. (1963). Der Nucleiotid-Abbau im Hertzmuskel bei Sauerstoffmangel und seine mögliche Bedeutung für die Coronardurchblutung. *Naturwissenschaften*, **50**, 228–229.

Gorczynski, R. I., and Duling, B. R. (1976). The role of O_2 lack in contraction induced arteriolar vasodilation in hamster striated muscle. *Fed. Proc.*, **35**, 448.

Granger, H. J., and Shepherd, A. P. (1973). Intrinsic microvascular control of tissue oxygen delivery. *Microvasc. Res.*, **5**, 49–72.

Grunewald, W. (1968). Theoretical analysis of the oxygen supply in tissue. In *Oxygen Transport in Blood and Tissue* (G. Thews and E. Witzleh, eds), G. Thieme Verlag, Stuttgart.

Grunewald, W. A., and Lübbers, D. W. (1975). Die Bestimmung der intracapillären HbO_2-Sättigung mit einer kryomikrofotometrischen Methode angewandte am Myokard des Kaninchens. *Pflügers Arch. Europ. J. Physiol.*, **353**, 255–273.

Grunewald, W. A., and Sowa, W. (1977). Capillary structures and O_2 supply to tissue. An analysis with a digital diffusion model as applied to the skeletal muscle. *Rev. Physiol. Biochem. Pharmacol.*, **77**, 149–209.

Haddy, F. J. and Scott, J. B. (1975). Metabolic factors in peripheral circulatory regulation. *Fed. Proc.*, **34**, 2006–2011.

Hester, R. L., Guyton, A. C., and Barber, B. J. (1982). Reactive and exercise hyperemia during high levels of adenosine infusions. *Amer. J. Physiol.*, **243**, H181–H186.

Hilton, R., and Eichholtz, E. (1925). The influence of chemical factors on the coronary circulation. *J. Physiol. (Lond.)*, **59**, 413–425.

Hoffman, J. I. E. (1980). Key references, coronary blood flow. *Circulation*, **62**, 187–198.

Honig, C. R., Odoroff, C. L. (1981). Calculated dispersion of capillary transit times: significant for oxygen exchange. *Amer. J. Physiol.*, **240**, H199–H208.

Knabb, R. M., Bacchus, A. N., Rubio, R., and Berne, R. M. (1980). Parallel changes in myocardial oxygen consumption and adenosine production. *Physiologist*, **23**, 5 (Abstr.).

Laird, J. D., and Spaan, J. A. E. (1982a). The effect of variations in coronary perfusion pressure and heart rate on coronary flow and oxygen extraction in the dog heart. *J. Physiol. (Lond.)*, **324**, 71P.

Laird, J. D., and Spaan, J. A. E. (1982b). A simple computer model of coronary flow based on interstitial oxygen tension. *J. Physiol. (Lond.)*, **324**, 1P.

Laird, J. D., and Spaan, J. A. E. (1982c). The mechanisms of coronary flow – some critical remarks. In *What is Angina?* (D. G. Julian, K. I. Lie, and L. Wilhelmsen, eds), A. B. Hasle, The Hague, pp. 42–49.

Laird, J. D., Breuls, P. N. W. M., van der Meer, P., and Spaan, J. A. E. (1981). Can a single vasodilator be responsible for both coronary autoregulation and metabolic vasodilation? *Basic Res. Cardiol.*, **76**, 354–358.

Lammerant, J., and Becsei, I. (1972). Response of the coronary circulation to hypoxia in the anesthetized intact dog infused with adenosine. *Arch. Internat. Pharmacodyn. Ther.*, **200**, 309–319.

Linder, F., and Rigler, R. (1931). Uber die Beeinflussing der Weite der Herzkranzgefässe durch Produkte des Zellkernstoffwechsels. *Pflügers Arch. Ges. Physiol.*, **226**, 697–708.

Lösse, B., Schuchardt, S., and Niederle, N. (1975). The oxygen pressure histogram in the left ventricular myocardium of the dog. *Pflügers Arch. Europ. J. Physiol.*, **356**, 121–132.

Markwalder, J., and Starling, E. H. (1913). A note on some factors which determine the blood-flow through the coronary circulation. *J. Physiol. (Lond.)*, **47**, 275–285.

Middleman, S. (1972). *Transport Phenomena in the Cardiovascular System*, John Wiley, New York.

Mild, K. H., and Linderholm, A. (1981). Some factors of significance for respiratory gas exchange. A mathematical analysis of a capillary model. *Acta Physiol. Scand.*, **112**, 395–404.

Moir, T. W., and Jones, P. K. (1973). Observations on the effect of changes in arterial oxygenation on adenosine induced coronary vasodilation. *Advanc. Exp. Med. Biol.*, **39**, 11–26.

Olsson, R. A. (1981). Local factors regulating cardiac and skeletal muscle blood flow. *Annu. Rev. Physiol.*, **43**, 385–395.

Riggs, D. S. (1976). *Control Theory and Physiological Feedback Mechanisms*, R. E. Krieger, Huntington, N.Y.

Schrader, J., Haddy, F. J., and Gerlach, E. (1977). Release of adenosine, inosine, and hypoxanthine from the isolated guinea pig heart during hypoxia, flow-autoregulation and reactive hyperemia. *Pflügers Arch. Europ. J. Physiol.* **369**, 1–6.

Schubert, R. W., Whalen, W. J., and Nair, P. (1978). Myocardial p_{O_2} distribution: relationship to coronary autoregulation. *Amer. J. Physiol.*, **234**, H361–H370.

Spaan, J. A. E., and Laird, J. D. (1981). Coronary vasoconstriction in long diastoles. *Circulation*, **64**, IV-39 (Abstr.).

Sparks, H. V. (1981). Effect of local metabolic factors on vascular smooth muscle. In *Handbook of Physiology, The Cardiovascular System, II Peripheral Circulation*, (D. F. Bohr, ed.), Bethesda, Md, American Physiological Society, Chapter 17.

Steenbergen, C., and Williamson, J. R. (1980). Heterogenous coronary perfusion during myocardial hypoxia. *Advanc. Myocardiol.*, **2**, 271–284.

Steinhausen, M., Tillmanns, H., and Thederan, H. (1978). Microcirculation of the epimyocardial layer of the heart. *Pflügers Arch. Europ. J. Physiol.*, **378**, 9–14.

Stowe, D. (1980). Vasodilator responses to moderate hypoxia after submaximal adenosine injection or coronary occlusion in isolated perfused guinea pig hearts. *Circulation Res.*, **47,** 392–399.

Tillmanns, H., Steinhausen, M., Leinberger, H., Thederan, H., and Kubler, W. (1981). Coronary microcirculatory hemodynamics during myocardial ischemia. *Europ. Heart J.* **2,** Suppl. A, 159 (Abstr. 303).

Verveen, A. A. (1978). Silent endocrine tumors: a steady-state analysis of the effects of changes in cell number for biological feedback systems. *Biol. Cybernet.*, **31,** 49–54.

Verveen, A. A. (1979). Left- and right-regulating systems: a steady-state analysis of function and structure of simple feedback systems. *Biol. Cybernet.*, **35,** 131–136.

Whalen, W. J. (1971). Intracellular p_{O_2} in heart and skeletal muscle. *Physiologist*, **14,** 69–82.

Wieringa, P. A., Spaan, J. A. E., Stassen, H. G., and Laird, J. D. (1982). Heterogeneous flow distribution in a three-dimensional network simulation of the myocardial microcirculation. *Microcirculation*, **2,** 195–216.

Williamson, J. R., Jamieson, D., Joseph, S. K., Davis, K., and Seeholzer, S. (1982). Quantitative analysis of tissue oxygen heterogeneity in perfused hearts. *Fed. Proc.*, **41,** 1530.

Cardiac Metabolism
Edited by A. J. Drake-Holland and M. I. M. Noble
© 1983 John Wiley & Sons Ltd

CHAPTER 13

High Energy Phosphate Compounds

L. H. Opie

Department of Medicine, University of Cape Town, Observatory 7925, Cape Town, South Africa

INTRODUCTION

The mechanisms and determinants of synthesis of high energy phosphates are reviewed extensively elsewhere in this book and will be only briefly mentioned. The possibility that cardiac high energy phosphate compounds are compartmentalized receives special attention. Thereafter, pathways for degradation and synthesis of high energy compounds are analysed. Mention is made of the possible function of adenosine triphosphate (ATP) as a neurotransmitter. Finally, non-adenine nucleotides are briefly examined.

AEROBIC METABOLISM

Substrates for the Normal Heart

Current knowledge of myocardial metabolism is a directly result of the pioneering work of Bing, who introduced coronary sinus catheterization in man. Detailed consideration of this subject is given in a separate chapter (Drake-Holland, Chapter 9 in this volume).

Effect of Circulating Levels of Non-esterified Fatty Acids (NEFAs = FFAs)

The spontaneous elevation of NEFAs in the blood, which occurs during fasting, leads to inhibition of glucose uptake and oxidation. Conversely, the decrease in blood levels of NEFAs during glucose and insulin administration leads to decreased fatty acid and increased glucose oxidation. The uptake of NEFAs by the heart is thought to depend on the circulating levels of NEFAs; the uptake does not require energy and is governed to a large extent by the rate of cellular oxidation of fatty acids. In addition, the molar ratio of NEFAs to albumin is important. NEFAs are carried in the blood by albumin. When the NEFA:albumin molar ratio is less than 2:1, tight binding sites on the albumin molecule are involved. Some workers think that at higher molar ratios it is easier for the fatty acid binding sites within the heart cell to free the circulating fatty acids from the circulating albumin. At normal albumin concentrations, NEFA can rise to about $1200 \, \mu\text{Eq} \, \text{l}^{-1}$ (1.2 mM) before exceeding the ratio of 2:1. Thus, as the circulating NEFA level rises, two conflicting factors are at work: the myocardial uptake processes become saturated and the rates of uptake of NEFA reach a plateau; at the same time progressively 'less tight' albumin binding sites are involved, with a tendency to increase the uptake of NEFAs (Opie, 1980).

Storage of NEFAs as intracellular products, such as triglycerides is reviewed by van der Vusse and Reneman (Chapter 10 in this volume).

Lactate Metabolism and Pyruvate Dehydrogenase

Lactate utilization by the heart is discussed by Drake-Holland, in Chapter 9 this volume. Pyruvate dehydrogenase activity, which regulates the rate of entry from glycolysis or from lactate (via pyruvate) into the Krebs' cycle is governed by a kinase–phosphatase cycle. The percentage of pyruvate dehydrogenase in the active form falls with fasting, or provision of NEFA or ketone bodies as alternate fuels or in diabetes or decreased cardiac activity (Randle, 1976). On the other hand, the percentage in the active form rises with provision of pyruvate, and when the $\text{NADH}:\text{NAD}^+$ ratio falls, as may occur with increased heart work. The activity of pyruvate dehydrogenase may limit glycolysis during ischaemia, but it may stay active in ischaemia, despite the higher mitochondrial ratios of $\text{NADH}:\text{NAD}^+$, because of the very low ATP/ADP ratio. The exact relation of these activating and inhibiting factors to the kinase-phosphatase cycle is not yet known.

Non-Esterified Fatty Acids and Mitochondrial Energy Production

There is an important relationship between fatty acid metabolism and mitochondrial oxidative phosphorylation. Normally acyl-CoA helps to regulate transfer of adenine nucleotides in and out of the mitochondria by the translocase.

During ischaemia acyl-CoA accumulates and the effects may include the following: (1) competitive inhibition of the nucleotide translocase with respect to ADP and ATP; (2) acyl-CoA may inhibit its own oxidation; (3) acyl-CoA may inhibit Na^+, K^+-ATPase activity of the cardiac sarcolemma; (4) acyl-CoA may inhibit acyl-CoA synthase activity and thereby inhibit its own formation and regulate the rate of fatty acid metabolism by the heart. Acyl-CoA also accumulates in starvation or alloxan diabetes and during provision of excess exogenous NEFA. An additional abnormality in ischaemia is the accumulation of acyl-carnitine, which inhibits the Na^+,

K$^+$-ATPase of the heart. The latter enzyme is more sensitive to acyl-carnitine than it is to acyl-CoA.

The simple hypothesis that long chain acyl-CoA inhibits mitochondrial oxidative phosphorylation in ischaemia has recently been challenged by Lochner *et al.* (1981). First, in dog hearts with coronary artery ligation, the tissue acyl-CoA level rises even in the non-ischaemic tissue, yet mitochondrial function in that zone is normal (Shug *et al.*, 1975). Secondly, Lochner (Table 13.1) was able to show in a hypoxic, low-flow model of ischaemia in the rat heart, that addition of glucose to perfusates containing palmitate increased mitochondrial acyl-CoA while decreasing adenine nucleotide activity and O$_2$ uptake, as predicted (Lochner *et al.*, 1981). However, in control non-ischaemic hearts, much higher mitochondrial acyl-CoA levels were reached in the presence of glucose, while the adenine translocase activity was unchanged and oxygen uptake was higher. Thus elevation of acyl-CoA, by itself, is not inhibitory to mitochondrial metabolism *in situ*. Possibly when there is combined accumulation of both intracellular NEFAs and acyl-CoA then the capacity of the intracellular fatty acid binding proteins is exceeded and acyl-CoA becomes inhibitory.

Table 13.1 Effect of variations in mitochondrial acyl-CoA on mitochondrial oxidative metabolism in ischaemic rat hearts

Substrate	Mitochondrial acyl-CoA (nmol (mg protein)$^{-1}$)	Adenine nucleotide translocase activity (nmol ATP mg^{-1} per 14 min)	Mitochondrial oxidative phosphorylation rate (nmol ATP mg^{-1} min^{-1})
1. None	0.269 ± 0.031 (6)	0.063 ± 0.008 (8)	40.1 ± 3.30 (16)
2. Glucose + insulin	0.341 ± 0.030 (4)	0.150 ± 0.015 (16)	104.1 ± 15.3 (5)
P vs. 1	NS	<0.001	<0.001
3. Glucose + insulin + propranolol	0.490 ± 0.028 (4)	0.229 ± 0.021 (8)	125.2 ± 9.9 (6)
P vs. 1	<0.001	<0.001	<0.001
4. Palmitate + albumin	0.322 ± 0.024 (4)	0.207 ± 0.013 (7)	126.5 ± 10.7 (4)
P vs. 1	NS	<0.001	<0.001
5. Palmitate + albumin + glucose	0.881 ± 0.072 (4)	0.157 ± 0.014 (8)	51.8 ± 4.6 (6)
P vs. 1	<0.001	<0.001	NS
P vs. 4			

Reproduced with permission from A. Lochner, I. van Niekerk, and J. C. N. Kotze, *J. Mol. Cell. Cardiol.*, **13**, 991–997 (1981).

ANAEROBIC ENERGY METABOLISM

Anoxia versus Ischaemia

In very primitive cells, with the absence or only rudimentary mitochondrial respiration, a major source of energy is from glycolysis. When such cells are deprived of oxygen, glycolysis is accelerated to produce increased amounts of anaerobic energy (Pasteur effect). A similar pattern of response of glycolysis to hypoxia can be found even in cells with high rates of mitochondrial metabolism, as in the heart. The Pasteur effect in the heart deprived of oxygen comprises: acceleration of glycolysis, especially at the level of the enzyme phosphofructokinase, by the metabolic consequences of hypoxia; loss of adenosine triphosphate and creatine phosphate; increase of inorganic phosphate and adenosine monophosphate; and a decrease in the level of citrate.

When ischaemia is also present (low-flow hypoxia), there are the superimposed effects produced by (1) a build-up of products of glycolysis and (2) persistent residual oxidative metabolism of varying degree and duration (Gevers, 1977).

Possible Contribution of Anaerobic Glycolysis to Energy Demands of the Well Perfused, Anoxic Heart

Because both anoxia and the acute onset of left atrial perfusion with a sudden increase in heart work increase glycolytic flux and at the same time lower the tissue contents of the substrates of phosphofructokinase (glucose-6-phosphate, fructose-6-phosphate, and ATP), the increased activity of phosphofructokinase must be caused by factors other than the substrate concentration. (This conclusion only holds if the concentration of substrate presented to the enzyme changes in a similar direction to the overall tissue content). Both anoxia and acute heart work appear to activate phosphofructokinase, probably by changes in adenine nucleotides. Opie (1971/72) subjected Langendorff-perfused hearts to the acute onset of left atrial perfusion with an anoxic perfusate, i.e. in condition of 'anoxic work'. The peak rates of glycolytic flow observed during the initial period of glycogenolysis could provide only about 30% of the energy needs of the working heart for less than 1 min.

Even with optimal conditions (high coronary perfusion rates and near maximal rates of membrane transport and flow through phosphofructokinase), anaerobic glycolysis could not sustain the energy required by the working heart should sudden, total deprivation of oxygen occur. Rather, it is necessary to conserve the available ATP by a reduction in heart work, such as can be achieved by (1) a medium high in K^+ or low in Ca^{++} or (2) a 'cardioplegic' medium low in Na^+ and containing procaine, or hypothermia. It is of interest that 'cardioplegia' and hypothermia also reduce ATP demand and are also associated with changes in the tissue contents of hexose monophosphates which are consonant with increased inhibition of phosphofructokinase activity.

The addition of citrate cycle intermediates to the medium, even in concentrations (10–15 mM) which are a great many times higher than those ever found in the circulation *in vivo*, were unable to maintain more than one-quarter of the normal heart rate of the 'non-working', Langendorff-perfused rat heart. It would be most unlikely that the energy demands of the working rat heart could be met in this way.

Further consideration of this problem is given by Drake-Holland and van der Vusse and Reneman (Chapters 9 and 10 in this volume).

HEART WORK AND ATP

Neely *et al.* (1972) found no overall change in adenine nucleotides with increased heart work and concluded that 'the particular approach utilized in this study is inadequate for the purpose of investigating mechanisms controlling cycle turnover'. Yet in 1976 Neely *et al.* conclude that 'the energy stores decreased with increased cardiac work at all concentrations of glucose studied' and in 1977 Hochachka *et al.*, state that 'there is general agreement that activation of respiration is associated with a decrease in cytosolic phosphate potential as defined by $[ATP]/[ADP][P_i]$'. Although these later conclusions are in accord with the earlier proposition of Opie and Mansford (1971) that adenine nucleotide changes as a result of increased heart work have a role in regulation of respiration (Opie *et al.* 1971a), and do not simply reflect tissue hypoxia, nevertheless it seems as if the earlier observations of Neely *et al.* (1972) cannot be dismissed.

Two possibilities present themselves. First, there may be beat to beat control with variations of high energy phosphate compounds during the heart cycle (see next section). Secondly, the adenine nucleotide changes reported by Neely *et al.* (1976) occurred in glucose-perfused hearts during the onset of atrial perfusion, as did the changes reported by Opie and Mansford (1971) and Opie *et al.* (1971a). There seems to be no repudiation of the findings with the Langendorff heart as presented in Neely *et al.* (1972). Therefore, a preculiarity of the Langendorff preparation seems a possibility; as already argued, it may be that respiration is coronary flow dependent in this unphysiological way of increasing the heart work. Thus, a primary increase in the coronary flow rate and perfusion pressure increases the contractile activity and oxygen uptake of the normal myocardium.

The phenomenon was apparently first described by Opie in 1965, but the

Table 13.2 Effect of increased heart work on high energy phosphate compounds of perfused rat heart

	ATP (μmol g^{-1})†	ADP (μmol g^{-1})	AMP (μmol g^{-1})	CP (μmol g^{-1})	ATP:ADP	ATP turnover (μmol g^{-1} min^{-1})‡
Opie et al. *(1971b), overall tissue values*						
Low work	4.84	0.96	0.071	8.27	5.0	33
Work, 5 s	4.58	1.13	0.147	4.75	4.1	83
Work, 15 s	4.27	1.26	0.192	3.86	4.2	83
Work, 5 min	5.00	1.17	0.052	5.86	4.3	83
Williamson et al. *(1976), overall tissue values*						
Low work	4.28	0.64	—	—	6.7	30
Work 20–30 s	4.01	0.74	—	—	5.4	120
Williamson et al. *(1976), cytosolic values*						
Low work	3.86	0.02	—	—	193	30
Work 20–30 s	3.68	0.04	—	—	92	120

† These units are micromoles per gram fresh weight (dry weight $\times$ 5).
‡ Calculated from oxygen uptake with a P:O ratio of 3.

mechanism of the effect still remains unknown. Arnold *et al.* (1968) have described the 'garden hose' phenomenon whereby an increased coronary perfusion pressure distends the coronary arteries, as does water filling a garden hose. As the hose stiffens, more contractile activity is required by the heart. Bacaner *et al.* (1971) have suggested that a certain amount of the normal myocardium is underperfused and when the coronary flow rate is increased, the tissue oxygenation improves. Hence respiration would be 'oxygen-driven' and not 'ADP-driven' (see Owen and Wilson, 1974). That would explain why Neely *et al.* failed to find adenine nucleotide changes with an increased perfusion pressure.

Further information on the problem as studied by NMR techniques is given by Dawson (Chapter 14 in this volume).

Beat-to-beat Control

Neely *et al.* (1972), expecting but failing to find adenine nucleotide changes when the coronary perfusion pressure was increased, supposed that there could be beat-to-beat changes with fluctuations in the overall tissue content of adenine nucleotides measured over some seconds by the Wollenberger freezing technique (Wollenberger *et al.*, 1960). Support for this contention is derived from Wollenberger's and his collaborators' observation (quoted by Wollenberger *et al.*, 1973) that the phosphate potential decreased at the initiation of systole. However, these data were obtained on the slowly beating frog heart. In the meantime, however, informative calculations could be made. With an increased perfusion pressure, the oxygen uptake of the Langendorff heart increased from 25 to 61 μmol O$_2$ min^{-1} per gram dry weight (Neely *et al.*, 1972) i.e. an increase of about 7 μmol O$_2$ min^{-1} per gram fresh weight; this represents an increased turnover of about 40 μmol ATP min^{-1} per gram fresh weight, or of about 0.1–0.2 μmol ATP min^{-1} per beat, compared with the tissue ATP content of 5 μmol per gram fresh weight. It is difficult to see how beat-to-beat variations in ATP could be measured as also suggested by a consideration of the turnover per beat versus total ATP content (Neely *et al.*, 1972). If *all* the ATP broken down formed ADP (which is unlikely) the free cytosolic ADP would have to rise by 0.1–0.2 μmol per beat to account for a doubling of respiration. In fact, the cytosolic content of ADP at a low workload is about 1/33 of the total ADP content according to Williamson *et al.* (1976b), i.e. about 0.025 μmol per gram fresh weight and therefore only about one-quarter of the calculated ATP breakdown would need to form cytosolic ADP to drive respiration during each beat, i.e. the changes are in the right order of magnitude. The problem could be examined by measuring beat-to-beat changes with NMR (Dawson, Chapter 14 in this volume).

Similar arguments for a similar increase in oxygen uptake obtained by left atrial filling should then suggest that ATP (and creatine phosphate, CP) should *not* be broken down in large amounts during increased heart work, whatever the means of induction of increased work might be. The most probable explanation of the change in ATP, and especially in CP, is that there is a transient period of ischaemia at the onset of heart work, according to the Anrep effect as stressed by Monroe *et al.* (1972). It could be speculated that such temporary ischaemia could lead to a compensatory rise in the coronary flow rate by the Berne adenosine mechanism, a sequence of events which could explain the large initial decreases in the high energy phosphate compounds (Opie *et al.*, 1971a) and the later restitution virtually to normal. Even in some normal subjects, ECG changes of ischaemia occur at the start of an abrupt increase in heart work (Barnard *et al.*, 1973).

Two other explanations for an excessive initial fall of ATP are advanced by Opie *et al.* (1971a). First, catecholamine stimulation could have occurred, because catecholamines are released from the actutely working heart (Monroe *et al.*, 1966). Secondly, an acute influx of Ca^{++} could have occurred (Nayler *et al.*, 1970) and Ca^{++} is known to break down high energy phosphate compounds (Schildberg and Fleckenstein, 1965).

It should be noted that myocardial *hypoxia*, sometimes thought to occur in the isolated perfused heart, is excluded because the mitochondrial $NAD^+ : NADH$ ratio changes in favour of NAD^+ (Opie and Owen, 1975; Achs *et al.*, 1982).

In summary, first principles suggest that there must be adenine nucleotide changes with increased heart work, and if the free cytosolic ADP is as low as estimated by Williamson *et al.* (1976b), then there is little prospect of detecting overall myocardial adenine nucleotide changes even if beat-to-beat changes could be measured. Thus the overall changes in adenine nucleotides reported in the working rat heart model are, therefore, best explained as occurring in response to the complex haemodynamic changes occurring in a work jump at the onset of heart work, (Achs *et al.*, 1982).

CREATINE PHOSPHATE

Creatine Phosphate and Energy Transfer

Creatine phosphate (CP) is only formed from ATP by the direct enzymatic transfer of a high energy phosphate compound group at the expense of ATP. Conversely, degradation occurs only by reversal of this reaction:

$$ATP + creatine \rightleftharpoons CP + ADP.$$

The enzyme concerned in this reaction is creatine phosphokinase (or creatine kinase). Thus it has been reasonable to regard CP as an energy reservoir (Lehninger, 1970, p. 305), especially because the equilibrium of the reaction favours ATP formation. Hence, during a prolonged stimulus, ATP will and does fall before CP.

More recently, however, interest in the breakdown products of CP has developed. Thus Newsholme and Start (1974) propose a role for CP in the genesis of inorganic phosphate (P_i) – which then stimulates glycolysis, especially at the level of phosphofructokinase. But CP–P_i may also act as an amplification system in P_i formation. The basis of this proposal is that the activity of phosphofructokinase, a regulator of glycolysis, is inhibited by CP (Krzanowski and Mutchinsky, 1969) among other factors and relieved by P_i. Thus changes in the ratio CP:P_i would have significance for the regulation of glycolysis.

The other breakdown product of CP, creatine, may help regulate the rate of production of CP (Seraydarian and Artaza, 1976) by stimulating oxidative phosphorylation, a function which could have been predicted on the basis of the mitochondrial creatine phosphokinase reaction, and the role of ADP formed from ATP and creatine (Jacobus and Lehninger, 1973).

An even more important role for CP has emerged. Now CP has come to be regarded not only as a storer but also a carrier of high energy phosphate. Early German workers made two important observations. First, the existence of isoenzymes of creatine phosphokinase (CPK) in relation to the mitochondrial and the myofibrils was shown (Jacobs and Heldt, 1964). Secondly, heart failure could be produced by the compound 1-fluoro-2,4-dinitrobenzene which inactivates CPK (Gercken and Schlette, 1968). At the time of failure, ATP and CP were both relatively well maintained with decreases of only 15–20%. Gercken and Schlette (1968) concluded that inhibition of CPK had in some way blocked energy transfer rather than causing an absolute deficiency. They proposed that high energy phosphate produced as ATP by oxidative phosphorylation was temporarily transferred by a mitochondrial CPK isoenzyme to creatine phosphate and then to cytoplasmic ATP by the cytoplasmic CPK isoenzyme. (see Opie, 1978).

Creatine Phosphokinase Isoenzymes

Thus evidence for the existence of a separate *mitochondrial CPK isoenzyme* came to be of importance. A major problem has been that of contamination. Sobel *et al.* (1972) achieved a relatively pure preparation from the rabbit heart with many properties differing from cytoplasmic isoenzymes. The enzyme was less susceptible than the cytoplasmic enzyme to inhibition by fluorodinitrobenzene, explaining why Gercken and Schlette (1968) failed to find total inhibition of energy transfer. Supportive evidence for a functional role of the mitochondrial isoenzyme was that, in mitochondria producing ATP as a result of ADP addition, creatine (which is not thought to penetrate the mitochondria) stimulated the oxygen uptake, presumably by the generation of more external ADP under the influence of mitochondrial CPK (Seraydarian and Artaza, 1976). Ogunro *et al.* (1977) could also distinguish a mitochondrial isoenzyme with specific qualities on electrophoresis, and probably localized to the outer aspect of the inner mitochondrial membrane (Ogunro *et al.*, 1979).

Further weight is given to the role of mitochondrial CPK in energy transfer by the finding that it is situated on the outside of the inner mitochondrial membrane (Scholte *et al.*, 1973) where it might be spatially close to the translocase, although firm evidence for this much quoted supposition is still lacking (the creatine phosphokinase and the translocase could theoretically be on different parts of the inner membrane). The kinetic properties of mitochondrial CPK are consonant with a role of this enzyme in synthesis of CP from ATP transported out of the mitochondria by the translocase (Farrell *et al.*, 1972; Saks *et al.*, 1975; Ogunro *et al.*, 1977).

However, the above studies were on animal tissue and some caution is required in extrapolating to man because one preliminary study (Kleine, 1965) found virtually no CPK activity in human mitochondria.

The existence of *cytoplasmic CPK* isoenzyme is not in doubt, being established by cell fractionation techniques (Kleine, 1965) and by electrophoresis (Ogunro *et al.*, 1977). Ogunro *et al.* (1979) and Kleine (1965) described CPK activity in cytoplasmic and in microsomal fractions of the cell. Gudbjarnason *et al.* (1970) visualized one cytoplasmic isoenzyme as acting at two sites respectively to transfer energy from CP to ATP available for contractile purposes, and to pick up CP from ATP made by glycolysis. In the absence of glycolytic ATP production it is evident that a reverse flow of high energy phosphate from CP could regenerate ATP in the glycolytic pool.

Evidence from chromatographic studies confirm that there is one cytoplasmic enzyme composed of one muscle (M) and one brain (B) type subunit (Jacobus, 1975). This enzyme, although found in some other tissues, is the only realistic source of blood MB-CPK elevation in developing myocardial infarction and is, therefore, termed a 'cardio-specific enzyme'. In addition, the MM isoenzyme and a trace of the BB isoenzyme are found in the cytosol (Ogunro *et al.*, 1977). The MM isoenzyme is found only in the cytosol but the MM isoenzyme can also occur in association with the myofibrils and the microsomes (Ogunro *et al.*, 1977). CPK isoenzyme localization to the myofibrils had previously been found by Ottaway (1967), Turner *et al.*, (1973), and Scholte (1973), and to the sarcoplasmic reticulum by Jacobus (1975).

Thus the overall evidence is compatible with the role of CPK isoenzymes in the compartmentalization of cellular ATP (Jacobus and Lehninger, 1973; Saks *et al.*, 1975, 1976). The existence of energy compartmentalization on the basis of CPK isoenzymes is compatible with but does not prove the concept of a pool of ATP in relation to the cell membrane.

ATP COMPARTMENTS

Mitochondrial versus Cytoplasmic ATP

Compartmentalization means that certain compounds are not uniformly distributed throughout the cell; rather, different concentrations are found in different compartments within the cell. Compartmentalization of ATP between its site of production in mitochondria and its site of utilization in the cytoplasm is well accepted. Ninety per cent or more of the ATP is found in the cytosol (Table 13.2). During actute heart work, it is the ATP in the cytosol which is broken down so that the very small amount of cytosolic ADP doubles. Cytosolic ADP will therefore rise with increased work to drive mitochondrial respiration, according to the classic concept that the rate of mitochondrial respiration is set by ADP.

Cytoplasmic Subcompartments

Are there also subcompartments of ATP within the cytoplasm? Here controversy abounds. Evidence *favouring* cytoplasmic subcompartmentalization is as follows. First, unequal distribution of creatine phosphokinase isoenzymes throughout the cytoplasm could form more ATP from creatine phosphate in specific cytosolic sites. Secondly, the existence of a small subcompartment of 'rapid turnover' ATP would explain those situations in which small changes in total ATP occur, but appear to have large effects – for example, the abrupt loss of contractile activity in ischaemic hearts while the ATP is still relatively high (Gudbjarnason *et al.*, 1970). Such low rates of fall of ATP in regional ischaemia, compared with the much faster fall of CP, have been shown by numerous workers. Hearse proposes that in the early seconds of ischaemia, more ATP than CP is lost. Depletion of only a small pool of ATP could cause contractile failure but it is equally possible that other factors such as a rise of tissue p_{CO_2} could cause the failure. Thirdly, ATP produced by glycolysis appears to have a special function in protecting the cell membrane (Bricknell and Ophie, 1978) and in promoting relaxation of the heart. When ischaemic contracture develops in underperfused hearts, it is the source of ATP and not the total ATP which is important in preventing contracture. Thus ATP made by glycolysis is effective, while ATP from residual mitochondrial metabolism is not (Bricknell *et al.*, 1981).

'Contraction' ATP

Arguments for a pool of 'contraction 'ATP were developed in 1969 (Opie, 1969). Although about two-thirds or more of the myocardial ATP utilization occurred by the contractile process, and although the available evidence showed that it was ATP and not CP that was used by the contractile apparatus, nevertheless, in a variety of models, impaired contractile activity occurred with only mild depletion of ATP stores. For example, during ischaemia, contraction ceased when the ATP had fallen from only 5.7 to 4.5 μmol g^{-1} (Gudbjarnason *et al.*, 1970). However, in non-ischaemic tissue ATP could fall as low as 2.0 μmol g^{-1} and still contract. Part of the explanation is probably the presence, in ischaemia, of factors inhibiting contraction such as the lactate ion or protons (Katz and Hecht, 1969) or of factors inhibiting energy transfer from the mitochondria outwards such as acyl-CoA. However, the different rate of decline in ATP and CP during ischaemia suggests that equilibrium does not exist, i.e. either ATP or CP is compartmentalized. The low rate of ATP fall compared with the much faster CP fall suggests that it is only a small ATP pool which is in equilibrium with CP. A similar phenomenon has been observed in tetanized skeletal muscle (Hohorst *et al.*, 1962). The complexities of the ischaemic situation lay the above data open to interpretation with reservations. However, in isolated, cultured rat heart cells (Harary, 1967) a small change in the ATP content causes spontaneous contractions to decrease.

At present a reasonable explanation for differential rates of change of ATP and CP in various condition would be the existence of ATP compartmentalization, partially based on anatomical factors (mitochondria, sarcoplasmic reticulum) and partially functional (CPK isoenzymes).

Glycolytic ATP and Electrogenesis

The hypothesis that ATP produced by glycolysis could be related to electrogenesis merits careful consideration in explaining the effects of glucose and of fatty acids on the infarcting myocardium. More specifically, the ATP concentration in or near the plasma membrane may play a role in the promotion of the slow inward calcium current associated with the plateau of the action potential. Such ATP is thought to exist in a compartment not exchanging readily with mitochondrially produced ATP, but rather to be generated by glycolysis. The rates of glycolytically generated ATP in the normally oxygenated heart are negligible from the point of view of the overall energy requirements of the heart, but this hypothesis would nevertheless accord a special role to such glycolytic ATP. The hypothesis was referred to in my review but could not be discussed in depth because of limited space (Opie, 1976).

In a truly anoxic cell, ATP can be made only by anaerobic production of lactate except under very exceptional circumstances, in which mitochondrial electron flow can be reversed. In the experiments of Prasad and MacLeod (1969), anoxic papillary muscle was used and the rate of lactate production correlated with the duration of the action potential. But in the well oxygenated muscle by far the major part of ATP is made in the mitochondria and then transported to the cytoplasm (Figure 13.1). Some data of Prasad and MacLeod suggest that, in the adult heart, mitochondrially produced ATP

GLYCOLYTIC ATP & LDH RELEASE

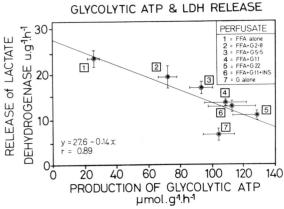

Figure 13.1 Relationship between rate of production of glycolytic ATP and release of lactate dehydrogenase from coronary ligated rat heart perfused with various substrates. Non-esterified fatty acids (NEFA) alone = palmitate 0.5 mmol l^{-1}, albumin 0.1 mmol l^{-1}, (G) = 2.8 mmol l^{-1}. G alone = 11 mmol l^{-1} glucose. All groups had coronary ligation. Note inverse relationship between production of glycolytic ATP and relese of enzyme. [Redrawn with permission from L. H. Opie and O. L. Bricknell, *Cardiovasc. Res.*, **13**, 693–702 (1979).]

enters the same compartment as glycolytically produced ATP to maintain the action potential. To establish whether mitochondrially produced ATP could maintain the action potential, Girardier and I compared the action potential obtained by a floating microelectrode from the isolated perfused rat heart when it was perfused with pyruvate with that obtained during glucose perfusion (Opie *et al.*, 1980); there were essentially no major differences except that the conduction velocity and heart rate were accelerated by pyruvate. No arrhythmias developed. In the presence of pyruvate, glycolytic flux from glycogen was totally inhibited and thus the production of glycolytic ATP was severely limited. Thus normal electrical activity of the oxygenated perfused heart could be maintained in the absence of glycolytic flux. However, in whole heart underperfusion causing ischaemia, glucose inhibited and pyruvate promoted the incidence of reperfusion arrhythmias and enzyme release, and the difference could be related to the rate of anaerobic ATP production during the ischaemic period. The earlier experiments of Cheneval *et al.* (1972) used foetal cultured cells, which generally are more dependent on glycolytic metabolism than is the adult heart; thus the result may not be extrapolated directly to the different metabolic pattern in the adult heart.

Glycolytic ATP and Enzyme Release

Opie and Bricknell (1979) showed that coronary ligated rat hearts released enzymes lactate dehydrogenase (LDH) and CPK and that such release was decreased when glucose was added to fatty acid perfusates. The protective effect of glucose could be related to the calculated rate of glycolytic flux in the heart (Figure 13.1) but not to changes in the high energy phosphate compounds. The rate of production of glycolytic ATP during the ischaemic period also appears to be a factor in the prevention of enzyme release from the 'non-working' underperfused rat heart upon reperfusion (Bricknell and Opie, 1978). Thus, in that model, changing the medium from glucose to pyruvate gave similar values for tissue contents of ATP and creatine phosphate at the end of the period of underperfusion, but release of LDH and arrhythmias during reperfusion were much less in glucose-perfused hearts (Bricknell and Opie, 1978).

Recently, Higgins *et al.* (1981) have shown that the resistance of cardiac cell plasma membrane to attack by phospholipases is dependent on the energy status. Possibly ATP may play a role in organizational changes in membrane proteins.

In another model (whole heart underperfusion), Bricknell and Opie (1978) described three groups of hearts: (1) glucose-perfused hearts with a relatively high glycolytic flux; (2) pyruvate-perfused hearts with inhibited

Table 13.3 Effects of substrate on enzyme release and comparison of content of tissue metabolites in infarcting zone with non-infarcting zone in hearts perfused with glucose, palmitate–albumin, or palmitate–albumin plus glucose and insulin. Biopsies taken by drill method 60 min after coronary artery ligation. Biopsies taken at the end of 15 min initial Langendorff perfusion gave ATP values of 3.66 ± 0.51 (8); after 15 min work (immediately preligation), ATP values were 3.50 ± 0.24 (4); values $\pm$ S.E.M. in micromoles per gram. Concentrations of substrates: glucose 11 mmol l^{-1}; palmitate 0.5 mmol l^{-1} (bound to albumin 0.1 mmol l^{-1}; insulin added as 2 mU cm^{-3}). Units: grams fresh weight ($=$ dry weight $\times 5$)

Enzyme release and tissue metabolite	Tissue zone	Glucose	P	Palmitate	P	Pyruvate + glucose + insulin
LDH release	Whole heart					
($g^{-1} h^{-1}$)		6.6	≪0.001	23.5	<0.001	12.8
ATP	Ischaemic	0.72	NS	0.69	NS	0.88
(μmol g^{-1})	Non-ischaemic	2.89	NS	2.35	NS	2.23
Creatine phosphate	Ischaemic	0.88	NS	1.15	NS	0.91
(μmol g^{-1})	Non-ischaemic	4.16	NS	3.48	NS	2.76
Lactate	Ischaemic	7.32	NS	5.03	<0.001	16.03
(μmol g^{-1})	Non-ischaemic	3.88	NS	2.81	<0.001	5.72
Glycogen	Ischaemic	2.97	NS	2.84	<0.005	8.4
(μmol C6 g^{-1})	Non-ischaemic	8.68	NS	8.93	<0.001	23.9

Reproduced with permission from L. H. Opie and O. L. Bricknell, *Cardiovasc. Res.*, **13**, 693–702 (1979).

glycolysis, probably due to the high intracellular citrate content and inhibition of phosphofructokinase; (3) acetate-perfused hearts with virtual cessation of the glycolytic flux at the end of ischaemia after initial stimulation. These data suggest that the rate of glycolytic flux during ischaemia may prevent enzyme release during reperfusion. Aerobically produced ATP may supply energy for contraction, whereas glycolytically produced ATP may be linked to transmembrane electrical activity and the ionic pumps (Figure 13.2). ATP but not ADP is absorbed and firmly bound to the cell membrane proteins in both hearts and other excitable tissue. A submembrane non-diffusible ATP pool may be supplied preferentially by strategically positioned glycolytic enzymes, especially membrane-bound phosphoglycerate kinase, as in the case of erythrocytes. Gudbjarnason *et al.* (1970) postulate an inhibition of intracellular energy transfer in ischaemic muscle which might be explained by a breakdown of the unidirectional phosphocreatine energy shuttle and exaggeration of ATP compartmentalization. The cardiac sarcoplasmic reticulum has associated with it a system of glycogenolytic enzymes and, because this membrane is impermeable to ATP, glycolysis in this organelle may be important in the control of intracellular calcium ion concentrations. Glycolytically formed ATP may be available for membrane functions such as ionic pumps and the maintenance of the

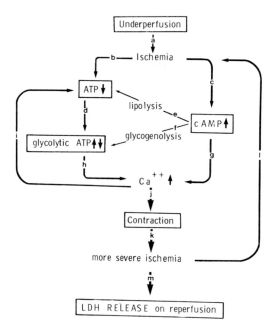

Figure 13.2 A hypothetical scheme of events leading to release of enzymes during reperfusion is proposed. (a) Underperfusion limits oxygen delivery and results in ischaemia. In ischaemia there is a fall (b) in total tissue ATP and in the non-glucose hearts a rise (c) in cAMP. (d) Glycolysis (glycolytic ATP production) is: (1) maintained with glucose as substrate, (2) inhibited with pyruvate as substrate, and (3) first increased, then decreased with acetate. The modulation of LDH release by nicotinic acid, insulin, and propranolol in pyruvate-perfused hearts could be mediated through lipolysis (e) by causing the accumulation of acyl-CoA which inhibits adenine nucleotide translocase. The depletion of glycogen in acetate- and palmitate-perfused hearts could be by cAMP-mediated glycogenolysis (f). Both the limitation of glycolytic ATP and the increase in cAMP could allow a rise (g and h) in free intracellular calcium. Increased free Ca^{++}, as evidenced by ischaemic contracture (j), could further reduce ATP by calcium overload (i), Hypercontraction of the heart (k) as in the case of acetate- and palmitate-perfused hearts, could further exaggerate ischaemia by (l) the reduction of small vessel perfusion. Enzyme washout on reperfusion (m) would, therefore, reflect severity of the ischaemic process. [Reproduced with permission from O. L. Bricknell and L. H. Opie, *Circulation Res.*, **43**, 102–115 (1978).]

phosphatidic acid cycle, thereby preventing the accumulation of lysophospholipids which are highly membrane-active and might cause cell lysis, thus allowing leakage of macromolecules such as enzymes.

A speculative but unifying hypothesis may be that entry of calcium ions could be the connecting link. High rates of cytoplasmic ATP production may be required for optimal function of the membrane ion pumps (see above).

Hypoxic damage and depletion of cytoplasmic ATP could allow greater ingress of sodium and calcium ions, as would accumulation of cyclic AMP. Hearts with greater acculation of calcium ions would exhibit an increased diastolic tension and would arrest earlier in contraction (as in acetate hearts); this would result in lower coronary flows in the ischaemic period (as in acetate hearts) and would also limit reactive hyperaemia and the heart rate in the reperfusion period (as in acetate hearts).

As a consequence of increased intracellular ionized calcium, two vicious circles could be created (Figure 13.2): (1) greater ATP demand and respiratory accumulation of calcium by the mitochondria may occur at the expense of phosphorylation and (2) the hypercontracted state could reduce coronary perfusion of the small vessels leading to more severe ischaemia. It should be noted that global ischaemia is not homogeneous and some intercapillary areas are more vulnerable to anoxia. Therefore, substrates may have variable effects in various areas, even in global ischaemia.

Glycolytic ATP and Ischaemic Contracture

The onset of ischaemic contracture is thought to be associated with the decline in ATP leading to calcium-independent rigor-complex formation. However, *in vitro* studies on skeletal muscle have shown that ATP concentrations as low as 0.01 mM are required for calcium-insensitive rigor-complex formation. There appears to be a 240-fold discrepancy between the ATP level required for the formation of calcium-insensitive rigor bonds and the measured levels of tissue ATP.

Katz and Tada (1977) have already emphasized the distinction between ATP content of the myocardium and the cytosolic ATP concentration surrounding the contractile proteins. ATP compartmentalization has been evoked as a possible explanation for the discrepancy. Cytosolic compartmentalization of ATP was proposed by Bricknell and Opie (1978) to explain why similar levels of tissue ATP in groups of hearts perfused with either glucose or pyruvate released different amounts of enzymes (indicative of membrane damage) on reperfusion. ATP produced by glycolysis was shown to be more effective than ATP produced from mitochondria in preserving membrane functions which could include maintenance of calcium ion homeostasis.

Bricknell *et al.* (1981) investigated the relationship between tissue ATP, ischaemic contracture, and glycolysis. Comparisions were made of the effect of varying the source of ATP production from either glycolysis or from the mitochondrial sources (Figure 13.3) using a similar approach to that used previously (Bricknell and Opie, 1978; see above). ATP produced by glycolysis was better able to delay or prevent contracture than ATP produced by oxidative phosphorylation. Three possibilities suggest themselves.

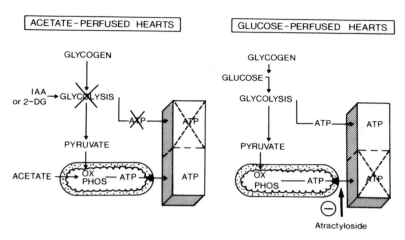

Figure 13.3 A simplified scheme of the energy-producing metabolic pathways and the points where the inhibitors are thought to act. IAA, iodoacetic acid, sodium salt; 2-DG, 2-deoxyglucose; ATP, adenosine triphosphate; OX PHOS, oxidative phosphorylation (intramitochondrial). The 'box' represents the cytosolic ATP while the division represents the hypothetical comparmentalization. Total tissue ATP is the sum of the cytosolic ATP and the mitochondrial ATP. (a) Acetate-perfused hearts; (b) glucose-perfused hearts. Acetate-perfused hearts with blocked glycolysis developed ischaemic contracture more readily than glucose-perfused hearts with blocked mitochondrial production of ATP. Thus it is the source of the ATP and not the total ATP level that is of importance in this model. [Reproduced with permision from O. L. Bricknell, P. S. Daries, and L. H. Opie, *J. Mol. Cell. Cardiol.*, **13**, 941–945 (1981).]

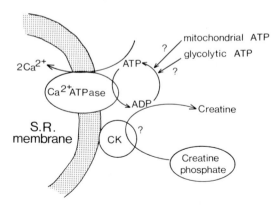

Figure 13.4 Hypothetical role of glycolysis in providing ATP for uptake of calcium by sarcoplasmic reticulum (SR). CK = creatine phosphokinase = creatine kinase

First, there could be strict cytosolic compartmentalization of ATP so that glycolysis provides a small but crucial supply of cytosolic ATP that is accessible to the contractile proteins but does not influence the total tissue ATP content. Secondly, glycolytically produced ATP may meet the energy requirements for calcium uptake by the sarcoplasmic reticulum, thus maintaining relaxation (Figure 13.4). Thirdly, during glycolysis other metabolites might be formed, such as hydrogen ions. However, there was no substantial difference in the measured tissue pH before and after contracture. Bing and Fishbein (1979) showed that added glycolytic inhibition produced more severe electron microscopic damage than hypoxia only, a result in general agreement with our findings.

Evidence against ATP Compartments

Not all evidence favours the existence of ATP compartments in the cytoplasm. When studying a variety of injuries to the cell, various other workers have concluded that the degree of fall of the total ATP level may help indicate whether or not the cell could recover. Thus Kübler and Spieckermann (1970) found that as myocardial ATP fell below 3.5 μmol per gram wet weight in hearts arrested by ischaemia at 15 °C, lactate production ceased because of ATP lack for the conversion of fructose-6-phosphate to fructose-1,6-diphosphate (phosphofructokinase reaction), and that ATP level was also the theoretical limit of myocardial ischaemia that could be tolerated. (By toleration they mean recovery of adequate cardiac function after rewarming the heart.)

Hearse (1977) has claimed a similar limit for recovery from whole heart ischaemia induced by aortic clamping. And Trump (Laiho and Trump, 1975; Trump *et al.*, 1976) has shown that the decline in the level of ATP during cell injury could be correlated with the development of mitochondrial swelling. However, Gudbjarnason *et al.* (1970) found that in the non-infarcted zone after coronary ligation in the dog, ATP could drop as low as 1.5 to 2.0 μmol g^{-1} and the heart could contract and survive. It may be that the studies of Trump *et al.* (1976) on Ehrlich tumour cells are not directly applicable to the heart.

Most studies on ischaemia show that CP is depleted before ATP. It is not unreasonable to suppose that there must be some overall correlation between life and death of the cell and the presence or absence of ATP (taking extremes) and hence some correlation of ATP decrease with irreversibility. Also, it is easy to see that when the heart cells are deprived of glycolysis as in the data of Haworth *et al.* (1981), that it will be total ATP and not glycolytic ATP production that is of prime importance. Thus the evidence from the studies cited above does not disprove the concept of compartmentalization.

Further considerations provided by NMR studies are given by Dawson (Chapter 14 in this volume).

DEGRADATION AND SYNTHESIS OF ADENINE NUCLEOTIDES

Control of Degradation of Adenine Nucleotides

Degradation of myocardial adenine nucleotides during oxygen deficiency is a well established phenomenon. The critical steps are

$$ATP \rightarrow ADP + P_i, \tag{13.1}$$

then by the myokinase reaction

$$2\ ADP \rightarrow ATP + AMP; \tag{13.2}$$

thus

$$\left.\begin{array}{l} ATP \rightarrow 2\ ADP + 2\ P_i, \\ 2\ ADP \rightarrow ATP + AMP. \end{array}\right\} \tag{13.3}$$

Therefore, ATP yields ADP, AMP, and P_i when broken down. Resynthesis of ATP could take place by reversal of the above reactions. When the reaction proceeds further than AMP, to release of adenosine, hypoxanthine, and inosine, the total adenine nucleotide content of the cell will fall because the dephosphorylated nucleotide breakdown products can pentrate the cell membrane. Adenosine is an important mechanism whereby the coronary flow is regulated in response to ischaemia (Berne, 1963) and, possibly, increased heart work (Foley *et al.*, 1978; Olsson, Chapter 23 in this volume).

The dephosphorylation of AMP to adenosine is accomplished by the enzyme *5'-nucleotidase* which is regulated in turn by adenine nucleotides and by magnesium (Edwards and Maguire, 1970; Sullivan and Alpers, 1971). The enzyme is inhibited by ATP and ADP and AMP is its substrate. Hence during ischaemia, when ATP falls (and ADP and AMP stay virtually constant), relief of 5'-nucleotidase inhibition might occur. Rubio *et al.* (1974) have suggested that, during hypoxia, it is a fall in the energy charge of the cell which activates 5'-nucleotidase, where the energy charge is given by

$$\frac{ATP + \frac{1}{2}ADP}{ATP + ADP + AMP}. \tag{13.4}$$

Table 13.4   Effect of regional ischaemia on energy charge

Time	Total adenine nucleotide ATP+ADP+AMP (μmol g^{-1})	AMP content (μmol g^{-1})	Energy charge
Control	6.59	0.08	1.56
1 min post-ligation	6.28	0.13	1.16
80–40 min	3.47	0.07	1.14
6 h, peripheral zone	2.27	0.12	1.14
6 h, central zone	1.32	0.12	1.28

Calculation of the energy charge for the onset of regional ischaemia pro-voked by coronary ligation (Opie *et al.*, 1972; Opie, 1976) is shown in Table 13.4.

Thus according to that concept, 5'-nucleotidase is activated within 1 min of coronary ligation and stays activated at the same level for at least 6 h. Because there is no consistent rise in the cardiac AMP content throughout the period of ischaemia (Table 13.4), the proposal that the drop in energy charge activates the enzyme breaking down AMP has obvious merit, ex-plaining both why AMP fails to rise and why the enzyme activity increases even though the substrate level does not increase. If, however, all the cellular ATP and ADP were bound to magnesium ions, which relieve the nucleotide inhibition, then control of the 5'-nucleotidase by the energy charge becomes unlikely (see Dawson, Chapter 14 in this volume).

Adenosine can either (1) be reconverted to AMP by the enzyme adenosine kinase or (2) form inosine under the influence of adenosine deaminase (by loss of ammonia); inosine in turn can form hypoxanthine and finally xanthine forms under the influence of xanthine oxidase. The factors governing the relative activities of these two pathways are not well under-stood but, as reviewed by de Jong (1978), the limiting step for phosphoryla-tion of adenosine is the rate of the carrier-mediated uptake of adenosine into the cell. Because adenylate kinase requires ATP, the kinase may be less active in states of energy depletion. However, even a concentration of MgATP of only 0.4 mM causes much more activity of the enzyme (de Jong and Kalkman, 1973). For whatever reason, soon after coronary occlusion there is a well documented, rapid rise in the adenosine content of the left ventricle (Olsson, 1970).

Functions of Adenosine

Adenosine is discussed elsewhere (Olsson, Chapter 23 in this volume). It could have a very important function in ischaemia, both increasing the oxygen supply (vasodilation) and decreasing the oxygen demand (decreased calcium entry; catecholamine antagonism).

Adenosine versus Inosine 5'-monophosphate (IMP)

Another pathway for adenosine degradation is via the enzyme adenosine deaminase to yield IMP (Baer *et al.*, 1966; Burger and Lowestein, 1967; de Jong, 1972) followed by dephosphorylation to yield inosine. The relative activity of this pathway versus that of the dephosphorylation pathway forming adenosine, is difficult to predict because of the large species differences (de Jong, 1978). During ischaemia both the amination and dephosphorylation may be increased (de Jong, 1978). The responses of the nucleotidase and the deaminase to ATP/P_i suggest that during ischaemia, adenosine formation is increased and IMP formation is decreased (Burger and Lowenstein, 1967; Rubio and Berne, 1969). However, other evidence suggests that the nucleotidase is so sensitive to ADP inhibition that it would always be inhibited unless ADP concentration is very low as a result of protein binding or chelation with metal ions; furthermore, inorganic phosphate is ineffective in relieving ATP or ADP inhibition (Sullivan and Alpers, 1971). Thus the factors regulating adenosine formation versus that of IMP remain an open question.

Functions of IMP

Apart from acting as a source of inosine and hypoxanthine (see Lehninger, 1970, p. 741), IMP might participate in the purine nucleotide cycle described by Lowenstein for skeletal muscle (see Lehninger, 1970, p. 743):

$$AMP + H_2O \rightarrow IMP + NH_3;$$

$$IMP + aspartate + GIP \rightarrow Adenylosuccinate + GDP + P_i;$$

$$Adenylosuccinate \rightarrow AMP + fumarate.$$

This cycle, not yet established for the heart, would yield fumarate, which could replenish citrate cycle intermediates of conditions of sudden accelerated activity of the citrate cycle, as for example follows intense heart work.

Salvage Pathways

It is possible to distinguish between 'salvage' pathways which resynthesize the adenine nucleotides from preformed precursors (Goldthwait, 1957; Maguire *et al.*, 1972), and *de novo* synthesis from precursors such as ribose 5-phosphate and glycine (Zimmer *et al.*, 1973; Zimmer and Gerlach, 1974). The rate of net synthesis (salvage and *de novo*) of adenine nucleotides in the rabbit heart is estimated at 80–100 nmol g^{-1} h^{-1} by the technique of labelling α-P groups with ^{32}P (Rossi, 1975), of which the largest part in near physiological conditions is due to activity of the salvage pathway (Rossi,

1975). There are distinct limitations to the estimation of the activity of a pathway by incorporation of radioactive tracers because of the problems of exchange reactions (shuttling) as opposed to true synthesis. Nevertheless, if Rossi's data are taken at face value, there must be a constant input into the salvage pathway, and a probable source is the re-uptake by myocardial cells of adenosine which is continuously released (Rubio *et al.*, 1969; Rubio *et al.*, 1974). In that case detailed knowledge of the regulation of the enzyme adenosine kinase, which rephosphorylates adenosine to AMP, would be of importance.

De novo Synthesis

Gerlach's group has elucidated some of the factors controlling *de novo* synthesis (Zimmer *et al.*, 1972, 1973; Zimmer and Gerlach, 1974). Using the specific activity of glycine as a marker of *de novo* synthesis, they found the basal rate to be about 6 nmol g^{-1} h^{-1}. During hypertrophy the rate doubled, probably due to stimulation of the activity of the pentose phosphate pathway, thereby producing ribose 5-phosphate and then forming 5-phosphoribosyl-1-pyrophosphate (PRPP) by the activity of the enzyme, PRPP synthetase. The next step in the synthetic pathway is the conversion of PRPP to 5-phosphoribosylamine and the enzyme PRPP amidotransferase controls this step. The concentration of cardiac nucleotides is thought to control this enzyme (Wyngaarden and Ashton, 1959).

These observations could explain increased purine biosynthesis in the heart after an ATP decrease induced by hypoxia (Zimmer *et al.*, 1973), isoproterenol (Zimmer and Gerlach, 1974), or the development of cardiac hypertrophy (Zimmer *et al.*, 1972). *De novo* synthesis of adenine nucleotide during cardiac hypertrophy lends support to the concept of Meerson, who proposed that the signal giving rise to the activation of the genetic apparatus of the cell is a deficiency of high energy phosphate compounds (Meerson and Pomoinitsky, 1972). However, the Meerson hypothesis did not fit the data for isoproterenol (Zimmer *et al.*, 1980) and there are further reservations (Gevers, 1972).

Adenine Nucleotide Turnover

The probable existence of the salvage pathway in the normal heart is explicable by continuous formation of adenosine and resynthesis of AMP. However, adenine nucleotides are used in the synthesis of RNA which would explain the physiological functioning of the pathway of *de novo* synthesis. *De novo* synthesis is also required when there is demand for increased RNA synthesis as in hypertrophy (Zimmer *et al.*, 1972) and to help replenish net loss of adenine nucleotides as after oxygen deprivation or isoproterenol stimulation (Zimmer and Gerlach, 1974).

ATP, ADENOSINE, AND PURINERGIC RECEPTORS

In 1972 Burnstock described a type of neurotransmitter, being non-adrenergic, non-cholinergic but 'purinergic' (Burnstock, 1980). The neurotransmitter was held to be ATP or a related purine nucleotide. On the basis of the relative potency of agonists (and other criteria), the purinergic receptors are now divided into (1) the P_1 receptors, which respond best to adenosine, are inhibited by methylxanthines, and modulate production of cyclic AMP and (2) the P_2 receptors, which respond best to ATP, are inhibited by quinidine and imidazolines, and provoke synthesis of prostaglandins. The effects of adenosine could be postulated to act via the P_1 receptors by vasodilation of the coronary arteries, inhibition of adenyl cyclase, reduction of sinus rate, decreased force of contraction, and inhibition of transmembrane Ca^{++} influx.

The P_2 receptors respond best to ATP. Generally ATP has been regarded as an intracellular compound, not able to cross the cell wall. Burnstock, however, proposed that purinergic nerve terminals were able to release ATP by exocytosis of ATP-containing vesicles. ATP released in this way and from hypoxic cells (Forrester, 1972; Forrester and Williams, 1977) may cause vasodilatation and release prostaglandins. Indomethacin reduces the vasodilation caused by ATP (Minkes *et al.*, 1973). Thus ATP, produced either by purinergic nerves or by hypoxic cells, may vasodilate via prostaglandins. Such prostaglandin-induced coronary vasodilation may be enhanced by nitrates (Morcillio *et al.*, 1980).

NON-ADENINE NUCLEOTIDES

While the existence of non-adenine nucleotides in the heart, as in other tissues, has been long established, their functions are only now becoming clearer. Such nucleotides are generally formed from ATP by the enzyme nucleotide diphosphokinase, with guanyl triphosphate as example:

$$ATP + GDP \rightleftharpoons ADP + GTP.$$

GTP is also formed in the Krebs' cycle by a substrate-level phosphorylation during the formation of succinate from succinyl-CoA. GTP functions relevant to this review are (1) as a modulator of the activity of glutamate dehydrogenase (Lehninger, 1970) which it inhibits (as does ATP); (2) as a stimulator of adenyl cyclase activity through binding to nucleotide regulatory sites (Lefkowitz, 1975); (3) as a carrier of high energy phosphate energy, e.g. substrate level phosphorylation of succinyl-CoA; and (4) GIP-specific protein kinases, activated by cyclic AMP-dependent kinases, may exist (Kuo, 1972).

Regulation of cardiac levels of GTP is very imperfectly understood but of potential importance. Cytosine compounds (CIP and CDP) function in synthesis of phospholipids, e.g. lecithin (Lehninger, 1970), whereas uridine triphosphate (UTP) functions in the synthesis of glycogen.

REFERENCES

Achs, M. J., Garfinkel, D., and Opie, L. H. (1982). Computer simulation of glucose-perfused rat heart in a work jump. *Amer. J. Physiol.*, **243**, R389–R399.

Arnold, G., Kosche, F., Miessner, E., Neitzert, A., and Lochner, W. (1968). The importance of the perfusion pressure in the coronary arteries for the contractility and the oxygen consumption of the heart. *Pflügers Arch. Ges. Physiol.*, **299**, 339–356.

Bacaner, M. B., Lioy, F. and Visscher, M. B. (1971). Coronary blood flow, oxygen delivery rate and cardiac performance. *J. Physiol. (Lond.)*, **216**, 111–127.

Baer, H. P., Drummond, G. I., and Duncan, E. L. (1966). Formation and deamination of adenosine by cardiac muscle enzymes. *Mol. Pharmacol.*, **2**, 67–76.

Barnard, R. J., MacAlpin, R., Kattus, A. A., and Buckberg, G. D. (1973). Ischemic response to sudden strenuous exercise in healthy men. *Circulation*, **48**, 936–942.

Berne, R. M. (1963). Cardiac nucleotides in hypoxia: possible role in regulation of coronary blood flow. *Amer. J. Physiol.*, **204**, 317–322.

Bing, O. H. L., and Fishbein, M. C. (1979). Mechanical and structural correlates of contracture induced by metabolic blockade in cardiac muscle from the rat. *Circulation Res.*, **45**, 298–308.

Bricknell, O. L., and Opie, L. H. (1978). Effects of substrates on tissue metabolic changes in the isolated rat heart during underperfusion and on release of lactate dehydrogenase and arrhythmias during reperfusion. *Circulation Res.*, **43**, 102–115.

Bricknell, O. L., Daries, P. S., and Opie, L. H. (1981). A relationship between adenosine triphosphate, glycolysis and ischaemic contracture in the isolated rat heart. *J. Mol. Cell. Cardiol.*, **13**, 941–945.

Burger, R., and Lowenstein, J. (1967). Adenylate deaminase. III. Regulation of deamination pathways in extracts of rat heart and lung. *J. Biol. Chem.*, **242**, 5281–5288.

Burnstock, G. (1980). Purinergic receptors in the heart. *Circulation Res.*, **46**, Suppl. 1, 175–182.

Cheneval, J.-P., Hyde, A., Blondel, B., and Girardier, L. (1972). Heart cells in culture. Metabolism, action potential and transmembrane ionic movements. *J. Physiol. (Paris)*, **64**, 413–430.

Edwards, M. J., and Maguire, M. H. (1970). Purification and properties of rat heart 5′-nucleotidase. *Mol. Pharmacol.*, **6**, 641–648.

Farrell, E. C., Baba, N., Brierley, G. P., and Grumer, H. D. (1972). On the creatine phosphokinase of heart muscle mitochondria. *Lab. Invest.*, **27**, 209–213.

Foley, D. H., Herlihy, J. T., Thompson, C. J., Rubio, R., and Berne, R. M. (1978). Increased adenosine formation by rat myocardium with acute aortic constriction. *J. Mol. Cell. Cardiol.*, **10**, 293–300.

Forrester, T. (1972). An estimate of adenosine triphosphate release into the venous effluent from exercising human forearm muscle. *J. Physiol. (Lond.)*, **224**, 611–628.

Forrester, T., and Williams, C. A. (1977). Release of adenosine triphosphate from isolated adult heart cells in response to hypoxia. *J. Physiol. (Lond.)*, **268**, 371–390.

Gercken, G., and Schlette, U. (1968). Metabolite status of the heart in acute insufficiency due to 1-fluoro-2,4-dinitrobenzene. *Experientia*, **24**, 17–19.

Gevers, W. (1972). The stimulus of hypertrophy in the heart. *J. Mol. Cell. Cardiol.*, **4**, 537–541.

Gevers, W. (1977). Generation of protons by metabolic processes in heart cells. *J. Mol. Cell. Cardiol.*, **9**, 867–874.

Goldthwait, D. A. (1957). Mechanisms of synthesis of purine nucleotides in heart muscle extracts. *J. Clin. Invest.*, **36**, 1572–1578.

Gudbjarnason, S., Mathes, R., and Ravens, K. G. (1970). Functional compartmentation of ATP and creatine phosphate in heart muscle. *J. Mol. Cell. Cardiol.*, **1**, 325–339.

Harary, I., Seraydarian, M., and Gerschenson, L. E. (1967). Effect of lipids on contractility of cultured heart cells. In *Factors Influencing Myocardial Contractility* (R. Tanz, F. Kavaler, and J. Roberts, eds), Academic Press, New York, pp. 231–244.

Haworth, R. A., Hunter, D. R., and Berkoff, H. A. (1981). Contracture in isolated adult rat heart cells. Role of Ca^{2+}, ATP and compartmentation. *Circulation Res.*, **49**, 1119–1128.

Hearse, D. J., Garlick, P. B., and Humphrey S. M. (1977). Ischemic contractive of the myocardium: mechanism and prevention. *Amer. J. Cardiol.*, **39**, 986–993.

Higgins, T. J. C., Bailey, P. J., and Allsopp, D. (1981). The influence of ATP depletion on the action of phospholipase C on cardiac myocyte membrane phospholipids. *J. Mol. Cell. Cardiol.*, **13**, 1027–1030.

Hochachka, D. W., Neely, J. R., and Driedzic, W. R. (1977). Integration of lipid utilization with Krebs cycle activity in muscle. *Fed. Proc.*, **36**, 2009–2014.

Hohorst, H. J., Reim, M., and Bartels, H. (1962). Studies on the creatine kinase equilibrium in muscle and the significance of ATP and ADP levels. *Biochem. Biophys. Res. Commun.*, **7**, 142–146.

Jacobs, H., and Heldt, H. W. (1964). High activity of creatine kinase in mitochondria from muscle and brain and evidence for a separate mitochondrial isoenzyme of creatine kinase. *Biochem. Biophys. Res. Commun.*, **16**, 516–521.

Jacobus, W. E. (1975). Heart creatine kinase: heterogeneous composition of the mammalian MB isoenzyme. *J. Mol. Cell. Cardiol.*, **7**, 783–791.

Jacobus, W. E., and Lehninger, A. L. (1973). Creatine kinase of rat heart mitochondria: coupling of creatine phosphorylation to electron tranport. *J. Biol. Chem.*, **248**, 4803–4810.

de Jong, J. W. (1972). Phosphorylation and deamination of adenosine by the isolated, perfused rat heart. *Biochim. Biophys. Acta*, **286**, 252–259.

de Jong, J. W. (1978). Biochemistry of acutely ischemic myocardium. In *Pathophysiology of Myocardial Perfusion* (W. Schapter, ed.), Elsevier/North Holland Biomedical Press, Amsterdam.

de Jong, J. W., and Kalkman, C. (1973). Myocardial adenosine kinase: activity and localization determined with rapid, radiometric assay. *Biochem. Biophys. Acta*, **320**, 388–396.

Katz, A. M., and Hecht, H. H. (1969). The early 'pump' failure of the ischemic heart, *Amer. J. Med.*, **47**, 497–502.

Katz, A. M., and Tada, M. (1977). The 'stone heart' and other challenges to the biochemist. *Amer. J. Cardiol.*, **39**, 1073–1077.

Kleine, T. O. (1965). Localization of creatine kinase in microsomes and mitochondria of human heart and skeletal muscle and cerebral cortex. *Nature*, **207**, 1393–1394.

Krzanowski, J., and Matschinsky, F. M. (1969). Regulation of phosphofructokinase by phosphocreatine and phosphorylated glycolytic intermediates. *Biochem. Biophys. Res. Commun.*, **34**, 816–823.

Kübler, W., and Spieckermann, P. G. (1970). Regulation of glycolysis in the ischemic and the anoxic myocardium. *J. Mol. Cell. Cardiol.*, **1**, 351–357.

Kuo, J. F. (1972). On the question of the existence of a guanosine triphosphate-specific protein kinase activated by adenosine 3′:5′-monophosphate-dependent protein kinase. *J. Biol. Chem.*, **249**, 1755–1759.

Laiho, K. U., and Trump, B. F. (1975). Studies on the pathogenesis of cell injury – effects of inhibitors of metabolism and membrane function on the mitochondria of Ehrlich ascites tumor cells. *Lab. Invest.*, **32**, 163–182.

Lefkowitz, R. J. (1975). Catecholamine stimulated myocardial adenylate cyclase: effects of nucleotides. *J. Mol. Cell. Cardiol.*, **7**, 237–248.

Lehninger, A. L. (1970). *Biochemistry*, Worth, New York.

Lochner, A., van Niekerk, I., and Kotze, J. C. N. (1981). Mitochondrial acyl CoA, adenine nucleotide translocase activity and oxidative phosphorylation in myocardial ischaemia. *J. Mol. Cell. Cardiol.*, **13**, 991–997.

Maguire, M. H., Lukas, M. C., and Rettie, J. F. (1972). Adenine nucleotide salvage synthesis in the rat heart; Pathways of adenosine salvage. *Biochem. Biophys. Acta*, **262**, 108–115.

Meerson, F. Z., and Pomoinitsky, V. D. (1972). The role of high-energy phosphate compounds in the development of cardiac hypertrophy. *J. Mol. Cell. Cardiol.*, **4**, 571–597.

Minkes, M. S., Douglas, J. R., and Needleman, P. (1973). Prostaglandin release by the isolated perfused rabbit heart. *Prostaglandins*, **3**, 439–445.

Monroe, R. G., LaFarge, W. J., Hammond, R. P., and Morgan, C. L. (1966). Norepinephrine release and left ventricular pressure in the isolated heart. *Circulation Res.*, **19**, 774–790.

Monroe, R. G., Gamble, W. J., LaFarge, C. C., Kumar, A. E., Stark, J., Sanders, G. L., Phornphutkul, C., and Davis, M. (1972). The Anrep effect reconsidered. *J. Clin. Invest.*, **51**, 2573–2584.

Morcillio, E., Reid, P. R., Dubin, N., Ghodgaonkar, R., and Pitt, B. (1980). Myocardial prostaglandin E release by nitroglycerin and modification by indomethacin. *Amer. J. Cardiol.*, **45**, 53–57.

Nayler, W. G., McInnes, I., Chipperfield, D., Carson, V., and Jurtz, J. B. (1970). Ventricular function and the calcium-accumulating activity of the sarcoplasmic reticulum. *J. Mol. Cell. Cardiol.*, **1**, 307–324.

Neely, J. R., Denton, R. M., England, P. J., and Randle, P. J. (1972). The effects of increased heart work on the tricarboxylate cycle and its interactions with glycolysis in the perfused rat heart. *Biochem. J.*, **128**, 147–159.

Neely, J. R., Whitmer, K. M., and Mochizuki, S. (1976). Effects of mechanical activity and hormones on myocardial glucose and fatty acid utilization, *Circulation Res.*, **38**, Suppl. 1, 22–29.

Newsholme, E. A., and Start, C. (1974). *Regulation in Metabolism*, John Wiley, London.

Ogunro, E. A., Peters, T. J., and Hearse, D. J. (1977). Subcellular compartmentation of creatine kinase isoenzymes in guinea pig heart. *Cardiovasc. Res.*, **11**, 250–259.

Ogunro, R. A., Peters, T. J., Wells, G., and Hearse, D. J. (1979). Submitochondrial and submicrosomal distribution of creatine kinase in guinea pig myocardium. *Cardiovasc. Res.*, **13**, 562–567.

Olsson, R. A. (1970). Changes in content of purine nucleoside in canine myocardium during coronary occlusion. *Circulation Res.*, **26**, 301–306.

Opie, L. H. (1965). Coronary flow rate and perfusion pressure as determinants of mechanical function and oxidative metabolism of isolated perfused rat heart, *J. Physiol.* (*Lond.*), **180,** 529–541.

Opie, L. H. (1969). Metabolism of the heart in health and disease, Part 2. *Amer. Heart J.*, **77,** 100–122.

Opie, L. H. (1971/72). Substrate utilization and glycolysis in the heart. *Cardiology,* **56,** 2–21.

Opie, L. H. (1976). Effects of anoxia and regional ischaemia on metabolism of glucose and fatty acids. Relative rates of aeroboic and anaerobic energy production during first 6 hours of experimental myocardial infarction. *Circulation. Res.,* **38,** Suppl. 1, 52–68.

Opie, L. H. (1978). Myocardial metabolism and heart disease. *Jpn. Circulation J.,* **42,** 1223–1247.

Opie, L. H. (1980). Nutrition and the heart. In *Hearts and Heart-like Organs* (G. H. Bourne, ed.), Academic Press, New York, pp. 101–118.

Opie, L. H., and Bricknell, O. L. (1979). Role of glycolytic flux in effect of glucose in decreasing fatty acid-induced release of lactate dehydrogenase from isolated coronary ligated rat heart. *Cardiovasc. Res.,* **13,** 693–702.

Opie, L. H., and Mansford, K. R. L. (1971). The value of lactate and pyruvate measurements in the assessment of the redox state of free nicotinamide-adenine dinucleotide in the cytoplasm of the perfused rat heart, *Europ. J. Clin. Invest.,* **1,** 295–306.

Opie, L. H., and Owen, P. (1975). Assessment of mitochondrial free $NAD^+/NADH$ ratios and oxaloacetate concentrations during increased mechanical work in isolated perfused rat heart during production or uptake of ketone bodies. *Biochem. J.,* **148,** 403–415.

Opie, L. H., and Owen, P. (1976). Effect of glucose–insulin–potassium infusions on arteriovenous differences of glucose and of free fatty acids and on tissue metabolic changes in dogs with developing myocardial infarction, *Amer. J. Cardiol.,* **38,** 310–321.

Opie, L. H. Owen, P., and Mansford, K. R. L. (1971a). Effects of increased heart work on glycolysis and adenine nucleotides in the perfused heart of normal and diabetic rats. *Biochem. J.,* **124,** 475–490.

Opie, L. H., Owen, P., Mansford, K. R. L. (1971b). Metabolic adjustments to acute heart work: observations on the isolated perfused rat heart. *Cardiovasc. Res.,* **5,** Suppl. 1, 87–95.

Opie, L. H., Thomas, M., Owen, P., and Shulman, G. (1972). Increased coronary venous inorganic phosphate concentrations during experimental myocardial ischemia. *Am. J. Cardiol.,* **30,** 503–513.

Opie, L. H., Tuschmidt, R., Bricknell, O. L., and Girardier, L. (1980). Role of glycolysis in maintenance of the action potential duration and contractile activity in isolated perfused rat heart. *J. Physiol.* (*Paris*)*.* **76,** 821–829.

Ottaway, J. H. (1967). Evidence for the binding of cytoplasmic creatine kinase to structural elements in heart muscle. *Nature,* **215,** 521–522.

Owen, C. S., and Wilson, D. F. (1974). Control of respiration by the mitochondrial phosphorylation state. *Arch. Biochim. Biophys.,* **161,** 581–591.

Prasad, K., and MacLeod, D. P. (1969). Influence of glucose on the transmembrane action potential of guinea-pig papillary muscle. *Circulation Res.,* **24,** 939–950.

Randle, P. J. (1976). Regulation of glycolysis and pyruvate oxidation in cardiac muscle. *Circ. Res.,* **38,** I-8–I-15.

Rossi, A. (1975). ^{32}P labelling of nucleotides in α-position in the rabbit heart. *J. Mol. Cell. Cardiol.*, **7**, 891–896.

Rubio, R., and Berne, R. M. (1969). Release of adenosine by the normal myocardium in dogs and its relationship to the regulation of coronary resistance. *Circulation Res.*, **25**, 407–415.

Rubio, R., Berne, R. M., and Katori, M. (1969). Release of adenosine in reactive hyperemia of the dog heart. *Amer. J. Physiol.*, **216**, 56–62.

Rubio, R., Wiedmeier, V. T., and Berne, R. M. (1974). Relationship between coronary flow and adenosine production and release. *J. Mol. Cell. Cardiol.*, **6**, 561–566.

Saks, V. A., Chernousova, G. B., Gukovsky, D. E., Smirnov, V. N., and Chazov, E. I. (1975). Studies of energy transport in heart cells. Mitochondrial isoenzymes of creatine phosphokinase; kinetic properties and regulatory action of Mg^{2+} ions. *Europ. J. Biochem.*, **57**, 273–290.

Saks, V. A., Lipina, N. V., Smirnov, V. N., and Chazov, E. I. (1976). Studies of energy transport in heart cells. The functional coupling between mitochondrial creatine phosphokinase and ATP–ADP translocase: kinetic evidence. *Arch. Biochem. Biophys.*, **173**, 34–41.

Schildberg, F. W., and Fleckenstein, A. (1965). Die bedeutung der extremcellulären Calciumkonzentration für die Spaltung von energiereichen Phosphat in rahendem und tätigem Myokardgewebe. *Pflügers Arch. Ges. Physiol.* **283**, 137–150.

Scholte, H. R. (1973). On the triple localization of creatine kinase in heart and skeletal muscle cells of the rat: evidence for the existence of myofibrillar and mitochondrial isoenzymes. *Biochim. Biophys. Acta*, **305**, 413–427.

Scholte, H. R., Weijers, P. J., and Wit-Peeters, E. M. (1973). The localization of mitochondrial creatine kinase, and its use for the determination of the sidedness of submitochondrial particles. *Biochim. Biophys. Acta*, **291**, 764–773.

Schrader, J., Baumann, G., and Gerlach, E. (1977). Adenosine as inhibitor of myocardial effects of catecholamines. *Pflugers Arch. Europ. J. Physiol.*, **372**, 29–35.

Seraydarian, M. W., and Artaza, L. (1976). Regulation of energy metabolism by creatine in cardiac and skeletal muscle cells in culture. *J. Mol. Cell. Cardiol.*, **8**, 669–678.

Shug, A. L., Shrago, E., Bittar, N., Folts, J. D., and Kokes, J. R. (1975). Long chain fatty acid CoA inhibition of adenine nucleotide translocase in the ischemic myocardium. *Amer. J. Physiol.*, **228**, 689–692.

Sobel, B. E., Shell, W. E., and Klein, M. S. (1972). An isoenzyme of creatine phosphokinase associated with rabbit heart mitochondria. *J. Mol. Cell. Cardiol.*, **4**, 367–380.

Sullivan, J. M., and Alpers, J. B. (1971). *In vitro* regulation of rat heart 5′-nucleotidase by adenine nucleotides and magnesium. *J. Biol. Chem.*, **246**, 3057–3063.

Trump, B. F., Mergner, W. J., Kahng, M. W., and Saladino, A. J. (1976). Studies on the subcellular pathophysiology of ischemia. *Circulation* **53**, Suppl. 1, 17–26.

Turner, D. C., Walliman, T., and Eppenberger, H. M. (1973). A protein that binds specifically to the M-line of skeletal muscle is identified as the muscle form of creatine kinase. *Proc. Natl. Acad. Sci.*, **70**, 702–705.

Williamson, J. R., Ford, C., Illingworth, J., *et al.*, (1976a). Co-ordination of citric acid cycle activity with electron transport flux. *Circulation Res.*, **38**, Suppl. 1, 39–51.

Williamson, J. R., Safer, B., Rich, T., Schaffer, S., and Kobayashi, K. (1976b). Effects of acidosis on myocardial contractility and metabolism. *Acta Med. Scand.*, **587**, 95–112.

Wollenberger, A., Ristau, O., and Schoffa, G. (1960). Eine einfache Technik der extrem schnellen Abkühlung grösserer Gewebestücke. *Pflügers Arch. Ges. Physiol.*, **270**, 399–412.

Wollenberger, A., Babskii, E. B., Krause, E. G., Genz, S., S., Blohm, D., and Bogdanova, E. V. (1973). Cyclic changes in levels of cyclic AMP and cyclic GMP in frog myocardium during the cardiac cycle. *Biochem. Biophys. Res. Commun.*, **55**, 446–452.

Wyngaarden, J. B., and Ashton, D. M. (1959). Regulation of activity of phosphoribosylpyrophosphate amidotransferase by purine ribonucleotides: potential feedback control of purine biosynthesis. *J. Biol. Chem.*, **234**, 1492–1496.

Zimmer, H.-G., and Gerlach, E. (1974). Effect of beta-adrenergic stimulation on myocardial adenine nucleotide metabolism. *Circulation Res.*, **35**, 536–543.

Zimmer, H.-G., Steinkopff, G., Ibel, H., and Koschine, H. (1980). Is the ATP decline a signal for stimulating protein synthesis in isoproterenol-induced cardiac hypertrophy? *J. Mol. Cell. Cardiol.*, **12**, 421–426.

Zimmer, H.-G., Trendelenburg, C., and Gerlach, E. (1972). Acceleration of adenine nucleotide synthesis de novo during development of cardiac hypertrophy. *J. Mol. Cell. Cardiol.*, **4**, 279–282.

Zimmer, H.-G., Trendelenburg, C., Kammermeier, H., and Gerlach, E. (1973). *De novo* synthesis of adenine nucleotides in the rat: acceleration during recovery from oxygen deficiency. *Circulation Res.*, **32**, 635–642.

CHAPTER 14

Nuclear Magnetic Resonance

M. J. Dawson

Department of Physiology, University College London, Gower Street, London WC1E 6BT, UK

'What an enormous revolution would be made in biology, if physics or chemistry could supply the physiologist with a means of making out the molecular structure of living tissues comparable to that which the spectroscope affords to the inquirer into the nature of the heavenly bodies. At the present moment the constituents of our own bodies are more remote from our ken than those of Sirius, in this respect.' [From the Royal Society Presidential Address given by T. H. Huxley (1885). The relevance of this remark to recent developments in nuclear magnetic resonance was noticed by Sir Andrew Huxley while preparing his own Presidential Address, 1980.]

INTRODUCTION

Nuclear magnetic resonance (NMR) techniques are non-invasive, have no known toxicity, and can be applied to the study of intact tissues or whole animals, including man. NMR is a form of spectroscopy which detects the presence and electromagnetic environment of particular atomic nuclei. Depending upon how the experiments are done, the physical data yield a wide variety of structural, biochemical, and physiological information, much of which cannot be obtained by any other method available at present. For this reason NMR promises to revolutionize important areas of scientific research and clinical medicine. The potential applications of NMR techniques to the study of the heart are among the most exciting: it may well be possible in the future to obtain by NMR a three-dimensional image of the beating heart of a human subject, together with an analysis of biochemical composition and the kinetics of metabolic reactions as these vary from one location to another and from systole to diastole. Even if no more technical innovations were forthcoming, NMR techniques, as they are available today, supply the physiologist with an extremely powerful tool for the study of the metabolism and metabolic control of cardiac tissue.

The Range of NMR Applications to Study of Intact Tissue

The first applications of NMR methods to studies of intact tissue appeared in the early 1970s; these can be roughly divided into two major categories:

(1) Imaging methods, or zeugmatography, which use information about the protons in water to produce a two-dimensional image, similar to that obtained by computerized X-ray tomography. Two new books on the application of NMR imaging techniques to medicine are now available (Kaufman *et al.*, 1981; Mansfield and Morris, 1982).

(2) NMR can be used to study tissue metabolism non-invasively. The concentrations of particular metabolites can be measured together with intracellular pH and changes in these variables as a result of experimental intervention can be observed. In addition to measuring *net* reaction rates, in some instances unidirectional flux rates for equilibrium reactions can be determined. A number of reviews of NMR studies of tissue metabolism are available (Radda and Seeley, 1979; Burt *et al.*, 1979; Griffiths and Iles, 1980; Gadian and Radda, 1981; Shaw, 1981).

At present efforts are being made to combine these two branches of NMR in order to obtain spatially resolved metabolic information. The recent development of surface coils (Ackerman *et al.*, 1980a) and of topical magnetic resonance (Gordon *et al.*, 1980; Cresshull *et al.*, 1980, 1981) to observe the chemical composition of known localized volumes are a step in this direction. A third, specialized type of biological NMR which may well become clinically important is the measurement of blood flow (reviewed by Singer, 1981). It may be possible to combine blood flow measurements with NMR imaging or metabolic measurements.

NMR Studies of Cardiac Metabolism

The first study of cardiac metabolism by NMR was accomplished only 6 years ago (Gadian *et al.*, 1976) when small unperfused rat hearts were fitted into a 7 mm diameter sample tube and ^{31}P spectra obtained at 4 °C and then 30 °C. The presence of the metabolically important phosphorus-containing metabolites (P-metabolites), adenosine triphosphate (ATP), phospho-creatine (PCr), and inorganic phosphate (P_i) were clearly observed. Methods of perfusing hearts within the spectrometer were quickly developed (Garlick *et al.*, 1977; Jacobus *et al.*, 1977) and in response to the growing need to accommodate large tissues and thus increase the signal obtained, wide-bore spectrometers (25–100 mm sample diameter) are becoming widely available. These machines have been used in studies of cardiac P-metabolites in rat (e.g. Garlick *et al.*, 1979), rabbit (e.g. Hollis *et al.*, 1978), and guinea-pig (see, for example, Figure 14.1) under normal, ischaemic, and hypoxic conditions.

The range of NMR techniques that can be applied to the heart is rapidly being extended. Development of gating and averaging methods has allowed

^{31}P NMR estimation of the variation in P-metabolites between systole and diastole (Fossel *et al.*, 1980). A specialized NMR technique, called 'saturation transfer' has been used to determine the unidirectional flux rates for the creatine kinase reaction in beating rat hearts (Brown *et al.*, 1978; Matthews *et al.*, 1981a). It has been shown possible to obtain useful ^{13}C spectra and thus derive information about metabolites that do not contain phosphorus (Bailey *et al.*, 1981).

In most of these studies the heart is placed within either a Helmholtz or a solenoidal receiver coil so that the signals received represent the average condition of the whole tissue. Recently (Nunnally and Bottomley, 1980) surface coils have been used to focus on a regional ischaemic area. Another important technical development has been to wrap a solenoidal coil around the heart within the chest of an intact, artificially ventilated rat (Ackerman *et al.*, 1980b).

While the rate of development of methodology appropriate for study of cardiac metabolism has been truly astounding, general acceptance of NMR as an experimental or clinical tool requires that the results obtained be demonstrated to be accurate and reliable. The present chapter will focus on this problem. I shall first describe the principles of NMR and their application to biological problems, and then go on to review NMR studies of cardiac tissue and how these relate to studies by more established experimental methods. It will not have escaped the notice of cardiologists or of investigators of cardiac metabolism just how difficult it is to obtain reliable information on the heart and it cannot be surprising that NMR studies of skeletal muscle metabolism are, for the moment at least, more advanced than those of cardiac tissue. For this reason I will in several instances discuss the NMR studies on the heart with reference to the more developed literature on skeletal muscle.

PRINCIPLES OF NUCLEAR MAGNETIC RESONANCE

The use of NMR to study tissue metabolism imposes constraints which are quite different from those encountered in conventional physiological or NMR experiments. In order to appreciate these constraints it is necessary to know something about the physical principles of NMR, and for this reason a brief account is given below. Those who are interested in a more detailed description of NMR principles and methods are referred to a recent book on NMR studies of intact tissues (Gadian, 1982).

Almost all studies of intact tissues are done by 'pulse and Fourier transform' spectroscopy, the techniques for which were developed in the late 1960s and early 1970s. The spectrometer is made up of three parts: (1) a magnet which produces a static field (B_0) to polarize the magnetic nuclei in the sample; (2) a probe which contains the sample and a radiofrequency coil whose magnetic field (B_1) oscillates at right angles to B_0; this coil acts both as a transmitter and a detector of magnetic radiation; (3) a computer which controls the data acquisition, and which stores and processes the results.

NMR techniques are based upon the fact that while all atomic nuclei have positive charge and mass, only some of them, including ^1H, ^{13}C, and ^{31}P, possess the additional quantum characteristic of spin. Only nuclei which possess spin give rise to NMR signals; Table 14.1 lists some of these together with relevant characteristics. The rotating charge causes the nucleus to behave like a tiny magnet and the spinning mass endows it with the properties of a gyroscope. When an external magnetic field is applied, the nuclear magnets do not line up with it in the same way that non-spinning magnets would. Instead, they precess like tops around the direction of the field at a characteristic frequency, the Larmor frequency, ν_L, which is directly proportional to the flux density, B, experienced by the nucleus ($\nu_L = kB$, where B is very slightly but importantly shifted from B_0 as described below). The proportionality constant, k, depends upon the nucleus, as shown in Table 14.1. For example, in the 4.7 T (T stands for tesla; 1 tesla = 47 kilogauss) magnetic field in which the data shown in Figure 14.1 were obtained, the ^{31}P nuclei precess at 81 MHz and ^1H at 200 MHz. (A spectrometer with this field strength is known as a 200 MHz machine, since it is customary to express magnetic flux density as the resonance frequency for protons.)

If a transverse pulse of electromagnetic energy of a few microseconds duration (B_1) is applied at the resonance frequency (Larmor frequency) for a particular type of atomic nucleus, some of these nuclei absorb energy and

Table 14.1 Characteristics of some atomic nuclei of biological interest which give rise to NMR signals

Nucleus	$k = \nu_L/B_0$	Natural abundance (%)	Relative sensitivity at constant field[†]
^1H	42.6	99.98	1
^2H	6.5	0.016	1.5×10^{-6}
^{13}C	10.7	1.1	1.6×10^{-4}
^{15}N	10.7	0.37	3.7×10^{-6}
^{19}F	40.1	100	0.83
^{23}Na	11.3	100	9.3×10^{-2}
^{31}P	17.2	100	6.6×10^{-2}

† Relative sensitivity is sensitivity of the nucleus relative to that of protons, multiplied by the percentage of natural abundance.

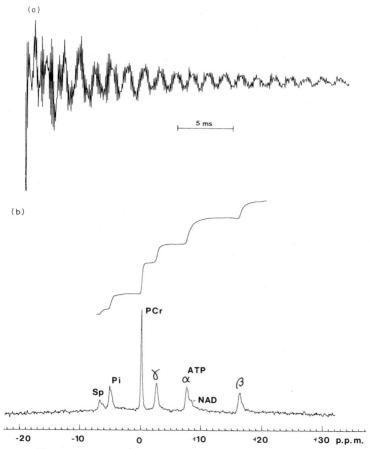

Figure 14.1 ^{31}P NMR study of a beating guinea-pig heart perfused by the Langendorff method; simulating electrodes and force transducer are in place. (a) Free-induction decay (FID), which contains exponentially decaying signals from all of the mobile P-nuclei. The x-axis is time and the y-axis is signal intensity. This FID represents the average response to 400 pulses of 50 μs duration, repeated at 8 s intervals. These conditions ensure that little signal saturation occurs (see text). Total accumulation time is 53.3 min. Four hertz line broadening was applied in order to increase the signal-to-noise ratio (i.e. the FID was multiplied by a 4 Hz decaying exponential). (b) The spectrum obtained by Fourier transformation of the FID shown above. The x-axis is frequency and the y-axis is signal intensity. The basis of identification of the resonances is described in the text. The narrow spike on the left side of the P_i resonance represents P_i in the external medium (pH = 7.26). The internal pH is approximately 7.03. The stepped function is the integral of the spectrum calculated by the computer. Note the convention now universally accepted that the chemical shift becomes more negative from left to right, though the frequency actually increases. In much of the earlier work from the Oxford laboratories, the opposite convention was adopted. [Unpublished data of P. Morris, A. S. V. Burgin and C. J. Harbird, National Institute of Medical Research, London.]

this becomes the basis of their detection. When the pulse is switched off, the excited nuclei return to thermodynamic equilibrium and in doing so re-radiate the energy they had absorbed. A portion of this re-radiated energy is detected and measured as shown in Figure 14.1(a) which illustrates a *free induction decay* (FID; the decline in signal as a function of time) obtained from a perfused rat heart when excited at the appropriate frequency range for ^{31}P.

The resonance frequencies for different types of atomic nuclei are widely separated from each other. In addition, the magnetic flux density (B) experienced by any *particular* nucleus is altered slightly by the effects of local circulating electrons, neighbouring magnetic nuclei, etc., which are characteristic of different compounds. Since $\nu_L = kB$, this results in a reso-nance frequency shift, called the chemical shift, which is detected and used to identify the different compounds present. Therefore, in the experiment shown in Figure 14.1, the applied radiofrequency pulse contains a band of frequencies spanning a few kilohertz and the FID contains contributions from all of the Larmor frequencies for all of the phosphorus compounds present in the sample. Analysis of the FID shown in Figure 14.1(a) into its frequency components by Fourier transformation yields the spectrum shown in Figure 14.1(b), in which the areas under the peaks are related to the concentrations of P-metabolites present. The x-axis is frequency expressed as parts per million (ppm) shift from the resonance frequency of a standard reference compound. When expressed in this way the chemical shifts ob-tained at different field strengths and in different spectrometers are directly comparable.

Nuclei present in immobile compounds exhibit a wide band of resonances instead of a single Larmor frequency and therefore do not give rise to sharp spectral peaks. For this reason conventional NMR methods only detect the presence of compounds which are free in solution, or which are bound to molecules that can themselves rotate freely. The usefulness of this charac-teristic is made apparent in a later section of this chapter.

Sensitivity and Time Resolution

Unfortunately NMR is an insensitive technique and in a single FID the interesting signals are usually buried in the noise. The signal-to-noise ratio is improved by averaging many signals or 'scans', typically several hundred, in order to obtain useful spectra. (The term 'scan' has been carried over from the older and less sensitive, continuous-wave NMR method in which the spectrum is scanned for signal at each individual frequency.) Although, as shown in Figure 14.1, the FID for ^{31}P decays within 10–50 ms (determined by T_2, the spin–spin relaxation time), it takes several seconds (determined by T_1, the spin–lattice relaxation time) for ^{31}P nuclei to revert to their unexcited state. Thus the radiofrequency pulses can only be repeated every few seconds.

Because of variations in nuclear properties, spectrometer sensitivity, sample size, relaxation times, and the relation between the period of accumulation and the amount of signal obtained, no single answer can be given concerning the sensitivity of the technique or its time resolution. The sensitivity increases with field strength, B_0 (but some artefacts are also a direct function of B_0) and in proportion to the volume of sample and to the square root of the number of scans. Sensitivity (at constant field) to ^{1}H is 15 times that of ^{31}P and 63 times that of ^{13}C. While ^{1}H and ^{31}P are naturally occurring isotopes in almost 100% abundance, the natural abundance of ^{13}C is only 1.1% and therefore isotopic enrichment is sometimes used to detect the presence of ^{13}C metabolites in tissue. In general, it is difficult to detect the presence of compounds whose concentration is less that about $0.5\ \mathrm{mmol\,l^{-1}}$.

The theoretical limit on time resolution is determined by T_2, the time constant for the decay of the FID, since after each pulse the observation is made with a 'window' of approximately this duration. In fact, because of the necessity to build-up an acceptable signal-to-noise ratio, the time required to obtain a spectrum varies from several seconds to several minutes. Time resolution can be improved by maintaining the tissue in a steady state of activity which is synchronized with repeated sampling. We have used this technique to observe the metabolic state of frog muscles undergoing 1 s contraction (Dawson *et al.*, 1977) and a similar technique has been used (Fossel *et al.*, 1980) to make four observations on beating rat hearts within a 214 ms cycle (minimum period between samples was 40 ms).

Topical Magnetic Resonance

The recent development of topical magnetic resonance (TMR) has allowed spectra to be obtained from localized volumes in intact small animals (e.g. rabbit) and adult human limbs. Several studies of skeletal muscle in normal individuals (Chance *et al.*, 1981; Wilkie *et al.*, 1983) and patients with various muscle disorders (reviewed by Edwards *et al.*, 1982) have already been undertaken. The technical problems associated with non-invasive investigation of human cardiac metabolism are considerable, in particular because of the continuous movements of the heart and the need for a very large spectrometer; however, it is very likely that these can be overcome.

TMR studies are made possible by two technical advances:

(1) The magnets have a 20 cm bore which is large enough to admit an adult human arm or leg, or a new-born baby. Magnets of 60 cm bore large enough for an adult torso, are now in production.

(2) The magnetic field is shaped so that signals are received from a localized volume.

Because of the dependence of resonance frequency on B_0, high resolution NMR requires that the field strength be as homogeneous as possible throughout the sample volume, which is normally a cross-section through a sample tube. In TMR spectroscopy the magnet bore contains an additional set of profiling coils which (together with a surface coil) modify the field so that within the sensitive volume it is uniform and outside this volume it changes rapidly. The resulting spectrum consists of two components, the high resolution spectrum from within the sensitive volume and a broad component from peripheral regions; this is removed by computer manipulation of the FID.

INFORMATION CONTAINED IN A ^{31}P SPECTRUM

Most of the metabolic studies so far accomplished in cardiac and skeletal muscle have used the ^{31}P nucleus, because of the simplicity of the spectrum, the relatively large signals and the importance of P-metabolites. Unless otherwise stated the technical points made in this section refer to NMR spectroscopy of other atomic nuclei as well.

Identification of Resonances

The assignment of the resonance peaks in the spectrum shown in Figure 14.1(b) is made by comparing the resonance positions with those of metabolites free in solution. Because resonances overlap, positive identification requires independent evidence that the metabolites in question are indeed present in the tissue being studied. In this way the resonances of ATP, PCr, P_i, and sugar phosphates (sugar-P) can be unequivocally assigned in spectra from skeletal muscle (Hoult *et al.*, 1974; Burt *et al.*, 1967a) and cardiac muscle (Gadian *et al.*, 1976; Jacobus *et al.*, 1977). Adenosine diphosphate (ADP) resonates in the α and γ adenosine–phosphate positions; however, in skeletal muscle (Dawson *et al.*, 1977) the amount of ADP that is free in solution is too low to be detected by NMR. Whether or not ADP can be detected in cardiac muscle is a controversial question which will be taken up in a later section. Nicotinamide adenine dinucleotide (NAD; i.e. total NAD and NADH) resonates near the α-adenosine phosphate and therefore appears as a shoulder on this peak. Resolution of individual sugar-P resonances is difficult since they are closely grouped at physiological pH. The region of the spectrum around +7.5 ppm includes resonances from species of the form: $-CH_2-O-PO_3^-$, such as glucose-6-phosphate, fructose-6-phosphate, fructose-1,6-diphosphate, adenosine monophosphate (AMP), and some triose phosphates.

A small and interesting resonance appears in the phosphodiester region (+3.2 ppm) of the ^{31}P spectrum from some hearts; this peak may be glycerophosphoryl choline, although the identification requires confirmation by chemical methods. In skeletal muscle three closely spaced resonances appear in the phosphodiester region, two of which have been chemically identified as glycerolphosphoryl choline (Burt *et al.*, 1976b) and serine-ethanolamine phosphodiester (Chalovich *et al.*, 1977). Barany and coworkers are investigating a possible link between these compounds and muscular dystrophy (Chalovich *et al.*, 1979).

Measurement of Concentrations

It is likely that, in the near future, non-invasive ^{31}P NMR studies will replace chemical analysis as a means of measuring energetically important P-metabolites. In addition to the obvious advantages of non-invasive methods in clinical investigations or in studies of the time-course of metabolic changes, we have also found that in some circumstances ^{31}P NMR studies of intact tissue yield more accurate results than can be obtained on extracts. Calibration methods have been devised for measuring absolute concentrations of P-metabolites in frog (Dawson *et al.*, 1977) and human (Dawson, 1982) skeletal muscle. Fossel *et al.* (1980) have used a different method in studies of beating rat heart.

There are two important problems which must be handled carefully if useful measurements of metabolite levels are to be made by NMR. The first is to maintain the tissue in a physiologically and biochemically normal state. The special constraints that NMR poses in this respect are that the materials used in the life-support system must interfere as little as possible with the homogeneity of the magnetic field and should not introduce radiofrequency noise nor be a means of magnetic loss.

The second problem is to assess accurately the relation between signal intensity and concentration of metabolite. The main difficulty in this regard is signal saturation resulting from inadequate delays between pulses. The areas of the various resonances are proportional to the quantities of metabolite within the volume enclosed by the radiofrequency coil, provided that the field is completely homogeneous and that the radiofrequency pulses are applied at time intervals much greater than the T_1 of the resonances, or the pulse duration is kept very short. In order to optimize the signal-to-noise ratio of the spectra it is usual to use a shorter duration pulse at a faster repetition rate, under which conditions the areas of the resonance peaks are reduced, an effect known as 'saturation', by factors determined by the T_1 values. The T_1 values are different for the nuclei in different metabolites and conceivably alter as a result of experimental interventions. For this reason the peak areas in most of the spectra of cardiac muscle now in the literature are *not* proportional to the concentrations of metabolites present.

Concentrations of Phosphorus Metabolites in Skeletal Muscle

Undoubtedly the most accurate estimates of P-metabolites by chemical methods have been obtained on frog sartorius and semitendinosus muscles maintained at 0 °C, and subjected to very fast freezing to terminate chemical reactions. It is now well known that freezing must be accomplished in less than 100 ms if no artefactual breakdown of PCr is to occur (Kretzschmar and Wilkie, 1969; Kretzschmar, 1970). Increasingly sophisticated methods of freezing, based on the 'hammer apparatus' designed by Kretzschmar and Wilkie allow very precise chemical measurements to be made, e.g. statistically significant changes in [ATP] of $0.1 \, \text{mmol kg}^{-1}$ have been observed during contraction (Gilbert *et al.*, 1971).

NMR measurements of P-metabolites in aerobic skeletal muscle were first published in 1976 (Dawson *et al.*, 1976, 1977). In this study the muscles were maintained in a good physiological state by perfusion with oxygenated Ringer's solution at 4 °C. We corrected for the effect of signal saturation by comparing the ratios of peak areas with their ratios at a much slower pulse repetition rate in which saturation does not occur. Table 14.2 shows that the concentrations of P-metabolites obtained in this way agree within experimental error with those determined by ultra-fast freezing followed by chemical analysis, a result which tends to confirm the accuracy of both techniques.

Table 14.2 Relative concentration of P compounds in resting frog sartorius as determined by NMR and by chemical analysis

		NMR	Chemical	*P*
PCr / βATP	$\bar{x}$	6.74	8.14	
	S.E.	±0.309	±0.744	n.s.
	(*n*)	(6)	(18)	
PCr / P₁	$\bar{x}$	16.02	13.10	
	S.E.	±1.58	±3.03	n.s.
	(*n*)	(6)	(17)	

Rough estimates of actual concentrations may be made by assuming that the resting PCr content is $27 \, \text{mmol kg}^{-1}$.
From Dawson *et al.* (1977).

Table 14.3 Composition of resting human muscle

P-metabolite	Concentration of P-metabolite (mmol kg^{-1} wet weight)		
	(1) Biopsy†	(2) ^{31}P TMR‡	(3) ^{31}P TMR§
ATP	5.5 ± 0.07 (81)	5.5	5.1 ± 0.10
PCr	17.4 ± 0.19 (81)	29.0 ± 0.69	27.4 ± 0.23
Pi	≈10 ± ? (3)	4.4 ± 0.33	4.3 ± 0.27
PCr + Cr	28.6 ± 0.28 (81)	—	—
PCr + P$_i$	31.6 ± 3.27 (11)	33.4 ± 0.77	31.7 ± 0.29
PdiE‖	—	0.7 ± 0.09	0.8 ± 0.09
NAD + NADH	0.7	1.0 ± 0.09	0.9 ± 0.07

Calibration of ^{31}P TMR peak integrals in terms of millimoles per kilogram wet weight was done by two essentially independent methods. In column (2) the ATP concentration was assumed to equal that obtained by needle biopsy while in column (3) the total mobile phosphorus was taken as the reference. The general agreement between columns (2) and (3) attests to the reliability of the results. See Wilkie *et al.* (1983) or Dawson (1982) for further information. [NAD + NADH] seems not to have been reported in human biopsies; that given in column (1) is from fast glycolysing porcine muscle.

† Mean values ± s.e.m. Values in parentheses are numbers of samples (*n*).

‡ Mean values ± s.e.m. [ATP] is assumed constant at 5.5 mmol kg^{-1}. *n* = 7.

§ Mean values ± s.e.m. Total integral assumed constant at 49.5 mmol kg^{-1}. *n* = 7.

‖ PdiE = phosphodiesters; see 'Identification of resonances' in text.

Table 14.3 shows a comparison of P-metabolite concentrations in human skeletal muscle obtained by needle and open biopsy with those obtained by ^{31}P TMR on normal subjects. Unlike the case of frog muscle there are differences in the results obtained by the two techniques, and the differences tend to confirm long-held suspicions that PCr is hydrolysed during the minimum of 6 s required to freeze the needle biopsy samples. Although the sensitive volume contains other tissue in addition to muscle, it was found that under the experimental conditions that pertained, no corrections were required for the presence of non-muscle phosphorus. The TMR results show a higher [PCr] and a lower [P$_i$] than is obtained by needle biopsy, but the total [PCr] + [P$_i$] is not significantly different by the two methods. Thus, it appears that in needle biopsies of resting human skeletal muscle approximately 20% of the total PCr is artefactually broken down during the sampling procedure.

Concentrations of Phosphorus Metabolites in Cardiac Muscle

There appears to be widespread agreement that in normal cardiac muscle maintained in a good physiological state [ATP] is roughly the same as it is in skeletal muscle, approximately 5 mmol l^{-1}, and while the reported values for [PCr] are much more variable they are often as much as double [ATP]. A rigorous comparison of absolute concentration of P-metabolites obtained by ^{31}P NMR with those obtained by chemical analysis, taking account of the limitations and strengths of both methods, is required before the reliability of ^{31}P NMR studies of this tissue will be generally accepted. This cannot be undertaken on the basis of presently available evidence, and so Table 14.4 and the following discussion are inevitably somewhat inconclusive.

Artefactual PCr breakdown during sampling, freezing, and extraction is a major problem in chemical studies of all tissues, including the heart, and demands urgent critical and experimental appraisal. It has been claimed that in cardiac muscle the measured [PCr] is not affected by sampling times of up to 30 s (Allison *et al.*, 1978), a remarkable discrepancy with the results on skeletal muscle which requires explanation. Variation during the cardiac cycle introduces scatter in the measurements, and since these results were analysed by *unpaired* t-test small changes in concentration could not be detected. In a study of sequential biopsies from the same animal, Drake (1980) has shown that a significant amount of PCr breakdown occurs after a 5 s delay in taking the biopsy to actual freezing. Therefore, PCr breakdown during sampling must be related to freezing time, as for skeletal muscle, but it is not always readily apparent in some of the relatively imprecise chemical studies on cardiac muscle.

There exist only two published studies in which absolute concentration of

Table 14.4 Concentrations of P-metabolites measured in rat heart by chemical analysis in comparison to ^{31}P NMR

P-metabolite	Concentration of P-metabolite (μmol g^{-1} dry weight)		
	Chemical[†]	^{31}P NMR[‡]	^{31}P NMR[§]
ATP	21.2 ± 0.3 (8)	23.7 ± 1.0 (5)	—
PCr	40.4 ± 1.2 (8)	30.5 ± 0.5 (5)	28.4 ± 1.7 (5)
P$_i$	10.1 ± 0.1 (6)	24.5 ± 0.6 (5)	9.7 ± 1.1 (5)
ADP	3.8 ± 0.2 (6)	0	—

All values are means ± S.E.M.; values in parentheses indicate numbers of samples. Perfusion methods differ in these 3 studies
[†] From Dhalla *et al.* (1972).
[‡] From Fossel *et al.* (1980).
[§] From Matthews *et al.* (1981b).

P-metabolites have been measured by ^{31}P NMR (Fossel *et al.*, 1980; Matthews *et al.*, 1981a). Fossel and coworkers measured the *changes* in ATP, PCr, and Pi within a single cardiac cycle in working rat hearts, a feat which has not been accomplished by chemical analysis. For comparison with chemical estimates, their mid-diastolic values are given in Table 14.4. While [ATP] determined by ^{31}P NMR is in good agreement with that obtained by highly regarded conventional studies, [PCr] is rather lower than the chemical estimate shown in Table 14.4. It is tempting to attribute the low [PCr] determined by NMR to the fact that in these studies P_i was not present in the perfusion fluid, a condition which is well known to cause rapid deterioration of mechanical activity, and which is associated with phosphate leakage from the tissue (Salhany *et al.*, 1979). In their early study with no P_i present in the perfusion fluid Garlick *et al.* (1977) have published concentration ratios for P-metabolites obtained by ^{31}P NMR; they find that the APT:PCr:P_i ratio is 1:1.8:1.

The measurement by Fossel and coworkers of changes in [PCr], [ATP], and [P_i] within a cardiac cycle is an advance of major significance. The signal from an aortic pressure transducer was used to synchronize the radio frequency observation pulse with the heart beat. Peak aortic pressure was sensed and after a preprogrammed delay the NMR pulse was initiated. The resulting FIDs from identically placed pulses were signal-averaged until sufficient signal was obtained.

Figure 14.2 shows that [ATP] and [PCr] vary during the cardiac cycle,

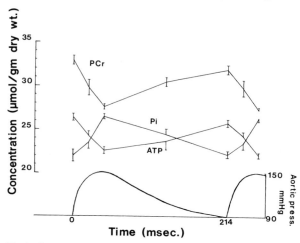

Figure 14.2 Variations of P-metabolites in rat heart within a single cardiac cycle. The data is from Figures 4 and 5 of Fossel *et al.* (1980). It is plotted here on an absolute time scale to make clear that the metabolite changes are not sinusoidal, as they appear in the original figures. (This point was made to me by G. Dawkins, a medical student at University College London.)

being maximal at minimal aortic pressure and minimal at maximal aortic pressure: [P_i] varies inversely with [ATP] and [PCr]. One caveat to these results is that it is extremely difficult to eliminate artefacts associated with the heart moving, with each beat, into areas of higher or lower NMR sensitivity within the volume bounded by the receiver coil. As is discussed later, it is difficult to reconcile these results with information now available about the creatine kinase reaction. Verification of the data shown in Fig. 14.2 by the same, and other laboratories is therefore urgently necessary.

Because of the relative difficulty of determining absolute concentrations of metabolites and because often one is really interested in the *changes* in metabolite levels as a result of experimental intervention, it is usual in NMR studies of the heart to plot percentage change in a particular resonance as a function of time. However, it is disappointing to see how often this is done by measuring peak *heights* which are used as an index of *areas*. This practice is invalid because the resonance peaks obtained from intact tissue are broadened for a variety of reasons and their width can vary as a result of experimental intervention. Such variations have been observed in ^{31}P NMR studies of the heart (Jacobus *et al.*, 1977; Nunnally and Bottomley, 1981).

Measurement of Intracellular pH

Intracellular pH measurements on cardiac tissue have recently been reviewed (Poole-Wilson, 1978) as has the use of NMR to measure intracellular pH (Gadian *et al.*, 1982). Although like other techniques NMR has its limitations, its advantages are such that it greatly extends the scope of experimental possibilities:

(1) It is harmless; non-invasive measurements of skeletal muscle pH are now made in patients as well as in normal human subjects.
(2) It is, or can be made to be, extremely rapid. The theoretical limit to time resolution approximates T_2 for P_i (approx. 10–50 ms). The most rapid ^{31}P NMR measurement of cardiac pH so far published is 30 s, similar to the time required for microelectrode measurements and very favourable in comparison to the 15–20 min required for distribution techniques.
(3) Under appropriate circumstances NMR can be used to measure both mean and distribution of pH (see below).
(4) pH can be measured simultaneously with measurements of concentrations of ^{31}P or ^{13}C metabolites and mechanical function. The advantages of this in establishing correlations is obvious; in addition, however, the ability to measure [H^+] together with the concentrations of P-metabolites allows calculation, under particular controlled conditions, of other quantities of interest. In skeletal muscle these include free [ADP], free energy change for

ATP hydrolysis, rate of lactic acid formation, and rate of ATP utilization (Dawson *et al.*, 1978).

In principle any resonance signal whose position is sensitive to $[H^+]$ can be used to measure pH. Those that have been used in studies of intact tissue include the ^{31}P resonances of P_i (very common), 2-deoxyglucose-6-phosphate (Bailey *et al.*, 1981), and the ^1H of haemoglobin histidine (Brown *et al.*, 1977). The P_i signal is often the most suitable since it is clearly observable and P_i has a pK_a in the region of biological interest:

$$H_2PO_4^- \rightleftharpoons H^+ + HPO_4^{--}, \quad pK_a = 6.9 \text{ at } 37\,°C. \tag{14.1}$$

If chemical exchange could be prevented these two species would give rise to two signals separated by approximately 2.3 ppm. However, in solution the two species exchange with each other rapidly (10^9–$10^{10}\,s^{-1}$) and as a result the observed spectrum is a single peak, the frequency of which is determined by the relative amounts of the two species present.

The pH of the solution can then be determined from the frequency of this single peak, in relation to a reference peak, provided that a calibration curve is determined under similar conditions. Figure 14.3 shows one such calibration curve; it is apparent that the chemical shift of P_i with respect to PCr can be used to measure pH in the region of about 6.0–7.7, although precision is

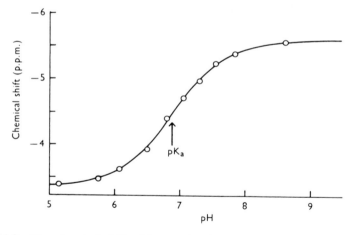

Figure 14.3 The chemical shift of inorganic phosphate as a function of pH under physiological conditions of ionic strength and at 4 °C (zero $[Mg^{++}]$). Abscissae, pH; ordinates, chemical shifts in parts per million (ppm) related to the resonance of phosphocreatine. The circles are experimental; the continuous line is drawn from the equation $pH = 6.88 + \log_{10}(\sigma - \sigma_1)/(\sigma_2 - \sigma)$, where σ is the observed chemical shift and σ_1 and σ_2 are the shifts of $H_2PO_4^-$ and HPO_2^{--}, -3.35 and -5.6 respectively. [Reproduced with permission from M. J. Dawson, D. G. Gadian, and R. D. Wilkie, *J. Physiol. (Lond).* **267**, 465–484 (1977), Copyright © 1977 *J. Physiol. (Lond).*]

reduced at the extreme ends of this range. It is usual to use the position of PCr as a reference, since this practice provides an automatic correction for any magnetic susceptibility differences between the intracellular and extracellular environments. The resonance position of P_i is remarkably insensitive to biological variables (Burt *et al.*, 1976a; Garlick *et al.*, 1979; Hollis, 1979; Jacobus *et al.*, 1982), but the factors influencing the PCr resonance position are not as well characterized, although known to include $[Mg^{++}]$ (Burt *et al.*, 1967a). The position of the calibration curve on the x-axis is also affected by temperature (as is the pH neutrality). The differences in tissue pH values obtained by NMR in different laboratories are in part due to differences in the composition of the calibration solutions, notably $[Mg^{++}]$, which can cause variations in the estimation of pH of up to 0.2 pH units. This problem is analogous to interference effects that also plague both the distribution and microelectrode techniques. Measurements of *changes* in pH are unaffected, unless intracellular $[Mg^{++}]$ also changes.

Clearly, it is necessary to know the cellular location of the P_i if pH measurements by this method are to be valid. This was pointed out by Poole-Wilson (1978) who suspected that the early NMR measurements reported for perfused heart (pH = 7.4; Jacobus *et al.*, 1977; Hollis *et al.*, 1977; Garlick *et al.*, 1977) were too alkaline to represent cytoplasmic pH. It now appears that Poole-Wilson's analysis was correct; in fact the most likely explanation for these alkaline pH values, suggested by Salhany *et al.* (1979), is that there was significant loss of P_i from the hearts perfused with phosphate-free buffer and that the pH measured was that of the bathing medium.

A technically painstaking study of cardiac pH is that of Garlick *et al.* (1979) on perfused rat hearts. They used a phosphate-buffered perfusion fluid to improve tissue viability and showed that the internal and external P_i peaks could be easily distinguished so that the extracellular P_i did not interfere with intracellular pH measurements. In seven normal hearts at 37 °C they found internal pH = 7.05 ± 0.02 (S.E.M.) when external pH = 7.38. Further justification for the accuracy of pH measurements by NMR was given in a follow-up paper by the same group (Bailey *et al.*, 1981). In this study the resonance position of accumulated deoxyglucose-6-phosphate ($pK_a = 6.16$) was used in addition to that of internal P_i. There was no significant difference between the pH values obtained with reference to these two markers, either in the normal or the ischaemic heart. Since deoxyglucose-6-phosphate is expected to be exclusively in the cytoplasm, these results show that both under normoxic and ischaemic conditions the P_i resonance also reflects the cytoplasmic pH. The results also establish that binding of P_i to proteins or membranes can be excluded as being responsible for the measured chemical shifts of intracellular P_i. The pH value obtained for four normal rat hearts was 7.01 ± 0.01 (S.D.). The values obtained in the two last quoted studies are in reasonably good agreement with those obtained for normal rat heart cytoplasmic pH by use of microelectrodes (pH = 7.14; Ellis and Thomas, 1976) and DMO (pH = 7.05; Steenbergen *et al.*, 1977).

Mg⁺⁺ Binding to P-Metabolites and Intracellular free Mg⁺⁺

The importance of this subject for accurate determination of pH by NMR was discussed above. It is also of more general importance because it is Mg-ATP rather than free ATP that is the substrate for the actomyosin ATPase and other energy-requiring reactions. Additionally, as a result of Mg binding to various reactants, free intracellular $[Mg^{++}]$ affects the equilibrium constants for enzymes such as creatine kinase and adenylate kinase, and the free energy change for ATP hydrolysis.

Since ATP binds to H^+ and Mg^{++}, the positions of the adenosine phosphate peaks are sensitive to both of these ions; this is shown for the β-peak in Figure 14.4. All of the ^{31}P NMR studies of both cardiac and skeletal muscle now in the literature agree that ATP is predominantly (more than 90%) bound to Mg^{++}. From a knowledge of the extent of Mg^{++} binding to ATP, together with the binding constant, it is theoretically possible to determine the concentration of free intracellular Mg^{++}. On this basis, Gupta and Moore (1980) have concluded that the concentration of

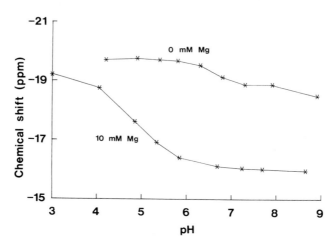

Figure 14.4 The chemical shift of the β adenosine phosphate peak of 5 mmol l⁻¹ ATP plotted as a function of pH in the absence of Mg^{++} and in the presence of 10 mmol l⁻¹ MgCl₂, when the ATP is almost fully complexed to Mg^{++}. These data are from Figure 2.10 of Gadian (1982), which also includes information on the α and γ adenosine peaks

free Mg^{++} in muscle is about 0.6 mM. There are, however, a number of uncertainties associated with this calculation: the chemical shift must be measured with unrealistically high precision, and may well be affected by factors that have not yet been explored; estimates for the binding constant of Mg^{++} to ATP vary. Uncertainty about the binding constant of Mg^{++} to ATP also plagues the work of Cohen and Burt (1977). On the basis of the effect of $[Mg^{++}]$ on the T_2 relaxation rate of PCr in solution, these authors concluded that the concentration of free Mg^{++} in muscle is about 3 mM. Again, however, it is impossible to prove that the muscle is completely analogous to the model solutions.

These results are comparable with those of studies of muscle by other methods, which range from 1.1 mM (Gilbert, 1960) to 4.2 mM (Brinley *et al.*, 1977). A recent Mg^{++} ion-sensitive electrode study (Hess and Weingart, 1981) indicates a concentration of free Mg^{++} of 3.1 ± 0.3 mM (S.E.M.), $n = 8$, for ventricular muscle of sheep and ferret.

The Creatine Kinase Reaction and Metabolic Compartmentalization in Skeletal and Cardiac Muscle

An early, although rather crude, example of the ability of NMR to detect compartmentalization was the demonstration (Hollis *et al.*, 1977) that two P_i peaks can be observed in regionally ischaemic hearts: one representing the pH of the normally perfused tissue and a second, in a more acid position, which must arise from the ischaemic region. As all NMR enthusiasts have been quick to point out, the possibility of detecting and evaluating the size of ischaemic regions has potentially important diagnostic value.

Another, equally important compartmentalization problem for which NMR has yielded useful information is the question of the availability of PCr and ATP to take part in energetically critical reactions. Much indirect evidence has been put forward in favour of these metabolites being confined in two or more different compartments in cardiac muscle. On the other hand, it is becoming increasingly clear that no such compartmentalization exists in skeletal muscle.

Compartmentalization and Binding of P-metabolites in Skeletal Muscle

It has long been assumed by most investigators that the creatine kinase reaction is in equilibrium in resting skeletal muscle and that [ATP] and [PCr] measured by chemical analysis represent the pool of high energy phosphate that is readily available for contraction. There are many indirect reasons for making these assumptions (see Carlson and Wilkie, 1974), and direct experimental evidence has recently been obtained (Veech *et al.*, 1979; Gadian *et al.*, 1981).

As discussed earlier the [ATP], [PCr], and [P$_i$] obtained by ^{31}P NMR in frog skeletal muscle agree within experimental error with those obtained by chemical analysis, indicating that there is no significant binding of these substances to large immobile molecules. In the case of ADP, the situation is quite different: in studies of both frogs and human muscle (Dawson 1982) paired *t*-tests show no significant difference between the γ- and β-adenosine phosphate peaks, in spite of the fact that the γ-peak contains a contribution from ADP while the β-peak does not. Although [ADP] determined by chemical analysis is near the limit of observation by NMR (about 0.5 mmol kg^{-1} in resting frog muscle), our inability to detect its presence suggests that *in vivo* it is largely bound to macromolecules. This is consistent with the fact that there are known binding sites for ADP on actin and myosin (see Ferenczi *et al.*, 1978) which together account for virtually all of the ADP present in resting muscle.

For this reason, [ADP] determined by chemical analysis is not directly relevant to metabolic studies. The concentration of ADP that is free in solution *in vivo* can only be determined by calculation from the creatine kinase reaction (Dawson *et al.*, 1978; Veech *et al.*, 1979), which at physiological pH and [Mg^{++}] can be written in the following form:

$$ADP + PCr + H \rightleftharpoons ATP + \text{creatine}. \tag{14.2}$$

When the creatine kinase reaction is in equilibrium, [ADP] can be determined from

$$[ADP] = \frac{[ATP][Cr]}{K[PCr][H^+]}. \tag{14.3}$$

This yields a value for the concentration of ADP that is free to take part in the creatine kinase reaction of approximately 20 μmol l^{-1}, in well maintained resting frog skeletal muscles. The demonstration that the concentration of ADP which is free in solution is much less than that determined by chemical analysis has profound consequences: it can be shown quantitatively that suggestions of compartmentalization of the creatine kinase reaction in skeletal muscle arise from failure to take this difference into account (see Wilkie, 1981a). Widespread failure to appreciate the extent and significance of ADP binding in skeletal muscle has led to generally incorrect assumptions about the *in vivo* environment by biochemists studying enzyme control systems *in vitro* (Wilkie, 1981b).

Calculation of [ADP] by equation (14.3) can only be correct if all of the measured reactants are in the same pool and the creatine kinase reaction is in equilibrium, conditions which have been tested using combined enzyme systems (Veech *et al.*, 1979) and saturation transfer NMR (Gadian *et al.*,

1981). The latter technique depends upon continuously irradiating a particular nucleus, e.g. the γ-phosphorus of ATP, so that it is saturated and yields no signal in response to the regular radiofrequency pulse. When the γ-phosphorus of ATP exchanges with the P of PCr through the creatine kinase reaction it takes its saturation with it and the PCr peak is diminished as well. In the reverse experiment the PCr peak is irradiated and the resulting diminution of the γ-adenosine peak is determined. The unidirectional flux rates for the creatine kinase reaction can then be calculated from the extent of transfer of saturation, the T_1, and concentrations of the nuclear species involved.

In resting frog gastrocnemii we have found that the forward and backward flux rates for the creatine kinase reaction are about 1.6×10^{-3} mM s^{-1}, i.e. roughly one-third of the total [ATP] is turned over in each second (Gadian *et al.*, 1981). This result is consistent with the creatine kinase reaction being in equilibrium and all of the ATP and PCr being available to react. During contraction, this equilibrium is disturbed by the rapid ATP hydrolysis, and reaction (14.2) is driven from left to right. In the above experiments, when the muscles were stimulated and the net rate of ATP hydrolysis determined as well as the creatine kinase unidirectional flux rates, the results were consistent with the well established observation that during contraction [ATP] falls by less that 2–3%.

The results relating to compartmentalization in skeletal muscle can be summarized as follows: The [ATP], [PCr], and [P$_i$] measured either by chemical analysis or ^{31}P NMR represent the concentrations of these reactants which are free in the cytoplasm and available to both creatine kinase and actomyosin ATPase. Most of the [ADP] that is measured by chemical analysis after tissue extraction is ADP that was stripped off from its *in vivo* binding sites, mainly actin and myosin; ^{31}P NMR offers a method of determining [ADP] that is free in solution. The creatine kinase reaction is at equilibrium in resting muscle, and during contraction it is driven from left to right mainly by the large relative increase in [ADP].

Metabolic Compartmentalization in Cardiac Muscle

A large proportion of cardiac creatine kinase is found in the mitochondria (Scholte, 1973) as an isoenzyme which is different from the one in the cytoplasm. These and other findings have led to the suggestion that creatine kinase does not function solely to buffer the supply of ATP, but may serve as a high energy phosphate transport system and thus regulate the supply of energy made available from respiration across the mitochondrial membrane. ^{31}P NMR yields direct methods for assessing some of these ideas, although the full capability of the technique has not been realized.

One of the arguments for metabolic compartmentalization in the heart is based upon the fact that the mass action ratio

$$K' = \frac{[\text{PCr}][\text{ADP}][\text{H}^+]}{[\text{ATP}][\text{Cr}]} \tag{14.4}$$

is not the same as the equilibrium constant for the creatine kinase reaction (Kubler and Katz, 1977). A more plausible explanation for this result is that the value obtained by chemical analysis does not reflect the true *in vivo* concentration of free ADP. Since [ADP] measured by chemical analysis and the content of actin and myosin are similar in the two tissues, one must conclude that in the heart, as in skeletal muscle, it is likely that most of the ADP is bound to these two proteins and unavailable to take part in chemical reactions.

The NMR results concerning the concentration of free ADP have changed as techniques have improved. There were reports that the area of the γ adenosine phosphate is larger than the β, both in normal (γ : β = 1.4; Gadian *et al.*, 1976) and ischaemic rat hearts (Hollis *et al.*, 1978); however, the relatively poor signal-to-noise ratio achieved in these early experiments throws doubt on the validity of the measurements. Fossel *et al.* (1980) found no significant difference between the integrals of the γ and β adenosine phosphate resonances of normal beating rat hearts, indicating that [ADP] that is free in solution is too low to be detected. The Oxford group (Matthews *et al.*, 1982) now agree with this conclusion.

Another type of evidence often put forward for metabolic compartmentalization is the fact that, during cardiac ischaemia, contractility declines to very low values while [ATP] remains nearly normal (e.g. Gudbjarnason *et al.*, 1970). However, the same phenomenon also occurs in fatiguing skeletal muscle where there is good reason to believe that nearly all of the ATP is present in the myofibrils (see CIBA Foundation Symposium, 1981). In a ^{31}P NMR study of repetitively stimulated frog gastrocnemius muscles we found that force declined to 10% of its initial value in the absence of any significant change in [ATP] (Figure 3 in Dawson *et al.*, 1978). The decline in force was strongly correlated with a rise in levels of products of ATP hydrolysis, including H^+; these substances could affect either the activation of contraction or the actomyosin ATPase.

There is thus reason to doubt the validity of some of the most often-quoted evidence for metabolic compartmentalization in the heart. This is not, of course, to say that such compartmentalization cannot exist. The NMR results are conflicting: some results have been interpreted in terms of metabolic compartmentalization (Nunnally and Hollis, 1979; Fossel *et al.*, 1980) while others (Matthews *et al.*, 1981b, 1982) have been interpreted to indicate a single compartment for P-metabolites.

It is not generally possible in studies of the heart to separate the metabolic events of systole from those of diastole. The ^{31}P NMR studies that average these events over periods of several minutes yield results which are consistent with the simple, single compartment model, together with high creatine kinase activity, that prevails in skeletal muscle. For example, the equilibrium constant for the creatine kinase reaction is such that, unless there is restricted access to substrates, there can be no detectable change in [ATP] until PCr is almost completely depleted. This is always observed in skeletal muscle, and a similar result has often been reported for ischaemic and anoxic hearts. Saturation transfer studies in the heart have been more equivocal since the results show that the forward flux rate (PCr → ATP) for the creatine kinase reaction is somewhat larger than the reverse rate (ATP → PCr) under steady state conditions (Brown *et al.*, 1978; Nunnally and Hollis, 1979; Ackerman *et al.*, 1980b; Brown, 1980). This apparent discrepancy could result either from (1) competition for ATP by other reactions or from (2) compartmentalization of the metabolites involved in the creatine kinase reaction. The Oxford group has recently presented evidence in favour of the first explanation (Matthews *et al.*, 1982) and therefore feel justified in using equation (14.3) to calculate the concentration of free ADP in the heart (Matthews *et al.*, 1981a,b).

However, an example of significant changes in [ATP] in the presence of apparently ample PCr buffer is illustrated in Figure 14.2, which shows that changes in [ATP] within the cardiac cycle are roughly equal to the changes in [PCr]. These results of Fossel *et al.* (1980) are inconsistent with the body of evidence presented by the Oxford group and discussed above. If cyclic variation in [ATP] in the presence of normal [PCr] is confirmed, it must be explained either by sequestration of PCr, or low creatine kinase activity.

NMR Studies of Ischaemia and Hypoxia

A great deal of interest has been focused on metabolic studies of the ischaemic or hypoxic myocardium by NMR, in part because of the importance of the subject and in part due to the ease with which the resulting metabolic changes can be detected. All of these studies show the well documented decline in [PCr], [ATP], and pH associated with ischaemia. In those studies in which the time course of metabolic changes could be clearly followed, [PCr] was observed to decline substantially before any fall in [ATP] (e.g. Hollis *et al.*, 1977; Garlick *et al.*, 1979; Matthews *et al.*, 1981a; Jacobus *et al.*, 1982) a result which is consistent with a number of earlier studies of tissue extracts (cf. Gibbs, 1978). Depolarization of the heart with KCl before the ischaemic period tends to diminish the metabolic and pH changes observed by ^{31}P NMR (Hollis *et al.*, 1977; Nunnally and Bottomley, 1981), a result which supplies at least a partial explanation for the well known protective effect of K depolarization on the ischaemic myocardium.

Of great practical as well as theoretical importance are ^{31}P NMR studies of conditions which facilitate recovery of stressed hearts. For example Nunnally and Bottomley (1981) showed that verapamil administration dramatically improves the metabolic status of the ischaemic heart while chlorpromazine is less effective. Garlick *et al.* (1979) showed that inclusion of $100 \, \text{mmol} \, l^{-1}$ HEPES buffer in the perfusion fluid considerably lessened the pH and P-metabolite changes associated with global ischaemia of rat hearts and promoted better recovery upon reperfusion. They concluded that the effect of HEPES is to decrease the inhibition of glycolysis by increased H^+. Bailey and Seymour (1981) have also studied recovery of rat hearts from total global ischaemia. They found that if reflow commenced after 6 min the heart recovered normal metabolite levels and mechanical function, but that recovery after 14 min of ischaemia was not complete.

Study of the link between metabolic status and mechanical function is another area where NMR studies can make a substantial contribution. It has been possible to establish correlations between mechanical and metabolic changes in fatiguing skeletal muscle (Dawson *et al.*, 1978, 1980) and to postulate hypotheses concerning the mechanism of the decline in force production and relaxation rate. A very similar approach can be used in the heart. Matthews *et al.* (1981b) have found that in the hypoxic heart the decline in contractility significantly precedes changes in [ATP] and intracellular pH. In a more recent, and more extensive study of ischaemic rabbit hearts, Jacobus *et al.* (1982) used ^{31}P NMR to measure metabolite levels and mass spectrometry to determine blood p_{O_2} and p_{CO_2}. They found that down to a 50% reduction in flow, pH, [PCr], [ATP], and p_{O_2} all remained normal, in spite of a 40% reduction in left ventricular developed pressure.

It is evident that ^{31}P NMR can be used to answer many of the outstanding questions in this area of cardiac research. Because the technique is still very new only a small amount of its potential has yet been realized; however, this is an area of intense activity and it is likely that there will be further significant advances before these words are printed. In addition, since the biochemical changes in ischaemic or otherwise stressed myocardium are not limited to alterations in P-metabolites and pH, interest is now being focused on studies using ^1H and ^{13}C NMR.

Other Nuclei and Heteronuclear Studies of Metabolism

^1H is the naturally occurring nucleus and yields a large signal, factors which make it ideal for the production of two-dimensional images by the NMR technique known as zeugmatography (see Introduction). However, for metabolic studies the very abundance of ^1H leads to a complicated spectrum which is difficult to analyse, and the presence of an extremely large water peak can obliterate nearby resonances from interesting metabolites. The use of 'spin-echo' NMR (a technique which uses the timing of radiofrequency pulses to separate signals having the same resonance frequencies but different T_1 relaxation rates) can help to overcome these problems. The technique has been used to follow the transport of alanine into red cells and, together with exchange of protons from lactate and pyruvate with D_2O, to measure the equilibrium unidirectional flux rates across lactate dehydrogenase in red cells (Brown and Campbell, 1980). The results so far suggest that ^1H and ^2H can be used in studies of metabolism but that this requires continued development of sophisticated pulsing techniques.

Applications of ^{13}C NMR to metabolic studies have recently been reviewed (Scott and Baxter, 1981). The low natural abundance and sensitivity (see Table 14.1) are severe limitations; however, natural abundance ^{13}C studies have been done on intact skeletal muscle (Fung, 1977; Doyle *et al.*, 1981) and rat heart (Bailey *et al.*, 1981). The heart spectra show resonances from fatty acyl esters and phospholipids. Natural abundance ^{13}C spectra have also been obtained from localized volumes of whole animals, including man (Alger *et al.*, 1981). These show the distribution of carbon in different types of fat, suggesting that the technique may be of use in studying disorders of fat metabolism.

^{13}C enrichment allows particular metabolic pathways to be followed. Shulman and coworkers (Ugurbil *et al.*, 1978) followed [^{13}C]glucose metabolism in *Escherichia coli*, and studied perfused mouse liver using [^{13}C]alanine and [^{13}C]ethanol (Cohen *et al.*, 1979). Recently, they have monitored the conversion of [1-^{13}C] glucose introduced into the stomach of a living rat to 1-^{13}C-labelled liver glycogen (Alger *et al.*, 1981). Bailey *et al.* (1981) studied rat heart metabolism using [^{13}C]acetate and concluded that this method can be used to investigate the rate of transport of reducing equivalents between mitochondria and cytosol. A major practical problem is that ^{13}C-labelled substrates are rather expensive.

The important possibility has also emerged of obtaining spectra from two (or perhaps more) nuclei in the same experiment, or even simultaneously, by using doubly tuned radiofrequency coils, or more than one coil. Styles *et al.* (1979) have studied red cell metabolism by obtaining ^{13}C and ^{31}P signals in alternate scans. In topical magnetic resonance studies (Edwards *et al.*, 1982) we have obtained ^1H and ^{13}C, or ^1H and ^{31}P, spectra using the same coil and are using the results from all three nuclei to obtain a quantitative estimate of muscle replacement by fatty-fibrous tissue in muscular diseases such as Duchenne dystrophy.

CONCLUSIONS

As a review of the NMR studies of cardiac metabolism, this chapter is complete at the time of writing, but no review of a rapidly growing subject can be up to date for long. I have tried to point out the extraordinary potential of NMR to contribute to our knowledge of cardiac metabolism and also to point out important sources of experimental artefact. The contributions of NMR to our knowledge of the heart and other tissues lag behind technical developments. This situation is inevitable given the rapid advances, and will be rectified when a larger number of competent physiologists and biochemists begin to regard NMR as one of the techniques available to them.

ACKNOWLEDGEMENTS

I wish to thank Dr P. Morris and Professor D. R. Wilkie for useful discussion, Mr K. J. Brooks and Mrs V. Vokes for assistance, and A. S. V. Burgin, C. J. Harbird, and P. Morris for permission to use their unpublished spectrum in Figure 14.1.

REFERENCES

Ackerman, J. J. H., Grove, T. H., Wong, G. G., Gadian, D. G., and Radda, G. K. (1980a). Mapping of metabolites in whole animals by ^{31}P NMR using surface coils. *Nature*, **283**, 167–170.

Ackerman, J. J. H., Bore, P. J., Gadian, D. G., Grove, T. H., and Radda, G. K. (1980b). N.m.r. studies of metabolism in perfused organs. *Phil. Trans. Roy. Soc. Lond. B*, **289**, 425–436.

Alger, J. R., Sillerud, L. O., Behar, K. L., Gillies, R. J., Shulman, R. G., Gordon, R. E., Shaw, D., and Hanley, P. E. (1981). In vivo carbon-13 nuclear magnetic resonance studies of mammals. *Science*, **214**, 660–662.

Allison, T. B., Ramey, C. A., and Holsinger, J. W., Jr (1978). Effects on labile metabolites of temporal delay in freezing biopsy samples of dog myocardium in liquid nitrogen. *Cardiovasc. Res.*, **12**, 162–166.

Bailey, I. A., and Seymour, A. M. (1981). The effect of reperfusion on the ^{31}P NMR spectrum of ischaemic rat hearts. *Biochem. Soc. Trans.*, **9**, 234–236.

Bailey, I. A., Gadian, D. G., Matthews, P. M., Radda, G. K., and Seeley, P. J. (1981). Studies of metabolism in the isolated, perfused rat heart using ^{13}C NMR. *FEBS Lett.*, **123**, 315–318.

Brinley, F. J., Jr, Scarpa, A., and Tiffert, T. (1977). The concentration of ionized magnesium in barnacle muscle fibres. *J. Physiol. (Lond.)*, **266**, 545–565.

Brown, F. F., and Campbell, I. D. (1980). N.m.r. studies of red cells. *Phil. Trans. Roy. Soc. Lond. B*, **289**, 395–406.

Brown, F. F., Campbell, I. D., Kuchel, P. W., and Rabenstein, D. C. (1977). Human erythrocyte metabolism studies by ^{1}H spin echo NMR. *FEBS Lett.*, **82**, 12–16.

Brown, T. R. (1980). Saturation transfer in living systems. *Phil. Trans. Roy. Soc. Lond. B*, **289**, 441–444.

Brown, T. R., Gadian, D. G., Garlick, P. B., Radda, G. K., Seeley, P. J., and Styles, P. (1978). Creatine kinase activities in skeletal and cardiac muscle measured by saturation transfer NMR. In *Frontiers of Biological Energetics: Electrons to Tissues*, Vol. 2 (L. Dutton, J. Leight, and A. Scarpa, eds), Academic Press, New York, pp. 1341–1349.

Burt, C. T., Glonek, T., and Bárány, M. (1976a). Analysis of phosphate metabolites, the intracellular pH and the state of adenosine triphosphate in intact muscle by phosphorus nuclear magnetic resonance. *J. Biol. Chem.*, **251**, 2584–2591.

Burt, C. T., Glonek, T., and Bárány, M. (1967b). Phosphorus-31 nuclear magnetic resonance detection of unexpected phosphodiesters in muscle. *Biochemistry*, **15**, 4850–4853.

Burt, C. T., Cohen, S. M., and Bárány, M. (1979). Analysis of intact tissue with ^{31}P NMR. *Annu. Rev. Biophys. Bioeng.*, **8**, 1–25.

Carlson, F. D., and Wilkie, D. R. (1974). *Muscle Physiology*, Prentice-Hall, Englewood Cliffs, N.J.

Chalovich, J. M., Burt, C. T., Cohen, S. M., Glonek, T., and Barany, M. (1977). Identification of an unknown ^{31}P nuclear magnetic resonance from dystrophic chicken as L-serine ethanolamine phosphodiester. *Arch. Biochem. Biophys.*, **182**, 683–689.

Chalovich, J. M., Burt, C. T., Danon, M. J., Glonek, T., and Barany, M. (1979). Phosphodiesters in muscular dystrophies. *Ann. N.Y. Acad. Sci.* **317**, 649–668.

Chance, B., Eleff, S., Leigh, J. S., Sokolow, D., and Sapega, A. (1981). Mitochondrial regulation of phosphocreatine inorganic phosphate ratios in exercising human muscle: a gated ^{31}P NMR study. *Proc. Natl Acad. Sci.* **78**, 6714–6718.

CIBA Foundation Symposium No. 82 (1981). *Human Muscle Fatigue: Physiological Mechanisms* (R. Porter and J. Whelan, eds), Pitman Medical, London.

Cohen, S. M., Shulman, R. G., and McLaughlin, A. C. (1979). Effects of ethanol on alanine metabolism in perfused mouse liver studied by ^{13}C NMR. *Proc. Natl Acad. Sci.*, **76**, 4808–12.

Cohen, S. M., and Burt, C. T. (1977). ^{31}P nuclear magnetic relaxation studies of phosphocreatine in intact muscle: determination of intracellular free magnesium. *Proc. Natl Acad. Sci.*, **74**, 4271–4275.

Cresshull, I. D., Gordon, R. E., Hanley, P. E., Shaw, D., Gadian, D. G., Radda, G. K., and Styles, P. (1981a). Localization of metabolites in animal and human tissues using ^{31}P topical magnetic resonance. *Bull. Mag. Reson.* **2**, 426.

Cresshull, I., Dawson, M. J., Edwards, R. H. T., Gadian, D. G., Gordon, R. E., Radda, G. K., Shaw, D., and Wilkie, D. R. (1981b). Human muscle analysed by ^{31}P nuclear magnetic resonance in intact subjects. *J. Physiol. (Lond.)*, **317**, 18P.

Dawson, M. J. (1982). Quantitative analysis of metabolite levels in normal subjects by ^{31}P topical magnetic resonance. *Bioscience Reports*, **2**, 727–733.

Dawson, M. J., Gadian, D. G., and Wilkie, D. R. (1976). Living muscle studied by ^{31}P nuclear magnetic resonance. *J. Physiol. (Lond.)*, **258**, 82–83P.

Dawson, M. J., Gadian, D. G., and Wilkie, D. R. (1977). Contraction and recovery of living muscle studied by ^{31}P nuclear magnetic resonance. *J. Physiol. (Lond.)*, **267**, 703–735.

Dawson, M. J., Gadian, D. G., and Wilkie, D. R. (1978). Muscular fatigue investigated by phosphorus nuclear magnetic resonance. *Nature*, **274**, 861–866.

Dawson, M. J., Gadian, D. G., and Wilkie, D. R. (1980). Mechanical relaxation rate and metabolism studied in fatiguing muscle by phosphorus nuclear magnetic resonance. *J. Physiol. (Lond.)*, **299**, 465–484.

Dhalla, N. S., Yates, J. C., Walz, D. A., McDonald, V. A., and Olson, R. E. (1972). Correlation between changes in the endogenous energy stores and myocardial function due to hypoxia in the isolated perfused rat heart. *Canad. J. Physiol. Pharmacol.*, **50**, 333–345.

Doyle, D. D., Chalovich, J. M., and Bárány, M. (1981). Natural abundance ^{13}C NMR spectra of intact muscle. *FEBS Lett.*, **131**, 147–150.

Drake, A. J. (1980). *The effect of intracellular pH, substrates and innervation on myocardial oxygen consumption and metabolism.* PhD thesis, London University.

Edwards, R. H. T., Dawson, M. J., Wilkie, D. R., Gordon, R. E., and Shaw, D. (1982). Clinical use of nuclear magnetic resonance in the investigation of myopathy. *Lancet, i*, 725–731.

Ellis, D., and Thomas, R. C. (1976). Direct measurement of the intracellular pH of mammalian cardiac muscle. *J. Physiol. (Lond.)*, **262**, 755–771.

Ferenczi, M. A., Homsher, E., Simmons, R. M., and Trentham, D. R. (1978). Reaction mechanism of the magnesium ion-dependent adenosine triphosphatase of frog muscle myosin and subfragment 1. *Biochem. J.*, **171**, 165–175.

Fossel, E. T., Morgan, H. E., and Ingwall, J. S. (1980). Measurement of changes in high energy phosphates in the cardiac cycle by using gated ^{31}P nuclear magnetic resonance. *Proc. Natl Acad. Sci.*, **77**, 3654–3658.

Fung, B. M. (1977). Carbon-13 and proton magnetic resonance of mouse muscle. *Biophys. J.*, **19**, 315–319.

Gadian, D. G. (1982). *Nuclear Magnetic Resonance and its Applications to Living Systems*, Clarendon Press, Oxford.

Gadian, D. G., and Radda, G. K. (1981). NMR studies of tissue metabolism. *Annu. Rev. Biochem.*, **50**, 69–83.

Gadian, D. G., Hoult, D. I., Radda, G. K., Seeley, P. J., Chance, B., and Barlow, C. (1976). Phosphorus nuclear magnetic resonance studies on normoxic and ischemic cardiac tissue. *Proc. Natl Acad. Sci.*, **73**, 4446–4448.

Gadian, D. G., Radda, G. K., Brown, T. R., Chance, E. M., Dawson, M. J., and Wilkie, D. R. (1981). The activity of creatine kinase in frog skeletal muscle studied by saturation-transfer nuclear magnetic resonance. *Biochem. J.*, **194**, 215–228.

Gadian, D. G., Radda, G. K., Dawson, M. J., and Wilkie, D. R. (1982). pH; measurements of cardiac and skeletal muscle using ^{31}P-NMR. in *Intracellular pH: Its Measurement, Regulation, and Utilization in Cellular Functions* (R. Nuccitelli and D. W. Deamer, eds), Alan R. Liss, New York, pp. 61–77.

Garlick, P. B., Radda, G. K., Seeley, P. J., and Chance, B. (1977). Phosphorus NMR studies on perfused heart. *Biochem. Biophys. Res. Commun.* **74**, 1256–1262.

Garlick, P. B., Radda, G. K. and Seeley, P. J. (1979). Studies of acidosis in the ischaemic heart by phosphorus nuclear magnetic resonance. *Biochem. J.*, **184**, 547–554.

Gibbs, C. L. (1978). Cardiac energetics. *Physiol. Rev.*, **58**, 174–254.

Gilbert, C., Kretschmar, K. M., Wilkie, D. R., and Woledge, R. C. (1971). Chemical change and energy output during muscular contraction. *J. Physiol. (Lond.)*, **218**, 163–193.

Gilbert, D. L. (1960). Magnesium equilibrium in muscle. *J. Gen. Physiol.*, **43**, 1103–1118.

Gordon, R. E., Hanley, P. E., Shaw, D., Gadian, D. G., Radda, G. K., Styles, P., Bore, P. J., and Chan, L. (1980). Localisation of metabolites in animals using ^{31}P topical magnetic resonance. *Nature*, **287**, 736–738.

Griffiths, J. R., and Iles, R. A. (1980). Nuclear magnetic resonance a 'magic eye' on metabolism. *Clin. Sci.*, **59**, 225–230.

Gudbjarnason, S., Mathes, P., and Ravens, K. G. (1970). Functional compartmentation of ATP and creatine phosphate in heart muscle. *J. Mol. Cell. Cardiol.* **1**, 325–339.

Gupta, R. K., and Moore, R. D. (1980). ^{31}P NMR studies of intracellular free Mg^{2+} in intact frog skeletal muscle. *J. Biol. Chem.*, **255**, 3987–3993.

Hess, P., and Weingart, R. (1981). Free magnesium in cardiac and skeletal muscle measured with ion-selective microelectrodes. *J. Physiol. (Lond.)*, **318**, 14P.

Hollis, D. P. (1979). Nuclear magnetic resonance studies of cancer and heart disease. *Bull. Magn. Reson.*, **1**, 27–37.

Hollis, D. P., Nunnally, R. L., Jacobs, W. E., and Taylor, G. J. (1977). Detection of regional ischemia in perfused beating hearts by phosphorus nuclear magnetic resonance. *Biochem. Biophys. Res. Commun.*, **75**, 1086–1091.

Hollis, D. P., Nunnally, R. L., Taylor, G. J., Weisfeldt, M. L., and Jacobus, W. E. (1978). Phosphorus nuclear magnetic resonance studies of heart physiology. *J. Magn. Reson.*, **29**, 319–330.

Hoult, D. I., Busby, S. J. W., Gadian, D. G., Radda, G. K., Richards, R. E. and Seeley, P. J. (1974). Observation of tissue metabolites using ^{31}P nuclear magnetic resonance. *Nature*, **252**, 285–287.

Huxley, T. H. (1885). Presidential address. *Proc. Roy. Soc., Lond.*, **39**, quotation from p. 294.

Jacobus, W. E., Taylor, G. J., Hollis, D. P., and Nunnally, R. L. (1977). Phosphorus nuclear magnetic resonance of perfused working rat hearts. *Nature*, **265**, 756–758.

Jacobus, W. E., Pores, I. H., Lucas, S. K., Kallman, C. H., Weisfeldt, M. L., and Flaherty, J. T. (1982). The role of intracellular pH in the control of normal and ischemic myocardial contractility: a ^{31}P nuclear magnetic resonance and mass spectrometry study. In *Intracellular pH: Its Measurement, Regulation, and Utilization in Cellular Functions* (R. Nuccitelli and D. W. Deamer, eds), Alan R. Liss, New York, pp. 537–566.

Kaufman, L., Crook., L. E., and Margulis, A. R. (eds) (1981). *Nuclear Magnetic Imaging in Medicine*, Igaku-Shoin, New York.

Kretzschmar, K. M. (1970). Energy production and chemical change during muscular contraction. PhD thesis, University of London, p. 216 and Table 3.

Kretzschmar, K. M., and Wilkie, D. R. (1969). A new approach to freezing tissues rapidly. *J. Physiol. (Lond.)*, **202**, 66–67P.

Kübler, W., and Katz, A. M. (1977). Mechanism of early 'pump' failure of the ischemic heart: possible role of adenosine triphosphate depletion and inorganic phosphate accumulation. *Amer. J. Cardiology*, **40**, 467–471.

Mansfield, P., and Morris, P. (1982). NMR imaging in biomedicine. *Advanc. Magn. Reson.*, Suppl. 2.

Matthews, P. M., Radda, G. K., and Taylor, D. J. (1981b). A ^{31}P n.m.r. study of metabolism in the hypoxic perfused rat heart. *Biochem. Soc. Trans.*, **9**, 236–237.

Matthews, P. M., Bland, J. L., Gadian, D. G., and Radda, G. K. (1981a). The steady-state rate of ATP synthesis in the perfused rat heart measured by ^{31}P NMR saturation transfer. *Biochem. Biophys. Res. Commun.*, **103**, 1052–1059.

Matthews, P. M., Williams, S. R., Seymour, A. M., Schwartz, A., Dube, G., Gadian, D. G., and Radda, G. K. (1982). A ^{31}P NMR study of some metabolic and functional effects of the inotropic agents epinephrine and ouabain, and the ionophore RO2-2985 (X537A) in the isolated, perfused rat heart. *Biochim. Biophys. Acta*, **721**, 312–317.

Nunnally, R. L., and Bottomley, P. A. (1981). Assessment of pharmacological treatment of myocardial infarction by phosphorus-31 NMR with surface coils. *Science*, **211**, 177–180.

Nunnally, R. L., and Hollis, D. P. (1979). Adenosine triphosphate compartmentation in living hearts: a phosphorus nuclear magnetic resonance saturation transfer study. *Biochemistry*, **18**, 3642–3646.

Poole-Wilson, P. A. (1978). Measurement of myocardial intracellular pH in pathological states. *J. Mol. Cell. Cardiol.*, **10**, 511–526.

Radda, G. K., and Seeley, P. J. (1979). Recent studies on cellular metabolism by nuclear magnetic resonance. *Annu. Rev. Physiol.*, **41**, 749–769.

Salhany, J. M., Pieper, G. M., Wu, S., Todd, G. L., Clayton, F. C., and Eliot, R. S. (1979). ^{31}P nuclear magnetic resonance measurement of cardiac pH in perfused guinea-pig hearts. *J. Mol. Cell. Cardiol.*, **11**, 601–610.

Scholte, H. R. (1973). On the triple localization of creatine kinase in heart and skeletal muscle cells of the rat: evidence for the existence of myofibrillar and mitochondrial isoenzymes. *Biochem. Biophys. Acta*, **305**, 413–427.

Scott, A. I., and Baxter, R. L. (1981). Applications of ^{13}C NMR to metabolic studies. *Annu. Rev. Biophys. Bioeng.*, **10**, 151–174.

Shaw, D. (1981). *In vivo* biochemistry. In *Nuclear Magnetic Resonance Imaging in Medicine* (L. Kaufman, L. E. Crooks, and A. R. Margulis, eds), Igaku-Shoin Medical Publishers, New York, pp. 147–183.

Singer, J. R. (1981). Blood flow measurements by NMR. In *Nuclear Magnetic Resonance Imaging in Medicine* (L. Kaufman, L. E. Crooks, and A. R. Margulis, eds), Igaku-Shoin Medical Publishers, New York, pp. 128–144.

Steenbergen, C., Deleeuw, G., Rich, T., and Williamson, J. R. (1977). Effects of acidosis and ischemia on contractility and intracellular pH of rat heart. *Circulation Res.*, **41**, 849–858.

Styles, P., Grathwohl, C., and Brown, F. F. (1979). Simultaneous multinuclear NMR by alternate scan recording of ^{31}P and ^{13}C spectra. *J. Magn. Reson.*, **35**, 329–336.

Ugurbil, K., Brown, T. R., Den Hollander, J. A., Glynn, P., and Shulman, R. G. (1978). High-resolution ^{13}C nuclear magnetic resonance studies of glucose metabolism in *Escherichia coli. Proc. Natl Acad. Sci.*, **75**, 3742–3746.

Veech, R. L., Lawson, J. W. R., Cornell, N. W., and Krebs, H. A. (1979). Cytosolic phosphorylation potential. *J. Biol. Chem.*, **254**, 6538–6547.

Wilkie, D. R. (1981a). Shortage of chemical fuel as a cause of fatigue: studies by nuclear magnetic resonance and bicycle ergometry. In *Human Muscle Fatigue: Physiological Mechanisms* (CIBA Foundation Symposium No. 82), Pitman Medical, London, pp. 102–119.

Wilkie, D. R. (1981b). The enzymes of glycolysis: structure, activity and evolution. Discussion at Royal Society Meeting. *Phil. Trans. R. Soc. Lond. B., Lond.*, **293**, 40–41.

Wilkie, D. R., Dawson, M. J. Edwards, R. H. T., Gordon, R. E., and Shaw, D. (1983). ^{31}P NMR studies of resting muscle in normal human subjects, in *Contractile Mechanisms in Muscle. Vol II, Mechanics, Energetics and Molecular Models*, Ed. Pollack, G. H. and Sugi, H.

Cardiac Metabolism
Edited by A. J. Drake-Holland and M. I. M. Noble
© 1983 John Wiley & Sons Ltd

CHAPTER 15

Contractile and Regulatory Proteins

R. Zak

Section of Cardiology, Department of Medicine, and Department of Pharmacological and Physiological Sciences

and

S. S. Galhotra

Physical Sciences Collegiate Division, The University of Chicago, Chicago, Illinois 60637, USA

INTRODUCTION

The contractile apparatus of the heart, as of other cross-striated muscles, consists of three classes of proteins: (1) contractile proteins – myosin and actin; (2) regulatory proteins – tropomyosin and troponin; (3) structural proteins – alpha-actinin, C-protein, M-protein, etc.

The term 'contractile' indicates that a process equivalent to muscle shortening, e.g. syneresis of actomyosin gel after addition of ATP, can be demonstrated when myosin and actin are present alone. However, without other proteins the interaction between myosin and actin cannot be regulated: once 'shortening' has been initiated by the addition of ATP, it proceeds until the ATP is depleted.

To regulate the interaction between the two contractile proteins, tropomyosin and troponin are required. A mixture of contractile and regulatory proteins mimics the behaviour of muscle cells, or their fragments, in that the rate of ATP hydrolysis is regulated by calcium. When the calcium ion concentration is high (10^{-4} M), ATP hydrolysis is increased ('shortening'); when it is low (10^{-8} M), ATP hydrolysis is inhibited ('relaxation').

Proteins of the third class form the structural components of the contractile apparatus. For example, α-actinin is believed to be part of the network which anchors thin filaments to the Z-line.

Within the muscle cell, proteins of the three classes constitute myofibrils. However, the term 'myofibril' has a somewhat different meaning in the case of the heart than in the case of fast, glycolytic, skeletal muscles. In the latter

339

Table 15.1   Protein composition of the rat left ventricle

Protein	Protein (mg) per gram wet weight
Total protein	150
Myofibrils†	87
Sarcoplasmic proteins‡	35
Myosin§	27

† Crude fraction containing nuclei, some membrane fragments, and cell debris.
‡ 100 000**g** supernatant fraction.
§ Determined by competitive radioimmunoassay and by isotope dilution methods (Everett *et al.*, 1982).

case, myofibrils are seen within the cytoplasm as discrete organelles. Although in the heart the double hexagonal mass of filaments forms a continuum within which nuclei, mitochondria, sarcoplasmic reticuli, and other organelles are interspersed, 'myofibrils' can nevertheless be isolated and purified by differential centrifugation.

Myofibrillar proteins contribute about 50% to the total protein mass of the heart, while mitochondrial proteins contribute 15%, and sarcoplasmic proteins contribute 25% (Table 15.1). Contractile proteins are the major constituents of myofibrils, with myosin making up 60%, and actin 15%, of myofibrillar mass. Regulatory proteins are next in abundance, with tropomyosin making up 10% and troponin 5%. Structural proteins contribute less than 10% to the myofibrillar mass. These estimates are crude, with the exception of those for total proteins, contractile proteins, and sarcoplasmic proteins, which can be measured with acceptable accuracy.

The pathways of ATP hydrolysis and the response of regulatory proteins to calcium are similar between muscles. However, the maximum speed of shortening and the corresponding myofibrillar ATPase activity vary widely between different muscles of the same individual, as well as between the same muscles of different animal species. This is true for both the heart and skeletal muscles because as a consequence of slight amino acid differences, termed microheterogeneity, the rate of biological activity of each member of a protein family differs from that of other members; this gives rise to the terms 'isozyme', 'isoprotein', 'isoform', 'isomysin' etc. The fraction of the protein family mass that each isoprotein makes up is not static, but changes with development and with the functional or hormonal state of the animal. For example, administration of thyroid hormone results in a marked change in the ratio of one ventricular isomyosin to another, due to reciprocal changes in their rates of synthesis. Analysis of unfractionated myosin, therefore, can be misleading or of limited value at best. The availability of isoproteins of cardiac proteins should eventually allow the preparation of probes for transcription of specific genes regulating the study of cardiac growth. More details concerning mixed proteins (i.e. myosin rather than isomyosin) can be found in an excellent review by Katz (1970).

STRUCTURE AND FUNCTION OF CONTRACTILE PROTEINS

Myosin

Prototype molecule

Myosin is one of the largest proteins known, having a molecular weight of 500 000 daltons. The typical molecule of myosin consists of two classes of subunits held together by non-covalent forces: heavy chains, HC (MW 200 000 daltons) and light chains, LC (MW 15 000–27 000 daltons). Each myosin molecule is a dimer of heavy chains, with dissimilar light chains attached to each of them. One of the light chains is found in every myosin molecule and undergoes a cycle of phosphorylation–dephosphorylation catalysed by specific light chain kinases and phosphatases. This light chain is called regulatory or LC-P. The second light chain varies depending on the type of myosin. Thus the general formula for myosin is

$$(HC)_2 \Big\langle {(LC\text{-}P)_2 \atop (LC\text{-}u)_2}$$

From its physicochemical properties (Lowey *et al.*, 1969) and from visualization by electron microscopy (Huxley, 1963), the myosin molecule is known to be highly asymmetrical, containing dissimilar domains. Its dimensions of $160\,nm \times 2.4\,nm$ give it a high axial ratio which is typical of fibrous proteins. However, the entire molecule is not rod-like, as the high axial ratio may suggest: at the N-terminus the heavy chain folds into a globular head, while at the C-terminus it is mostly an α-helix. So, the molecule is a 'Y' in which each 'arm' is the globular head of a heavy chain to which two light chains are non-covalently bound, and the 'trunk' is the interwined α-helical regions of the two heavy chains (Figure 15.1).

By selective and limited proteolytic attack, the molecule can be cleaved into several fragments (Figure 15.1) each having different properties (Table 15.2). The head, also called subfragment 1 (S-1), has low α-helical content, is soluble in solutions of low ionic strength, has ATPase activity, binds actin, and is the cross-bridge which propels the thin filament when the sarcomere shortens.

Adjacent to S-1 is subfragment 2 (S-2) which is highly α-helical, but, like S-1, is soluble at low ionic strength. This part of the molecule provides the point of flexibility which allows the head, the cross-bridge, to project out

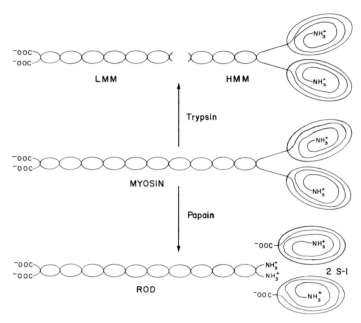

Figure 15.1 Scheme of myosin molecule and its fragmentation by proteolytic enzymes. LMM, light meromyosin; HMM, heavy meromyosin; S-1, subfragment 1. The light chains have been omitted for simplicity

Table 15.2

	Schematic of electron micrograph	MW (kilodaltons)	Length (nm)	α-Helix content (%)	No. amino acids
Myosin		500	140		1650
HMM		340	50	46	1200
LMM		150	90	90	450
Rod		220	130	94	900
S-1		110	10	33	750
S-2		60	40	87	400

This table is based on data of Huxley (1963) and Lowey *et al.* (1969). The approximate number of amino acids per polypeptide is based on a private communication from M. Elzinga.

from the long axis of the thick filament. For this reason, S-2 is also called the 'neck'.

The filamentous tail region of the myosin molecule, called light meromyosin (LMM), is highly α-helical and aggregates at ionic strengths like those found inside the muscle cell. Due to its tendency to aggregate, this portion of the molecule is responsible for the association of myosin molecules into the superstructure which is the thick filament. Due to the properties of the myosin molecule's α-helical coiled-coil portion, the thick filament acquires the rigidity required by the sliding filament theory.

By modifying the protocol for proteolytic digestion, one can also obtain larger fragments, mainly heavy meromyosin (HMM) which corresponds to S-1 plus S-2, and the rod which corresponds to LMM plus S-2, i.e. the entire α-helical coiled-coil portion.

The analysis of myosin properties at the level of the amino acid sequence is just beginning. Due to its large size (the heavy chain contains about 1600 amino acid residues) the sequence analysis is laborious and completed only for segments of the molecule. The active centre of myosin ATPase is thought to be localized in the N-terminal 25 000 dalton peptide of the heavy chain, i.e. in the head region, and has a complex tertiary structure (Chantler, 1980). The binding of the ATP occurs near an arginine residue. Also, two sulphydryl groups of cysteine residues, called SH-1 and SH-2 are intimately involved in ATP hydrolysis although they are far removed from the active site in sequence (perhaps the active site is folded back in the polypeptide).

The actin interaction with myosin takes place at the myosin head which also contains the active centre of ATPase. Inhibitors of ATPase bind to the enzymatic site without detaching actin (Marston *et al.*, 1979). Nevertheless, there is a co-operativity between the two domains of S-1 since nucleotide binding influences actin myosin interaction.

The third, not entirely understood property of myosin is the self-aggregation of individual molecules in a highly ordered fashion. The molecules assemble in pairs along the long axis of the aggregate, one on each side of the thick filament. Successive pairs are displaced by exactly 14.3 nm and are rotated relative to each other by 120°. The tails of adjacent molecules, more specifically the LMM regions, overlap each other for a distance of about 70 nm (Figure 15.2). To explain the aggregation properties of myosin, spatial models of α-helical coiled coils have been generated using the amino acid sequence determined for a segment of the myosin rod. These models support the views that the 14.3 nm spacing is due to the variation in the pitch of the coiled coil, and its stability is due to electrostatic interactions between clusters of opposite acidic and basic side chains (Elzinga and Trus, 1980).

It is not known why the aggregate of myosin molecules reverses its polarity in the middle of the thick filament (the 'bare' zone). This results in

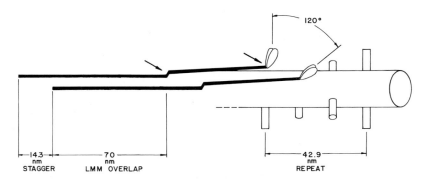

Figure 15.2 Arrangement of myosin molecules in the thick filament. Detail of the association between two myosin molecules is shown on the left. A helical array of cross-bridge pairs (schematized as cylinders) projecting from the thick filament is drawn on the right

the filament being bipolar with myosin molecules in an anti-parallel arrangement at both ends. This puzzling self-assembly process will be explained, perhaps, when more complete sequence data become available and are analysed. Rowe (1982) explains it on the basis of myosin assembling inwards from the two half-sarcomeres.

The role of the light chains in myosin function is as yet unclear, they can be divided into classes: regulatory and essential. The terminology, however, is neither universally accepted nor does it accurately reflect the function of various light chains. To avoid any confusion, the synonyms frequently used in the literature are listed in Table 15.3.

All light chains are globular proteins, as can be predicted from their α-helix content, which can be 30–40%. Their amino acid sequences suggest definite similarity. These two light chains have (137) identical residues at the C-terminal end (Frank and Weeds, 1974). The two proteins differ in that the larger light chain has 41 more residues at the N-terminal end and that

Table 15.3 Synonyms used for myosin light chains

Used in this chapter	Synonyma
LC-1	Essential LC, A-1
LC-2	Regulatory LC, LC-P, DTNB, Nbs$_2$
LC-3	Essential LC, A-2

The DTNB, Nbs$_2$, A-1, and A-2 is used for fast muscles only. P stands for 'phosphorylated'; DNTB and Nbs$_2$ stand for sulphydryl group reagent 5,5′-dithiobis(2-nitrobenzoic acid).

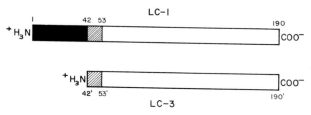

Figure 15.3 Scheme of amino acid sequences of alkali light chains. □, Invariable region; ▨, variable region; ■, Δ peptide. [Redrawn from Frank and Weeds (1974).]

adjacent to the difference peptide is a short, highly variable region in which five out of eight amino acids differ when compared to the corresponding N-terminal end of the smaller light chain (Figure 15.3).

The regulatory chains appear to have sequence homology, although limited, with both the Δ peptide and the common C-terminal portion of the essential light chains. Consequently, LC-2 shows immunological cross-reactivity with both LC-1 and LC-3, but the similarity with the Δ peptide is especially striking (Holt and Lowey, 1977). Phosphorylation of the light chains is discused by England (Chapter 16 in this volume).

The second class of light chains can be removed from intact myosin by a variety of denaturing procedures, including exposure to alkaline pH. For this reason, these chains in fast muscles, where this observation was made first, are referred to by some as alkaline light chains, A-1 and A-2. Hybridization of heavy chains with heterologous light chains does not have any effect on the resulting ATPase activity (Wagner 1981). In another experiment, light chains were removed under non-denaturing conditions; no change in ATP-ase activity occurred. The term 'essential', thus, is a misnomer. The heavy chains appear to be the sole determinant of myosin ATPase activity and at present we do not know what the function of 'essential' light chain is.

Isomyosins

Refined methods have revealed that myosin does not exist as the single prototype molecule described above. Rather, both the heavy and light chains exhibit polymorphism and at the time of writing 10 molecular variants of myosin have been identified in cross-striated muscles.

Two classes of myosin have been detected: one present in fast muscles, the other in slow and cardiac muscles. The ATPase activities of these myosins differ as evidenced by differences in their V_{max}, pH curve of inactivation, and the pattern of activation by sulphydryl reagents. Moreover, the two classes of myosin exhibit different rates of proteolytic cleavage into heavy and light meromyosins and also in the staining pattern of light meromyosin paracrystals (see Syrovy, 1979), suggesting that the primary structures of myosins are responsible for the observed differences. An example of this is that two 3-methylhistidine residues localized in subfragment 1 were found to be present in myosin of fast muscles but absent in slow and cardiac muscles (Huszar and Elzinga, 1972).

The amino acid sequence of the entire myosin heavy chain has not yet been reported for any species. Numerous studies of peptide fragments produced by proteolytic (Whalen *et al.*, 1979) and CNBr cleavage (Leger *et al.*, 1979) clearly demonstrate, however, that there are not merely two classes of myosin. Rather, *fast, slow,* and *cardiac* myosins are all different molecules, although the peptide maps of slow and cardiac myosins are quite similar. This interpretation of peptide maps is in agreement with sequence analysis of sulphydryl groups containing peptide produced by CNBr cleavage of subfragment 1 (Flink *et al.*, 1977). The determination of amino acid sequence is by far the most conclusive evidence for *fast, slow,* and *cardiac* myosins being products of three different genes.

The second line of evidence for the existence of multiple forms of myosin came from the analysis of their light chains. Electrophoresis of myosin on polyacrylamide gels in the presence of sodium dodecylsulphate revealed that the light chains of myosin obtained from *fast, slow,* and *cardiac* muscles are all different polypeptides (Sarkar *et al.*, 1971). Thus, there are three regulatory chains characteristic of a given type of muscle. In addition, myosins of fast and slow muscles contain two essential light chains each, while the cardiac myosin contains only one. This gives a total of five essential light chains (Figure 15.4).

Due to the low molecular weight of light chains their sequence analysis is

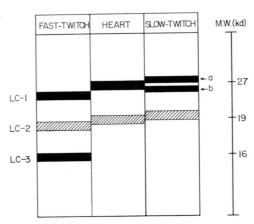

Figure 15.4 Schematic drawing of myosin light chains displayed by electrophoresis in the presence of sodium dodecylsulphate. [After Weeds (1976).]

Table 15.4 Some properties of myosin light chains

| | | Skeletal muscle | | |
| | Fast | Slow | | |
Class of light chain		LC-1a	LC-1b	Heart
LC-1	→ SH, Δ	SH, Δ	SH, Δ ⟷ SH, Δ	
LC-2	⌐ SH	No SH ⟷ No SH		
LC-3	∟→ SH	—		—

SH, contain sulphydryl group(s); Δ, difference peptide present; —, chain absent. The arrows indicate substantial homology.

more advanced than that of heavy chains. There are two distinct polypeptides in fast and slow twitch muscles which were previously indicated by the analysis of their relative electrophoretic mobilities (Weeds, 1976). Furthermore, in all three types of muscle the essential light chains contain sulphydryl groups and the LC-1 chains also contain the proline-rich difference peptide mentioned in the description of prototype myosin (Table 15.4), (e.g., Weeds, 1976). The regulatory chains of slow and cardiac muscles both lack sulphydryl groups. This contrasts with LC-2 from fast muscles in which sulphydryl groups are present (Weeds, 1976).

A new insight into myosin polymorphism was gained when electrophoresis under non-denaturing conditions was developed (d'Albis and Gratzer, 1973; Hoh *et al.*, 1976). Using non-denaturing electrophoresis of intact myosins, the three classes of myosin mentioned so far have been resolved into additional variants. Thus three isomyosins were detected in fast muscles, and two in slow muscles. Moreover, cardiac myosin has been resolved into two atrial isomyosins and one to three (depending on the animal species and age) ventricular isomyosins.

Pyrophosphate gel electrophoresis has not only detected new, as yet unresolved isomyosins, but has also eluciated the puzzling stoicheiometry of myosin subunits, especially in the case of fast muscles. Three light chains have been detected not only in myosin of entire muscles but also in individual fibres where the possibility of contamination due to multiple fibre types is eliminated (Pette and Schnez, 1977). Furthermore, the quantitation of light chains indicated that LC-1 and LC-3 chains are present in non-equimolar amounts with about twice as much of LC-1 as LC-3 (Lowey and Risby, 1971). The electrophoretic analysis of native myosin gave full support to the existence of multiple forms of myosin in fast muscle. In addition to the two variants mentioned above, a third species of myosin has been detected, and apparently contains both alkali light chains (d'Albis *et al.*, 1979).

For the heavy chains, the situation is somewhat less clear. Analysis of the N-terminal peptide produced by chymotryptic digestion of heavy chains

Table 15.5   Isomyosins of adult skeletal and cardiac muscles

Muscle	Myosin	HC	LC-1		LC-2	LC-3
Skeletal						
Fast	FM-1	f	f		f	—
	FM-2	f	f		f	f
	FM-3	f†	—		f	f
Slow			LC-1a LC-1b‡			
	SM-1	s	s —		s	—
	SM-2	s	— s		s	—
Heart						
Ventricle	VM-1	α	v		h	—
	VM-2	αβ	v		h	—
	VM-3	β	v		h	—
Atria	AM-1	α	a		h(?)	—
	AM-2	α	a′		h(?)	—

† Some fast muscles contain two classes of HCs.
‡ The light chain doublet is not present in all slow muscles.
The lower case letters indicate that the protein is specific for the following muscles: a = atria; f = fast; h = heart; s = slow; v = ventricle.

detected the presence of two amino acids at the same position. These two amino acids were present in the same ratio as were the LC-1 and LC-3 chains (Starr and Offer, 1973). It is conceivable that, as in some fast muscles, the heavy chains also exist in multiple forms. But, there is no further proof for this hypothesis yet.

In the heart, the family of myosins appears to be as complex as in the skeletal muscles, despite electrical coupling between individual cardiac cells. It has been known for some time that the myocardia of different animal species differ in their shortening velocities and the properties of their myosin ATPase. In general, the smaller the animal, the higher the myosin ATPase activity. Moreover, in animals of similar size the ATPase activity is higher in those whose survival requires sustained exertion rather than short bursts of activity (Schwarz *et al.*, 1981).

Most recently, it was shown that cardiac myosin differs not only between various animals but that in the same heart myosin exists in multiple molecular forms. Both atria and venticles contain distinct sets of isomyosin which differ in their ATPase activity, class of light chains, and primary structure of heavy chains.

In the ventricle multiple molecular forms of myosin have been identified by native gel electrophoresis in some species, namely rabbit and rat (Hoh *et al.*, 1978; Lompre *et al.*, 1981), while in other species such as guinea-pig, dog, and man only one band of myosin can be resolved by using this procedure (Clark *et al.*, 1982). Based on its electrophoretic behaviour, the variant having relatively high mobility is classified as VM-1 (also called V-1 by others) isomyosin, while the intermediate and low mobility isomyosins are referred to as VM-2 and VM-3 respectively. The ATPase activity of VM-1 isomyosin is about three times higher than that of VM-3; VM-2 appears to have activity which is in between these two.

Classification of myosins in animals whose ventricles yield only one band upon electrophoresis is difficult, since the procedure depends on the determination of relative electrophoretic mobilities of individual isomyosins. As can be seen in Figure 15.5, the electrophoretic mobility, reflecting the endogeneous charge of myosin at alkaline pH, differs between animals. Consequently, different isomyosins in the ventricles of different animals might have similar mobilities (compare VM-1 of rabbit with VM-3 of the rat). Thus, while electrophoretic analysis is a useful tool for classification of myosin in some species, it has to be supplemented by additional procedures for other species. In such cases, differences between myosin heavy chains can be detected by analysing the peptide produced either by CNBr or by proteolytic fragmentation and by immunochemical characterization. By these procedures, for example, ventricular myosins of guinea-pig and pig were identified as VM-1 and VM-3 despite identical electrophoretical mobilities (Clark *et al.*, 1982).

The observed differences in antigenic structure and proteolytic fragments displayed by isomyosins are probably a consequence of difference in amino

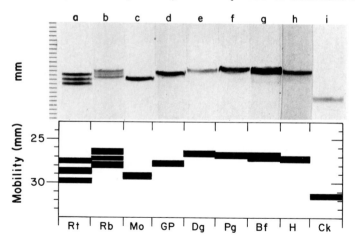

Figure 15.5 Pattern of ventricular isomyosins separated by electrophoresis under non-denaturing conditions. Rt, rat; Rb, rabbit; Mo, mouse; GP, guinea-pig; Dg, dog; Pg, pig; Bf, cattle; H, human; Ck, chicken. [Reproduced with permission from W. A. Clark, R. A. Chizzonite, A. W. Everett, M. Rabinowitz, and R. Zak, *J. Biol. Chem.*, **257**, 5449–5454 (1982).]

acid sequence and not a result of post-translational modification. No difference in the degree of phosphorylation or methylation – the only two known
post-translational modifications – has been detected in the myosin heavy
chains (Banerjee *et al.*, 1976).

The molecular diversity of ventricular myosin appears to reside in the
heavy chains, which are of two types, HC-α and HC-β, associated with
VM-1 and VM-3, respectively (Hoh *et al.*, 1978; Chizzonite *et al.*, 1982).
These two heavy chains differ in their peptide maps, and in several antigenic
determinants in both the LMM and HMM parts of the molecule. The amino
acid sequence analysis of the long peptide localized in the S-2 segment
shows 15% divergence. Clearly, HC-α and HC-β are products of different
genes.

In contrast, the sets of light chains associated with VM-1 and VM-3 are
identical as far as electrophoretic properties are concerned, based on both
molecular size and electric charge (Banerjee *et al.*, 1976). Ventricular
myosin thus differs from skeletal myosin in that the heavy chains rather than
the light chains are responsible for myosin multiplicity. With identical light
chains and two dissimilar heavy chains one can postulate the existence of
three distinct molecules: two homodimers, $(HC-α)_2$ and $(HC-β)_2$, and one
heterodimer (HC-α–HC-β), as suggested by the fact that both the relative
mobility on pyrophosphate gels and the ATPase activity of VM-2 is in
between that of VM-1 and VM-3 (Hoh *et al.*, 1978). Immunoaffinity studies
using monoclonal antibodies specific for either HC-α or HC-β (Everett *et
al.*, 1982) showed that when a preparation of ventricular myosin containing
all three isomyosins is passed through a column of immobilized antibody
specific for HC-α, both VM-1 and VM-2 were absorbed, while VM-3 passed
through freely. The column of HC-β antibody as immunoabsorbent removed VM-3 and VM-2, but not VM-1. These data are consistent with the
presence of both α and β heavy chains in VM-2.

Multiple forms of myosin have been detected not only in ventricles but
also in atria. It has been known for some time that the properties of myosin
ATPase in the two chambers of the heart differ (Syrovy *et al.*, 1979). Similar
to the rate of tension development, the ATPase activity of myosin in the atria
is about twice that in the ventricles (Long *et al.*, 1977; Yazaki *et al.*, 1979).
The affect of alkaline pH and of sulphydryl blocking agents is also different
(Yazaki *et al.*, 1979). It is of interest that in these two properties atrial myosin
resembles that of fast skeletal muscle. This is especially striking as far as the
effects of pH are concerned: atrial and fast muscle myosin both resist
inactivation at pH 9, while ventricular and slow muscle myosins rapidly lose
their activity.

Atrial and ventricular myosins also differ in their light chains (Wikman-
Coffelt and Srivastava, 1979). As in skeletal muscles, however, the light
chains do not exert any noticeable effect on myosin ATPase (Hollosi *et al.*,
1980) and their function still remains to be elucidated.

Within atria themselves, two isomyosins have been detected by electrophoresis under non-denaturing conditions. Their heavy chains are not distinguishable from those of ventricular HC-α. This has been shown by peptide mapping and analysis of antigenic properties (Libera and Sartore, 1981; Everett *et al.*, 1982). Moreover, when the light chains of atria were exchanged with those of ventricular myosin, the electrophoretic mobility of the hybrid atrial myosin became identical with that of VM-1, indicating that the electrical charge of atrial heavy chains is the same as that of ventricular HC-α.

Actin

In comparison to myosin, less is known about the properties of actin and of the regulatory proteins. This is especially true for their molecular variants.

Prototype molecule

Both myosin and actin are parts of highly asymmetrical filaments present in motile cells. However, at the molecular level, the building blocks of these filaments are vastly different (Taylor, 1972). While myosin (present in thick filaments) is a large asymmetrical molecule, actin (present in the thin filaments) is a globular protein of slightly ovoid shape with an axial ratio of about 1:2. Actin has a relatively low molecular weight of about 45 000 daltons. Actin is known to exist in two forms: monomeric, which is referred to as G-actin (G for globular), and polymerized, which is called F-actin (F for fibrous). In the muscle cell, however, all the actin exists only in the F form. In contrast, purified actin can readily be interconverted between the F and G forms. The polymerization of G-actin can be induced by adding salt solutions of physiological concentrations, while their removal by dialysis, on the other hand, results in F-actin depolymerization. Each monomer of F-actin contains one molecule of ADP and calcium, which, together with several SH groups, serves to maintain its proper molecular conformation. Neither the bound nucleotide, nor the cation can be exchanged with free molecules in solution. When F-actin becomes depolymerized, however, this steric hinderance is lost and both ADP and calcium become readily exchangeable. It is of interest that, when G-actin is prepared in a solution containing ADP, its terminal phosphate undergoes hydrolysis during polymerization. This phenomenon, however, has no bearing on muscle contraction or on the polymerization itself. Both relaxed and stimulated muscles contain actin exclusively in the F form and polymerization can be induced even with nucleotide-free actin, although the protein is prone to denaturation.

The structural features of F-actin, as well as the thin filament, are similar. Each is composed of two strands of G-actin wound around each other to form a double helical filament. The pitch of the helix is 38.5 nm and there are seven actins per turn. Besides being the structural component of the sarcomere, actin serves two important functions in muscle contraction:

(1) Actin dramatically increases the activity of myosin ATPase. At rest, the rate of ATP hydrolysis is very low, while stimulation of a muscle results in a several thousandfold activation of the ATPase (Barany and Burt, 1979). *In vitro*, for example, when actin is added to myosin in a solution of physiological ionic strength, in the presence of magnesium, such large activation had not been achieved until recently when S-1 and F-actin were covalently cross-linked (Mornet *et al.*, 1981). Under these conditions the myosin head enters into van der Waals contacts with neighbouring actins.

Interaction of actin with myosin (Marston and Taylor, 1980), causes a large decrease in the free energy of ATP binding and a release of one of the hydrolysis products, the inorganic phospate, takes place upon attachment of actin to the myosin head.

(2) Actin interacts with myosin allowing propulsion of the thin filament along the length of the stationary thick filament. Each actin monomer appears to have two myosin binding sites (Mornet *et al.*, 1981). The sites are localized in different domains of the molecule and each domain is specific for different portions of the myosin head. Consequently, each actin monomer interacts with two heads and each myosin head with two actin monomers (Figure 15.6).

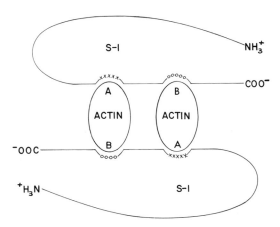

Figure 15.6 Scheme depicting actin binding to myosin head (S-1). The two G-actins represent two strands of the F-actin filament. Note the reversed polarity of the two binding sites. [After Mornet *et al.* (1981).]

The chemical nature of the actin–myosin interaction is not known, but the dependence on ionic strength, as well as the analysis of the product between S-1 and F-actin, suggests that electrostatic interactions betwen ionic pairs take place at the recognition sites of these two proteins (Mornet *et al.*, 1981). Possibly, a carboxyl group on the actin site comes into contact with a nucleophilic group on the myosin site, such as an amino group.

Isoactins

Actin is an ubiquitous cellular protein with a remarkably high degree of evolutionary conservation. With respect to a variety of properties such as molecular weight, kinetics of polymerization, activation of myosin ATPase, and binding to HMM, only minor, if any, differences have been found between actins isolated from different types of cells or from muscles of different animal species. Analyses of peptide maps and of amino acid sequences demonstrate that actin of various sources are indeed very similar in primary structure, but are not identical (Garrels and Gibson, 1976; Vanderkerchkove and Weber, 1978). The amino acid subsitution between actins is reflected in the electric charge which allows the resolution of three broad groups of actins on isofocusing gels (Garrels and Gibson, 1976; Whalen *et al.*, 1976). In order of decreasing isoelectric points, the actin classes are labelled as α, β, and γ. The α isoactins are typical of muscle cells while the β and γ forms are present in various cytoplasmic systems. Within α isoactins at least two variants are known: skeletal and cardiac (Elzinga and Lu, 1976). These two isoactins show only minor divergence in amino acid sequence which, nevertheless, is reflected in their antigenic properties (Morgan *et al.*, 1980).

In contrast to myosin, there is no significant divergence in biological activity of isoactins. Yet, the microheterogeneity in their primary structure clearly indicates that the members of the actin family are products of different genes.

STRUCTURE AND FUNCTION OF REGULATORY PROTEINS

Tropomyosin

Tropomyosin is thought to move from a position which blocks the interaction of actin with myosin. The unblocked actin then activates myosin ATPase and initiates contraction. However, it must be noted that this model is not universally accepted (see Perry, 1977).

Tropomyosin prototype molecule

Tropomyosin is a unique protein in the sense that it is completely helical. It is a dimer of α-helical polypeptides wound around each other forming a two-stranded coiled coil with molecular weight of about 65 000 daltons and length of 40 nm (Taylor, 1972). Tropomyosin is part of the thin filament where it lies in the groove created by the two strands of the actin helix. The tropomysin molecules are bonded head to tail, thus forming a long cable which spans the entire length of the thin filament.

The effect of troponin is highly amplified when tropomyosin is also present: tropomyosin extends the effect of troponin so that one molecule of troponin can influence more than one molecule of actin. This is rather important since it is known that during contraction all actins are unblocked. Troponin however, is localized along the thin filament with a periodicity of about 40 nm, which leaves seven actin monomers for each troponin complex. From this stoicheiometry it is clear that in the absence of tropomyosin full activation of actomyosin ATPase in the presence of calcium cannot occur.

Isotropomyosins

Two classes of tropomyosin subunits have been identified and isolated from cross-striated muscles which show heterogeneity in primary structure and consequently in charge distribution and antigenic properties (Cummins and Perry, 1973; Johnson, 1974). One class, labelled as α-tropomyosin, contains one sulphydryl group, while the β class contains two. Since tropomyosin is a dimer, it is conceivable that three isotropomyosins exist: α_2, β_2, and $\alpha\beta$. The evidence for homodimers is twofold. First, some muscles, such as rabbit heart, contain only the α form (Cummins and Perry, 1974). Moreover, in some muscles, such as the rabbit embryonic skeletal muscles, the β form predominates (Roy *et al.*, 1976). Second, antibodies specific for either α or β subunits, but not both, used to stain muscle sections, have shown that the α variant is present in fast glycolytic (type II) fibres, while slow oxidative (type I) fibres contain the β variant (Dhoot and Perry, 1979). So far there is no evidence for the presence of the putative $\alpha\beta$ heterodimer within one cell, although *in vitro* the two non-identical subunits readily associate into a fully functioning protein.

The tropomyosin of the myocardium is of the α class (like fast muscle) based on its amino acid composition and sequence (Lewis and Smillie, 1980). This is of great interest, since in most properties, such as the structure of myosin heavy and light chains, speed of contraction and metabolic pattern, the myocardium resembles slow muscles.

The pure α tropomyosin of heart is typical of small mammals only (Leger *et al.*, 1976). In more slowly contracting hearts of large mammals such as sheep, pig, and man, the tropomyosin has been resolved into two bands. However, to identify the second band conclusively as β-tropomyosin, additional studies are required since in some cases the observed heterogeneity has been shown to be caused by the presence of the phosphorylated form of tropomyosin (Lewis and Smillie, 1980).

Troponin

The second component of regulatory proteins which renders actomyosin ATPase sensitive to calcium is troponin, which actually consists of three proteins (hence called troponin complex). The three components of the complex differ in their primary structures and each one carries one of the three physiological functions of the whole: troponin-C, which is the calcium ligand (hence C); troponin-T, which binds tropomyosin (hence T); and troponin-I, which inhibits the activity of actomyosin ATPase (hence I).

The complex is localized in the thin filament, not along its entire length, but rather at regular intervals of about 40 nm (Perry, 1977).

Prototype molecule of the troponin complex

Troponin-C has a molecular weight of 18 000 daltons and in primary structure it is very closely related to other known calcium binding proteins, calmodulin and parvalbunin. There are four calcium binding sites located in different domains of the molecule. Only two of these sites, however, are physiologically important since they bind calcium specifically and with high affinity. The other two sites bind both calcium and magnesium with relatively low affinities and consequently under ionic conditions in the muscle cell are probably occupied by magnesium.

Troponin-T is the largest of the three proteins of the complex, having a molecular weight of about 38 000 daltons. Mixing experiments have shown that troponin-T readily forms complexes with troponin-C and tropomyosin. Consequently, its role is viewed by the proponents of the steric block model as anchoring troponin to the backbone of the thin filament. Troponin-T contains three serine residues which can be specifically phosphorylated by the phosphorylase kinase of actin. The physiological significance of this modification, however, is unknown.

Troponin-I has a molecular weight of about 27 000 daltons and serves as a specific inhibitor of magnesium-activated ATPase of actomyosin. Troponin-I complexes with troponin-C and can serve as a substrate for phosphorylation; as in the case of troponin-T, the role of phosphorylation remains to be elucidated.

Isoforms of troponin components

As individual components of the troponin complex, troponin-T and -I differ in amino acid sequence and antigenic properties between fast, slow, and cardiac muscles (Table 15.6), although the divergences are rather limited (Syska *et al.*, 1974; Wilkinson and Grands, 1978; Dhoot and Perry, 1979). Cardiac troponin-I differs in one additional feature, i.e. the presence of 26 amino acid residues at the amino terminus (Perry, 1977). This peptide contains a serine residue which is phosphorylated by a cAMP-dependent protein kinase at a much higher rate than is known for other serine residues of troponin-I molecules present in skeletal muscles. The significance of this intriguing difference in the contractile properties of cardiac and skeletal muscles is not entirely understood.

As far as troponin-C is concerned, the variants present in cardiac and slow muscles are identical (Wilkinson, 1980) but differ from troponin-C present in fast muscles (Dhoot *et al.*, 1979).

Table 15.6   Isoforms of tropomyosin–troponin complex

| | Skeletal muscle | | Ventricle |
	Fast	Slow	
Tropomyosin	$(\alpha)_2$	$(\beta)_2$	$(\alpha)_2$
Troponin-I	f	s	s
Troponin-C	f	s	v
Troponin-T	f	s	v

The lower case letters indicate that the protein is specific for the following muscles; f = fast; s = slow; v = ventricle.

METABOLISM OF CONTRACTILE AND REGULATORY PROTEINS

During the last decade it has been shown conclusively that all cellular constituents undergo turnover, i.e. are continuously being degraded and resynthesized. The half-life of different constituents varies widely from minutes (e.g. ornithine decarboxylase) to days (e.g. myosin heavy chain) to even weeks (e.g. collagen). Only nuclear DNA remains undegraded, although mitochondrial DNA does undergo turnover. In the latter case, the degradation of DNA reflects the short life-span of mitochondria themselves.

Synthesis and Turnover of Myofibrillar Proteins

Although the qualitative demonstration of protein turnover is quite convincing, the actual magnitude of protein half-life is a matter of controversy.

The main reason is that the rigorous use of tracer techniques require measurements of radioactivities both in the precursor and product pools. The direct precursor of protein synthesis, aminoacyl-tRNA, however, is very difficult to measure because its quantity in muscle is quite small. As a consequence of technical difficulties, there have at present been only a few studies in which the half-life has been measured rigorously.

The following conclusions can be made based on the limited data available so far. Skeletal muscle turnover is two to three times lower than that of the ventricle and fast muscle turnover is slower than that of slow oxidative muscle. Classified by the rate of turnover, the myofibrillar proteins of rat ventricle fall into two groups: those with half-lives of about 5 days (myosin heavy chain and α-actin) and those with half-lives ranging between 6 and 8 days (actin, tropomyosin, troponin, and the two myosin light chains). These data clearly show that not only individual myofibrillar proteins, but also their subunits, have uneven rates of turnover (Zak et al., 1977; Martin, 1981). The possible significance of such heterogeneity will be discussed later.

The above-mentioned studies of myofibrillar turnover have been carried out on animals with non-growing hearts. As for protein synthesis and degradation in growing hearts, unequivocal interpretation of the data is difficult because in most studies individual isoproteins have not been separated. The *in vivo* labelling of total proteins (Everett et al., 1977) and total myosins (Morkin et al., 1972) is increased during pressure-induced cardiac hypertrophy. Similarly, acute pressure overload of perfused hearts leads to elevated labelling of total myocardiac proteins (Kao et al., 1978).

In thyroid hormone-induced growth of the heart the synthetic rates have been determined for HC-α and HC-β after their fractionation by immuno-absorption columns using monoclonal antibodies specific for individual heavy chains (Everett et al., 1982). Administration of thyroid hormone results in a several-fold increase in the synthetic rate of HC-α and depression in the synthetic rate of HC-β. After 2 days of hormone treatment, the synthesis of HC-α represents 94% of the total myosin. These changes in synthetic rates are accompanied by the transformation of ventricular myosin from a population of mixed HC-α and HC-β to pure HC-α isomyosin. Simultaneous estimates of the levels of messenger RNA (mRNA) specific for the respective heavy chains revealed that there is a very close relationship between the relative synthetic rates and levels of mRNA of a given chain (Everett et al., 1982). These data suggest strongly that changes in transcription play a major role in the control of myosin heavy chain expression in the heart. No data are presently available for the period immediately after the induction of compensatory growth when additional mechanisms, such as control of translation or degradation, might determine the content of the two heavy chains.

Pathways of Myofibrillar Assembly and Degradation

Comparison of half-lives of individual proteins which constitute cellular organelles, offers an opportunity for the analysis of pathways of their assembly and degradation.

Uniform half-lives are consistent with a model in which myofibrils are degraded as a unit. This process might involve, for example, digestion by autophagic vacuoles. The model also implies co-ordination between synthesis and assembly of myofibrillar proteins. Uneven half-lives, on the other hand, suggest that individual myofibrillar components are synthesized and degraded independently of each other. The turnover of myofibrillar proteins is clearly heterogeneous, ranging from 5 to 8 days (Zak *et al.*, 1977). This uneven turnover is thus inconsistent with digestion of intact myofibrils within lysosomes being the major pathway of their degradation. As an alternative model, one possibility is that myofibrillar proteins are first released into the cytoplasm, perhaps with the participation of specific proteases. Several cytoplasmic neutral proteases have indeed been described in muscle tissues. One of them specifically removes α-actinin from Z-lines (Reddy *et al.*, 1975; Dayton *et al.*, 1976); another protease described in the literature is one which degrades myosin into large molecular weight fragments (Murakami and Uchida, 1978). Additional evidence for the existence of free intermediates in myofibrillar turnover came from the demonstration that the cytoplasm of cardiac cells contains a pool of unassembled light chains (Zak *et al.*, 1977). Also, the small population of filaments which is released from myofibrillar core by treatment with solutions containing Mg-ATP and a chelator of calcium may represent an intermediate between mature myofibrils and the site of their actual degradation (Etlinger *et al.*, 1975). Thus, the presently available data are consistent with a two-step model of myofibrillar degradation: release into the cytoplasm and/or partial fragmentation of large molecules and final degradation via the lysosomal pathway.

Electron microscopic examination indicates that lysosomes are not prominent structures in the heart. Nevertheless, all the classical elements of the lysosomal system have been clearly described in myocardial cells (Topping and Travis, 1974). Most of the lysosomes appear within the perinuclear region; a few are scattered throughout the cytoplasm, especially within the mitochondrial rows that divides the myofibrillar masses.

Biochemical studies of muscle are fully consistent with the vesicular, sequestered character of acidic proteases. Fractionation of heart tissue has revealed acidic hydrolases in all subcellular fractions (Tolnai and Beznak, 1971), with the highest specific activity found in fractions of mitochondria and membrane fragments.

The exact role of proteases in the turnover of myofibrillar proteins, however, still remain obscure. One of the difficulties is that the cellular origin of proteases is unknown. Besides myocytes, lysosomes are also present in large quantities in connective tissue cells, whereas mast cells have been shown to be rich in neutral proteases (see Everett and Zak, 1980).

Determinants of Isoprotein Profile of Myocardial Cells

One of the characteristics of muscle is its ability to match its size to the extent and type of work it is required to perform. Many examples of compensatory growth are known both for cardiac and skeletal muscles (Zak, 1981). Besides the workload, the differentiation and growth of muscle is also controlled by intrinsic, time-dependent factors, e.g., a single myogenic cell, when cultured, gives rise to a colony of myoblasts that will eventually undergo differentiation culminating in the formation of cross-striation in the absence of any nerve cells and hence of contractile activity.

During cardiac morphogenesis, the distinction between the endogeneous developmental programme and the effect of contractile activity is less clear than in skeletal muscle, since both heart and circulation develop simultaneously. Nevertheless, the existence of endogeneous factors is hinted by demonstration that cardiac looping proceeds normally when the contractile activity of chick embryo explants is abolished.

Studies of the control of gene expression during heart differentiation are just at their beginning because the markers of specific genes – i.e. molecular variants of muscle proteins – have been identified only recently. Molecular variants of these proteins are present in a variety of cells, including, for example, fibroblasts. Although The non-muscle variants of contractile proteins contribute very little to the total protein mass, but at the level of nuclear activity, such as transcription, they may be important.

The expression of isomyosins changes continuously during normal development. For example, in ventricles of rabbits in the late gestation period the VM-3 isomyosin predominates. At birth, when the ATPase activity of total myosin, as well as the heart rate, are high, the synthesis and consequent accumulation of VM-1 outstrips that of VM-3. With increasing age, however, this trend reverses itself and VM-1 is gradually replaced by VM-3 isomyosin until, in old animals, it is eliminated. These sequential changes have been demonstrated by native gel electrophoresis of myosin (Hoh *et al.*, 1978), by immunofluorescence staining of heart sections (Sartore *et al.*, 1981), and by immunochemical and peptide map analysis of ventricular myosin heavy chains (Chizzonite *et al.*, 1982).

The synthetic rate of VM-1 isomyosin during the neonatal period correlates with the surge in the serum level of thyroid hormone but later is independent of thyroid hormone declining with age (Everett *et al.*, 1982; Chizzonite *et al.*, 1982). Administration of thyroid hormone in pharmaceutical doses induces synthesis of HC-α with consequent transformation of ventricular myosin into pure VM-1 isomyosin (Morkin, 1979; Sartore *et al.*, 1981; Chizzonite *et al.*, 1982). In contrast, the hypothyroid state is associated with a shift towards the predominance of VM-3 isomyosin (Hoh *et al.*, 1978).

In addition to thyroid hormone, other determinants of the isomyosin profile in the heart are known. For example, swimming in rats induces replacement of VM-3 by VM-1, while pressure overload results in opposite changes (Gorza *et al.*, 1981).

The functional significance of isomyosin changes in the ventricle is not entirely understood at present. It is known, however, that VM-1 isomyosin has a higher ATPase activity than VM-3 (Pope *et al.*, 1980). Although the relationship between myosin ATPase and muscle function is certainly more complex in cardiac muscle than in skeletal muscle, the generalization that there is a correlation betwen the ATPase activity of myosin and the maximal speed of shortening holds true for both muscle types. Since it is also known that the efficiency of muscle shortening depends on contraction velocity (Hamrell and Alpert, 1977), it is conceivable that isomyosin shifts represent an adaptive response of the myocardium to altered haemodynamic load.

REFERENCES

d'Albis, A., and Gratzer, W. B. (1973). Electrophoretic examination of native myosins. *FEBS Lett.*, **29**, 292–296.

d'Albis, A., Pantaloni, C., and Bechet, J.-J. (1979). An electrophoretic study of native myosin isoenzymes and of their subunit content. *Europ. J. Biochem.*, **99**, 261–272.

Banerjee, S. K., Flink, I. L., and Morkin, E. (1976). Enzymatic properties of native and N-ethylmaleimide-modified cardiac myosin from normal and thyrotoxic rabbits. *Circulation Res.*, **39**, 319–326.

Barany, M., and Burt, C. T. (1979). The adenosine triphosphatase activity of myosin in intact muscle. *Fed. Proc.*, **38**, 338.

Chantler, P. (1980). Sails set for the myosin active site, *Nature*, **283**, 621.

Chizzonite, R. A., Everett, A. W., Clark, W. A., Jakovcic, S., Rabinowitz, M., and Zak, R. (1982). Isolation and characterization of two molecular variants of myosin heavy chains from rabbit ventricle: change in their content during normal growth and after treatment with thyroid hormone. *J. Biol. Chem.*, **257**, 2056–2065.

Clark, W. A., Chizzonite, R. A., Everett, A. W., Rabinowitz, M., and Zak, R. (1982). Species correlations between cardiac isomyosins. *J. Biol. Chem.* **257**, 5449–5454.

Cooke, R., and Stull, J. T. (1981). Myosin phosphorylation: a biochemical mechanism for regulating contractility. In *Cell and Muscle Motility* 1 R. M. Dowben and J. W. Shaw, eds), Plenum, New York, pp. 99–133.

Cummins, P., and Perry, S. V. (1973). The subunits and biological activity of polymorphic forms of tropomyosin. *Biochem. J.*, **133**, 765–777.

Cummins, P., and Perry, S. V. (1974). Chemical and immunochemical characteristics of tropomyosins from striated and smooth muscle. *Biochem. J.*, **141**, 43–49.

Dayton, W. R., Reville, W. J., Goll, D. E., and Stomer, M. H. (1976). A Ca^{2+}-activated protease possibly involved in myofibrillar turnover. Partial characterization of the purified enzyme. *Biochemistry*, **15**, 2159–2167.

Dhoot, G. K., and Perry, S. V. (1979). Distribution of polymorphic forms of troponin components and propomyosin in skeletal muscle. *Nature*, **278**, 714–718.

Dhoot, G. K., Fearson, N., and Perry, S. V. (1979). Polymorphic forms of troponin T and troponin C and their localization in striated muscle cell type, *Exp. Cell Res.*, **122**, 339–350.

Elzinga, M., and Lu, R. C. (1976). Comparative amino acid sequence studies on actins. In *Contractile Systems in Non-muscle Tissues* (S. V. Perry *et al.*, eds), Elsevier/North Holland Biomedical Press, Amsterdam, pp. 29–37.

Elzinga, M., and Trus, B. (1980). Sequence and proposed structure of a 17,000 dalton fragment of myosin. In *Methods in Peptide and Protein Sequence Analysis*, (C. Birr, ed.), Elsevier/North Holland Biomedical Press, Amsterdam, pp. 213–224.

Etlinger, J. D., Zak, R., Fischman, D. A., and Rabinowitz, M. (1975). Isolation of newly synthesized myosin filaments from skeletal muscle homogenates and myofibrils. *Nature*, **255**, 259–261.

Everett, A. W., and Zak, R. (1980). Protein synthesis and degradation in the normal and diseased myocardium. In *Drug-induced Heart Disease* (M. R. Bristow, ed.), Elsevier/North Holland, Amsterdam, pp. 63–80.

Everett, A. W., Clark, W. A., Chizzonite, R. A., and Zak, R. (1982). Change in synthesis rates of gamma- and beta-myosin heavy chains in rabbit heart after treatment with thyroid hormone, *J. Biol. Chem.*, in press.

Everett, A. W., Taylor, R. R., and Sparrow, M. P. (1977). Protein synthesis during right ventricular hypertrophy after pulmonary artery stenosis in the dog. *Biochem. J.*, **166**, 315–321.

Flink, I. L., Morkin, E., and Elzinga, M. (1977). Cyanogen bromide peptide from bovine cardiac myosin containing two essential thiols. *FEBS Lett.*, **84**, 261–266.

Frank, G., and Weeds, A. G. (1974). The amino-acid sequence of the alkali light chains of rabbit skeletal muscle myosin. *Europ. J. Biochem.* **44**, 317–334.

Garrels, J. I., and Gubson, W. (1976). Identification and characterization of multiple forms of actin. *Cell*, **9**, 798–805.

Gorza, L., Pauletto, P., Pessina, A. C., Sartore, S., and Schiaffino, S. (1981). Isomyosin distribution in normal and pressure-overloaded rat ventricular myocardium. *Circulation Res.*, **49**, 1003–1009.

Hamrell, B. B., and Alpert, N. R. (1977). The mechanical characteristics of hypertrophied rabbit cardiac muscle in the absence of congestive heart failure. The contractile and series elastic elements. *Circulation Res.*, **40**, 20–25.

Hoh, J. F. Y., McGrath, P. A., and White, R. I. (1976). Electrophoretic analysis of multiple forms of myosin in fast-twitch and slow-twitch muscles of the chick. *Biochem. J.*, **157**, 87–95.

Hoh, J. F. Y., McGarth, P. A., and Hale, P. T. (1978). Electrophoretic analysis of multiple forms of cardiac myosin: effect of hypophysectomy and thyroxine replacement. *J. Mol. Cell. Cardiol.*, **10**, 1053–1076.

Hollosi, G., Srivastava, S., and Wikman-Coffelt, J. (1980). Cross-hybridization of light chains of cardiac myosin isozymes: atrial and ventricular myosins. *FEBS Lett.*, **120**, 199–204.

Holt, J. C., and Lowey, S. (1977). Distribution of alkali light chains in myosin: isolation of isoenzymes. *Biochemistry*, **16**, 4398–4402.

Huszar, G., and Elzinga, M. (1972). Homologous methylated and non-methylated histidine peptides in skeletal and cardiac myosin. *J. Biol. Chem.*, **247**, 745–753.

Huxley, H. E. (1963). Electron microscope studies on the structure of natural and synthetic protein filaments from striated muscle. *J. Mol. Biol.*, **7**, 281–308.

Johnson, L. S. (1974). Non-identical tropomyosin subunits in rat skeletal muscle, *Biochim. Biophys. Acta*, **371**, 219–225.

Kao, R., Rannels, D. E., Whitman, V., and Morgan, H. E. (1978). Factors accounting for growth and atrophy of the heart, in *Recent Advanc. Studies Cardiac Struct. Metab.*, **12**, 105–113.

Katz, A. M. (1970). Contractile proteins of the heart. *Physiol. Rev.*, **50**, 63–158.

Leger, J., Bouveret, P., Schwartz, K., and Swynghedauw, B. (1976). A comparative study of skeletal and cardiac tropomyosins. *Pflügers Arch. Europ. J. Physiol.*, **362**, 271–277.

Leger, J. J., Klotz, C., Caville, F., and Marotte, F. (1979). Structural differences between the heavy chains of myosin subfragment-1 from bovine, porcine and human hearts. *FEBS Lett.*, **106**, 157–161.

Lewis, W. G., and Smillie, L. B. (1980). The amino acid sequence of rabbit cardiac tropomyosin. *J. Biol. Chem.* **251**, 6854–6859.

Libera, L. D., and Sartore, S. (1981). Immunological and biochemical evidence for atrial-like isomyosin in thyrotoxic rabbit ventricle. *Biochim. Biophys. Acta*, **669**, 84–92.

Lompre, A. M., Mercadier, J. J., Wisnewsky, C., Bouveret, P., Pantaloni, C., d'Albis, A., and Schwartz, K. (1981). Species- and age-dependent changes in the relative amounts of cardiac myosin isoenzymes in mammals. *Develop. Biol.*, **84**, 286–290.

Long, L., Fabian, F., Mason, D. T., and Wikman-Coffelt, J. (1977). A new cardiac myosin characterized from canine atria, *Biochem. Biophys. Res. Commun.*, **76**, 626–635.

Lowey, S., and Risby, D. (1971). Light chains from fast and slow muscle myosin. *Nature*, **234**, 81–85.

Lowey, S., Slayter, H. S., Weeds, A. G., and Baker, H. (1969). Substructure of the myosin molecule. *J. Mol. Biol.*, **42**, 1–29.

Marston, S. B., and Taylor, E. W. (1980). Comparison of the myosin and actomyosin ATPase mechanisms of the four types of vertebrate muscles. *J. Mol. Biol.*, **139**, 573–600.

Marston, S. B., Tregear, R. T., Rodger, C. D., and Clarke, M. L. (1979). Coupling between the enzymatic site of myosin and the mechanical output of muscle. *J. Mol. Biol.*, **128**, 111–126.

Martin, A. F. (1981). Turnover of cardiac troponin in subunits. *J. Biol. Chem.*, **256**, 964–968.

Morgan, J. L., Hollady, C. R., and Spooner, B. S. (1980). Immunological differences between actin from cardiac muscle, skeletal muscle, and brain. *Proc. Natl Acad. Sci.*, **77**, 2069–2073.

Morkin, E., Kimata, S., and Skillman, J. J. (1972). Myosin synthesis and degradation during development of cardiac hypertrophy in the rabbit. *Circulation Res.*, **30**, 690–702.

Mornet, D., Bertrand, R., Pantel, P., Audemard, E., and Kassab, R. (1981). Structure of the actin–myosin interface. *Nature*, **292**, 301–308.

Murakami, U., and Uchida, K. (1978). Purification and characterization of a myosin-cleaving protease from rat heart myofibrils. *Biochim. Biophys. Acta*, **525**, 219–229.

Perry, S. V. (1977). The regulation of contractile activity in muscle. *Biochem. Soc. Trans.*, **7**, 593–617.

Pette, D., and Schnez, U. (1977). Coexistence of fast and slow type myosin light chains in single muscle fibres during transformation as induced by long term stimulation. *FEBS Lett.*, **83**, 128–130.

Pope, B., Hoh, J. F. Y., and Weeds, A. (1980). The ATPase activities of rat cardiac myosin isoenzymes. *FEBS Lett.*, **118**, 205–208.

Reddy, M. K., Etlinger, J. D., Rabinowitz, M., Fischman, D. A., and Zak, R. (1975). Removal of Z-lines and α-actinin from isolated myofibrils by a calcium-activated neutral protease. *J. Biol. Chem.*, **250**, 4278–4284.

Rowe, A. (1983). Symmetry and self-assembly in vertebrate A-filaments. In *Cross-bridge Mechanisms in Muscle Contraction* (H. Sugi and G. Pollack, eds), Plenum Press, New York, (1983).

Roy, R. K., Potter, J. D., and Sarkar, S. (1976). Characterization of the regulatory complex of chick embryonic muscles: polymorphism of tropomyosin in adult and embryonic fibers. *Biochem. Biophys. Res. Commun.*, **70**, 28–36.

Sarkar, S., Sreter, F. A., and Gergely, J. (1971). Light chains of myosins from white, red, and cardiac muscles. *Proc. Natl Acad. Sci.*, **68**, 946–950.

Sartore, S., Gorza, L., Bormioli, S. P., Libera, L. D., and Schiaffino, S. (1981). Myosin types and fiber types in cardiac muscle. *J. Cell. Biol.*, **88**, 226–233.

Schwartz. K., Lecarpentier, Y., Martin, J. L., Lompre, A. M., Mercadier, J. J., and Swynghedauw, B. (1981). Myosin isoenzymic distribution correlates with speed of contraction. *J. Mol. Cell. Cardiol.*, **13**, 1071–1075.

Starr, R., and Offer, G. (1973). Polarity of the myosin molecule. *J. Mol. Biol.*, **81**, 17–31.

Syrovy, I. (1979). Polymorphism and specificity of myosin. *Internat. J. Biochem.*, **10**, 577–616.

Syrovy, I., Delcaye, C., and Swynghedauw, B. (1979). Comparison of ATPase activity and light subunits in myosins from left and right ventricles and atria in seven mammalian species. *J. Mol. Cell. Cardiol.*, **11**, 1129–1135.

Syska, H., Perry, S. V., and Trayer, I. P. (1974). A new method of preparation of troponin I (inhibitory protein) using affinity chromatography. Evidence for three different forms of troponin I in striated muscle. *FEBS Lett.*, **40**, 253–257.

Taylor, E. W. (1972). Chemistry of muscle contraction. *Annu. Rev. Biochem.*, **41**, 577–616.

Tolnai, S., and Beznak, M. (1971). Studies of lyosomal enzyme activity in normal and hypertrophied mammalian myocardium. *J. Mol. Cell. Cardiol.*, **3**, 193–208.

Topping, T. M., and Travis, D. F. (1974). An electron cytochemical study of mechanisms of lysosomal activity in the rat left ventricular mural myocardium, *J. Ultrastruct. Res.*, **46**, 1–22.

Vandekerchkove, J., and Weber, K. (1978). Mammalian cytoplasmic actins are the products of at least two genes and differ in primary structure in at least 25 identified positions from skeletal muscle actins. *Proc. Natl Acad. Sci.*, **75**, 1106–1110.

Wagner, P. D. (1981). Formation and characterization of myosin hybrids containing essential light chains and heavy chains from different muscle myosins. *J. Biol. Chem.*, **256**, 2493–2498.

Weeds, A. G. (1976). Light chains from slow-twitch muscle myosin. *Europ. J. Biochem.*, **66**, 157–173.

Whalen, R. G., Butler-Browne, G. S., and Gros, F. (1976). Protein synthesis and actin heterogenity in calf muscle cells in culture. *Proc. Natl Acad. Sci.*, **73**, 2018–2022.

Whalen, R. G., Schwartz, K., Bouveret, P., Sell, S., and Gross, F. (1979). Contractile protein isozymes in muscle development: identification of an embryonic form of myosin heavy chain. *Proc. Natl Acad. Sci.*, **76**, 5197–5201.

Wikman-Coffelt, J., and Srivastava, S. (1979). Differences in atrial and ventricular myosin light chains. *FEBS Lett.*, **106**, 207–212.

Wilkinson, J. M. (1980). Troponin C from rabbit slow and cardiac muscles is the product of a single gene. *Europ. J. Biochem.*, **103**, 179–188.

Wilkinson, J. M., and Grands, R. J. A. (1978). Comparison of amino acid sequence of troponin I from different striated muscles. *Nature*, **271**, 31–35.

Yazaki, Y., Ueda, S., Nagai, R., and Shimada, K. (1979). Cardiac atrial myosin adenosine triphosphatase of animals and humans. *Circulation Res.*, **45**, 522–527.

Zak, R. (1981). Contractile function as a determinant of muscle growth, In *Cell and Muscle Motility* 1 (R. M. Dowben and J. W. Shay, eds), Plenum, New York, pp. 1–33.

Zak, R., and Rabinowitz, M. (1979). Molecular aspects of cardiac hypertrophy. *Annu. Rev. Physiol.*, **41**, 539–552.

Zak, R., Martin, A. F., Prior, G., and Rabinowitz, M. (1977). Comparison of turnover of several myofibrillar proteins and critical evaluation of double isotope method. *J. Biol. Chem.*, **252**, 3430–3435.

Cardiac Metabolism
Edited by A. J. Drake-Holland and M. I. M. Noble
© 1983 John Wiley & Sons Ltd

CHAPTER 16

Phosphorylation of Cardiac Muscle Contractile Proteins

P. J. England

Department of Biochemistry, University of Bristol Medical School, Bristol BS8 1TD, UK

INTRODUCTION

A general scheme for the phosphorylation and dephosphorylation of proteins can be shown as

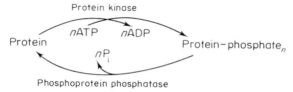

The importance of this as a regulatory mechanism is that covalent attachment of phosphate groups to serine, threonine, or tyrosine residues can induce conformational changes in the three-dimensional structure of proteins which cause changes in their expressed properties. Examples of such changes observed with contractile proteins include changes in calcium affinity, rates of enzyme reactions, and association with other proteins. In order for this mechanism to be of regulatory significance, it is necessary to control the activities of the kinase and phosphatase so as to vary the proportion of protein in the phosphorylated state. Many protein kinases are regulated by low molecular weight compounds which act as activitors. Well documented examples of relevance to the phosphorylation of contractile proteins are cyclic AMP-dependent protein kinase and several Ca^{++}-activated kinases. Changes in the concentrations of the regulator molecules by hormonal or other effects can then result in changes in the state of phosphorylation of target proteins. However, more complex regulatory mechanisms involving interaction of kinases with other proteins or membrane components are known. Generally, the regulation of phosphoprotein phosphatases is less well understood, although inhibition by specific regulator proteins appears to be of major importance.

In this chapter the phosphorylation of cardiac contractile proteins will be discussed in relation to changes in contractility induced by hormones, particularly catecholamines and acetylcholine. Phosphorylated intracellular proteins fall into two main categories. First, there are proteins in which the phosphate groups are in rapid equilibrium with intracellular ATP, and in which the level of phosphorylation can change rapidly following hormonal or neural stimulation. This indicates that the appropriate protein kinases and phosphoprotein phosphatases are active and under hormonal control in the cell. Three major contractile proteins are in this category: troponin-I, myosin P-light chain, and C-protein. Secondly, there are proteins in which the phosphate groups are not in equilibrium with ATP, and do not change in response to hormonal stimulus. The phosphorylation of these proteins will not be of significance for the acute regulation of contractility. Troponin-T, tropomyosin, and myosin heavy chains are examples of this type. This chapter will concentrate on the first category of phosphorylated proteins.

Three main experimental approaches are used to study protein phosphorylation. There are experiments on the phosphorylation of isolated proteins by specific kinases and phosphatases, which give information on which proteins are substrates for the interconverting enzymes, and the sites of phosphorylation on the proteins. A second type of experiment is to discover what are the effects of phosphorylation on the properties of the proteins. Thirdly, there are studies using intact tissues, to discover under what conditions and to what extent the proteins are phosphorylated in response to physiological stimulii. Data from all three approaches are necessary before a complete understanding of the physiological importance of the phosphorylation of a protein can be obtained. In this chapter the phosphorylation of contractile proteins will be discussed from an experimental viewpoint, and where possible hypotheses will be presented relating phosphorylation to mechanisms for the regulation of contractility.

PROTEIN KINASES AND PHOSPHOPROTEIN PHOSPHATASES

Protein kinases are usually classified according to the substances which cause their activation (Krebs and Beavo, 1979). There are about 20 protein kinases identified in eukaryotic cells, but only a few are known to phosphorylate contractile proteins. These are shown in Table 16.1, classified according to their activators.

Cyclic AMP-dependent Protein Kinase (cAMP–PK)

This enzyme is thought to be the main (or even only) target protein for cyclic AMP in eukaryotic cells (Krebs and Beavo, 1979), and is therefore a key link in the mechanism whereby hormones which elevate cyclic AMP

Table 16.1 Classification of protein kinases which phosphorylate muscle proteins

Activator	Name of kinase	Substrate specificity
Cyclic AMP	Cyclic AMP-dependent protein kinase	Broad range of proteins are phosphorylated
Cyclic GMP	Cyclic GMP-dependent protein kinase	Similar specificity to cyclic AMP-kinase
Ca^{++}	Phosphorylase kinase	Phosphorylase, glycogen synthetase
	Myosin light chain kinase	Myosin P-light chain
	Phospholamban-Ca kinase	Phospholamban
?	Troponin-T kinase	Troponin-T

cause changes in cell function. The subunit structure and mode of activation of cAMP–PK is shown by the equation

$$R_2C_2 + 4cAMP \rightleftharpoons R_2.cAMP_4 + 2 C, \qquad (16.1)$$

where R is the regulatory subunit which binds cyclic AMP and C is the catalytic subunit which will only phosphorylate proteins when disssociated from R (Corbin *et al.*, 1978; Krebs and Beavo, 1979; Walsh and Cooper, 1979; Builder *et al.*, 1980). There are two isoenzymes of cAMP–PK in mammalian tissues, differing only in their regulatory subunits (Reimann *et al.*, 1971; Hofmann *et al.*, 1975; Nimmo and Cohen, 1977). However, hearts from different species having widely different proportions of the two isoezymes show identical patterns of protein phosphorylation, suggesting little functional difference between them.

Although cAMP-PK will phosphorylate a considerable number of proteins, there is .a well defined specificity as to which serine (or occasionally threonine) residues are phosphorylated, determined by the primary sequence around the phosphorylation site (Krebs and Beavo, 1979). The two major patterns of sequences are (a) –Lys–Arg–X–X–Ser(P) and (b) –Arg–Arg–X–Ser(P) (Shenolikar and Cohen, 1978). In general the presence of at least two basic residues on the N-terminal side of the phosphorylated residues are required.

The reader is referred to several chapters in Rosen and Krebs (1981) for detailed accounts of recent work on this enzyme.

Cyclic GMP-dependent Protein Kinase (cGMP–PK)

This enzyme, originally discovered in arthropods (Kuo and Greengard, 1970) has been shown to be present in all mammalian tissues (see Nimmo and Cohen, 1977). It differs from cAMP-PK in its specificity for cyclic GMP as an activator, and that it is a dimeric molecule, each subunit carrying both the nucleotide binding and catalytic sites (Takhai *et al.*, 1975; Kuo *et al.*, 1976; Gill *et al.*, 1976; Lincoln and Corbin, 1977). Activation by cyclic GMP is not therefore accompanied by dissociation of the subunits. However, cGMP-PK and cAMP-PK have an almost identical specificity with respect to the proteins phosphorylated (Lincoln and Corbin, 1977; Krebs and Beavo, 1979), and to the amino acid requirements around the phosphorylated sites.

Several suggestions have been made that cyclic GMP and cyclic AMP may have antagonistic actions in many tissues (Goldberg and Haddox, 1977), including the heart (Chapter 17 in this volume). However, the identical specificities of cAMP–PK and cGMP–PK mean that an increase in either cyclic AMP or cyclic GMP will lead to phosphorylation of the same proteins. Any mechanisms to explain a possible antagonism between cyclic AMP and cyclic GMP must therefore involve systems other than the nucleotide-dependent protein kinases.

Calcium-activated Protein Kinases

Unlike cAMP–PK and cGMP–PK, which phosphorylate a wide range of proteins, the calcium-activated kinases form a group of relatively specific enzymes, each one phosphorylating a very restricted number of proteins. Three of these are of relevance to the phosphorylation of muscle proteins (a) phosphorylase kinase, which phosphorylates phosphorylase *b*, glycogen synthetase, and, although probably not of physiological significance, troponin subunits (Brostrom *et al.*, 1971; England *et al.*, 1973; Roach *et al.*, 1978; Soderling *et al.*, 1979); (b) myosin light chain kinase, which has as its only known substrate the P-light chain of myosin (Perrie *et al.*, 1973; Pires *et al.*, 1974); (c) a kinase which phosphorylates an 11 000 dalton protein of sarcoplasmic reticulum (phospholamban) (Namm *et al.*, 1972; Le Peuch *et al.*, 1979; Bilezikjian *et al.*, 1980; see Chapter 17 in this volume).

All these kinases are stimulated by Ca^{++} at concentrations of 0.1–1 μM, and either require or have as part of their structure the Ca^{++}-binding protein calmodulin. This was first discovered as being essential for the Ca^{++} activation of brain cyclic nucleotide phosphodiesterase (Cheung, 1970), but it has since become apparent that almost all cytoplasmic enzymes regulated by micromolar levels of Ca^{++} have calmodulin as an essential subunit. For a comprehensive discussion of calmodulin and its actions the reader is referred to Cheung (1980).

Calmodulin is a highly acidic protein of molecular weight 16 700 daltons, which contains four 'pockets' especially rich in acidic amino acids (Klee, 1980). These bind one Ca^{++} each with dissociation constants of approximately 1 μM, which induce conformational changes in the protein. For most calmodulin–enzyme systems, the calmodulin only binds to and activates the enzyme when complexed with Ca^{++} (Cheung, 1980), the only exception being phosphorylase kinase (Cohen *et al.*, 1978). This enzyme has four molecules of calmodulin tightly bound even in the absence of Ca^{++}, but interestingly, can be further activated by additional exogenous calmodulin (Shenolikar *et al.*, 1979). The one cytoplasmic system regulated by Ca^{++} in which calmodulin is not implicated is muscle contraction itself. Here, Ca^{++} binds to troponin-C, which has some 70% sequence homology with calmodulin (Vanamann, 1980), and three similar Ca^{++}-binding domains.

Phosphoprotein Phosphatases

Phosphoprotein phosphatases have been less well studied than protein kinases, but recent work has led to the emergence of a number of concepts which are generally applicable to most mammalian tissues (Lee *et al.*, 1981; Li, 1981; Cohen, 1982). The major phosphoprotein phosphatase activity, called phosphatase-1 (Cohen, 1982) or phosphatase-S (Li, 1981) has an active monomer molecular weight of 35 000 daltons, and has a broad protein substrate specificity. This enzyme will dephosphorylase glycogen synthetase, phosphorylase, phosphorylase kinase β-subunit, phosphatase inhibitor-1 (see below), histone, troponin-I, and several other proteins. It can exist in a number of aggregated forms with molecular weights up to 300 000 daltons, in which the specificity of the enzyme may be modified (e.g. Li, 1981). This enzyme may also exist in an inactive form which can be activated by incubation with ATP-Mg (Vandenheede *et al.*, 1981). The enzyme is inhibited by two heat-stable protein inhibitors, called inhibitor-1 and inhibitor-2 (Huang and Glinsmann, 1976). Inhibitor-1 will only function as an inhibitor when phosphorylated by cAMP–PK. Significantly for this chapter, however, is the observation that cardiac muscle does not appear to contain inhibitor-1 (P. J. England, unpublished observations; P. Cohen, personal communication).

A second group of at least three phosphoprotein phosphatases present in tissues generally have a narrower specificity for their protein substrates (e.g. Cohen, 1982), and are not inhibited by the phosphatase inhibitor proteins mentioned above. There may be little similarity between these enzymes, and they are best considered as an operationally defined group, rather than a set of homologous proteins. Within this group, the enzyme of most relevance to this chapter is myosin light chain phosphatase (Morgan *et al.*, 1976). This is a highly specific enzyme which will dephosphorylate myosin P-light chain but not a number of other muscle proteins. It has been isolated from smooth muscle (Pato and Adelstein, 1980) with a molecular weight of 150 000 daltons.

The control of these phosphatases in heart is not well understood. Indeed, it is not even established which proteins are dephosphorylated by which phosphatases, owing to their overlapping specificities. The absence of inhibitor-1 means that the general phosphoprotein phosphatase cannot be controlled through this cyclic AMP-dependent mechanism. In the following discussion a number of relevant points will be raised as to mechanisms for control of phosphoprotein phosphatases, but these should be viewed as speculations only, owing to the lack of relevant data.

PHOSPHORYLATION OF THIN FILAMENT PROTEINS

Phosphorylation of Troponin-I

Troponin is the protein complex which confers Ca^{++} sensitivity on striated muscle (Ebashi, 1966) (Chapter 15 in this volume). It is composed of three subunits: troponin-C, the Ca^{++}-binding subunit; troponin-I, which inhibits the interaction between actin and myosin; troponin-T, the tropomyosin binding subunit. These three subunits are present in whole troponin in a 1:1:1 ratio, and interact together tightly (Greaser and Gergely, 1971).

The first report of phosphorylation of troponin subunits was by Bailey and Villar-Palasi (1971), who found that troponin-I from skeletal muscle was phosphorylated by cAMP–PK. Both troponin-I and troponin-T from skeletal muscle could be phosphorylated by phosphorylase kinase (Stull *et al.*, 1971; England *et al.*, 1973), although the rates of phosphorylation were very low, especially when the whole troponin complex was used (Perry and Cole, 1974).

As isolated from muscle, skeletal troponin contained 1 mol of covalently bound phosphate per troponin-T subunit, and none bound to troponin-I (Perry and Cole, 1974). It quickly became apparent that troponin-I was not phosphorylated to any significant extent *in vivo* in skeletal muscle (Stull and High, 1977), and that the earlier results were an artefact arising from the use of isolated troponin subunits.

In contrast, when whole troponin isolated from cardiac muscle was incubated with cAMP-PK, a rapid phosphorylation of troponin-I was observed (Reddy *et al.*, 1973; Cole and Perry, 1975). This could also be demonstrated using cardiac myofibrils (Ray & England, 1976). Unlike the situation with skeletal muscle, troponin-T was not phosphorylated by cAMP-PK (Cole and Perry, 1975; Ray and England, 1976), and there was no phosphorphorylation of troponin-I by phosphorylase kinase (Cole and Perry, 1975). The difference in the phosphorylation of cardiac and skeletal troponin-I was found to be due to the presence in cardiac troponin-I of an additional 26 amino acid residues at the N-terminal end of the molecule (Grand *et al.*, 1976). This contains the sequence –Val–Arg–Arg–Ser(P)– (Moir and Perry, 1977) which is the serine (residue no. 20) phosphorylated by cAMP–PK. There was also a second serine residue (no. 146) which was slowly phosphorylated (Moir and Perry, 1977).

The rapid phosphorylation of cardiac troponin-I, coupled with the hormonal sensitivity of cardiac contraction, led to a series of experiments to show the *in vivo* phosphorylation of troponin-I in heart. It was discovered that troponin-I was phosphorylated to only a small extent in unstimulated hearts of several species, but that on perfusion with adrenaline a rapid increase in phosphorylation occurred (England, 1975, 1976, 1977; Solaro *et al.*, 1976; Stull, 1980). Between 1 and 1.5 mol of phosphate was incorporated per troponin subunit, predominantly into Ser-20 (Moir *et al.*, 1980) and there was a good correlation between the initial increase in contractile force and troponin-I phosphorylation. This phosphorylation was dependent on increases in intracellular cyclic AMP, as increase in the force of contraction induced by cardiac glycosides, increased rate of contraction and increased perfusate Ca^{++} did not result in increases in troponin-I phosphorylation (Solaro *et al.*, 1976; Ezrailson *et al.*, 1977). This suggested that phosphorylation *in vivo* was catalysed by cAMP-PK, and not phosphorylase kinase, this being confirmed later by direct measurements (England, 1977; Moir and Perry, 1980). However, increases in cardiac cyclic AMP do not always lead to phosphorylation of troponin-I. Brunton *et al.* (1979) found that perfusion of rat hearts with PGE_1 increased cyclic AMP, but did not cause phosphorylation of troponin-I or phosphorylase. This indicates an intracellular compartmentation of cyclic AMP, with some hormones (e.g. beta-adrenergic agonists, glucagon) increasing cyclic AMP in a pool which leads to phosphorylation of certain proteins, including troponin-I, and others (e.g. PGE_1) which increase cyclic AMP in a different pool.

The correlation between troponin-I phosphorylation and increased contraction observed during the initial period of stimulation with catecholamine (England, 1975, 1976) was not, however, seen under all circumstances. In particular, following a short pulse of catecholamine there was a dissociation between phosphorylation and contraction (England, 1976; Stull *et al.*, 1981). After the initial increase in contraction in response to the catecholamine there was a decrease back to the control level over a 2–3 min period. However, the phosphate content of troponin-I, which was increased by the catecholamine, remained elevated for at least 4 min. In contrast, phosphorylase, which was also phosphorylated in response to the catecholamine, was rapidly dephosphorylated again following removal of the hormones. This suggests that the phosphoprotein phosphatase which dephosphorylates troponin-I is virtually inactive in heart under these circumstances, whereas the enzyme that dephosphorylates phosphorylase is active. We have recently found that in rat heart there is a specific phosphorylase phosphatase, as well as a general phosphoprotein phosphatase which will dephosphorylate troponin-I and other proteins (D. Mills and P. J.

England, unpublished observations). These results supply a mechanism whereby phosphorylase and troponin-I dephosphorylation can occur at different rates, provided that the two phosphatases are under separate control. The actual control of troponin-I dephosphorylation is not understood, although there is an indication that cyclic GMP may be implicated. When hearts were pulsed with adrenaline as above, and the pulse followed by perfusion with acetylcholine, there was a rapid dephosphorylation of troponin-I which was accompanied by an increase in cyclic GMP (England, 1976). In isolated, skinned cardiac myofibrils, cyclic GMP reversed the effect of cyclic AMP on the .Ca^{++} sensitivity of the myofibrils, this being accompanied by a dephosphorylation of troponin-I (McClellan and Winegrad, 1980). A similar cyclic GMP stimulation of protein dephosphorylation is discussed below (Hartzell and Titus, 1982). These results suggest, although do not prove, that cyclic GMP may be activating a phosphoprotein phosphatase, possibly the general phosphatase-1.

The effect of phosphorylation of troponin-I on its properties has been investigated using isolated troponin, washed myofibrils and skinned fibre preparations. It was initially reported that phosphorylation of troponin-I in intact myofibrils by cAMP-PK caused an increase in the Ca^{++} sensitivity of cardiac myofibrils (Rubio *et al.*, 1975). However, subsequent studies (Ray and England, 1976; Reddy and Wyborny, 1976; Bailin, 1979; Holroyde *et al.*, 1979a) have shown that phosphorylation of troponin-I actually decreases the Ca^{++} sensitivity of cardiac myofibrils. Typically there is a threefold increase in concentration of Ca^{++} required for half-maximal activation when troponin-I is phosphorylated (Ray and England, 1976). In some of these studies (Reddy and Wyborny, 1976; Bailin, 1979) phosphorylation was also reported to cause a decrease in the maximum rate of myofibrillar ATPase at saturating Ca^{++}. However, as will be seen below, this latter effect is not observed in studies with skinned cardiac fibres. It is also difficult to reconcile a large decrease in maximal ATPase rate (indicative of a decreased actin–myosin interaction) with the increased tension development observed in intact heart on stimulation with catecholamine.

Studies with skinned fibres, in which the cell membranes are made permeable to Ca^{++} either by treatment with EGTA (McClellan and Winerad, 1978; Mope *et al.*, 1980) or glycerol (Herzig and Ruegg, 1980) have confirmed the above results in a more intact preparation. Following skinning, the tension developed by the fibre was measured at different Ca^{++} concentrations, before and after treatment with cyclic AMP and theophylline. There was an increase in the concentration of Ca^{++} required for half-maximal tension of up to threefold, which was correlated with the extent of troponin-I phosphorylation (Mope *et al.*, 1980). McClellan and Winegrad (1980) also reported that this treatment increased the maximal tension at saturating Ca^{++}, although this was not observed by Herzig and Ruegg (1980).

How can the above results, which show a decreased Ca^{++} sensitivity of the myofibrils when troponin-I is phosphorylated, be reconciled with the observed increase in contraction caused by catecholamine in the intact heart? The decrease in Ca^{++} sensitivity means that when troponin-I is phosphorylated it is necessary to increase the cytoplasmic Ca^{++} even to develop the same tension as when tropinin-I was not phosphorylated. Since cardiac troponin-I phosphorylation is often associated with increased tension development (e.g. with catecholamines), this implies an even larger increase in Ca^{++} concentration than would have been necessary without troponin-I phosphorylation. As discussed in Chapters 3 and 17 in this volume, the increase in cytoplasmic Ca^{++} in the heart on stimulation with catecholamines is well documented, and is presumably sufficient to cause the observed increase in tension.

Phosphorylation of troponin-I is more likely to be implicated in the increased rate of relaxation of the heart induced by catecholamines. As shown in Figure 16.1, the rate of removal of Ca^{++} from the troponin on the myofibrils is dependent on both the rate of Ca^{++} removal from the cytoplasm (k_2), and the rates of Ca^{++} binding and release from troponin (k_1 and k_{-1}).

If k_{-1} and k_2 are of the same order of magnitude, then either could be rate limiting in the overall relaxation of the muscle. Since catecholamines probably increase k_2, this could then make k_{-1} the rate-limiting step under these circumstances. However, the evidence suggests that phosphorylation of troponin-I results in an increase in k_{-1} to counteract this. The results with myofibrils and skinned fibres show a decreased affinity for Ca^{++} of troponin-I when phosphorylated. This can be brought about by a decrease in k_1 or an increase in k_{-1}. Preliminary observations have indicated that phosphorylation of troponin-I causes an increase in k_{-1} of approximately 50% (Robertson *et al.*, 1982), and that the rate of Ca^{++} release is slow enough to be a significant factor in determining the overall rate of relaxa-

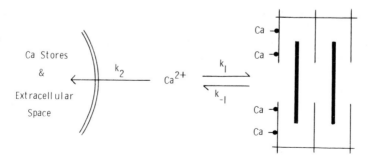

Figure 16.1 A model of the dissociation of Ca^{++} and troponin during relaxation of the heart. k_1, k_{-1}, and k_2 are rate constants for the relevant reactions. The dissociation constant for Ca^{++} and troponin is given by $K_d = k_{-1}/k_1$

tion. The most plausible explanation at the moment for the function of troponin-I phosphorylation is, therefore, that it is concerned with an increased rate of dissociation of Ca^{++} from troponin, contributing to the increased rate of relaxation caused by catecholamines.

A point of interest arises from the observation that following a pulse of catecholamine troponin-I phosphorylation remains elevated, even when the contractile response, including the rate of relaxation, has returned to normal (England, 1976; Stull *et al.*, 1981). It is clear from Figure 16.1 that if during this period k_2 returns to its normal value, then as long as it is the rate-limiting step, it is of no consequence that k_{-1} is still elevated, i.e. the rate of relaxation is determined solely by the rate of removal of Ca^{++} from cytoplasm. However, the fact that troponin-I is still phosphorylated means that the Ca^{++} sensitivity of the myofibrils remains decreased. Therefore to obtain a given contractile force under these conditions, the systolic cytoplasmic Ca^{++} must be elevated compared to that required before the catecholamine response. It is difficult to see the advantage of this to the myocardium, as more Ca^{++} has to be cycled at each beat, requiring an increased expenditure of energy which would be avoided if the dephosphorylation of troponin-I was more rapid.

Phosphorylation of Troponin-T

During the initial studies on troponin phosphorylation it was observed that troponin-T as isolated from skeletal and cardiac muscle contained covalently bound phosphate (England *et al.*, 1973; Perry and Cole, 1974; Stull and Buss, 1977). Troponin-T from cardiac muscle contained 0.2–0.5 mol phosphate per mole of troponin-T, depending on the extraction conditions used. Early work suggested that troponin-T could be phosphorylated by phosphorylase kinase (England *et al.*, 1973; Perry and Cole, 1974; Moir *et al.*, 1977). However, troponin-T isolated from mice deficient in phosphorylase kinase was still phosphorylated (Moir *et al.*, 1977), suggesting that a new, unidentified protein kinase could be present which would phosphorylate troponin-T. Starting with a crude phosphorylase kinase preparation, a highly specific troponin-T kinase has been purified from skeletal (Gusev *et al.*, 1978; Kumin and Villar-Palasi, 1979; Risnik *et al.*, 1980) and cardiac (Villar-Palasi & Kumon, 1981) muscle. The cardiac troponin-T kinase has a molecular weight of 130 000 daltons, composed of two subunits of molecular weight 37 000 daltons, and two of 28 000 daltons. It will phosphorylate casein and phosvitin at rates between five and six times slower than troponin-T, but has no activity towards typical cAMP–PK substrates.

The phosphate content of troponin-T is not changed during inotropic interventions in rat heart (P. J. England, unpublished observations), but may possibly increase in turtle heart (Barany *et al.*, 1981). In mammalian heart the bound phosphate also equilibrates very slowly with intracellular ATP, suggesting a low activity of the kinase/phosphatase couple. Phosphorylation of troponin-T is therefore unlikely to have any short term regulatory significance, and may have either a long term regulatory or a structural function.

Phosphorylation of Tropomyosin

Tropomyosin from both skeletal and cardiac muscle has been found to contain covalently bound phosphate (Ribolow and Barany, 1977; Stull and Buss, 1977), although cardiac tropomyosin only contained 0.21 mol phosphate per mole of tropomyosin. This is bound to a single site, serine 283 of the α-subunit of tropomyosin (Mak *et al.*, 1978). As with the phosphate on troponin-T, there is a very slow turnover of the phosphate, and no apparent changes in the phosphate content with inotropic interventions (P. J. England, unpublished observations). There is no information as to the protein kinase(s) or phosphatase(s) involved in phosphorylation of tropomyosin, or of the function of the phosphorylation.

THICK FILAMENT PROTEIN PHOSPHORYLATION

Myosin Light Chain Phosphorylation

The myosin molecule is composed of two heavy chains (molecular weight 200 000 daltons) and four light chains associated with the head region of the heavy chain. In heart these light chains are of two types, a loosely associated light chain of 19 000 daltons, and a tightly bound one of 27 000 daltons. The 19 000 dalton light chain is often referred to as the DTNB-light chain regulatory light chain, or LC2, but in this chapter will be called the phosphorylated light chain (P-LC). This name was given by Frearson and Perry (1975) when it was discovered that it could be phosphorylated in myosin from several muscle types. Subsequent work has shown that phosphorylation of P–LC occurs in all muscle and non-muscle cells containing myosin (see, for example, Stull, 1980). The P-LC is located on the outside of the myosin head region, as shown by its ease of removal with non-denaturing reagents (Gazith *et al.*, 1970), its reaction in intact myosin to P-LC antibodies (Holt and Lowey, 1975), and its specific digestion by proteases (Malhotra *et al.*, 1979).

There may be a regulatory role for P-LC not related to its phosphorylation. Morimoto and Harrington (1974) suggested that there could be a mechanism for the direct activation of myosin by Ca^{++}, separate from the troponin system. Lehman (1978) found an activation of skeletal actomyosin ATPase by Ca^{++} in the absence of troponin/tropomyosin, providing evidence for Ca^{++} control of myosin. Myosin has two high affinity sites for Ca^{++}, which are lost when the P-LC is removed (Holroyde et al., 1979b). These sites also have a much lower affinity for Mg^{++}. Any mechanism for a Ca^{++} switch on myosin would therefore probably involve Ca^{++} binding to P-LC. However, Bagshaw and Reed (1977) suggested that Ca^{++} association and dissociation were too slow to allow Ca^{++} regulation of myosin during single contractions.

As was discusssed earlier in the chapter, the kinase that phosphorylates myosin P-LC is a specific, Ca^{++}-dependent enzyme, myosin light chain kinase (MLC kinase). As the enzyme has slightly different properties depending on the tissue of origin, this discussion will concentrate on the enzyme from heart. The enzyme is composed of a catalytic subunit of molecular weight 90 000 daltons (Hofmann and Wolf 1981), which is only active when complexed with Ca-calmodulin. It has a K_m for P-LC of 15 μM, and phosphorylates the P-LC on one specific site, which has the sequence Ala–Ala–Ala–Glu–Gly–Gly(Ser, Ser(P))–Asn–Val (Perrie et al., 1973). This is totally dissimilar to sites phosphorylated by cAMP-PK or phosphorylase kinase, indicating the different specificity requirement of MLC kinase. The cardiac enzyme has a V_{max} of 20–30 μmol phosphate transferred per minute per milligram of enzyme (Hofmann and Wolf, 1981). These properties are very similar to those of the skeletal muscle enzyme. The enzyme can be phosphorylated by cAMP-PK, but this has little or no effect on its activity (Wolf and Hofmann, 1980; Walsh and Guilleux, 1981). This is in contrast to the smooth muscle enzyme, where phosphorylation by cAMP-PK causes a marked decrease in activity (Adelstein et al., 1978). The level of activity of MLC kinase in heart muscle is considerably lower than that observed in skeletal muscle, and is similar to the activity of the light chain phosphatase in heart (Frearson et al., 1976a). The significance of this will be discussed below in relation to the regulation of cardiac P-LC phosphorylation *in vivo*.

A regulatory function for the phosphorylation of myosin P-LC has been sought extensively since its intial discovery. Early reports using myosin from skeletal muscle indicated that phosphorylation of P-LC has no effect on its basal or actin-activated ATPase rate (Morgan et al., 1976). Recently, however, it has been reported that phosphorylation caused an increase in actomyosin ATPase activity (Pemrick, 1980), apparently by an increase in the affinity of myosin for actin. Bhan et al. (1981) discovered that cardiac myosin could be specifically depleted of P-LC and that this caused an increase in myosin or actomyosin ATPase activity. Addition of dephosphorylated P-LC reduced the ATPase activity back to the control level, while phosphorylated P-LC did not. Whether this reflects an effect of P-LC phosphorylation on reassociation, or a genuine effect on myosin ATPase, is not clear. It has also been reported that phosphorylation of P-LC causes an increase in Ca^{++} affinity of whole myosin (Kardami *et al.*, 1980). It would therefore appear that in striated muscle there is evidence for changes in myosin activity on phosphorylation of the P-LC, but that much work remains to be done.

In myosin from smooth muscle, the effect of phosphorylation of P-LC is better established (see, for example, Stull, 1980) Myosin can be prepared from smooth muscles in a low activity, dephosphorylated state, or a high activity, phosphorylated state (Aksoy *et al.*, 1976; Sobieszek, 1977; DiSalvo *et al.*, 1978; Mrwa *et al.*, 1980). The effect of phosphorylation is particularly noticeable in the presence of actin. Interconversion of the two forms, with corresponding changes in P-LC phosphorylation, can be brought about by incubation with MLC kinase and phosphate. These and similar results have led to the hypothesis that contraction in smooth muscle is regulated by phosphorylation of P-LC (Adelstein, 1978). In relaxed muscle the P-LC is dephosphorylated. On stimulation there is an increase in cytoplasmic Ca^{++}, causing an activation of MLC kinase and phosphorylation of P-LC. This then stimulates myosin–actin interaction leading to contraction. This hypothesis has been supported by measurement of P-LC phosphorylation in intact smooth muscle (Barron *et al.*, 1979; Driska and Murphy, 1979; Aksoy and Murphy, 1979). On stimulation there is a rapid phosphorylation of P-LC, which preceded the development in tension. However, it should be realized that not all workers agree with this hypothesis (Mikawa *et al.*, 1977; Ebashi, 1980), and there may be other control mechanisms involving Ca^{++} regulation of the thin filament (Marston *et al.*, 1980).

Most of the studies of phosphorylation in cardiac muscle have centred on the level of phosphorylation in intact tissue, and changes in this caused by inotropic interventions. Initial reports suggested that the adrenaline caused a decrease in P-LC phosphorylation (Frearson *et al.*, 1976b), although this has since been recognized as an artefact (Perry *et al.*, 1979). Studies in a number of laboratories (Holroyde *et al.*, 1979c; Jeacocke and England, 1980a; High and Stull, 1980; Westwood and Perry, 1981) have found that P-LC isolated from hearts of several species perfused under control conditions have a phosphate content of 0.5 mol phosphate per mole of P-LC. This value was unchanged by perfusion with adrenaline, increased medium Ca^{++}, or increased extracellular K^+. It was also unchanged in rabbits or rats with altered thyroid states (Litten *et al.*, 1981; P. J. England, unpublished observations), which cause changes in myosin isoenzyme patterns in the heart (Morkin, 1979). It would thus appear that with both short and long term changes in contractility there is no change in the phosphorylation state of P-LC in heart. However, perfusions with $^{32}P_i$ show that the phosphate in the P-LC is being rapidly turned over in rat heart under these conditions

(Jeacocke and England, 1980a). This indicates that the MLC kinase and phosphatase are both active in the heart. An explanation for these results has been suggested by Stull *et al.* (1981). Computer simulation has shown that once MLC kinase is activated by Ca-calmodulin, there is only a slow inactivation when the free Ca^{++} concentration falls. A half-time of inactivation of 1.3 s was calculated for skeletal muscle MLC kinase, and a similar value is likely for the heart enzyme. This suggests that in the intact heart, when the Ca^{++} concentration is fluctuating every beat, the MLC kinase does not have time to inactivate during diastole and so remains more or less fully activated. When the intracellular Ca^{++} is elevated by catecholamine or increased extracellular Ca^{++} there can be no further activation of the MLC kinase, and hence no change in P-LC phosphorylation. The exact level of phosphorylation will of course be determined by relative activities of MLC kinase and phosphatase in the tissue.

The lack of change in the level of P-LC phosphorylation with changes in the inotropic state of the heart indicate that P-LC phosphorylation cannot have a role in the regulation of contraction, at least over the short term. The results with altered thyroid states also suggest that longer term regulation is also unrelated to P-LC phosphorylation, although a wider variety of studies are required to substantiate this statement.

It should be pointed out that studies of P-LC phosphorylation in some laboratories have suggested changes during inotropic interventions. Kopp and Barany (1979) reported that in control perfusions of rat heart the P-LC has a phosphate content of 0.1 mol per mole, which was increased to 0.15 mol per mole with isoprenaline. These measurements were made indirectly from ^{32}P incorporation into P-LC measured by autoradiography. The very low control values suggest that this technique may lead to systematic errors in calculation of phosphate content. Resink *et al.* (1981a,b) found that in control rat heart perfusions the P-LC contained 0.07 mol phosphate per mole, and that this could be increased to 0.21 mol per mole with isoprenaline. Interestingly, if the rats had undergone a prior programme of exercise training, the level of phosphorylation of P-LC during perfusion with isoprenaline increased to 0.4 mol per mole. The low level of P-LC phosphorylation in control perfusions when compared to those obtained in most other laboratories is not readily explainable. However, if these results are not artefacts of the method of purifying light chains or assaying protein-bound phosphate, they do indicate a possible situation when changes in cardiac P-LC phosphorylation can occur.

Changes in P-LC phosphorylation have been well documented in fast-twitch skeletal muscle (Manning and Stull, 1979; Stull *et al.*, 1981). The level of phosphorylation of P-LC is low in resting extensor digitorum longus muscle. Following a 1 s tetanus there is an increase in phosphorylation of P-LC to 0.7 mol phosphate per mole, but this value was only reached 10 s

1976). Hartzell and Titus (1982) found that C-protein dephosphorylation in frog atria could also be stimulated by carbamylcholine, and that this appeared to be related to a cyclic GMP-stimulated mechanism (*vide supra*). These results suggest that troponin-I and C-protein are dephosphorylated by the same phosphoprotein phosphatase.

The function of C-protein phosphorylation is unknown. Indeed, because the function of C-protein itself is obscure it is not possible to make any definite suggestions at present. It is clear that when phosphorylation of C-protein occurs *in vivo* there will be a significant charge effect. If there are three C-protein molecules at each location, each with four phosphate groups attached, at pH 7 there will be 15–20 negative charges introduced at each 43 nm location on the thick filament. Whether this will affect thick filament structure, or myosin cross-bridge movement, or actin–myosin interaction is a matter for speculation at the moment.

GENERAL CONCLUSIONS

In Chapter 17 of this volume the role of protein phosphorylation in the control of Ca^{++} concentration will be discussed. This should probably be regarded as the fundamental point of regulation of contraction, with the phosphorylation of contractile proteins discussed in this chapter of subsidiary importance. Thus changes in contractility can be brought about by changes in intracellular Ca^{++} concentration without changes in phosphorylation of contractile proteins. However, particularly in terms of physiological changes in contractility induced by catecholamines and acetylcholine, changes in contractile protein phosphorylation are of real significance. Certainly in quantitative terms, contractile proteins represent the major proteins in heart in which the phosphate groups are being rapidly turned over (Jeacocke and England, 1980b; Onorato and Rudolph, 1981). Thus in hearts perfused with $^{32}P_i$ under control conditions the myosin P-LC accounts for 70–80% of protein-bound ^{32}P. After stimulation with adrenaline there is an increase in the ^{32}P bound to troponin-I and C-protein to roughly the same level as that for P-LC. These three proteins account for 90% of total protein-bound ^{32}P in the heart. Compared to these, the phosphate incorporated into an 11 000 dalton protein (probably phospholamban) (Chapter 17 in this volume) or phosphorylase is very small. It can be calculated that to phosphorylate troponin-I and C-protein at the rate observed in heart following stimulation with catecholamine requires more than 80% of the cAMP-PK present in the cell (England, 1976). Additionally, myosin LC kinase is a major Ca^{++}-stimulated kinase activity in the heart.

Krebs and Beavo (1979) put forward four criteria which must be satisfied before phosphorylation–dephosphorylation of a protein can be accepted as a physiological control mechanism. These may be stated as follows:

(1) The purified protein should be phosphorylated at a significant rate and in a stoicheiometric manner by an appropriate protein kinase, and dephosphorylated by a phosphoprotein phosphatase.

(2) The functional properties of the protein must undergo reversible, physiologically relevant changes *in vitro* which correlate with the degree of phosphorylation.

(3) The protein must be phosphorylated and dephosphorylated *in vivo* with accompanying physiological changes.

(4) A correlation should exist *in vivo* between the degree of phosphorylation of a protein and the cellular concentrations of effectors of the appropriate kinases and/or phosphatases.

In the case of the proteins discussed in this chapter, only troponin-I satisfies these criteria, and even then not completely. With myosin P-LC criterion (1) and part of (3) only have been satisfied, and with C-protein criterion (1), part of (3) and (4). Some of the problems arise because of the difficulty of establishing the exact function of a contractile protein which exists in the cell as one of many proteins in a highly ordered and complex system. It is therefore often impossible to make any meaningful measurements of physiological function on an isolated protein, and measurements on the whole assembly are not readily resolved into the effects of individual components. It should be noted these criteria have been satisfied in an even less satisfactory manner for phospholamban and other phosphorylated membrane proteins (Chapters 17 and 18 in this volume).

Proteins containing phosphate groups which are only slowly turned over, i.e. troponin-T and tropomyosin, were discussed briefly in this chapter. It is quite likely that other proteins also contain covalently bound phosphate groups of this type. There is some evidence that myosin heavy chains contain phosphate which has the same half-life as the protein itself (McPherson *et al.*, 1974). These phosphate groups are presumably of physiological significance, although not in short term regulation of contraction. It may be that for the correct tertiary structure of the protein, or the packing of proteins into organized filaments, the presence of negative charges are necessary. Changes in the level of phosphorylation could then affect filament assembly or function, giving a long term control which could be related to adaptive changes of the heart. However, few measurements of changes in phosphate content of such proteins have been made, and this hypothesis remains speculative. Indeed, it is quite probable that far more proteins than currently are known exist as phosphoproteins with slowly turning over phosphate groups, and a much wider role may exist for this type of phosphorylation than is realized at present.

REFERENCES

Adelstein, R. S. (1978). Myosin phosphorylation, cell motility and smooth muscle contraction. *Trends Biochem. Sci.*, **3,** 27–30.

Adelstein, R. S., Conti, M. A., Hathaway, D. R., and Klee, C. B. (1978). Phosphorylation of smooth muscle myosin light chain kinase by the catalytic subunit of adenosine 3′:5′ monophosphate-dependent protein kinase. *J. Biol. Chem.*, **253,** 8347–8350.

Aksoy, M. O., and Murphy, R. A. (1979). Temporal relationship betwen phosphorylation of the 20 000 dalton myosin light chain (LC) and force generation in arterial smooth muscle. *The Physiologist*, **22,** 2.

Aksoy, M. O., Williams, D., Sharkey, E. M., and Hartshorne, D. J. (1976). A relationship between Ca^{2+} sensitivity and phosphorylation of gizzard myosin. *Biochem. Biophys. Res. Commun.*, **69,** 35–41.

Bagshaw, C. R., and Reed, G. H. (1977). The significance of the slow dissociation of divalent metal ions from myosin regulatory light chains. *FEBS Lett.*, **81,** 386–390.

Bailey, C., and Villar-Palasi, C. (1971). Cyclic AMP-dependent phosphorylation of troponin. *Fed. Proc.*, **30,** 1147.

Bailin, G. (1979). Phosphorylation of a bovine cardiac actin complex. *Amer. J. Physiol.*, **236,** C41–C46.

Barany, M., Barany, K., Barron, J. T., Kopp, S. K., Doyle, D. D., Hager, S. R., Schlesinger, D. M., Homa, F., Sayers, S. T., and Janis, R. J. (1981). Protein phosphorylation in live muscle. *Cold Spring Harbor Conf. Cell Prolif.*, **8,** 869–886.

Barron, J. T., Barany, M., and Barany, K. (1979). Phosphorylation of the 20,000 dalton light chain of myosin of intact arterial smooth muscle in rest and in contraction. *J. Biol. Chem.*, **254,** 4954–4956.

Bhan, A., Malhotra, A., and Scheuer, J. (1981). Subunit function in cardiac myosin. *J. Biol. Chem.*, **256,** 7741–7743.

Bilezikjian, L. M., Kranias, E. G., Potter, J. D., and Schwartz, A. (1980). Calmodulin-dependent phosphorylation of cardiac sarcoplasmic reticulum. *Fed. Proc.*, **39,** 1663.

Brostrom, C. O., Hunkeler, F. L., and Krebs, E. G. (1971). The regulation of skeletal muscle phosphorylase kinase by Ca^{2+}. *J. Biol. Chem.*, **246,** 1961–1967.

Brunton, L. L., Hayes, J. C., and Mayer, S. E. (1979). Hormonally specific phosphorylation of cardiac troponin-I and activation of glycogen phosphorylase. *Nature*, **280,** 78–80.

Builder, S. E., Beavo, J. A., and Krebs, E. G. (1980). The mechanism of activation of bovine skeletal muscle protein kinase by cAMP. *J. Biol. Chem.*, **255,** 3514–3519.

Cheung, W. Y. (ed.) (1980). *Calcium and Cell Function*, Vol. 1, *Calmodulin*, Academic Press, New York.

Cohen, P. (1982). The role of protein phosphorylation in neural and hormonal control of cellular activity. *Nature*, **296,** 613–620.

Cohen, P., Burchall, A., Foulkes, G. J., Cohen, P. T. W., Vanamann, T. C., and Nairn, A. C. (1978). Identification of the Ca-dependent modulator protein as the fourth subunit of rabbit skeletal muscle phosphorylase kinase. *FEBS Lett.*, **92,** 287–293.

Cole, H. A., and Perry, S. V. (1975). The phosphorylation of troponin-I from cardiac muscle. *Biochem. J.*, **149,** 525–533.

Corbin, J. D., Sugden, P. M., West, L., Flockart, D. A., Lincoln, T. M., and McCarthy, D. (1978). Studies of the properties and mode of action of the purified regulatory subunit of bovine heart adenosine 3′:5′ monophosphate dependent protein kinase. *J. Biol. Chem.*, **253**, 3997–4003.

Craig, R., and Offer, G. (1976). The localisation of C-protein in rabbit skeletal muscle. *Proc. Roy. Soc. Lond. B*, **192**, 451–461.

DiSalvo, J., Gruenstein, E., and Silver, P. (1978). Ca^{2+} dependent phosphorylation of bovine aortic actomyosin. *Proc. Soc. Exp. Biol. Med.*, **158**, 410–414.

Driska, S. P., and Murphy, R. A. (1979). Phosphorylation of myosin light chain on stimulation of intact smooth muscle. *Biophys. J.*, **25**, 73a.

Ebashi, S. (1966). Excitation–contraction coupling, *Annu. Rev. Physiol.*, **38**, 293–313.

Ebashi, S. (1980). Regulation of muscle contraction. *Proc. Roy. Soc. Lond. B*, **207**, 259–286.

England, P. J. (1975). Correlation between contraction and phosphorylation of the inhibitory subunit of troponin in perfused rat heart. *FEBS Lett.*, **50**, 57–60.

England, P. J. (1976). Studies on the phosphorylation of the inhibitory subunit of troponin during modification of contraction in perfused rat heart. *Biochem. J.*, **160**, 295–304.

England, P. J. (1977). Phosphorylation of the inhibitory subunit of troponin in perfused hearts of mice deficient in phosphorylase kinase. *Biochem. J.*, **168**, 307–310.

England, P. J., Stull, J. T., Huang, T.-S., and Krebs, E. G. (1973). Phosphorylation and dephosphorylation of skeletal muscle troponin. *Metabolic Interconversions of Enzymes*, **3**, 175–184.

Ezrailson, E. G., Potter, J. D., Michael, L., and Schwartz, A. (1977). Positive inotropy induced by ouabain, by increased frequency, by X537A (R02-2985), by calcium and by isoproterenol: the lack of correlation with phosphorylation of Tn-I. *J. Mol. Cell. Cardiol.*, **9**, 693–698.

Frearson, N., and Perry, S. V. (1975). Phosphorylation of the light chain components of myosin from cardiac and red skeletal muscles. *Biochem. J.*, **151**, 99–107.

Frearson, N., Focant, B. W. W., and Perry, S. V. (1976a). Phosphorylation of light chain component of myosin from smooth muscle. *FEBS. Lett.*, **63**, 27–32.

Frearson, N., Solaro, R. J., and Perry, S. V. (1976b). Changes in phosphorylation of P light chain of myosin in perfused rabbit heart. *Nature*, **264**, 801–802.

Gazith, J., Himmelfarb, S., and Harrington, W. F. (1970). Studies on the subunit structure of myosin. *J. Biol. Chem.*, **245**, 15–22.

Gill, G. N., Holdy, K. E., Walton, G. M., and Kanstein, G. B. (1976). Purification and characterization of 3′:5′ cyclic GMP-dependent protein kinase. *Proc. Nat. Acad. Sci.*, **73**, 3918–3922.

Goldberg, N. D., and Haddox, M. K. (1977). Cyclic GMP metabolism and involvement in biological regulation. *Annu. Rev. Biochem.*, **46**, 823–896.

Grand, R. J. A., Wilkinson, J. M., and Mole, L. E. (1976). The amino acid sequence of rabbit cardiac troponin I. *Biochem. J.*, **159**, 633–641.

Greaser, M. L., and Gergely, J. (1971). Reconstitution of troponin activity from three protein components. *J. Biol. Chem.*, **246**, 4226–4233.

Gusev, N. B., Dobrovol'skii, A. B., and Severin, S. E. (1978). Skeletal muscle troponin and phosphorylation: site of troponin-T phosphorylated by specific protein kinase. *Biokhimiya*, **43**, 292–298.

Hartzell, H. C., and Titus, L. (1982). Effects of cholinergic and adrenergic agonists on phosphorylation of a 165,000-dalton myofibrillar protein in intact cardiac muscle. *J. Biol. Chem.* **257**, 2111–2120.

Herzig, J. W., and Ruegg, J. C. (1980). Investigation on glycinerated cardiac muscle fibres in relation to the problem of regulation of cardiac contractility-effects of Ca^{2+} and c-AMP. *Basic Res. Cardiol.*, **75**, 26–33.

High, C. W., and Stull, J. T. (1980). Phosphorylation of myosin in perfused rabbit and rat hearts. *Amer. J. Physiol.*, **239**, H756–H764.

Hofmann, F., and Wolf, H. (1981). Basic properties of myosin light chain kinase from bovine cardiac muscle. *Cold Spring Harbor Conf. Cell. Prolif.*, **8**, 841–848.

Hofmann, F., Beavo, J. A., Bechtel, P. J., and Krebs, E. G. (1975). Comparison of adenosine 3′:5′ monophosphate-dependent protein kinases from rabbit skeletal and bovine heart muscle. *J. Biol. Chem.*, **250**, 7795–7801.

Holroyde, M. J., Howe, E., and Solaro, R. J. (1979a). Modification of calcium requirements for activation of cardiac myofibrillar ATPase by cyclic AMP dependent phosphorylation. *Biochim. Biophys. Acta*, **586**, 63–69.

Holroyde, M. J., Potter, J. D., and Solaro, R. J. (1979b). The calcium binding properties of phosphorylated and unphosphorylated cardiac and skeletal myosins. *J. Biol. Chem.*, **154**, 6448–6482.

Holroyde, M. J., Small, D. A. P., Howe, E., and Solaro, R. J. (1979c). Isolation of cardiac myofibrils and myosin light chains with *in vivo* levels of light chain phosphorylation. *Biochim. Biophys. Acta*, **587**, 628–637.

Holt, J. C., and Lowey, S. (1975). An immunological approach to the role of the low molecular weight subunits in myosin. *Biochemistry*, **14**, 4600–4609.

Huang, F. L., and Glinsmann, W. M. (1976). Separation and characterisation of two phosphorylase phosphatase inhibitors from rabbit skeletal muscle. *Europ. J. Biochem.*, **70**, 419–426.

Jeacocke, S. A., and England, P. J. (1980a). Phosphorylation of myosin light chains in perfused rat heart. *Biochem. J.*, **188**, 763–768.

Jeacocke, S. A., and England, P. J. (1980b). Phosphorylation of a myofibrillar protein of M_r 150 000 in perfused rat heart, and the tentative identification of this as C-protein. *FEBS Lett.*, **122**, 129–132.

Kardami, E., Alexis, M., de la Paz, P., and Gratzer, W. (1980). Phosphorylation and the binding of calcium and magnesium to skeletal myosin. *Europ. J. Biochem.*, **110**, 153–160.

Klee, C. B. (1980). Calmodulin: structure–function relationships. In *Calmodulin and Cell Function*, Vol. 1 (W. Y. Cheung, ed.), Academic Press, New York, pp. 59–78.

Kopp, S. J., and Barany, M. (1979). Phosphorylation of the 19,000-dalton light chain of myosin in perfused rat heart under the influence of negative and positive inotropic agents. *J. Biol. Chem.*, **254**, 12007–12012.

Krebs, E. G., and Beavo, J. A. (1979). Phosphorylation–dephosphorylation of enzymes. *Annu. Rev. Biochem.*, **48**, 923–959.

Kumon, A., and Villar-Palasi, C. (1979). Purification and properties of troponin-T kinase from rabbit skeletal muscle. *Biochim. Biophys. Acta*, **566**, 305–320.

Kuo, J. F., and Greengard, P. (1970). Cyclic nucleotide dependent protein kinases. *J. Biol. Chem.*, **245**, 2493–2498.

Kuo, J. F., Kuo, W. N., Shoji, M., Davis, C. W., Seery, V. L., and Donnelly, T. E. (1976). Purification and general properties of guanosine 3′:5′-monophosphate dependent protein kinase from guinea pig fetal lung. *J. Biol. Chem.*, **251**, 1759–1766.

Lee, E. Y. C., Silberman, S. R., Ganapathi, M. K., Paris, H., and Petrovic, S. (1981). Properties of rabbit skeletal muscle protein phosphatases. *Cold Spring Harbor Conf. Cell Prolif.*, **8**, 425–440.

Lehman, W. (1978). Thin filament linked calcium regulation in vertebrate striated muscle. *Nature*, **274**, 80–81.

Le Peuch, C. H., Haiech, J., and Demaille, J. G. (1979). Concerted regulation of cardiac sarcoplasmic reticulum calcium transport by cyclic adenosine monophosphate dependent and calcium-calmodulin-dependent protein kinase. *Biochemistry*, **18**, 5150–5157.

Li, H.-C. (1981). Purification and properties of cardiac muscle phosphoprotein phosphatase and alkaline phosphatase isoenzymes. *Cold Spring Harbor Conf. Cell Prolif.*, **8**, 441–458.

Lincoln, T. M., and Corbin, J. D. (1977). Adenosine 3′ : 5′-cyclic monophosphate and guanosine 3′ : 5′-cyclic monophosphate-dependent protein kinases: possible homologous proteins. *Proc. Nat. Acad. Sci.*, **74**, 3239–3243.

Litten, R. Z., Martin, B. J., Howe, E. R., Alpert, N. R., and Solaro, R. J. (1981). Phosphorylation and adenosine triphosphatase activity of myofibrils from thyrotoxic rabbit hearts. *Circulation Res.*, **48**, 498–501.

McClellan, G. B., and Winegrad, S. (1978). The regulation of the calcium sensitivity of the contractile system in mammalian cardiac muscle. *J. Gen. Physiol.*, **72**, 737–764.

McCllellan, G. B., and Winegrad, S. (1980). Cyclic nucleoltide regulation of the contractile proteins in mammalian cardiac muscle. *J. Gen. Physiol.*, **75**, 283–296.

McPherson, J., Fenner, C., Smith, A., Mason, D. T., and Wikman-Coffelt, J. (1974). Identification of *in vivo* phosphorylated myosin subunits. *FEBS Let.*, **47**, 149–154.

Mak, A., Smillie, L. B., and Barany, M. (1978). Specific phosphorylation at serine-238 of α-tropomyosin from frog skeletal and rabbit skeletal and cardiac muscle. *Proc. Natl Acad. Sci.* **75**, 3588–3592.

Malhotra, A., Huang, S., and Bhan, A. (1979). Subunit function in cardiac myosin: effect of removal of LC2 (18 000 molecular weight) on enzymatic properties. *Biochemistry*, **18**, 461–467.

Manning, D. R., and Stull, J. T., (1979). Myosin-light chain phosphorylation and phosphorylase *a* activity in rat extensor digitorium longus muscle. *Biochem. Biophys. Res. Commun.*, **90**, 164–170.

Marston, S. B., Tervett, R. M., and Walters, M. (1980). Calcium ion-regulated thin filaments from vascular smooth muscle. *Biochem. J.*, **185**, 355–365.

Mikawa, T., Nonomura, Y., and Ebashi, S. (1977). Does phosphorylation of myosin light chain have direct relation to regulation in smooth muscle? *J. Biochem.*, **82**, 1780–1791.

Miyahara, M., and Noda, H. (1980). Interaction of C-protein with myosin. *J. Biochem.*, **87**, 1413–1420.

Moir, A. J. G., and Perry, S. V. (1977). The sites of phosphorylation of rabbit cardiac troponin I by adenosine 3′ : 5′-cyclic monophosphate-dependent protein kinase. *Biochem. J.*, **167**, 333–343.

Moir, A. J. G., and Perry, S. V. (1980). Phosphorylation of rabbit cardiac muscle troponin-I by phosphorylase kinase. *Biochem. J.*, **191**, 547–554.

Moir, A. J. G., Cole, H. A., and Perry, S. V. (1977). The phosphorylation sites of troponin-T from white skeletal muscle and the effects of interaction with troponin-C on their phosphorylation by phosphorylase kinase. *Biochem. J.*, **161**, 371–382.

Moir, A. J. G., Solaro, R. J., and Perry, S. V. (1980). The site of phosphorylation of troponin-I in the perfused rat heart. *Biochem. J.*, **185**, 505–513.

Moos, C., and Feng. I. M. (1980). Effect of C-protein on actomyosin ATPase. *Biochim. Biophys. Acta*, **632**, 141–149.

Moos, C., Offer, G., Starr, R., and Bennet, P. (1975). Interaction of C-protein with myosin, myosin rod and light meromyosin. *J. Mol. Biol.*, **97**, 1–9.

Moos, C., Mason, C. M., Besterman, J. M., Feng, I. M., and Dubin, J. H. (1978).

The binding of skeletal muscle C-protein to F-actin, and its relation to the interation of actin with myosin subfragment-1. *J. Mol. Biol.*, **124**, 571–586.

Mope, L., McClellan, G. B., and Winegrad, S. (1980). Calcium sensitivity of the contractile system and the phosphorylation of troponin in hyperpermeable cardiac cells. *J. Gen. Physiol.*, **75**, 271–282.

Morgan, J., Perry, S. V., and Ottaway, J. (1976). Myosin light chain phosphatase. *Biochem. J.*, **157**, 687–697.

Morimoto, K., and Harrington, W. F. (1974). Evidence for structural changes in vertebrate thick filament induced by calcium. *J. Mol. Biol.*, **88**, 693–709.

Morkin, E. (1979). Stimulation of cardiac myosin adenosine triphosphatase in thyrotoxicosis. *Circulation Res.*, **44**, 1–7.

Mrwa, U., Troschka, M., Gross, C., and Katzinski, L. (1980). Ca-sensitivity of pig carotid actomyosin ATPase in relation to phosphorylation of the regulatory light chain. *Europ. J. Biochem.*, **103**, 415–419.

Namm, D. H., Woods, E. L., and Zucker, J. L. (1972). Incorporation of the terminal phosphate of ATP into membrane protein of rabbit cardiac sarcoplasmic reticulum. *Circulation Res.*, **31**, 308–316.

Nimmo, H. G., and Cohen, P. (1977). Hormonal control of protein phosphorylation. *Advance. Cyclic Nucleotide Res.*, **8**, 145–266.

Offer, G., Moos, C., and Starr, R. (1973). A new protein of the thick filaments of vertebrate skeletal myofibrils. *J. Mol. Biol.*, **74**, 653–676.

Onorato, J. J., and Rudolph, S. A. (1981). Regulation of protein phosphorylation by inotropic agents in isolated rat myocarcial cells. *J. Biol. Chem.*, **256**, 10697–10703.

Pato, M. D., and Adelstein, R. S. (1980). Dephosphorylation of the 20,000 dalton light chain of myosin by two different phosphatases in smooth muscle. *J. Biol. Chem.*, **255**, 6535–6538.

Pemrick, S. M. (1980). The phosphorylated L2 light chain of skeletal muscle myosin is a modifier of the actomyosin ATPase. *J. Biol. Chem.*, **255**, 8836–8841.

Perrie, W. T., Smillie, L. B., and Perry, S. V. (1973). A phosphorylated light chain component of myosin from skeletal muscle. *Biochem. J.*, **135**, 151–164.

Perry, S. V., and Cole, H. A. (1974). Phosphorylation of troponin and the effects of interactions between the components of the complex. *Biochem. J.*, **141**, 733–743.

Perry, S. V., Cole, H. A., Frearson, N., Moir, A. J. G., Nairn, A. C., and Solaro, R. J. (1979). Phosphorylation of the myofibrillar proteins. *Proc. 12th FEBS Meeting*, **54**, 147–159.

Pires, E., Perry, S. V., and Thomas, M. A. W. (1974). Myosin light chain kinase, a new enzyme from striated muscle. *FEBS Lett.*, **41**, 292–296.

Ray, K. P., and England, P. J. (1976). Phosphorylation of the inhibitory subunit of troponin and its effect on the calcium dependence of myofibril adenosine triphosphatase. *FEBS Lett.*, **70**, 11–16.

Reddy, Y. S., and Wyborny, L. E. (1976). Phosphorylation of guinea pig cardiac natural actomyosin and its effect on ATPase activity. *Biochem. Biophys. Res. Commun.*, **73**, 703–709.

Reddy, Y. S., Ballard, D., Giri, N. Y., and Schwartz, A. (1973). Phosphorylation of cardiac native tropomyosin and troponin: inhibitory effect of actomyosin and the possible presence of endogenous myofibrillar-located cyclic AMP-dependent protein kinase. *J. Mol. Cell. Cardiol.*, **5**, 461–471.

Reimann, E. M., Walsh, D. A., and Krebs, E. G. (1971). Purification and properties of rabbit skeletal muscle adenosine 3′:5′-monophosphate-dependent protein kinases. *J. Biol. Chem.*, **246**, 1986–1995.

Resink, T. J., Gevers, W., Noakes, T. D., and Opie, L. H. (1981a). Increased cardiac myosin ATPase activity as a biochemical adaptation to running training: enhanced response to catecholamine and a role for myosin phosphorylation. *J. Mol. Cell. Cardiol.*, **13**, 679–694.

Resink, T. J., Gevers, W., and Noakes, T. D. (1981b). Effects of extracellular calcium concentration on myosin P light chain phosphorylation in hearts from running-trained rats. *J. Mol. Cell. Cardiol.*, **13**, 753–765.

Ribolow, H., and Barany, M. (1977). Phosphorylation of tropomyosin in live frog muscle. *Arch. Biochem. Biophys.*, **179**, 718–720.

Risnik, V. V., Dobrovol'skii, A. B., Gusev, N. B., and Severin, S. E. (1980). Phosphorylase kinase phosphorylation of skeletal muscle troponin-T. *Biochem. J.*, **191**, 851–854.

Roach, P. J., De Paoli-Roach, A. A., and Larner, J. (1978). Ca^{2+}-stimulated phosphorylation of muscle glycogen synthetase by phosphorylase kinase. *J. Cyclic Nucleotide Res.*, **4**, 245–266.

Robertson, S. P., Johnson, J. D. Holroyde, M. J., Kranias, E. G., Potter, J. D., and Solaro, R. J. (1982). The effect of troponin-I phosphorylation on the Ca^{2+}-binding properties of the Ca-regulatory site of bovine cardiac troponin. *J. Biol. Chem.*, **257**, 260–263.

Rosen, O. M., and Krebs, E. G. (eds) (1981). Protein phosphorylation. *Cold Spring Harbor Conf. Cell Prolif.*, **8**.

Rubio, R., Bailey, C., and Villar-Palasi, C. (1975). Effects of cyclic AMP-dependent protein kinase on cardiac actomyosin: increase in Ca^{2+} sensitivity and possible phosphorylation of Tn-I. *J. Cyclic Nucleotide Res.*, **1**, 143–150.

Shenolikar, S., and Cohen, P. (1978). The substrate specificity of cyclic AMP-dependent protein kinase. *FEBS Lett.*, **86**, 92–98.

Shenolikar, S., Cohen, P. T. W., Cohen, P., Nairn, A. C., and Perry, S. V. (1979). The role of calmodulin in the structure and regulation of phosphorylase kinase from rabbit skeletal muscle. *Europ. J. Biochem.*, **100**, 329–337.

Sobieszek, A. (1977). Ca-linked phosphorylation of a light chain of vertebrate smooth muscle myosin. *Europ. J. Biochem.*, **73**, 477–483.

Soderling, T. R., Sheorain, V. S., and Ericsson, L. M. (1979). Phosphorylation of glycogen synthetase by phosphorylase kinase. *FEBS Lett.*, **106**, 181–184.

Solaro, R. J., Moir, A. J. G., and Perry, S. V. (1976). Phosphorylation of troponin-I and the inotropic effect of adrenaline in perfused rabbit heart. *Nature*, **262**, 615–616.

Starr, R., and Offer, G. (1971). Polypeptide chains of intermediate molecular weight in myosin preparations. *FEBS Lett.*, **15**, 40–44.

Starr, R., and Offer, G. (1978). The interaction of C-protein with heavy meromyosin and subfragment-2. *Biochem. J.*, **171**, 813–816.

Stull, J. T. (1980). Phosphorylation of contractile proteins in relation to muscle function. *Advanc. Cyclic Nucleotide Res.*, **13**, 39–93.

Stull, J. T., and Buss, J. E. (1977). Phosphorylation of cardiac troponin by cyclic adenosine 3′:5′ monophosphate-dependent protein kinase. *J. Biol. Chem.*, **252**, 851–857.

Stull, J. T., and High, C. W. (1977). Phosphorylation of skeletal muscle contractile proteins *in vivo*. *Biochem. Biophys. Res. Commun.*, **77**, 1078–1083.

Stull, J. T. Brostrom, C. O., and Krebs, E. G. (1971). Phosphorylation of the inhibitor component of troponin by phosphorylase kinase. *J. Biol. Chem.*, **247**, 5272–5274.

Stull, J. T., Sanford, C. F., Manning, D. R., Blumenthal, D. K., and High, C. W. (1981). Phosphorylation of myofibrillar proteins in striated muscle. *Cold Spring Harbor Conf. Cell Prolif.*, **8**, 823–840.

Takhai, Y., Nishiyama, K., Yamamura, H., and Nishizuka, Y. (1975). Guanosine 3′:5′-monophosphate-dependent protein kinase from bovine cerebellum. *J. Biol. Chem.*, **250**, 4690–4695.

Vanamann, T. C. (1980). Structure, function and evolution of calmodulin. In *Calmodulin and Cell Function*, Vol. 1 (W. Y. Cheung, ed.), Academic Press, New York, pp. 41–58.

Vandenheede, J. R., Yang, S.-D. Goris, J., and Merleverde, W. (1981). Regulation of rabbit muscle MgATP-dependent protein phosphatase by the interaction with a cyclic AMP- and Ca^{2+}-independent synthetase kinase. *Cold Spring Harbor Conf. Cell Prolif.*, **8**, 497–512.

Villar-Palasi, C., and Kumon, A. (1981). Purification and properties of dog cardiac troponin-T kinase. *J. Biol. Chem.*, **256**, 7409–7415.

Walsh, D. A., and Cooper, R. H. (1979). The physiological regulation and function of cAMP-dependent protein kinases. *Biochem. Action Hormones*, **6**, 1–75.

Walsh, M. P., and Guilleux, J. C. (1981). Calcium and cyclic AMP-dependent regulation of myofibrillar calmodulin-dependent myosin light chain kinases from cardiac and skeletal muscles. *Advanc. Cyclic Nucleotide Res.*, **14**, 375–390.

Westwood, S. A., and Perry, S. V. (1981). The effect of adrenaline on the phosphorylation of the P light chain of myosin and troponin-I in the perfused rabbit heart. *Biochem. J.*, **197**, 185–193.

Wolf, H., and Hofmann, F. (1980). Purification of myosin light chain kinase from bovine cardiac muscle. *Proc. Natl Acad. Sci.*, **77**, 5852–5855.

Yamamoto, K., and Moos, C. (1981). A comparative study of C-proteins from heart and skeletal muscles. *Biophys. J.*, **33**, 237a.

Cardiac Metabolism
Edited by A. J. Drake-Holland and M. I. M. Noble
© 1983 John Wiley & Sons Ltd

CHAPTER 17

Modulation of Myocardial Membrane Function: Phosphorylation of Membrane Proteins

Angela J. Drake-Holland

Department of Medicine 1, St George's Hospital Medical School, London SW17, UK

and

Mark I. M. Noble

The Midhurst Medical Research Institute, Midhurst, West Sussex GU29 0BL, UK

INTRODUCTION

This chapter is intended to complement other sections in this book concerning calcium ions, excitation–contraction coupling, contractility, contractile proteins, and cyclic AMP. We discuss possible mechanisms whereby these functions can be carried out in sarcolemmal and sarcoplasmic reticulum membranes and their modification by metabolic alterations.

The principle physiological modulation of working ventricular myocardium is the control of contractility by the sympathetic nerves (noradrenaline release from sympathetic nerve terminals) and by circulating catecholamines. The interaction of these agonists with the cell membrane causes an increase in cyclic adenosine $3',5'$-monophosphate (cyclic AMP) which mediates some of the intracellular effects. The cyclic AMP-dependent processes affecting the membrane proteins will be reviewed; they have attracted considerable interest in recent years. However, it is probable that the Ca^{++}-dependent processes (calmodulin mediated) are of even greater importance, being essential for normal function. Catecholamines and cyclic AMP probably act merely as a booster for the basic system. However, owing to insufficient information, the calmodulin-dependent processes will take up less space in this account. Also taking up little space is a section on membrane lipid changes which may be very much more important than the protein changes; however, it is the latter which have received most attention in myocardium of late. Finally, we will attempt to give a very brief account of the influence of hydrogen ions.

THE THEORY OF CATECHOLAMINE ACTION VIA THE SECOND MESSENGER SYSTEM (CYCLIC AMP)

Many hormones, including catecholamines, interact with exterior cell-surface receptors to activate adenylate cyclase leading to an increase in intracellular cyclic AMP; the increase in cyclic AMP is held to be responsible for the intracellular effects of the hormone (Katz, 1979). There are many problems affecting the measurement of cyclic AMP and the interpretation of the literature (see Chapter 18 by van Belle in this volume). However, if we accept results as reported in the literature at their face value, we may question to what extent cyclic AMP may be responsible for the increased contractility and accelerated relaxation produced by catecholamines in mammalian ventricular myocardium. (In frog ventricle, contractility appears to depend on the ratio of cyclic AMP to cyclic GMP (Singh *et al.*, 1978).).

Cyclic AMP is thought to produce its effects by inducing phosphorylation of contractile proteins and membrane proteins. We will not be concerned with phosphorylation of contractile proteins in this chapter because this is dealt with by England (Chapter 16). In any case, the effect on the contractile proteins appears to be the induction of *decreased* sensitivity to calcium ions, (Ray and England, 1976; Allen and Blinks, 1978; Marban *et al.*, 1980; Herzig *et al.*, 1981). In the case of membrane proteins, phosphorylation might be expected to produce a positive inotropic effect. This possibility will be discussed together with the relative roles of cyclic AMP-dependent and cyclic AMP-independent mechanisms.

Before proceeding further we should dispense with the question of whether changes of cyclic AMP *during the cardiac cycle* are of importance. This feature has only been reported in frog myocardium (Brooker, 1973); this tissue may differ considerably from mammalian ventricle in which no oscillations in cyclic AMP have been shown (Dobson *et al.*, 1976), although further studies are required to settle this point. Even in frog, the evidence is dubious since the oscillations apparently do not occur in catecholamine-depleted tissue (Krause and Wollenberger, 1976). Isolated contractile proteins interact without the presence of cyclic AMP (e.g. Weber and Murray, 1973). Therefore we will assume that cyclic AMP does not have an obligatory role in the excitation–contraction cycle; our ideas on this process are summarized in Chapter 3 (in this volume). It seems to us more likely that cyclic AMP modulates certain cellular functions by change in its steady state concentrations.

Metabolic Mediation of Cyclic AMP Effects

Cyclic AMP increases the breakdown of tryglyceride and indirectly activates glycogen breakdown (Krebs, 1973; Mayer, 1974; van der Vusse and

Reneman, Chapter 10 in this volume). The effects of cyclic AMP are mediated by protein kinases (Walsh *et al.*, 1968; Kuo and Greengard, 1969). The enzymes concerned are substrate proteins for these kinases which catalyse the transfer of the terminal phosphate from ATP (protein phosphorylation; see also Chapter 16 by England in this volume). Since catecholamines produce (1) an increase in intracellular cyclic AMP, (2) increased contractility, and (3) more rapid relaxation, it is natural to postulate that (2) and (3) are caused by (1). However, it is equally possible that the increased cyclic AMP is solely concerned with increased breakdown of glycogen and triglyceride and that the effects of catecholamines on contractility and relaxation are mediated by other mechanisms. Entman *et al.* (1976) have shown that sarcoplasmic reticulum is a complex organelle containing enzyme complexes required for participation in glycogenolysis. Cyclic AMP-dependent protein kinase may only be present in sarcoplasmic reticulum and sarcolemmal vesicles (Wray *et al.*, 1973; Krause *et al.*, 1975) for this purpose and its presence does not therefore necessarily imply a role in other functions of these membranes, such as excitation–contraction coupling.

Dissociation of Effects of Catecholamines on Contractility and Relaxation

Catecholamines increase contractile force, shorten time to peak tension and induce earlier relaxation (Figure 17.1(a)). However, only the relaxant effect is completely blocked by the so-called beta-adrenergic blockers. In addition sympathomimetic amines lacking so called beta-adrenergic agonist activity, (i.e. alpha-adrenergic agonists) have a positive inotropic effect without shortening of time to peak force or production of earlier relaxation (Figure 17.1(b)), e.g. phenylephrine (Ledda *et al.*, 1975). This 'residual' positive inotropic effect is only blocked by so-called alpha-adrenergic blockade. What are we to make of this combination of facts?

We prefer not to be persuaded, just because both alpha and beta blockade are required to remove completely the positive inotropic effect of physiological catecholamines (a purely pharmacological aspect), that two *separate physiological mechanisms* for a positive inotropic effect exist. However we do conclude, since the inotropic and relaxing effects of catecholamines can be dissociated (Figure 17.1), that *these* two effects are subserved by different mechanisms.

Dissociation between the Positive Inotropic Effect of Catecholamines and Intracellular Cyclic AMP

As has been emphasized above, catecholamines produce both a positive inotropic effect and a transient rise in intracellular cyclic AMP. However,

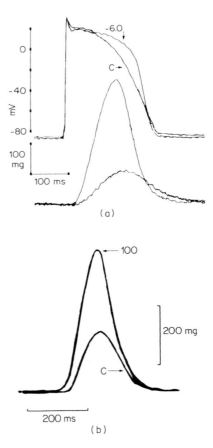

(a)

(b)

Figure 17.1 (a) Effect of isoprenaline on the action potential (above) and contraction (below) of dog papillary muscle. C and smaller twitch=control. −6.0 and larger
twitch = 10^{-6} M isoprenaline. Note elevation of action potential plateau voltage.
[Reproduced with permission from D. Nathan and G. W. Beeler, Jr, *J. Mol. Cell.
Cardiol.*, **7**, 1–15 (1975). Copyright: Academic Press Inc. (London) Ltd.] (b) Effect of
10^{-4} M phenylephrine (100) on contraction in guinea-pig ventricular muscle. C =
control. [Reproduced with permission from F. Ledda, P. Marchetti, and A. Mugelli,
Brit. J. Pharmacol., **54**, 83–90 (1975).]

such an association does not necessarily mean that one is the cause of the
other, and if the inotropic effect is sometimes not accompanied by an
increase in cyclic AMP, the logical conclusion is that they are not causally
linked.

The first point of disparity between the two effects is seen in published
accounts of the time courses of the effects (Figure 17.2; Tsien, 1977). It
seems clear that force development continues to rise after cyclic AMP levels

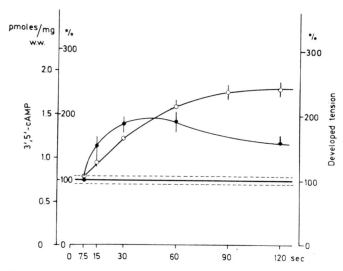

Figure 17.2 Time course of changes in contractile force (open circles) and cyclic AMP (closed circles) in rabbit papillary muscles exposed to 3×10^{-7} M isoproterenol. [Reproduced with permission from H. J. Schümann, M. Endoh, and O. E. Broddie, *Naunyn-Schmiedebergs Arch. Pharmacol.*, **289**, 291–302 (1975).]

have reached a peak and begun to decline. Furthermore, it was shown many years ago by Cheung and Williamson (1965) that an infusion of catecholamines in perfused whole hearts caused only a transient peak of cyclic AMP whereas, of course, the contractility increase is sustained throughout exposure to the drug. The immediate cause of the increased contractility (discussed later) is an increased influx of Ca^{++} across the sarcolemma and an increase in intracellular Ca^{++} (Katz, 1977). However, there is evidence that Ca^{++} actually *decreases* cyclic AMP levels (Namm *et al.*, 1968; Harary *et al.*, 1976). Furthermore, increased frequency of contractions which produces an increase of intracellular Ca^{++} and force (see Noble, Chapter 3 in this volume) is also associated with a decrease in cyclic AMP (Endoh *et al.*, 1976, Harary *et al.*, 1976). It seems reasonable to conclude that this results from stimulation of cyclic AMP phosphodiesterase (increasing the breakdown of cyclic AMP) by Ca^{++}. This effect of calcium is mediated by the 'modulator' or 'activator' protein, now called calmodulin (Cheung, 1971, 1980). We shall be returning to calmodulin later, but in the present context we are only concerned with the following questions: (1) Is the rise in intracellular calcium with catecholamines caused by the increase in cyclic AMP, or (2) is the rise in cyclic AMP incidental, and its subsequent fall as tension rises due to the rise in intracellular calcium?

The second idea is reinforced by the fact that positive inotropic effects of catecholamines can sometimes be dissociated completely from changes in cyclic AMP. One such circumstance is the 'alpha-adrenergic effect' discussed above (Schumann *et al.*, 1975). This non-cyclic AMP-related positive inotropic effect appears to be caused by increased Ca^{++} inflow, as judged by changes in action potential configuration; Giotti *et al.* (1973), showed that noradrenaline in the presence or absence of propranolol caused prolongation of the action potential in sheep Purkinje fibres.

Most important evidence for a dissociation between contractility and cyclic AMP comes from experiments by Venter *et al.* (1975) in which a catecholamine (isoprenaline) was administered to the surface of a papillary muscle while linked to glass beads' via a silicon–propylamido–phenyldiazo side chain. This produces a positive inotropic effect similar to that of soluble isoprenaline (the dose of soluble drug required being many orders of magnitude greater) but no change in cyclic AMP (Figure 17.3). The mechanism for this is controversial (Tsien, 1977). According to Venter's latest ideas (Venter, 1983) the catecholamine can influence the slow inward channel by an effect *within* the cell membrane. Whether these ideas are correct or not is immaterial to our argument, which is that if the positive inotropic effect can be obtained without the cyclic AMP effect, the former is not likely to be caused by the latter.

A dissociation in the other direction is obtained with papaverine, i.e. an increase in cyclic AMP without a positive inotropic effect (Henry *et al.*, 1975). A positive inotropic effect was found by others using higher concentrations of the drug (Endoh and Schumann, 1975). The argument that the

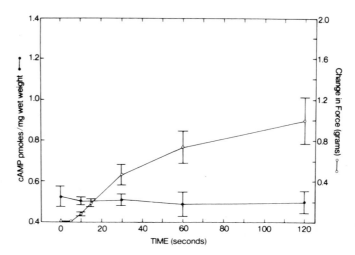

Figure 17.3   Effect of isoprenaline-glass beads on contractile force (open circles) and cyclic AMP (closed circles). [Reprroduced with permission from J. C. Ventner, J. Ross, and N. O. Kaplan, *Proc. Natl. Acad. Sci.*, **72**, 824–828 (1975).]

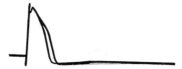

Figure 17.4 Effect of an isolated increase in intracellular cyclic AMP, produced by iontophoresis, on the transmembrane action potential. The plateau voltage (reflecting slow inward Ca^{++} current) is not affected. The action potential is shortened. [Redrawn with permission from R. W. Tsien, *Nature New Biol.*, **245,** 120–122 (1973). Copyright © 1973 Macmillan Journals Limited.]

negative inotropic effect of even higher doses of papaverine might have cancelled out the positive effect in Henry *et al.*'s experiments (Tsien, 1977) seems difficult to reconcile with the fact that these authors used the lowest concentrations. If Henry *et al.*'s results are correct, the hypothesis that cyclic AMP causes the positive inotropic effect of catecholamines seems to be disproved. The positive inotropic effect of catecholamines is produced by an increase in slow inward Ca^{++} current which increases the action potential plateau voltage (Figure 17.1(a)). Such an increase in plateau voltage does not occur if intracellular cyclic AMP is increased by iontophoresis (Figure 17.4).

In most tissues, alpha- and beta-adrenergic effects are distinct. There are pharmacologically distinct receptors causing biochemically different effects, i.e. non-cyclic AMP-mediated effects for alpha receptors and cyclic AMP-mediated effects for beta receptors. If we are correct in thinking that the balance of evidence in the literature favours a non-cyclic AMP mechanism for the inotropic response of the myocardium to catechomalimes (which is mainly beta-adrenergic), we are faced with a difficulty. The response does not fall into an otherwise tidy pharmacological-biochemical scheme. Is the general rule linking beta effects to cyclic AMP wrong or is our judgement of the evidence in this case wrong? One way round the difficulty would be to postulate that the cyclic AMP which matters for the inotropic effect is some small subcellular compartment, changes of which are undetectable in the presence of the total intracellular pool; this may be especially so in view of the difficulty of accurate and reproducible cyclic AMP measurements (Van Belle, Chapter 18 in this volume). Alternatively, it could be suggested that increased cyclic AMP turnover takes place without a change in cyclic AMP pool size. In either case, the apparently non-cyclic AMP positive inotropic effect of catecholamines, e.g. the isoprenaline–glass bead effect, should be accompanied by a detectable increase in adenylate cyclase activity. That cyclic AMP effects may occur in the absence of a detectable change in its concentration is shown by the isoproterenol-induced phosphorylation of troponin (England, Chapter 16 in this volume). This occurs at a much lower concentration of the drug than is required to increase the cyclic AMP (Onerato and Rudolph, 1981).

Lack of Dissociation between the Relaxant Effect of Catecholamines and Increases in Cyclic AMP

In our review of the literature we have not found a dissociation for the relaxant effect and cyclic AMP similar to that for the positive inotropic effect and cyclic AMP. For instance, with 'alpha-adrenergic' stimulation, there is no relaxant effect and no cyclic AMP increase. Conversely, glucagon produces enhanced relaxation with a non-adrenergic increase in cyclic AMP (Greef, 1976; Tsien, 1977).

Relaxation is generally held to be caused by sequestration of calcium ions (Ca^{++}) from the contractile proteins by the sarcoplasmic reticulum. Since Ca^{++} uptake by isolated sarcoplasmic reticulum is stimulated by cyclic AMP, adrenaline, and glucagon (Entman *et al.*, 1969), it seems reasonable to retain the hypothesis that this function of catecholamines is mediated by cyclic AMP.

THEORY OF ENHANCED RETICULAR Ca^{++} UPTAKE DUE TO PHOSPHORYLATION OF PHOSPHOLAMBAN

This idea has been put forward by Morkin and LaRaia (1974) and Katz *et al.* (1975) and is presented in Figure 17.5. Ca^{++} uptake by a microsomal (membrane vesicle) preparation rich in vesicles of sarcoplasmic reticulum was stimulated by cyclic AMP in the absence or presence of oxalate. (Oxalate precipitates Ca^{++} inside the vesicles and increases Ca^{++} uptake.) It was subsequently shown that a membrane-bound protein in sarcoplasmic reticulum vesicles, of molecular weight 22 000 daltons, is phosphorylated by cyclic AMP-dependent protein kinase. This occurs with the endogenous protein kinase within the microsomal preparation but can also be increased by adding more (exogenous) protein kinase (Figure 17.6). The protein which was phosphorylated by this reaction was called phospholamban by Katz (Tada *et al.*, 1973; Katz *et al.*, 1975). Dephosphorylation of phospholamban by treatment of the vesicles with phosphoprotein phosphatase decreases the rate of Ca^{++} uptake (Tada *et al.*, 1975). Phospholamban is separate from the Ca^{++}-dependent ATPase (molecular weight 90 000 daltons), but is thought to interact with and stimulate this enzyme when phosphorylated (Katz, 1977). It is now apparent that the 22 000 dalton protein is only obtained under certain preparative conditions and more consistently appears as 11 000 daltons; the 22 000 dalton unit may therefore be a dimer of two phopholamban molecules (Le Peuch *et al.*, 1980).

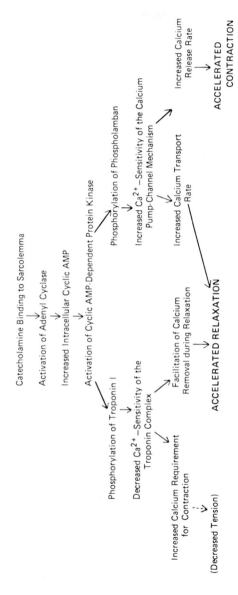

Figure 17.5 Scheme of Katz to explain the accelerated relaxation and contraction produced by catecholamines

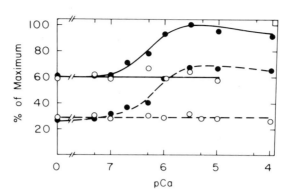

Figure 17.6 Phosphorylation of isolated cardiac sarcoplasmic reticulum as a function of pCa ($= -\log_{10}[Ca^{++}]$). O---O, catalysed by endogenous cAMP-protein kinase; ●--●, 10^{-7} M calmodulin also present; O—O, catalysed by exogenous cAMP-protein kinase; ●—●, 10^{-7} M calmodulin also present. [Reproduced with permission from L. M. Bilezikjian, E. G. Kranias, J. D. Potter, and A. Schwartz, *Circulation Res.*, **49**, 1356–1362 (1981)]

The hypothesis that these Ca^{++} uptake processes into sarcoplasmic reticulum could be responsible for relaxation depend on them having comparable time courses, i.e. 50–200 ms. The accumulation of Ca^{++} by microsomes, in the absence of oxalate, seems to be fast enough to account for the uptake of Ca^{++} during diastole (Will *et al.*, 1976). Stimulation of this rapid uptake by cyclic AMP-dependent protein kinase also seems to be sufficient to account for much of the decrease in relaxation time caused by catecholamines (Wollenberger and Will, 1978). These characteristics are all compatible with Katz's hypothesis, but it will be necessary to confirm them *in vivo*.

Can the Increased Ca^{++} Uptake by Sarcoplasmic Reticulum caused by Catecholamines lead to a Positive Inotropic Response?

Katz *et al.* (1975) also postulated that an increased rate of Ca^{++} uptake would lead to greater sarcoplasmic reticulum calcium content, to increased calcium release in subsequent contractions, and thus to enhanced contractility. According to the model of excitation–contraction coupling presented in Chapter 3 (see Figure 3.1 in this volume), this would not be the case. Ca^{++} would be sequestered more rapidly under the influence of cyclic AMP, leading to faster relaxation, but this does not increase the amount of Ca^{++} delivered to the release compartment. That can only occur through an increase in the *recirculated fraction* of Ca^{++}. In a recent study in our laboratory, this possibility was explored and disproved.

A further proposal of Katz (1979) is that phosphorylation of phospholamban could lead to accelerated contraction by stimulating Ca^{++} release. This is based on experiments over a time course of an hour (see Katz, 1979, Fig. 4) and implies a steady state change in background function of the membrane. By this mechanism, the release store (see Chapter 3 in this volume) could be discharged more rapidly each cycle.

Phosphorylation of Sarcolemmal Protein

Very similar results to those for sarcoplasmic reticulum vesicles have been obtained with sarcolemmal vesicles, namely: (1) accumulation of Ca^{++} in the presence of oxalate in an ATP-dependent process (Sulakhe *et al.*, 1976), (2) acceleration of this process by cyclic AMP (Sulakhe *et al.*, 1976), (3) stimulation of this acceleration by exogenous added protein kinases (Sulakhe *et al.*, 1976), (4) a resultant phosphorylation of membrane protein (Dowd *et al.*, 1976), (5) stimulation of Ca^{++} uptake in the absence of oxalate by cyclic AMP and protein kinase (Will *et al.*, 1973), and (6) phosphorylation of a sarcolemmal protein estimated to be of molecular weight 11 500–11 700 daltons (Wollenberger and Will, 1978) or 24 000 daltons (Krause *et al.*, 1975). A most important finding, which establishes this mechanism in a way which has not been done for sarcoplasmic reticulum, is that the process occurs *in vivo* (Walsh *et al.*, 1979). The proteins phosphorylated in this study included one of 27 000 daltons which had a distinctly separate mobility peak from that of phospholamban. This is not confirmed by more recent work which suggests that sarcolemma contains the same 11 000 dalton unit which many now identify as the phospholamban monomer.

The importance of these results is shown by the finding of Lullmann and Peters (1976) that sarcolemmal vesicles can form inside out. These vesicles can be identified by careful disruption to reveal the cell surface receptors within (Jones *et al.*, 1980). It is possible that such vesicles form a not inconsiderable portion of sarcoplasmic reticulum vesicles as a contaminant. This means that binding of calcium by such vesicles represents sequestration of Ca^{++} from the cell interior by the T-tubules, and that transport into the lumen by the Ca^{++} ATPase of these vesicles represents active extrusion of Ca^{++} into the extracellular space. The finding that these processes are accelerated by cyclic AMP-dependent protein kinase implies that this is a mechanism whereby catecholamines accelerate both Ca^{++} sequestration and Ca^{++} efflux by the sarcolemma. The balance between this Ca^{++} efflux and Ca^{++} binding and re-release intracellularly will determine the recirculation fraction. As stated in the previous section, this is found not to change in model analysis of physiological experiments.

A further feature of the experiments of Walsh *et al* (1979) is of interest. Phosphorylation of sarcolemmal protein in hearts perfused with adrenaline occurred more slowly than the increase in contraction. The increase in contraction had reached a maximum before a significant increase in phosphorylation had occurred. Therefore the phosphorylation of sarcolemmal proteins is unlikely to be the mechanism whereby adrenaline causes an increase in cytoplasmic Ca^{++}. This view is not altered by the fact that such phosphorylation may occur with right side out vesicles *in vitro* (Rinaldi *et al.*, 1981).

PHOSPHORYLATION OF CARDIAC MEMBRANES BY CALMODULIN-DEPENDENT PROTEIN KINASE

Ca^{++}-dependent, cyclic AMP-independent phosphorylation of microsomes (vesicles formed from cardiac membranes *in vitro*) was found by Namm *et al.* (1972). Katz and Remtulla (1978) reported that incubation of sarcoplasmic reticulum vesicles with calmodulin in the absence of cyclic AMP resulted in an enhancement of both Ca^{++} binding and Ca^{++} transport. Le Peuch *et al.* (1979) reported that, in the presence of Ca^{++}, calmodulin stimulates phosphorylation of phospholamban, a process which is totally inhibited by removing the Ca^{++} with EGTA. The reaction is unaffected by a cyclic AMP–protein kinase inhibitor. Similar results were obtained by Bilezikjian *et al.* (1980, 1981) who showed, in their 1981 paper, that the Ca^{++} ion concentrations required were in the range compatible with levels (10^{-7}–10^{-5} M) postulated to occur during the contraction–relaxation cycle of the heart (Katz, 1977).

Figure 17.6, taken from Bilezikjian *et al.* (1981), summarizes the present position regarding phosphorylation of phospholamban. At zero Ca^{++} concentration, phosphorylation proceeded at 30% of maximum under the influence of endogenous cyclic AMP-dependent protein kinase. This was increased to 60% by addition of exogenous cyclic AMP-dependent protein kinase. As Ca^{++} concentration was increased above 10^{-7} M (pCa 7), no difference was found in the absence of calmodulin (open circles). However in the presence of calmodulin, phosphorylation rose by a further 40% regardless of whether exogenous cyclic AMP-dependent protein kinase was present or not. With 1 μM free Ca^{++} present, the system was activated by calmodulin at a concentration of 10^{-7} M. The calmodulin-stimulated phosphorylation was inhibited by trifluoperazine, a calmodulin inhibitor.

What is the physiological significance of calmodulin-dependent phosphorylation of phospholamban (which is completely independent of cyclic AMP and the extent of saturation of the cyclic AMP-specific sites)? In a previous section, the case was made that relaxation could be due to calcium binding by the sarcoplasmic reticulum mediated by phospholamban phosphorylation. The finding that this phosphorylation is calmodulin-dependent means that sarcoplasmic reticulum Ca^{++} uptake will be stimulated by the rise in intracellular Ca^{++} which occurs during activation of contraction, because calmodulin is activated by Ca^{++} (Cheung, 1980). In Chapter 3 in this volume (Figure 3.9) is shown the possible time course of Ca^{++} binding to calmodulin. There must be some delay (not known as yet) between this process and the subsequent activation of calmodulin and phosphorylation of phospholamban. Assuming that there is enough phospholamban for this function, we may ask whether there is enough calmodulin-dependent protein kinase to phosphorylate it (and enough phosphatase – see below – to dephosporylate it). Figure 17.6 suggests that the Ca^{++}-activated phosphorylation could produce 35% of the maximum possible effect and this maximum must be way in excess of that occurring *in vivo*. If the system is quantitatively adequate, a dynamic delay in the processes of calmodulin, contractile protein, and phospholamban activations is all that would be required to produce automatic relaxation following contraction. Possibly the calmodulin-mediated process provides the basic mechanism for relaxation and this is only modulated by the addition of the cyclic AMP-dependent process which provides modifications of the speed of relaxation. This perspective has not been possible before because the cyclic AMP-dependent process was discovered first.

Two questions arise from these new findings:

(1) To what extent is the microsomal preparation used in these studies contaminated with inside-out vesicles of sarcolemma? For instance, Namm *et al.* (1972) took precautions to prevent mitochondrial contamination but did not determine what proportion of their 'sarcoplasmic reticulum' was inside-out sarcolemma.

(2) Would similar results be obtained with microsomal preparations enriched with such sarcolemmal vesicles?

It does not seem improbable that calmodulin might phosphorylate a similar protein on the plasma membrane causing it to bind Ca^{++}. This would imply a similar role in relaxation for the T-tubules to that of sarcoplasmic reticulum. Furthermore if the finding of calmodulin-mediated increased Ca^{++} transport by Ca^{++}-ATPase in sarcoplasmic reticulum (Katz and Remtulla, 1978, Lopaschuk *et al.*, 1980) can be extrapolated to the sarcolemma, it would imply that calmodulin not only plays a vital role in relaxation but also in active extrusion of Ca^{++} from the cell with each contraction–relaxation cycle, i.e. beat-dependent Ca^{++} efflux (Chapter 3 in this volume).

Ca-ATPase of Sarcolemmal and Sarcoplasmic Reticulum Membranes

As mentioned in previous sections, there is a Ca^{++} transport system in sarcoplasmic reticulum vesicles which is closely associated with Ca-dependent ATPase activity (Suko, 1973). It appears that this enzyme protein acts by transfer of phosphate from ATP to a phosphorylated intermediate (Namm *et al.*, 1972; Pang and Briggs, 1973) which is distinct from phospholamban, having a molecular weight of 90 000–100 000 (Fanburg and Matsushita, 1973). Its formation is sensitive to Ca^{++} concentration over the range 10^{-8}–10^{-5} M (Suko and Hasselbach, 1975). The activity of the enzyme appears to be controlled by phosphorylation of phospholamban (see previous section).

> 'Plasma membrane Ca^{++}-ATPase is generally believed to be the Ca^{++} pump responsible for extruding Ca^{++} from the cytoplasmic compartment. An increase of intracellular Ca^{++} activates the Ca^{++}-ATPase and increases the Ca^{++} efflux; this action would constitute a self-regulating device for maintaining a low steady-state level of intracellular Ca^{++}. Thus, Ca^{++} modulates not only the activity of Ca^{++}-ATPase, but also its own cellular concentration' (Cheung, 1980).

The presence of a sarcolemmal ATP-dependent Ca^{++}-pumping system in heart has been confirmed by Caroni and Carafoli (1980). In heart muscle the Ca^{++} pump might be expected to extrude the Ca^{++} bound by the sarcolemma during relaxation in proportion to the quantity of Ca^{++}, i.e. a beat-dependent Ca^{++} efflux which is so vital for long term stability of the excitation–contraction–relaxation cycle (Chapter 3 in this volume; Noble, 1979). Na^+–Ca^{++} exchange (Chapter 6 in this volume) would also be expected to cause Ca^{++} efflux proportional to intracellular Ca^{++} (this would be electrogenic). However, the increased Ca^{++} flux associated with catecholamines does not appear to be accompanied by increased Na^+–Ca^{++} exchange (Jundt *et al.*, 1975).

Dephosphorylation of phospholamban and the Ca^{++} ATPase intermediate

If phosphorylation of membrane proteins is thought to mediate relaxation, they must be dephosphorylated before the next following relaxation. This function may be subserved by the phosphoprotein phosphatase activity in sarcoplasmic reticulum vesicles (LaRaia *et al.*, 1973; LaRaia and Morkin, 1974). Further characterization of the microsomal phosphatase was carried out by Tada *et al.* (1975). However, it remains to be seen whether this and other similar processes are quantitatively adequate and sufficiently rapid to carry out complete dephosphorylation within diastole.

Modulation of Ionic Conductances of the Cell Membrane

This subject is also discussed in Chapter 3 (in this volume), particularly in relation to the dependence of slow inward calcium current on interval between beats and intracellular calcium. In the present context, the influence of catecholamines is the first to be examined. The positive inotropic effect of catecholamines appears to be solely due to this effect. In our own experiments mentioned in a previous section where we found no change in 'recirculated calcium fraction', we consistently found an increase in the residual contractility during adrenaline infusion.

According to the model presented in Chapter 3 (in this volume), this residual contractility depends upon the action potential duration (*shortened* by adrenaline in our preparation), the calcium conductance, and the sensitivity of the contractile proteins to Ca^{++} (*decreased* by adrenaline). Thus there must have been a very large increase in calcium conductance, i.e. catecholamines increase contractility by increasing Ca^{++} entry during the action potential, leading to an accumulation of Ca^{++} in the internal stores.

Evidence that cyclic AMP mediates this effect is weak in that it depends upon a correlation between intracellular cyclic AMP increases produced by dibutyryl cyclic AMP (a synthetic cyclic AMP derivative) and the positive inotropic effect produced by this agent (Tsien, 1977). In a previous section we explained that the many instances of lack of correlation between cyclic AMP rises and the positive inotropic effect of catecholamines negate such correlations. We must therefore search for a non-cyclic AMP-dependent mechanism.

Promotion of Ca^{++} entry into cardiac cells by catecholamines has been demonstrated by tracer flux studies using ^{45}Ca (Grossman and Furchgott, 1964; Reuter, 1965) and by measurements of slow inward current (Reuter, 1967; Vassort *et al.*, 1969; Reuter, 1974). An increase in slow inward current appears on the first depolarization after exposure to noradrenaline (Figure 17.7) while the increased force appears on the second depolarization. This is because the extra Ca^{++} entering on beat 1 must enter the uptake compartment and only becomes releasable subsequently (see Chapter 3 in this volume). The characterization of the behaviour of adrenaline in relation to slow inward current, internal calcium stores, and the relaxant effect has been carried out in a series of papers by Morad (Kavaler and

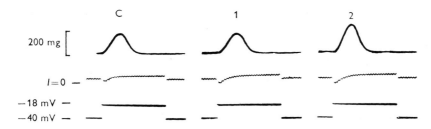

Figure 17.7 Voltage clamp studies of cat papillary muscle. Traces: upper = tension; middle = slow inward current; lower = membrane potential. C = control. 1 and 2 = first and second depolarizations after exposure to noradrenaline. [Reproduced with permission from H. Reuter, *J. Physiol.* (*Lond.*), **242**, 429–451 (1974)]

Morad, 1966; Morad, 1969; Morad and Rolett 1972; Morad *et al.*, 1978; Morad, 1983).

The increase in slow inward current with catecholamines appears to be a true increase in conductance because the reversal potential (membrane potential at which current is zero) is not affected, nor is the voltage and time-dependent opening and closing of the channels (Reuter, 1974). The mechanism is, at present, conjectural (Venter, 1982).

The effect of catecholamines on the action potential is consistent as far as elevation of the plateau is concerned (Figure 17.1(a)) but inconsistent with regard to action potential duration. In some species the duration is prolonged, e.g. rabbit, whereas in others it is shortened, e.g. dog (Figure 17.1(a)). This suggests a species-dependent increase in outward current. One possibility is an increase in slow potassium current as described in Purkinje fibres, which is stimulated by adrenaline (Tsien *et al.*, 1972).

There is evidence in the same tissue (Purkinje fibre) that the shortening of the action potential (but not the elevation of potential on the plateau which is due to Ca^{++} current) is mediated by cyclic AMP (Figure 17.4). Tsien (1973) investigated this by increasing intracellular cyclic AMP by iontophoresis. Figure 17.4 is redrawn from Tsien's Figure 1A and shows the shortening effect. After prolonged exposure there is a decline in the plateau voltage the significance of which is unclear.

MODULATION OF MEMBRANE LIPIDS – PHOSPHATIDYLINOSITOL AND PHOSPHATIDYLSERINE

We have paid greatest attention in this chapter to membrane proteins. This gives an unbalanced view because the basic membrane structure is a lipid bilayer, the lipid component being of primary importance in membrane function. The anionic lipids phosphatidylinositol and phosphatidylserine, for instance, bind Ca^{++} avidly. The ratio of Ca^{++} bound to lipid reaches a maximum when the spacing between phospholipid molecules is most favourable for the electrostatic attachment of Ca^{++}, i.e. the spacing between the phospholipid approaches the diameter of hydrated Ca^{++} (Hauser *et al.*, 1969). The possible role of phosphatidylserine in excitation–contraction coupling is outlined in the chapter by Lüllman *et al.* (Chapter 1 in this volume). The emphasis on proteins in this chapter reflects the predominance work on this subject has been given in the literature (Tsien, 1977; Katz, 1979; England, 1980).

In tissues other than myocardium, the importance of inositol phospholipids is well recognized (Mitchell, 1975). They appear to be involved in the responses to a number of agonists, e.g. muscarinic, cholinergic, beta-adrenergic, and insulin; these responses are not associated with an increase

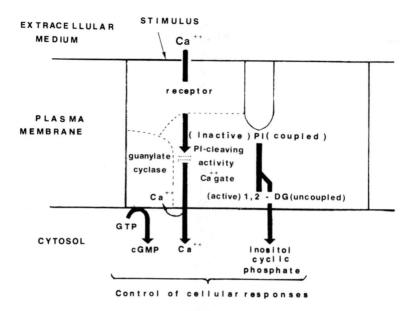

Figure 17.8 Hypothetical scheme of Michell (1975) for phosphatidylinositol-linked phenomena in the cell membrane. PI, phosphatidylinositol; 1,2-DG, 1,2-diacylglycerol

in cyclic AMP but are associated with an increase in cyclic GMP (Mitchell, 1975). The role of cyclic GMP in mammalian myocardial cells is unclear; it may control the effects of the beta-adrenergic agonists–receptor interaction (Watanabe *et al.*, 1982). In Figure 17.8 we reproduce Michell's suggested model for the events in lipid metabolism in a cell exposed to an appropriate stimulus. This process of phosphatidylinositol cleavage may control Ca^{++} movements at the plasma membrane, e.g. in smooth muscles Ca^{++} entry by inward current is enhanced. Although cardiac muscle could be expected to differ, there is sufficient in common between the Ca^{++} channels of the two tissues (e.g. both blocked by verapamil) to indicate that a response of the kind illustrated in Figure 17.8 could be responsible for the increased Ca^{++} conductance produced by catecholamines.

One of the intermediate metabolites in the phosphatidylinositol breakdown and resynthesis cycle (Figure 17.9) is phosphatidic acid. It has recently been suggested that this acts as an ionophore (Putney *et al.*, 1980; Salmon and Honeyman, 1980; Harris *et al.*, 1981), i.e. it produces an increase in Ca^{++} conductance. This may provide the mechanism whereby phosphatidylinositol turnover, stimulated by an external hormone, may produce increased Ca^{++} entry.

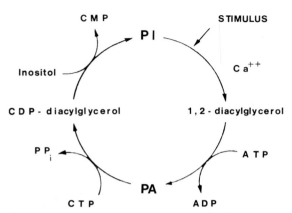

Figure 17.9 The phosphatidylinositol breakdown and resynthesis cycle. PI = phosphatidylinositol; PA = phosphatidic acid

In smooth muscles which contract in response to acetylcholine, the early tension rise is dependent on Ca^{++} which is released from binding to the plasma membrane (the later maintained response requires Ca^{++} entry from the exterior) (Chang and Triggle, 1972). This idea of membrane-bound pools of Ca^{++} from which Ca^{++} is released to the interior is applied to myocardium by Lüllman *et al.* (Chapter 1 in this volume) so that the plasma membrane (sarcolemma) is a possible site for the intracellular Ca^{++} store in excitation–contraction coupling (Chapter 3 in this volume).

If Mitchell's ideas on cells in general are of any relevance to heart cells, it will also be necessary to consider the possibility that the adenylate cyclase in plasma membranes is dependent on its interactions with anionic lipids, particularly phosphatidylinositol and phosphatidylserine (Mitchell, 1975). In addition, phosphatidylinositol cleavage will also probably lead to an increased intracellular concentration of inositol cyclic phosphate which may act synergistically with Ca^{++} (Mitchell, 1975).

Hydrogen Ions and Membrane Function

The influence of pH on membranes is a more basic problem than the foregoing, but may not be relevant in physiological circumstances. It has been established that acidosis has a negative inotropic effect which is greater for a respiratory acidosis (hypercapnia) than for a metabolic acidosis (Noble *et al.*, 1967; Johannsson and Nilsson, 1975, I; Poole-Wilson and Langer, 1975), i.e. a fall in intracellular pH (caused by hypercapnia) is a more potent depressor than a fall in extracellular pH. It is also established that this effect is much greater in cardiac than in skeletal muscle (Pannier and Leusen, 1968; Pannier *et al.*, 1970).

Hydrogen ions decrease the sensitivity of the contractile proteins by interacting with the calcium-binding site of troponin (Fuchs *et al.*, 1970) and reducing myofibrillar ATPase activity (Williams *et al.*, 1975). However, this would not cause the difference between cardiac and skeletal muscle (Fabiato and Fabiato, 1978) which is presumably due to a greater effect on cardiac membranes. Pang (1980) showed that acidosis decreased Ca^{++} uptake by fragmented sarcoplasmic reticulum and Mandel *et al.* (1982) showed slowed rates of formation and decomposition of the phosphorylated intermediate of the ATPase; a major role for this organelle in the effect is proposed by Fabiato and Fabiato (1978). However, the way this is postulated to effect contractility is by a mechanism which is the inverse of that proposed by Katz for increased contractility due to cyclic AMP (above), i.e. decreased uptake into the sarcoplasmic reticulum results in less Ca^{++} in the release compartment. As explained in connection with cyclic AMP, this implies a change in the recirculated fraction of Ca^{++} (Chapter 3 in this volume). Recent experiments in our laboratory showed that this was 0.86 before and 0.83 during hypercapnia, a non-significant change. We suggest that this result reduces the likelihood of a dominant sarcoplasmic reticulum-mediated mechanism.

The other possibility is for hydrogen ions to reduce sarcolemmal calcium conductance during the action potential. Acidosis has been shown by Kohlhardt *et al.* (1976) to depress slow inward Ca^{++} current in myocardium. In our experiments, the residual contractility was significantly lower (134 mmHg s^{-1} compared to 178 mmHg s^{-1}) during hypercapnia. This term is dominated by the duration of the action potential (unchanged; Johannsson and Nilsson, 1975, II) and a coefficient named B_{AP} (see Chapter 3 in this volume). In a preliminary experiment B_{AP} was reduced from 14.6 to 6.6 (mmHg s^{-1} ms^{-1}) by hypercapnia. B_{AP} is determined by the calcium conductance of the cell membrane and the sensitivity to Ca^{++} of the contractile proteins (see Figure 3.1(d) in this volume). If the effect on the contractile proteins is comparable in skeletal and cardiac muscle, it follows that the greater effect on contractility in cardiac muscle is likely to be caused by the decreased calcium conductance of the cell membrane. Such an effect is not surprising since hydrogen ions would be expected to bind to anionic lipids in the cell membrane. Williamson *et al.* (1975) could not demonstrate clear-cut competititon between H^+ and Ca^{++} in isolated sarcolemma. However, Na^+–Ca^{++} exchange in this preparation is inhibited by acidity (Philipson *et al.*, 1982).

REFERENCES

Allen, D. G., and Blinks, J. R. (1978). Calcium transients in aequorin-injected frog cardiac muscle. *Nature*, **273**, 509–513.
Bilezikjian, L. M., Kranias, E. G., Potter, J. D., and Schwartz, A. (1980). Calmodulin-stimulated phosphorylation of cardiac sarcoplasmic reticulum. *Fed. Proc.*, **39**, 1663 (Abstr.).

Bilezikjian, L. M., Kranias, E. G., Potter, J. D., and Schwartz, A. (1981). Studies on phosphorylation of canine cardiac sarcoplasmic reticulum by calmodulin-dependent protein kinase. *Circulation Res.*, **49**, 1356–1362.

Brooker, G. (1973). Oscillation of cyclic adenosine monophosphate concentration during the myocardial contraction cycle. *Science*, **182**, 933–934.

Caroni, P., and Carafoli, E. (1980). An ATP-dependent Ca^{++}-pumping system in dog heart sarcolemma. *Nature*, **283**, 765–767.

Chang, K. J., and Triggle, D. J. (1972). In *The Role of Membranes in Metabolic Regulation*. (M. A. Mehlman and R. W. Hauson, eds). Academic Press, New York, pp. 59–110.

Cheung, W. Y. (1971). Cyclic 3',5'-nucleotide phosphodiesterase. Evidence for and properties of a protein activator. *J. Biol. Chem.*, **246**, 2859–2869.

Cheung, W. Y. (1980). Calmodulin plays a pivotal role in cellular regulation. *Science*, **207**, 19–27.

Cheung, W. Y., and Williamson, J. R. (1965). Kinetics of cyclic adenosine monophosphate changes in rat heart following epinephrine administration. *Nature*, **207**, 979–981.

Dobson, J. G., Ross, J., and Mayer, S. E. (1976). The role of cyclic adenosine 3',5'-monophosphate and calcium in the regulation of contractility and glycogen phosphorylase activity in guinea pig for papillary muscle. *Circulation Res.*, **39**, 388–395.

Dowd, F. J., Pitts, B. J. R., and Schwartz, A. (1976). Phosphorylation of a low molecular weight polypeptide in beef heart Na^+,K^+-ATPase preparations. *Arch. Biochem. Biophys.*, **175**, 321–331.

Endoh, M., Brodde, O. E., Reinhardt, D., and Schumann, H. J. (1976). Frequency dependence of cyclic AMP in mammalian myocardium. *Nature*, **261**, 716–717.

Endoh, M., and Schumann, H. J. (1975). Effects of papaverine on isolated rabbit papillary muscle. *Europ. J. Pharmacol.*, **30**, 213–220.

England, P. J. (1980). Protein phosphorylation in the regulation of muscle contraction. In *Recently Discovered Systems of Enzyme Regulation by Reversible Phosphorylation* (P. Cohen, ed.), Elsevier North-Holland Biomedical Press, Amsterdam.

Entman, M. L., Levey, G. S., and Epstein, S. E. (1969). Mechanism of action of epinephrine and glucagon on the canine heart. *Circulation Res.*, **25**, 429–438.

Entman, M. L., Kaniike, K., Goldstein, M. A., Nelson, T. E., Bornet, E. P., Futch, T. W., and Schwartz, A. (1976). Association of glycogenolysis with cardiac sarcoplasmic reticulum. *J. Biol. Chem.*, **251**, 3140–3146.

Fabiato, A., and Fabiato, F. (1978). Effects of pH on the myofilaments and the sarcoplasmic reticulum of skinned cells from cardiac and skeletal muscles. *J. Physiol. (Lond.)*, **276**, 233–255.

Fanburg, B. L., and Matsushita, S. (1973). Phosphorylated intermediate of ATPase of isolated cardiac sarcoplasmic reticulum. *J. Mol. Cell. Cardiol.*, **5**, 111–115.

Fuchs, F., Reddy, Y., and Briggs, F. N. (1970). The interaction of cations with the calcium-binding site of troponin. *Biochim. Biophys. Acta.* **221**, 407–409.

Giotti, A., Ledda, F., and Mannioni, P. F. (1973). Effects of noradrenaline and isoprenaline in combination with α and β receptor blocking substances, on the action potential of cardiac Purkinje fibres. *J. Physiol. (Lond.)*, **229**, 99–113.

Greef, K. (1976). Einfluss von Pharmaka auf die Kontraktilitat des Herzems. *Verh. Deut. Ges. Kreislauforsch.*, **42**, 80–92.

Grossman, A., and Furchgott, R. F. (1964). The effect of various drugs on calcium exchange in the isolated guinea pig left auricle. *J. Pharmacol. Exp. Ther.*, **145**, 162–172.

Harary, I. Renaud, J.-F., Sato, E., and Wallace, G. A. (1976). Calcium ions regulate cyclic AMP and beating in cultured heart cells. *Nature*, **261,** 60–61.

Harris, R. A., Schmidt, J., Hitzemann, B. A., and Hitzemann, R. J. (1981). Phosphatidate as a molecular link between depolarization and neurotransmitter release in the brain. *Science*, **212,** 1290–1291.

Hauser, H., Chapman, D., Dawson, R. M. C. (1969). Physical studies of phospholipids. XI. Ca^{++} binding to monolayers of phosphatidylserine and phosphatidylinositol. *Biochim. Biophys. Acta*, **83,** 320–333.

Henry, P. D., Dobson, J. G., and Sobel, B. E. (1975). Dissociations between changes in myocardial cyclic adenosine monophosphate and contractility. *Circulation Res.*, **36,** 392–400.

Herzig, J. W., Kohler, G., Pfizer, G., Ruegg, J. C., Woffle, G. (1981). Cyclic AMP inhibits contractility of detergent-treated glycerol extracted cardiac muscle. *Pflügers Arch. Europ. J. Physiol.*, **391,** 208–212.

Johannsson, M., and Nilsson, E. (1975). Acid–base changes and excitation–contraction coupling in rabbit myocardium. I. Effects on isometric tension development at different contraction frequencies. II. Effects on resting membrane potential, action potential characteristics and propagation velocity. *Acta. Physiol. Scand.*, **93,** 295–317.

Jones, L. R., Maddock, S. W., and Besch, H. R., Jr (1980). Unmasking effect of alametnicin on the (Na^+, K^+)-ATPase, β-adrenergic receptor-coupled adenylate cyclase, and cAMP-dependent protein kinase activities of cardiac sarcolemmal vesicles. *J. Biol. Chem.*, **255,** 9971–9980.

Jundt, H., Porzig, H., Reuter, H., and Stucki, J. W. (1975). The effect of substances releasing intracellular calcium ions on sodium-dependent calcium efflux from guinea-pig auricles. *J. Physiol. (Lond.)*, **246,** 229–253.

Katz, A. M. (1977). *Physiology of the Heart*, Raven Press, New York.

Katz, A. M. (1979). Role of the contractile proteins and sarcoplasmic reticulum in the response of the heart to catecholamines: an historical review. *Advanc. Cyclic Nucleotide Res.*, **11,** 303–343.

Katz, S., and Remtulla, M. A. (1978). Phosphodiesterase protein activator stimulates calcium transport in cardiac microsomal preparations enriched in sarcoplasmic reticulum. *Biochem. Biophys. Res. Commun.*, **83,** 1373–1379.

Katz, A. M., Tada, M., and Kirchberger, M. A. (1975). Control of calcium transport in the myocardium by the cyclic AMP–protein kinase system. *Advanc. Cyclic Nucleotide Res.*, **5,** 453–472.

Kavaler, F., and Morad, M. (1966). Paradoxial effects of epinephrine on excitation–contraction coupling in cardiac muscle. *Circulation Res.*, **18,** 492–501.

Kohlhardt, M., Haap, K., and Figulla, H. R. (1976). Influence of low extracellular pH upon Ca inward current and isometric contractile force in mammalian ventricular myocardium. *Pflügers Arch. Europ. J. Physiol.*, **366,** 31–38.

Krause, E. G., Will, H., Schirpke, B., and Wollenberger, A. (1975). Cyclic AMP-enhanced protein phosphorylation and calcium binding in a cell membrane-enriched fraction from myocardium. *Advanc. Cyclic Nucleotide Res.*, **5,** 473–490.

Krause, E. G., and Wollenberger, A. (1976). Cyclic nucleotides and heart. In *Cyclic Nucleotides: Mechanism of Action* (H. Cramer and J. Schultz, eds), John Wiley, New York.

Krebs, E. G. (1973). The mechanism of hormonal regulation by cyclic AMP. In *Endocrinology: Proceedings of the 4th International Congress*, Excerpta Medica, Amsterdam.

Kuo, J. F., and Greengard, P. (1969). Cyclic nucleotide-dependent protein kinase.

IV. Widespread occurrence of adenosine 3′,5′-monophosphate dependent protein kinase in various tissues and phyla of the animal kingdom. *Proc. Natl Acad. Sci.*, **64**, 1349–1355.

La Raia, P. J., and Morkin, E. (1974). Phosphorylation-dephosphorylation of cardiac microsomes; a possible mechanism for control of calcium uptake by cyclic AMP. *Recent Advanc. Stud. Cardiac Struct. Metab.*, **4**, 417–426.

La Raia, P. J., Zwerling, L. J., and Morkin, E. (1973). Phosphorylation–dephosphorylation of cardiac microsomes; a possible mechanism for control of calcium uptake by cyclic AMP. *Fed. Proc.*, **32**, 346.

Ledda, F., Marchetti, P., and Mugelli, A. (1975). Studies on the positive inotropic effect of phenylephrine. A comparison with isoprenaline. *Brit. J. Pharmacol.*, **54**, 83–90.

Le Peuch, C. J., Haiech, J., and Demaille, J. G. (1979). Concerted regulation of cardiac sarcoplasmic reticulum calcium transport by cyclic adenosine monophosphate dependent and calcium-calmodulin-dependent phosphorylation. *Biochemistry*, **18**, 5150–5157.

Le Peuch, C. J., Le Peuch, D. A. M., and Demaille, J. G. (1980). Phospholamban, activator of the sarcoplasmic reticulum calcium pump; physicochemical properties and diagonal purification. *Biochemistry*, **19**, 3368–3373.

Lopaschuk, G., Richter, B., and Katz, S. (1980). Characterization of calmodulin effects on calcium transport in cardiac microsomes enriched in sarcoplasmic reticulum. *Biochemistry*, **19**, 5603–5607.

Lüllman, H. and Peters, T. (1976). *Recent Advanc. Stud. Cardiac Struct. Metab.*, **9**, 311–328.

Mandel, F., Kranias, E. G., Grassi de Geude, A., Sumida, M., and Schwartz, A. (1982). The effect of pH on the transient-state kinetics of Ca^{++}–Mg^{++}-ATPase of cardiac sarcoplasmic reticulum. *Circulation Res.*, **50**, 310–317.

Marban, E., Rink, T. J., Tsien, R. W., and Tsien, R. Y. (1980). Free calcium in heart muscle at rest and during contraction measured with Ca^{++} sensitive microelectrodes. *Nature*, **286**, 845–850.

Mayer, S. E. (1974). Effect of catecholamines on cardiac metabolism. *Circulation Res.*, **34–35**, Suppl. III, 129–137.

Mitchell, R. H. (1975). Inositol phospholipids and cell surface receptor function. *Biochem. Biophys. Acta*, **415**, 81–147.

Morad, M. (1969). Contracture and catecholamines in mammalian myocardium. *Science*, **166**, 505–506.

Morad, M. (1983). Inotropic and relaxant effects of adrenaline: possible mechanism(s). In *Catecholamines in the Non-ischaemic and Ischaemic Myocardium* (R. Riemersma and M. Oliver, eds), Princess Liliane Foundation Symposium, Elsevier, Amsterdam, in press.

Morad, M., and Rolett, E. L. (1972). Relaxing effect of catecholamines on mammalian heart. *J. Physiol. (Lond.)*, **224**, 537–558.

Morad, M., Weiss, J., and Cleeman, L. (1978). The inotropic action of adrenaline on cardiac muscle: Does it relax or potentiate tension. *Europ. J. Cardiol.*, **7**, Suppl., 53–62.

Morad, M., Sanders, C., and Weiss, J. (1981). The inotropic actions of adrenaline on frog ventricular muscle: relaxing versus potentiating effects. *J. Physiol. (Lond.)*, **311**, 585–604.

Morkin, E., and La Raia, P. J. (1974). Biochemical studies on the regulation of myocardial contractility. *New Eng. J. Med.*, **290**, 445–451.

Namm, D. H., Mayer, S. E., and Maltbie, M. (1968). The role of potassium and calcium ions in the effect of epinephrine on cardiac cyclic adenosine 3',5'-mono-phosphate, phosphorylase kinase and phosphorylase. *Mol. Pharmacol.*, **4**, 522–530.

Namm, D. H., Woods, E. L., and Zucker, J. L. (1972). Incorporation of the terminal phosphate of ATP into membranal protein of rabbit cardiac sarcoplasmic reticulum. *Circulation Res.*, **31**, 308–316.

Nathan, D., and Beeler, G. W., Jr (1975). Electrophysiologic correlates of the inotropic effects of isoproterenol in canine myocardium. *J. Mol. Cell. Cardiol.*, **7**, 1–15.

Noble, M. I. M. (1979). *The Cardiac Cycle*, Blackwell Scientific Publications, Oxford.

Noble, M. I. M., Trenchard, D. and Guz, A. (1967). Effect of changes in $PaCO_2$ and PaO_2 on cardiac performance in conscious dogs. *J. Appl. Physiol.*, **22**, 147–152.

Onerato, J. J., and Rudolph, A. (1981). Regulation of protein phosphorylation by inotropic agents in isolated rat myocardial cells. *J. Biol. Chem.*, **256**, 1697–1703.

Pang, D. C. (1980). Effect of inotropic agents on the calcium binding to isolated cardiac sarcolemma. *Biochim. Biophys. Acta*, **598**, 528–542.

Pang, D. C., and Briggs, F. N. (1973). Reaction mechanism of the cardiac sarcotubule calcium (II) dependent adenosine triphosphatase. *Biochemistry*, **12**, 4095–4911.

Pannier, J. L. and Leusen, I. (1968). Contraction characteristics of papillary muscle during changes in acid–base composition of the bathing fluid. *Arch. Internat. Physiol. Biochem.*, **76**, 624–634.

Pannier, J. L., Weyne, J., and Leusen, I. (1970). Effects of PCO_2, bicarbonate and lactate on the isometric contractions of isolated soleus muscle of the rat. *Pflügers Arch. Ges. Physiol.*, **320**, 120–132.

Philipson, K. D., Bersohn, M. M., and Nishimoto, A. Y. (1982). Effects of pH on Na^+–Ca^{++} exchange in canine cardiac sarcolemmal vesicles. *Circulation Res.*, **50**, 287–293.

Poole-Wilson, P. A., and Langer, G. A. (1975). Effect of pH on ionic exchange and function in rat and rabbit myocardium. *Amer. J. Physiol.*, **229**, 570–581.

Putney, J. W., Weiss, S. J., van de Walle, C. M., and Haddas, R. A. (1980). Is phosphatidic acid a calcium ionophore under neurohumoral control? *Nature*, **284**, 345–347.

Ray, K. P., and England, P. J. (1976). Phosphorylation of the inhibitory subunit of troponin and its effects on the calcium dependence of cardiac myofibrillar ATPase. *FEBS Lett.*, **70**, 11–16.

Reuter, H. (1965). Uber die Wirkung von Adrenalin auf den cellularen Ca-Umsatz des Meerschweinchenvorhofs. *Naunyn-Schmeidebergs Arch. Pharmacol.*, **251**, 401–412.

Reuter, H. (1967). The dependence of slow inward current in Purkinje fibres on the extracellular calcium concentration. *J. Physiol. (Lond.)*, **192**, 479–492.

Reuter, H. (1974). Localization of β-adrenergic receptors, and effects of noradrenaline and cyclic nucleotides on action potentials, ionic currents and tension in mammalian cardiac muscle. *J. Physiol. (Lond.)*, **242**, 429–451.

Rinaldi, M. L., Le Peuch, C. J., and Demaille, J. G. (1981). The epinephrine-induced activation of the cardiac slow Ca^{++} channel is mediated by the cAMP dependent phosphorylation of calciductin, a 23,000 M_r sarcolemmal protein. *FEBS Lett.*, **129**, 277–281.

Salmon, D. M. and Honeyman, T. W. (1980). Proposed mechanism of cholinergic action in smooth muscle. *Nature*, **284**, 344–345.

Schümann, H. J., Endoh, M. and Brodde, O. E. (1975). The time course of the effects of α- and β-adrenoreceptor stimulation by isoprenaline and methoxamine on the contractile force and cAMP level of the isolated rabbit papillary muscle. *Naunyn-Schmiedebergs Arch. Pharmacol.*, **289**, 291–302.

Singh, J., Flitney, F. W., and Lamb, J. F. (1978). Effects of isoprenaline on contactile force and intracellular cyclic 3',5'-nucleotide levels in the hypodynamic frog ventricle. *FEBS Lett.*, **91**, 269–272.

Suko, J. (1973). The calcium pump of cardiac sarcoplasmic reticulum. Functional alterations at different levels of thyroid state in rabbits. *J. Physiol.*, **228**, 563–582.

Suko, J., and Hasselbach, W. (1975). Phosphoprotein formation and ADP–ATP exchange of cardiac sarcoplasmic reticulum. *Recent Advanc. Stud. Cardiac Struct. Metab.*, **5**, 117–123.

Sulakhe, P. V., Leung, N. L.-K., and St Louis, P. J. (1976). Stimulation of calcium accumulation in cardiac sarcolemma by protein kinase. *Canad. J. Biochem.*, **54**, 438–445.

Tada, M., Kirchberger, M. A., Iorio, J. M., and Katz, A. M. (1973). Phosphorylation of a low molecular weight component (phospholamban) in cardiac sarcoplasmic reticulum catalyzed by cyclic AMP-dependent protein kinase. *Circulation*, **48**, Suppl. 4, 25.

Tada, M., Kirchberger, M. A., and Li, H.-C. (1975). Phosphoprotein phosphatase-catalyzed dephosphorylation of the 22,000 dalton phosphoproteins of cardiac sarcoplasmic reticulum. *J. Cyclic Nucleotide Res.*, **1**, 329–338.

Tsien, R. W. (1973). Adrenaline-like effects of intracellular iontophoresis of cyclic AMP in cardiac Purkinje fibres. *Nature New Biol.*, **245**, 120–122.

Tsien, R. W. (1977). Cyclic AMP and contractile activity in heart. *Advanc. Cyclic Nucleotide Res.*, **8**, 363–420.

Tsien, R. W., Giles, W. R., and Greengard, P. (1972). Cyclic AMP mediates the action of adrenaline on the action potential plateau of cardiac Purkinje fibres. *Nature New Biol.*, **240**, 181–183.

Vassort, G., Rougier, O., Garnier, D., Sauviat, M. P., Coraboeuf, E., and Gargouil, Y. M. (1969). Effects of adrenaline on membrane inward currents during the cardiac action potential. *Pflügers Arch. Ges. Physiol.*, **309**, 70–81.

Venter, J. C. (1983). β-adrenergic receptors and the adrenergic control of cardiac positive inotropic responses. In *Catecholamines in the Non-ischaemic and Ischaemic Myocardium* (R. Riemersma and M. Oliver, eds), Princess Liliane Foundation Symposium, Elsevier, Amsterdam, in press.

Venter, J. C., Ross, J., and Kaplan, N. O. (1975). Lack of detectable change in cyclic AMP during the cardiac inotropic response to isoproterenol immobilized on glass beads. *Proc. Natl Acad. Sci.*, **72**, 824–828.

Walsh, D. A., Perkins, J. P., and Krebs, E. G. (1968). An adenosine 3',5'-monophosphate-dependent protein kinase from rabbit skeletal muscle. *J. Biol. Chem.*, **243**, 3763–3765.

Walsh, D. A., Clippinger, M. S., Sivaramakrishnan, S., and McCullough, T. E. (1979). Cyclic adenosine monophosphate dependent and independent phosphorylation of sarcolemma membrane proteins in perfused rat heart. *Biochemistry*, **18**, 871–877.

Watanabe, A. M., Jones, L. R., Manalan, A. S., and Besch, H. R., Jr (1982). Cardiac autonomic receptors: recent concepts from radio labeled ligand-binding studies. *Circulation Res.*, **50**, 161–174.

Weber, A., and Murray, J. M. (1973). Molecular control mechanisms in muscle contraction. *Physiol. Rev.*, **53**, 613–673.

Will, H., Blanck, J., Smeltan, G., and Wollenberger, A. (1976). A quench-flow kinetic investigation of calcium ion accumulation by isolated cardiac sarcoplasmic reticulum. Dependence of initial velocity on free calcium ion concentration and influence of preincubation with a protein kinase, MgATP, and cyclic AMP. *Biochim. Biophys. Acta*, **449**, 295–303.

Will, H., Schirpke, B., and Wollenberger, A. (1973). Binding of calcium to a cell membrane-enriched preparation from pig myocardium: increase in calcium affinity upon membrane protein phosphorylation enhanced by a membrane-bound cyclic AMP-dependent protein kinase. *Acta Biol. Med. Germ.*, **31**, K45–52.

Williams, G. J., Collins, S., Muir, J. R., and Stephens, M. R. (1975). Observations on the interaction of calcium and hydrogen ions on ATP hydrolysis by the contractile elements of cardiac muscle. *Recent Advanc. Stud. Cardiac Struct. Metab*, **5**, 273–280.

Williamson, J. R., Woodrow, M. L., and Scarpa, A. (1975). Calcium binding to cardiac sarcolemma. *Recent Advanc. Stud Cardiac Struct. Metab.*, **5**, 61–71.

Wollenberger, A., and Will, H. (1978). Protein kinase-catalyzed membrane phosphorylation and its possible relationship to the role of calcium in the adrenergic regulation of cardiac contraction. *Life Sci.*, **22**, 1159–1178.

Wray, H. L., Gray, R. R., and Olsson, R. A. (1973). Cyclic adenosine 3',5'-monophosphate stimulated protein kinase and substrate associated with cardiac sarcoplasmic reticulum. *J. Biol. Chem.*, **248**, 1496–1498.

Cardiac Metabolism
Edited by A. J. Drake-Holland and M. I. M. Noble
© 1983 John Wiley & Sons Ltd

CHAPTER 18

A Critical Review on cyclic AMP and its Role in Cellular Metabolism and Heart Muscle Contractility

H. Van Belle

Department of Biochemistry, Janssen Pharmaceutica Research Laboratories, B-2340 Beerse, Belgium

'Once written, statements (data, results, hypotheses, etc.) tend to take on an excessive air of certainty, not easily shaken by later questioning.'

Cohen (1981)

INTRODUCTION

The cyclic AMP story is one of the best examples of Cohen's statement. It all began when Cook *et al.* (1957) and Sutherland and Rall (1957) almost simultaneously described a compound which later on (Lipkin *et al.*, 1959) was identified as adenosine 3',5'-cyclic adenosine monophosphate (cAMP). The former group found it as a degradation product of ATP, when boiled in a barium hydroxide ($Ba(OH)_2$) solution, whereas the latter group discovered it as a cofactor in the conversion of phosphorylase *b* to *a*. The description of adenylate cyclase, the enzyme responsible for cAMP formation *in vivo*, followed shortly afterwards (Sutherland, *et al.*, 1962; Rall and Sutherland, 1962). There then began a whole era of intensive studies on cAMP, with an explosion of experiments resulting in the almost universal acceptance of cAMP as the second messenger for a great variety of hormonal and drug actions (Sutherland *et al.*, 1968). It looked as if cAMP was involved in anything and everything. The enthusiasm was so great that many times the involvement of cAMP was assumed without paying much attention to the four rules devised by Sutherland to accept a substance as a second messenger. Those rules are as follows: (1) the response to a first messenger should be accompanied by an increase in intracellular cAMP; (2) exogenously applied cAMP or an analogue mimics the effects of the first messenger; (3) methylxanthines mimic or potentiate the action of the first messenger; and (4) adenyl cyclase in broken cell preparations should respond to the same hormones.

In 1972, Rasmussen *et al.*, in a review on the role of cAMP and Ca^{++} in cell activation, mentioned several additional assumptions which have been

417

made by other investigators: (a) the inhibition of phosphodiesterase (PDE) is the only important action of methylxanthines; (b) large extracellular concentrations of cAMP or its analogue(s) are equivalent to small intracellular concentrations; (c) the only action of cAMP in the cell is through protein kinase activation; (d) first messenger receptors and adenylate cyclase are synonymous; (e) cAMP is the sole second messenger; (f) adenylate cyclase and the first messenger receptors are located at the plasma membrane; and (g) the physiological response is inhibited when adenylate cyclase is blocked. The authors warned against premature conclusions on the role of cAMP by stating: 'A survey of nearly any specific system in which cAMP has been implicated served to demonstrate that many of the criteria and assumptions are not fulfilled'. More recently, Stoclet (1978), making a reassessment of the criteria, found it obvious that the conclusions of many early studies should be re-examined using improved methodology. In fact, the absolute involvement of cAMP has been questioned in the cell cycle (Coffino *et al.*, 1975), control of protein synthesis (Horak and Koschel, 1977), DNA synthesis (Hilfiker and Higgins, 1980), lipolysis (Zapf *et al.*, 1981), smooth muscle contraction (Diamond, 1978), heart muscle contraction (Tsien, 1977), gluconeogenesis (Garrison and Borland, 1979), hormone release (Sen and Menon, 1979), and glucagon activation of glycogenolysis (Cote and Epand, 1979), to mention some processes which were (and still are) widely accepted as being cAMP-dependent.

The lack of criticism about the assumptions, together with the availability of extremely sensitive, specific, and relatively easy methods for the detection of cAMP, has led to the situation that in many experiments changes in cAMP have been looked for at the nanomolar level, whilst changes in other cellular components which may have accompanied the response, and possibly occurred at a much higher level, have been disregarded.

The first aim of this paper is to take a critical look at the methodological pitfalls (analytical and enzymological) in assessing the role of cAMP in many processes. In a second part, the role of cAMP in heart contractility will be briefly discussed. The intention is to provide the reader with some detailed information from existing reports. These 'details' are rarely stressed, because they do not fit into what is generally accepted, but it may be worthwhile to keep them in mind whenever one has to decide about the involvement of cAMP in the process under study.

PITFALLS IN ASSESSING THE ROLE OF cAMP

Analytical Problems

In the early 1960s the only way to determine cAMP was through its catalytic effect on the conversion of phosphorylase *b* to phosphorylase *a*, i.e.

the system devised by Sutherland and his group and also the reaction upon which they based the idea of the physiological role of cAMP. Since then, many other procedures have been reported using chromatographic systems, protein kinases, protein binding, and radioimmunoassay. It is beyond the scope of this article to review them all – only a few will be briefly discussed.

When reading reports on novel assays one always wonders how it was possible to get exact results with the older methods. A typical example comes from Sutherland's group, where they got a tenfold increase in sensitivity of their phosphorylase system, simply by preincubating the reaction mixture at 0 °C for 30 min (Butcher *et al.*, 1965). If such a mild treatment was able to provoke that marked change, what other factors could then affect the reaction besides cAMP, and what is the probability that this also happened in the earlier experiments?

A method based on luciferase luminescence has been reported by Sutherland's group (Johnson *et al.*, 1970) to be very specific, sensitive, and linear over a broad concentration range, but apparently the method has never been widely used. The same applies to a gas–liquid chromatographic procedure published by Krishna (1968). A quantitative determination with linearity between 0.3×10^{-9} and 6×10^{-9} mol was feasible. This relatively simple and sensitive method, if valid, should also give an idea about what changes in the other nucleotides occur under conditions where cAMP metabolism is affected. The same benefit is afforded by electrophoresis on cellulose acetate (Delaage *et al.*, 1974). cAMP was clearly separated from the other components of the reaction mixture and quantitated by its labelling (^{3}H-labelled ATP as substrate). However, when applied to adenylate cyclase from the rat hypothalamus, the results are rather confusing (see below).

A frequently used method is the one described by Kuo and Greengard (1970), based on the activation by cAMP of a protein kinase phosphorylating a histone mixture. In this assay system, cAMP is not essential but merely accelerates the reaction. Upon prolonged incubation the histones are phosphorylated by ATP and Mg^{++} to a similar extent, even in the complete absence of cAMP. Since it is now known that the role of cAMP is to displace the regulatory subunit from the kinase, leaving the catalytic subunit free for enzyme activity, the question remains what other conditions besides cAMP affect the dissociation (see below under protein kinases).

The acetylation radioimmunoassay, fully described and discussed recently by Brooker *et al.* (1979) is based upon competitive ligand binding to endogenous proteins with affinity for cAMP. When compared with Gillman's procedure (1970), the acetylation step increases sensitivity considerably. If the detailed procedure is carefully followed, it should be the most sensitive and least troublesome method now available. Apart from its sensitivity and specificity, a major advantage is that crude samples can be applied – no purification, with concomitant losses, is necessary.

To determine the few nanomoles, or even picomoles, of cAMP formed upon the action of adenylate cyclase, $[\alpha\text{-}^{32}P]ATP$ is the substrate of choice. The $[^{32}P]cAMP$ thus released has to be separated completely from the many other labelled ATP breakdown products (see below under adenylate cyclase). In their original procedure for prepurification, Krishna *et al.* (1968) reported a recovery of 70%, but others, using the same technique, achieved a recovery of only 28–40%. Using columns of hydrous aluminium oxide, the recovery could be increased to 90% (Ramachandran, 1971). Many variations on Krishna's method have been tried. They have been thoroughly discussed by Salomon (1979) in a recent paper presenting full details on his version of a sensitive and reliable assay for adenylate cyclase.

Detailed experimental data from comparative studies in one particular system with several different methods for measuring changes in cAMP are not available. Apparently, sentences such as 'The results are comparable to those found with other methods' or 'Increases in cAMP upon treatment with a hormone or sodium fluoride could be detected' have to convince the reader. When looking at some details in the method, one is also worried to find that every new method introduces a step to correct the shortcomings of the existing procedures, but in the meantime the conclusions drawn from the experiments in which the earlier (= incorrect) methods were applied, are not challenged.

It may be worthwhile to look in more detail at some of the major shortcomings which may have disturbed the 'earlier' methods.

First, to stop all enzymatic activities and to extract cAMP, several procedures have been proposed with varying success:

(1) Boiling for 3–5 min, as first applied by Sutherland's group, is by far the most widely used procedure. However, when applied to a radioimmunoassay, it was shown (Larner and Rutherford, 1978) that boiling (for up to 5 min) produces a linear decrease in the percentage of bound radioactivity, due to non-enzymatically formed cAMP. On the other hand, using column elution chromatography, heating was also found to generate an undesirably high background because of extensive destruction of cAMP, particularly at pH 7.5 or above (Sinha and Colman, 1981).

(2) In the case of trichloroacetic acid or perchloric acid extraction, both compounds interfere with the protein binding and radioimmunoassays and have to be removed. The removal of trichloroacetic acid with water-saturated ether is rather inconvenient and even then interference could still be detected (Cooper *et al.*, 1972; Arner and Ostman, 1975). A more rapid procedure for the removal of trichloroacetic acid was proposed by Tihon *et al.* (1977), who neutralized the extracts by the addition of calcium carbonate in excess. However, when applied to a protein binding assay instead of a radioimmunoassay, it resulted in erroneously high cAMP values, as did the

removal of perchloric acid with either calcium carbonate, or potassium carbonate and potassium hydroxide (KOH) (Meurs *et al.*, 1980).

(3) Dilute hydrochloric acid (HCl) and boiling for 3 min (Meurs *et al.*, 1980), or trichloroacetic acid containing 0.1 M HCl followed by ether extraction and neutralization (Døskeland and Haga, 1978), have been used for protein binding assays. In an adenylate cyclase assay using [α-^{32}P]ATP, it was necessary to stop the reaction by heating for 4 min at 95 °C in 0.165 N HCl, in order to eliminate contaminants in the ATP which interfered in the subsequent chromatographic system (Counis and Mongongu, 1978). On the other hand, HCl extracts of brain tissue were found to contain a factor (or factors) that inhibited the protein binding (Nahorski and Rogers, 1973). Others found it necessary to apply a double treatment with barium hydroxide (Ba(OH)$_2$) and zinc sulphate (ZnSO$_4$) after perchloric acid extraction and neutralization with KOH–KCl (Nahorski and Rogers, 1973). Cooper *et al.* (1973) preferred using sulphuric acid (H$_2$SO$_4$) and sonication, followed by barium acetate. However, using a luciferin–luciferase system, it was shown (Ebadi *et al.*, 1971) that exposure to Ba^{++} ions for 1 h at room temperature resulted in a non-enzymatic conversion of 0.1% of ATP into cAMP. A 0.1% conversion is much more than the basal adenylate cyclase activity in many experiments. Summarizing, it may be concluded that the extraction procedure may need a more careful examination for any particular system used. In this respect, a remarkable statement can be found in (Cooper *et al.*, 1972):

'Both the recovery and dilution experiments, and the assay of standard cAMP solutions in extracted buffer, suggested that perchloric acid (HClO$_4$) and probably also trichloroacetic acid were *not suitable* for preparation of extracts. It was observed, however, that *identical* tissue contents of cAMP were obtained when slices incubated under control conditions were extracted by boiling and in HClO$_4$'

Secondly, the column-chromatographic procedures for the determination of cAMP require strictly controlled conditions and materials in order to be reproducible, and recovery experiments must be performed for any particular application. A prominent example was reported by Salomon *et al.* (1974) from his experiments on adenylate cyclase using [α-^{32}P]ATP as substrate. Using an alumina column to remove ATP and other contaminants, the cAMP, *non-enzymatically* produced, was as high as 39 pmol. This was drastically reduced to 2.1 pmol for Dowex + barium sulphate and to 0.3 pmol for Dowex + alumina. The basal adenylate cyclase activity resulted in a formation of 2.9, 3.3, and 3.2 pmol respectively of cAMP in 5 min.

Thirdly the protein binding assays and radioimmunoassays should also be applied with caution. Because of their extreme sensitivity, part of the changes they detect are not necessarily due to activation of adenylate cyclase, but may also originate from displacement of cAMP from non-specific cAMP binding sites. Thus yeast glyceraldehyde 3-phosphate dehydrogenase is known (Brownlee and Polya, 1980) to bind cAMP as well as all other adenosine derivatives, including nicotinamide adenine dinucleotide (NAD). A variety of antimitotics, adrenergic receptor antagonists, and non-steroidal anti-inflammatory agents are able to displace the bound cAMP. It is evident that these overlapping ligand specificities may compromise simple interpretations of experiments on the effects of pharmacologically active compounds, when using extremely sensitive methods.

The factors affecting the binding of cAMP are also poorly understood. Thus a sensitive saturation assay has been described using a relatively crude adrenal protein as the specific binding protein. The technique becomes considerably less sensitive when a more highly purified protein is used (Brown *et al.*, 1971).

Omission of protein kinase inhibitor in Gilman's protein binding assay leads to underestimation of intracellular cAMP by 60–70% in human adipose tissue (Arner and Östman, 1975). This was ascribed to a falsely low standard curve, since addition of protein kinase inhibitor increased the binding of cAMP only in the samples from the standard curve and not in tissue samples. In the same report it is also shown that intracellular cAMP is underestimated by 30% when incubating the tissue *in vitro* in a medium with 1% albumin, as compared with incubation in the absence of albumin. Activation by albumin of the binding capacity was also shown, amongst other investigators, by Meurs *et al.* (1980). The effect of albumin and protein kinase inhibitor was clearly demonstrated in an assay using competitive binding to salt-dissociated protein kinase, where both were necessary for the stabilization of the protein during the time needed for the binding reaction (Døskeland and Haga, 1978). In the absence of albumin, only 10% could be recovered, increasing to 80% when albumin was added and 97% when both albumin and crude heat-stable inhibitor preparations were present.

These few remarks, as well as some others mentioned below (under the heading 'Adenylate cyclase'), are not intended to deny the merits of the many efforts for improving the quantitative assay of cAMP. When cautiously applied, several of the more recent procedures may provide valuable results. The question, however, is how many important conclusions have been drawn from experiments using methods where, besides cAMP, so many other factors could have interfered.

The application of a sensitive and specific technique may provide useful information as to changes in one particular component, but if this change is only one out of a chain of events occurring in the system, then a causal relationship cannot be established as long as changes in the other components are neglected. This is what happened with many experiments on

Table 18.1 Effect of corticosterone on nucleotides and nucleosides in rat hypothalamus adenylate cyclase preparation. The values are recalculated from the results of Delaage *et al.* (1974) and are expressed as percentages of the total radioactivity added as [³H]ATP

Time (min)	cAMP Control	+Hormone	Adenosine Control	+Hormone	Inosine Control	+Hormone	AMP Control	+Hormone	ADP+ATP Control	+Hormone
0	0.012		0.84		0.034		0.49		98.7	
5	0.120	0.22	1.38	1.00	0.30	0.22	2.49	0.81	95.7	97.7
12	0.135	0.42	1.76	1.76	0.20	1.56	1.68	13.61	96.2	82.0

cAMP, as may be illustrated with a few examples. Thus Delaage *et al.* (1974), using an electrophoretic procedure to separate and quantitate nucleosides and nucleotides, including cAMP, looked for the effect of 2.2×10^{-6} M corticosterone on rat hypothalamus adenylate cyclase. The substrate was [³H]ATP (2×10^{-3} M) and phosphoenol pyruvate–pyruvate kinase (PEP–PK) was added as regenerating system. The amount of metabolites, recalculated as percentage of the total radioactivity of added ATP is shown in Table 18.1.

A rather similar experiment was reported (Verbert and Cacan, 1972) on rat liver adenylate cyclase and stimulation with sodium fluoride. From the curves, the radioactivity found in nucleotides and adenosine can be estimated. The figures are shown in Table 18.2.

When looking at both tables, it is evident that adenylate cyclase activity is stimulated. However, the changes (absolute and relative) induced in the other components are much more dramatic and it may be questioned why adenylate cyclase should be the target for the hormone or sodium fluoride action.

Table 18.2 Radioactivity (percentage of total) in nucleotides and adenosine in rat liver adenylate cyclase with and without 20 mM NaF (recalculated from Verbert and Cacan, 1972)

	ATP	AMP	cAMP	Adenosine
Control	58	28	0.05	14
+NaF	62	7	0.25	31

The Enzymes Involved in cAMP Formation and Metabolism

Adenylate cyclase

Analytical problems As already mentioned, soon after the discovery of the catalytic effect of cAMP on the phosphorylase *b* to *a* conversion Sutherland's group described adenylate cyclase, the enzyme responsible for the production in the cell of cAMP (Sutherland *et al.*, 1962; Rall and Sutherland, 1962). The stoicheiometry is very simple:

$$1 \text{ ATP} \rightleftharpoons 1 \text{ cAMP} + 1 \text{ PP}_i \text{ (pyrophosphate)}.$$

It is surprising that, apart from a study by Hirata and Hayashi (1967) on the adenylate cyclase from *Brevibacterium liquefaciens*, the stoicheiometric evidence provided by Sutherland and his collaborators was not further questioned. At first glance, the results are indeed convincing: on three different cyclase preparations there is a simultaneous formation of cAMP and PP_i from ATP. There are, however, a few remarks to be made: (1) as stated in the text, it was found essential to remove ATP with charcoal when isolating PP_i, because 'intolerable' amounts of PP_i were formed from ATP during the isolation procedure (= non-enzymatically); (2) when looking at the formation of $[^{32}P]PP_i$ from $[\alpha,\beta,\gamma\text{-}^{32}P]$ATP by soluble skeletal muscle adenylate cyclase, it is remarkable that at zero time the PP_i, already present, is higher than the amount subsequently formed by the enzyme upon incubation for 20 min; (3) the addition of $ZnSO_4$ (1.2×10^{-4} M) strongly inhibited the cAMP formation (more than 80% inhibition) but much less the PP_i formation (the PP_i formed by the soluble skeletal muscle adenylate cyclase or the soluble calf brain adenylate cyclase under these conditions was three times and eight to 13 times respectively the cAMP produced); and (4) it was admitted by the authors that 'the data do not warrant firm conclusions concerning the stoichiometry of the reaction'.

The experiments on the enzyme from *Brevibacterium liquefaciens* look more convincing. The purified enzyme is almost free of ATPase, pyrophosphatase, and phosphodiesterase and the cAMP formation measured after 60 min equals the production of PP_i and the loss of ATP. However, the enzyme markedly differs in many aspects from the mammalian one in that (1) it has an absolute requirement for an α-keto acid (pyruvate); (2) it is linear for at least 60 min; (3) it has a pH optimum between 9 and 10; and (4) it is not stimulated by epinephrine. Where, in general, the ATP → cAMP conversion rarely exceeds 0.1% of the substrate in most adenylate cyclase preparations, the bacterial enzyme converted 50% of the ATP within 60 min. Unfortunately, no details are given on blanks which should be considered under the rather extreme conditions of the incubation (8.16 mM ATP; 61 mM Mg^{2+}; 100 mM Tris *pH 9.0*; and 2 mM pyruvate).

It must be admitted that studies on the stoicheiometry are hampered by the lack of stable pure enzyme preparations. Indeed, all the many efforts up to now have been rather unsuccessful. The only highly purified preparation known is that of Homcy *et al.* (1978), who used a hydrophobic resolution before chromatography on an ATP-Sepharose affinity resin. They succeeded in a 5000-fold purification, but data on stability or kinetics of this enzyme were not mentioned.

The lack of a highly purified enzyme makes it necessary to be very cautious in the interpretation of the results from an adenylate cyclase assay for several reasons:

(1) *The non-enzymatic formation of cAMP from ATP*   As already mentioned, the first report on cAMP (Cook *et al.*, 1957) described its formation from ATP upon boiling for 30 min in 0.4 N Ba(OH)$_2$. The amount thus formed (5–15%) is enormous when compared with the amounts usually detected with adenylate cyclase preparations and which rarely exceed 0.1% (Salomon, 1979). Since, in most of the assays, the reaction is terminated by boiling the incubation mixture for at least 3 min, one wonders how much cAMP is formed non-enzymatically. Many authors have looked for this and have concluded that, from their blanks, it is only a few per cent of the amount produced by the enzyme. The blank is either ATP without enzyme or ATP with boiled enzyme. However, due to the action of a variety of contaminating enzymes on ATP, the incubation mixture is not ATP but a mixture of ATP, ADP, AMP, PP$_i$, P$_i$, adenosine, and its catabolites together with metal ions, proteins, and possibly an ATP regenerating system. Apparently attempts were never made to measure how much cAMP is formed non-enzymatically by boiling such a mixture. It is also worthwhile to mention that the non-enzymatic conversion of ATP into cAMP does not necessarily require the drastic conditions used by Cook *et al.* (1957). Indeed, it has been shown recently (Brooker *et al.*, 1979) that *14%* of ATP was converted into cAMP after 5 min at 90°C in 0.1 M Ba(OH)$_2$ and 10 mM EDTA. This reaction is so reproducible that it could be applied to the determination of ATP using a sensitive assay for cAMP. Even a slight excess of Ba^{++}, as present in the Ba(OH)$_2$–ZnSO$_4$ prepurification system, is able to convert 0.1% of ATP into cAMP *at room temperature* in 1 h (Ebadi *et al.*, 1971). Simple storage of [α-^{32}P]ATP was reported (Counis and Mongongu, 1978) to lead to the formation of a cAMP-like radioactive material seriously increasing the blanks in the assay system used. It may also be relevant here to mention the paper by Kimura and Murad (1974) on the non-enzymatic formation of cyclic guanosine monophosphate (cGMP) from GTP. If GTP is kept for 3 min at 100 °C in 50 mM Tris, pH 7.6, very little cGMP is formed. The addition of 10 mM Ca^{++} increased that amount by a factor of 12 without creatine phosphate (CP) and by 125 with CP (15 mM). The addition of 2 mM potassium phosphate to 1 mM GTP, 10 mM MnCl$_2$, and 50 mM Tris resulted in an eight times greater formation of cGMP upon boiling for 3 min. It is quite surprising that the ATP → cAMP conversion has not been studied under the same conditions. The authors only mention that there is no formation of cAMP from ATP in 40 mM Tris pH 7.4 in the presence of 6 mM Mg^{++} after heating for 3 min at 100 °C.

(2) *The presence of many contaminating enzymes acting on both the substrate and the product*   Stansfield and Franks (1970) isolated a rat luteal

adenylate cyclase free of phosphodiesterase activity. However, a strong ATPase activity was still present. The addition of NaF (10 mM) maximally stimulated the adenylate cyclase but even then the ATPase activity was more than 1000-fold higher (10^{-6} mol min^{-1} mg^{-1} for the ATPase versus 0.66×10^{-9} mol min^{-1} mg^{-1} for adenylate cyclase). At 100 mM sodium fluoride the ATPase was inhibited by 80% but the adenylate cyclase activity was also lost. NaN$_3$ effectively inhibited both enzymes. Recently (Kiss, 1979) rat liver plasma membranes were shown to contain an enzyme (alcohol–AMP synthesizing enzyme) which, when incubated under the conditions usually employed for adenylate cyclase (Tris, pH 7.5; 0.4mM [α-^{32}P]ATP; CP; CPK; and Mg^{++}) converts 2.5% of the ATP into Tris-AMP within 10 min. It seems rather unlikely that this compound interferes with the newer specific assays for cAMP (although it has not been tested) but it may well alter the results using ^{32}P measurements after isolation on resins. In fact, the compound is a phosphodiester and it is produced in quantities at least one order of magnitude higher than cAMP. The presence of cAMP-binding proteins (similar to the yeast GAPDH mentioned above; Brownlee and Polya, 1980) may complicate the interpretation of experiments on adenylate cyclase and the effect of pharmacologically active compounds. They could indeed displace cAMP and thus increase the levels of free cAMP or the apparent adenylate cyclase activity. The presence of phosphodiesterase (PDE) may also strongly affect the determination of adenylate cyclase activity. This problem is usually solved in two ways. Either cold cAMP is added to the incubate in large excess to saturate the PDE, or PDE inhibitors (methylxanthines) are used. From an enzymological point of view, addition of an excess of cold cAMP is likely to affect the enzyme's kinetics. Thus, looking at the data from Salomon *et al.* (1974), it can be calculated that upon maximal stimulation with sodium fluoride the adenylate cyclase activity in their preparation resulted in the formation of 15 pmol of labelled cAMP per 5 min per incubate in the presence of 100 000 pmol of cold cAMP. The problem with using PDE inhibitors is the diversity of PDE activities (for a review see Wells and Hardman, 1977). Papaverine, caffeine, theophylline, and methylisobutylxanthine are the most frequently used inhibitors but they leave the calmodulin-dependent PDE activity unaffected. Inhibitors of the latter have not yet been applied. Recently it was shown (Stockton and Turner, 1981) that caffeine and theophylline competitively displace cAMP from the binding protein used in Gilman's procedure and it is open to question just how much this may have affected the earlier experiments.

(3) *Contaminating ATPases and anomalous adenylate cyclase-kinetics* The contaminating enzymes, especially the ATPases, are claimed to be responsible for the poor linearity of adenylate cyclase with time and protein concentration. For instance, the specific activity of a rat kidney

adenylate cyclase preparation decreased from 933 over 533 to 400 pmol per 10 min per milligram of protein by increasing the protein concentration from 0.25 mg to 1 and 2 mg per incubate. On incubating 1.8 mg per incubate for 1, 5, 10, and 20 min, the specific activities were found to be 556, 278, 222 and 185 respectively (Dousa and Rychlik, 1970). Another remarkable result was reported on rat adrenal adenylate cyclase (Ramachandran, 1971): irrespective of the protein content, which ranged from 30 to 125 μg per incubate, the cAMP produced in 15 min was 4–5 pmol per incubate under basal conditions. When 1×10^{-5} M ACTH was added, a direct proportionality to the enzyme concentration was claimed for 60 μg protein per incubate or less but only one concentration below 60 μg was tested. Above 60 μg, a doubling of the protein content did not result in any additional formation of cAMP.

To obtain linearity, an ATP regenerating system is frequently used, either PEP–PK or, more frequently, CP–CPK. For rat fat cell ghosts it was shown (Schwabe *et al.*, 1974) that without a regenerating system 0.3 mM ATP was decreased by 95% within 5 min but remained at 75–80% when CP–CPK was included. The same authors report on inhibition of the basal, but not of the hormone-stimulated, activity by CP concentrations above 10 mM. Nevertheless, several investigators continued to use CP as high as 25 mM (Table 3 in Salomon, 1979; Birnbauer and Yang, 1974; Wattiaux-De Coninck *et al.*, 1981). Anyway, it is now generally accepted that the addition of regenerating systems markedly improves linearity. However, it would be interesting to look in every preparation if the regenerating system is indeed effective. For instance, Katz and Tenenhouse (1973) utilizing PEP–PK, showed an almost complete disappearance of ATP upon incubation at 37 °C for 10 min of a cerebral cortex adenylate cyclase preparation, whereas in a synaptic membrane adenylate cyclase preparation almost 50% of ATP was left under similar conditions but without PEP–PK. Even in the presence of an ATP regenerating system Schwabe *et al.* (1979) found a complete flattening within 4 min of the cAMP production in a preparation from isolated fat cells. The addition of 1 mM vanadate (a well known inhibitor of many – if not all – ATPases at this concentration) resulted in an almost linear reaction for 10 min.

Johnson and Welden (1977) recently reported stimulatory and inhibitory effects of ATP regenerating systems on adenylate cyclase from liver. The inhibition by PEP-PK could be accounted for by the formation of metal–PEP complexes while activation of guanine nucleotide-stimulated activity (see further) might be due to GTP sparing. CP also had stimulatory and inhibitory effects, but these were attributable to impurities in the commercially available preparations.

Another way to minimize substrate exhaustion is by the use of 5′-adenylylimidophosphate (AMP-PNP), an ATP analogue that resists phosphohydrolase activities. However, its resistance depends on the source of the enzyme, as shown recently (Johnson, 1980; Johnson and Welden, 1977). It is readily hydrolysed to 5'-AMP and adenosine by partially purified plasma membranes from rat liver, less rapidly by membranes from fat cells, and indeed very poorly with detergent-dispersed preparations from rat cerebellum. The adenosine, thus formed, might well be sufficient to inhibit the hepatic adenylate cyclase activity – this inhibition being most pronounced on the stimulated enzyme (sodium fluoride–glucagon–GTP). The same enzymatic activity, that of a pyrophosphatase, was also found to attack GTP or GMP-PNP, both modulator nucleotides of adenylate cyclase (see later). Using AMP-PNP, the rat fat cell ghost adenylate cyclase activity was shown (Schwabe *et al.*, 1974) to be only 30% of the activity with ATP and a stimulatory effect of 10 μM noradrenaline could no longer be detected, in contrast with a threefold stimulation with ATP as substrate.

The problems with linearity of adenylate cyclase may also partly be due to the activation of adenylate cyclase by its own substrate, as has recently been described in two papers for liver plasma membranes. If true, one wonders whether it is even possible to get a linear course of the reaction. However, both reports show conflicting results. Kiss (1980), preincubating the membranes for 12 min at 33 °C with Mg^{++} or Mg^{++} plus ATP, found a three- or fourfold stimulation respectively, but only of the fluoride-activated adenylate cyclase. A phosphorylation by Mg–ATP could be excluded. On the other hand, Richards *et al.* (1981), preincubating similarly prepared liver plasma membranes with comparable amounts of Mg–ATP, but for 24 h at 4 °C, found a four- to sevenfold activation, but only of the basal activity. In fact, when the incubation-induced activation of the basal activity had reached its maximum, the basal and fluoride-stimulated activities were indistinguishable.

In conclusion, it seems highly desirable to reconsider many experiments and their conclusions in the light of our present knowledge of the multiple factors which may affect an estimation of the true level of cAMP and/or of the activity of adenylate cyclase with or without stimulation.

The hormone sensitivity of adenylate cyclase and the role of guanine nucleotides The involvement of the guanine nucleotides in the regulation of adenylate cyclase activity was shown in the early 1970s. 5'-Guanylylimidophosphate (GMP-PNP), a GTP analogue, stimulated adenylate cyclase in a variety of eukaryotic cells. It may even stimulate it to maximal activity in the absence of hormones or of functional hormone receptors (Londos *et al.*, 1974). Intensive studies during the last 5 years have now begun to unravel the whole system. For details, the reader is referred to two recent reviews (Ross and Gilman, 1980; Limbird, 1981).

According to Limbird (1981), the recognition of the obligatory role of

GTP relied on three major improvements: (1) the preparation of membranes devoid of endogenous guanine nucleotide contaminants; (2) the availibility of ATP free of contaminating GTP or GDP; and (3) the utilization of the ATPase-resistant ATP analogue AMP-PNP to inhibit the membrane transphosphorylation of GDP → GTP.

Adenylate cyclase appears to be composed of at least three interacting proteins:

(1) The catalyst, which *per se* is relatively inactive (basal activity).

(2) A guanine nucleotide and/or fluoride binding protein (G-protein), which, in the presence of GTP, leads to stimulation of the catalyst by hormones. The activation is terminated if GTP is converted into GDP.

(3) A regeneration system of the G-protein, whereby, due to the formation of a receptor–hormone complex, GDP is reconverted into GTP.

The general scheme for stimulation of adenylate cyclase by hormones is

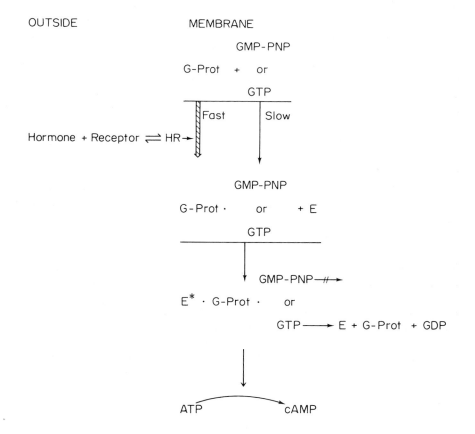

According to this scheme, there is no direct interaction of the hormone receptor with the catalytic unit: the GTP binding protein (or proteins) is the macromolecular messenger in receptor–cyclase coupling. The interaction of the G-protein with the receptor occurs only in relatively unperturbed membranes which may explain why the extent of hormonal activation assayed *in vitro* is generally much less than in intact cells or tissues. Solubilized adenylate cyclase no longer responds to catecholamine stimulation, despite the presence of the beta-adrenergic receptor (Limbird, 1981).

Pike and Lefkowitz (1980) did studies in frog and turkey erythrocyte membranes, applying stimulation by beta-adrenergic agents, agonist-induced desensitization and modification with group-specific reagents. All data were consistent with the hypothesis that guanine nucleotide regulation of adenylate cyclase activity and beta-receptor binding are mediated through the same protein (G-protein), which shows GTPase activity. The pharmacological specificity and intrinsic stimulatory activity on adenylate cyclase of several beta-adrenergic agonists closely parallels their effects on the GTPase. The conclusions from the experiments on the GTPase activity should, however, be taken with caution and would require confirmation on a purified, reconstituted system if ever possible. Indeed, in order to find any effect of isoproterenol, several tricks had to be applied. Thus the non-specific GTPase activity ($= 100\%$) was inhibited with 0.5 mM AMP-PNP to 9.78%. Upon further addition of CP-CPK, the GTPase rose to 10.56%. With AMP-PNP + CP-CPK + 0.1 mM ATP the GTPase was again reduced to 8.06%. It is on the latter system that isoproterenol shows a stimulatory effect in a dose-dependent way, but the maximal stimulation (at 10^{-4} M) still resulted in only 11.37% of the original GTPase. Instead of 'stimulation' it may be better to call this effect 'dis-inhibition'.

Very recently the functions of the subunits were studied in reconstituted adenylate cyclase from bovine brain (Neer and Salter, 1981). The catalytic unit was activated two- to threefold by calmodulin (this activation does not require the G-protein) and also directly inhibited by adenosine. The G-protein and the GTPase activity eluted at the same position. The hormone receptor did not activate the catalytic unit directly but regulated the *state* of the G-protein. The release of tightly bound GDP was found not to be the rate-limiting step in activation of the adenylate cyclase. Activation should merely be caused by a slow conformational or structural change in the G-protein due to the dissociation from an inactive (190 000 dalton) to an active (80 000 dalton) form. GMP-PNP is thought to stabilize the dissociated form.

It would certainly be worthwhile to reconsider or even repeat earlier fundamental experiments on adenylate cyclase and cAMP in the light of our present knowledge on its regulation by a guanyl nucleotide binding (or metabolizing) protein. On the one hand, it is known that the guanine nucleotides are required for stimulation of adenylate cyclase by virtually all hormones and drugs investigated today (Limbird, 1981). On the other hand, as will be mentioned further, several hormone-induced processes, once thought to be solely mediated by increases in cAMP, are now known to occur without any change in cAMP. Is it possible that, by focusing on cAMP, the metabolism of the guanine nucleotides has been overlooked and that in fact this metabolism is more important for the regulation of cellular activities than is the formation of cAMP? In this respect a recent paper (Sharif and Roberts, 1981) should be mentioned, where it is shown that guanine derivatives markedly affect the binding of glutamate to synaptic membrane vesicles by reducing the apparent affinity for the receptor.

Phosphodiesterase (PDE)

In elucidating the second messenger role of cAMP, the existence of PDE, specific for cAMP, has played a crucial role. The existence of many PDE isoenzymes in many tissues is well documented and relatively potent inhibitors, some of them with marked tissue specificity, have been developed. It is beyond the scope of this paper to discuss in detail the available knowledge which the reader may find in recent reviews (Wells and Hardman, 1977; Stoclet, 1979). However, a few critical comments seem justified.

(a) The 'classical' PDE inhibitors have been applied to systems, supposedly involving cAMP, in many instances without much criticism. Their potential pharmacological activities, besides inhibition of PDE, have been overlooked. Furthermore, it is quite surprising that most frequently theophylline has been utilized, which for many PDEs is far less inhibitory than papaverine and is even ineffective in several systems (Schwabe *et al.*, 1974). Generalizations about pharmacological effects of PDE inhibitors and cAMP should be avoided, as is illustrated by the findings that theophylline at 5×10^{-4} M inhibits spontaneous contractions in the isolated rat uterus without any effect on the levels of cAMP (Mitznegg *et al.*, 1974), or that the ability of methylxanthines to increase tension of rat diaphragms shows no apparent relationship to their inhibition of PDE acting on cAMP or cGMP (Kramer and Wells, 1980).

Whenever these inhibitors are called upon to prove that a particular process is mediated by cAMP, one also has to prove that the compound effectively inhibits PDEs from that particular system, which is the correct interpretation of Sutherland's rule.

(b) The fact that PDEs exist is not necessarily proof of the fact that their substrate *in vivo* is cAMP and their only role is to destroy cAMP. Many other phosphodiesters exist *in vivo*, some of them being certainly very important, such as the phospholipids and especially phosphatidylinositol, which is involved in many processes (Michell, 1975). It may be worthwhile to study the effect of isolated PDEs on this and other substrates.

(c) An important group of PDEs are those stimulated by calmodulin and Ca^{++}. It may be relevant to know whether the more specific inhibitors of this class of PDE (trifluoperazine, penfluriodol, or calmidazolium – R 24 571) are able to raise the cAMP of a given preparation and to see whether the final result on metabolism is comparable to that of the methylxanthines.

In conclusion, one of Sutherland's criteria, i.e. the ability of methylxanthines either to mimic or to potentiate the action of the first messenger, should be more strictly and critically applied. Otherwise strange flights of logic may occur, such as the one encountered in a discussion in a 1973 paper (Long *et al.*, 1973): '... Thus theophylline appears to relax vascular smooth muscle by inhibiting the enzymatic inactivation of cAMP levels. The opposite effect of theophylline seen in man is probably not due to this mechanism ...'.

The protein kinases

The most important – if not the only – role for cAMP is its catalytic effect on protein kinases. The most prominent example is the phosphorylase b to a conversion, which is accelerated by 10^{-6}–10^{-7} M cAMP. Originally the $b \rightarrow a$ conversion was thought to be due to activation by cAMP of the phosphorylase b kinase directly. In the meantime it has become apparent that cAMP is activating a protein kinase, phosphorylase b kinase-kinase, which in turn phosphorylates (= activates) phosphorylase b-kinase.

In the late 1960s and early 1970s, a great deal of research was carried out on cAMP-dependent protein kinases and on the importance of protein phosphorylation for cellular processes (for a review see Krebs and Beavo, 1979). It is nowadays generally accepted that the cAMP-dependent protein kinases exist as a catalytic (= active, C) subunit and a regulatory (= inhibitory, R) subunit. The general reaction scheme is

$$R_2C_2 + 4\, cAMP \rightleftharpoons R_2cAMP_4 + 2\, C.$$

Two holoenzymes, only differing in their R subunits, are known to exist. Their respective amounts differ from tissue to tissue and from species to species. Thus the rabbit heart contains 48% of Type I ($R_2 = 86\,000$ daltons) and 52% of Type II ($R_2 = 98\,000$ daltons). The bovine heart has 10% of Type I and 90% of Type II, and the rat heart 80% of Type I and 20% of Type II (Nimmo and Cohen, 1977). The catalytic subunits are functionally identical and the R subunits have two high affinity cAMP binding sites per R monomer. The cAMP-dependent protein kinases are also known to be specific enzymes in that only relatively few proteins are phosphorylated at significant rates.

The hormonal control of protein phosphorylation is thought to occur according to the following (simplified) scheme:

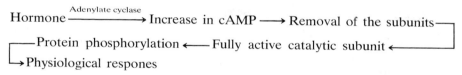

In 1973, Krebs defined five criteria to be fulfilled for accepting the mediation of an effect of cAMP by phosphorylation of a protein. In their review on the hormonal control of protein phosphorylation Nimmo and Cohen (1977) redefined these criteria as follows:

(a) A protein substrate must exist for a cAMP-dependent protein kinase with functional relationship to the process under study. The rate of phosphorylation of that protein should be adequate to account for the speed at which the process occurs *in vivo* in response to cAMP.

(b) The function of the protein should undergo a reversible alteration *in vitro* by phosphorylation–dephosphorylation.

(c) A reversible change in the function of the protein should occur *in vivo* in response to cAMP.

(d) Phosphorylation *in vivo* in response to a hormone should occur at the same site, phosphorylated by cAMP-dependent protein kinase *in vitro*.

The authors conclude: '. . . These criteria have been rigorously met only for phosphorylase kinase and even then many questions still exist. A number of authors have reported an activation *in vivo* of the cAMP-dependent protein kinase in response to hormones but quantitatively reliable data are lacking . . .'.

A few other comments may be added to show that the role of cAMP-dependent protein phosphorylation *in vivo* is not as evident as it looks at first glance.

(1) In the enthusiasm about the cAMP-dependent protein kinases, the protein kinases not catalysed by cAMP have almost completely been ignored. The role of the latter has become obscure because protein phosphorylation and cAMP function were considered to be almost synonymous, as stated by Walsh and Ashby in 1973. The finding that cAMP-independent protein kinase may result from dissociation of the R subunit has further helped the suggestion that all protein kinases are regulated *in vivo* by cAMP.

Van den Berg *et al.* (1980) recently studied phosphorylation of rat liver soluble proteins by endogenous protein kinases. The heat-stable inhibitor protein, specific for cAMP-dependent kinase (see also later), almost completely inhibited the phosphorylation of seven proteins. The phosphorylation of eight proteins was not affected, and the phosphorylation of six proteins, including phosphorylase, was only partially inhibited. Micromolar Ca^{++} stimulated phosphorylation of three proteins, including phosphorylase.

Two other cAMP-independent protein kinases are now coming more and more into focus as candidates for regulation of protein phosphorylation:

(a) *The calmodulin–Ca^{++}-dependent protein kinases*   With the recent explosion of research on calmodulin, it becomes evident that several protein kinases exist which are exclusively dependent on Ca^{++} + calmodulin (for reviews see Klee *et al.*, 1980; Brostrom and Wolff, 1981; Stoclet, 1981). Phosphorylase *b* kinase and the myosin light chain kinase from the smooth muscle have been studied most extensively. The role of calmodulin on muscle phosphorylase *b* kinase has been largely unravelled by Cohen and his group in recent years (see review by Picton *et al.*, 1981). In short, the kinase has calmodulin as a fourth (δ) subunit conferring Ca^{++} sensitivity to the enzyme. In addition it can be further stimulated by binding another molecule of calmodulin (or the related troponin-C in the skeletal muscle).

(b) *The Ca^{++}-phospholipid-dependent protein kinase*   In 1979 Takai *et al.* described a protein kinase, the C-kinase, which was able to phosphory-late five histone fractions as well as muscle phosphorylase kinase. The kinase is only active in the presence of Ca^{++} and phosphatidylserine and it is strongly stimulated by unsaturated diacylglycerol. The enzyme could be clearly differentiated from the cAMP-dependent and the Ca^{++}–calmodulin-dependent kinases (see Nishizuka and Takai, 1981, for a review). It is suggested that this protein kinase, occurring in a wide variety of tissues and species (Kuo *et al.*, 1980), plays a crucial role in the transmission of information of a large number of extracellular signals which involve the phosphatidic acid–phosphatidylinositol turnover response (Michell, 1975):

(2) A heat-stable inhibitor protein of molecular weight around 11 000 daltons (thus clearly different from the R subunit) can easily be isolated from several tissues, especially brain, heart, and skeletal muscle. It is known specifically to inhibit the catalytic subunit of cAMP-dependent protein kinases. Although it is of great help in differentiating protein kinases *in vitro*, its function *in vivo* is not known. In rat hearts it has been calculated that 21% of the cAMP protein kinase(s) activity is blocked by the inhibitor (Walsh and Ashby, 1973).

(3) The binding and activation constants of the R subunits, as determined by conventional Lineweaver–Burke plots and Scatchard plots, are in the range 10^{-8}–5×10^{-8} M. This is well below the cAMP concentrations in unstimulated cells. This would mean either that even in these cells the protein kinases are fully activated, or that, as proposed by Swillens *et al.* (1974), the constants as determined are almost worthless as evidence of an *in vivo* role for cAMP and protein kinase.

(4) The existence of polyphosphate in probably every living cell has been evidenced by Gabel and Thomas (1971). In a proposal Gabel (1972) wondered whether the rapidly exchangeable phosphoproteins are in fact not polyphosphate–protein complexes. In his opinion it seems unreasonable that phosphate ester bonds, such as in the phosphoserine or phosphothreonine from phosphoproteins, could participate in any rapid cyclic phosphate exchange mechanism because of their relative stability and their low free energy of hydrolysis. On the other hand, polyphosphates are noted for their constant reorganization and state of flux and they are known to form tightly bound ionic complexes with proteins. The finding that in several conditions proteins are phosphorylated in their serine or threonine moieties may well be an artefact, produced by either the acidic isolation procedure or by thermal phosphorylation of the protein through polyphosphate. The same authors showed (Gabel and Thomas, 1976) that chicken intestinal alkaline phosphatase incorporates phosphate into its phosphoserine moiety under acidic conditions, and that it contains a considerable amount of polyanionic phosphorus. The enzyme, as well as the abiogenic inorganic polyphosphate, incorporates ^{32}P-labelled phosphate under similar experimental conditions. The role of polyphosphate in protein phosphorylation (cAMP-dependent or independent) merits further investigation.

(5) Although it is now generally accepted that cAMP exerts its effect on protein kinase by releasing the inhibitory R subunit from the active catalytic (= cAMP-independent) subunit, other factors affecting this system have been insufficiently studied. One example, mentioned above, is the marked increase in sensitivity towards cAMP of the phosphorylase system simply by a preincubation at low temperature. More recently, Weinhold and Amrhein (1977) have shown that saturating concentrations of cAMP stimulated their protein kinase from the rabbit skeletal muscle 23-fold. However, agitation with a vortex mixer of the incubation mixture for 30–40 s before the addition of ATP stimulated the kinase activity 15–16-fold and this in a very reproducible way. Subsequent assays in the presence of cAMP have shown an activity not exceeding the activation by cAMP alone, indicating that mechanical agitation and cAMP produce the same effect. Inclusion of 0.1% Triton X-100 during agitation totally prevented the activation by agitation, but left the activation by cAMP unaffected. A sevenfold activation of rat liver phosphorylase kinase has been shown (Chrisman *et al.*, 1981) to occur upon incubation in the presence of submicromolar concentrations of heparin. The stimulation was rapid (within 15 s), and inversely proportional to the concentration of phosphorylase *b*. The degree of activation was similar to that found by phosphorylation.

(6) In 1971, Stull and Mayer did experiments on the regulation of phosphorylase activation in the skeletal muscle *in vivo*. They measured the responses of cAMP, phosphorylase *b* kinase, and phosphorylase *a* to muscle

contraction and to isoproterenol. Tetanic electrical stimulation alone rapidly stimulated phosphorylase *a* formation without any change in cAMP or phosphorylase *b* kinase. Administration of isoproterenol (4×10^{-12} mol) increased phosphorylase *a* activity without changing cAMP content or the *b* kinase activity. The application of 4×10^{-10} mol resulted in an increase in phosphorylase *a* which *preceded* the increase in cAMP and phosphorylase *b* kinase. Beta-adrenergic blockade partially inhibited both cAMP and phosphorylase *a* responses to isoproterenol, but not the formation of activated phosphorylase *b* kinase. The authors conclude that phosphorylase *a* formation is not exclusively a consequence of an increase in cAMP and transformation of non-activated *b* kinase but involves regulation by more complex mechanisms. The cAMP system may be brought into action only by epinephrine released *in high concentrations* from the adrenal medulla.

(7) Villar-Palasi and Wai (1970) calculated that the amount of non-activated phosphorylase kinase ($=$cAMP-independent), present in the skeletal muscle would convert, under the usual conditions of assay, all the phosphorylases in the muscle into the *a* form in less than 0.2 s. The fact that in the resting muscle phosphorylase is in the *b* form indicates that some type of metabolic control restrains the activity of the kinase rather than that the non-activated kinase is essentially inactive. They found ATP strongly to repress the kinase, whereas free Mg^{++} stimulates it. The *in vivo b* to *a* conversion during muscle contraction may be triggered by the breakdown of ATP, resulting in increases in the Mg^{++}:ATP ratio.

(8) Although cAMP is by far the most efficient in stimulating protein kinase at the micro- or submicromolar level, one should not forget that *all* purine and pyrimidine derivatives *maximally* stimulate the enzymatic activity at 5×10^{-4} M (Schorderet, 1974). I know of no *living* cell where the sum of ATP, ADP and AMP is below this level.

Note on dibutyryl-cAMP

One of the criteria proposed by Sutherland for presuming an agent to act through cAMP is that exogenous cyclic nucleotide should mimic the agent's pharmacological effect.

This turned out to be rather hard to prove in cells or intact tissues – an effect can only be induced by nearly millimolar concentrations of exogenous cAMP. The explanation looked simple: cell membranes are poorly permeable to the nucleotide. With the synthesis of the dibutyryl derivative and the early findings that on several occasions this compound was more active than cAMP, it became generally accepted that it is much more easily taken up by intact cells. Actual measurements are, however, scarce and the available information casts doubt on experiments using extracellularly added cyclic nucleotides. Thus McManus *et al.* (1971), incubating thymus lymphocytes with ³H- or ³²P-labelled cAMP, recovered 0.5% of the ³²P label and 3–6% of the ³H label from the cell interior, but only in inorganic phosphate, ADP, and ATP and not in cAMP. Pearlmutter *et al.* (1973), superfusing rat adrenals with ³H-labelled cAMP and dibutyryl-cAMP, showed a more rapid uptake of label from cAMP than from its derivative. However, dibutyryl-cAMP was taken up intact, whereas cAMP was completely degraded. Nevertheless, maximal stimulation of steroidogenesis by dibutyryl-cAMP is 30% lower than by comparable amounts of cAMP. This single experiment clearly illustrates the several problems in interpreting results from experiments with exogenously added cyclic nucleotides in that the following factors are evident:

(a) Dibutyryl-cAMP is less rapidly taken up by cells than is cAMP, contrary to what is generally believed.

(b) Extracellular cAMP stimulates steroidogenesis, although it is completely degraded when reaching the cell interior.

(c) Dibutyryl-cAMP, which slowly enters the cell and is left intact (it is not a substrate for PDE), stimulates steroidogenesis, but by 30% less than similar concentrations of cAMP, which is completely degraded. The derivative even decreases the rate of steroidogenesis that is maximally stimulated by cAMP.

(d) It is known from other studies (Schorderet, 1974) that dibutyryl-cAMP does not activate cAMP-dependent protein kinases at doses at which cAMP is maximally active. How then could unchanged dibutyryl cAMP stimulate steroidogenesis, assuming that all actions of cAMP are due to a stimulation of protein kinases?

(e) When using dibutyryl-cAMP as a substitute for cAMP, possible effects of butyric acid should also be kept in mind. This compound, either present as a contaminant or formed during metabolism, shows peculiar effects on cells, effects which, in earlier studies, have been ascribed to the cAMP-moiety (for a review, see Fiszman, 1978).

General conclusion

That cAMP does exist is beyond any doubt. The way of its formation in the cell is, however, not yet firmly established because of the lack of a pure enzyme preparation and the apparent ease of its formation *non-enzymatically* at the levels occurring *in vivo*. That its formation can be drastically enhanced by the addition of several hormones or sodium fluoride does not necessarily mean that cAMP is *causally* related to the response of the cell – it may well be a *symptom*, accompanying other, possibly more dramatic, induced changes. Examples do exist where similar responses can be provoked without any change in cAMP-levels or where increased levels of cAMP do not result in any response. That cAMP enhances protein kinase activities at very low concentrations is no absolute argument for an essential role in response to hormonal stimulation. Therefore, the importance *in vivo* of phosphorylation of any particular protein should be firmly established and, if so, cAMP-independent protein kinase activities should be absolutely excluded.

cAMP AND HEART CONTRACTILITY

In the late 1960s, the hypothesis that the positive inotropic response to the catecholamines is mediated by cAMP was generally accepted (Sutherland *et al.*, 1968). Since then, however, the relationship has become more and more obscure. Benfey *et al.* (1974) were able to dissociate cardiac inotropic and adenylate cyclase-activating adrenoceptors and they suggested that many reported correlations between myocardial cAMP-production and inotropic responses to sympathomimetic amines may reflect *parallel* processes rather than a cause and effect relationship. In 1977, Tsien, in an excellent review, to which the reader is referred for more details, concluded that the same experimental philosophy, which was used to suggest a *causal* relationship between an increase in cAMP and increased contractile force, has been used by other investigators to demonstrate the opposite. This problem is dealt with by England and by Drake-Holland and Noble (Chapters 16 and 17 in this volume).

The more recent work has not added any more evidence of a causal relationship between cAMP and heart muscle contractility. A definite answer must await a more clear-cut answer into the following questions:

(1) What other changes, besides cAMP, occur in response to extracellular signals?

(2) What is the exact role of phosphorylation?

(3) What, if phosphorylation of a particular protein is important, is the exclusivity of cAMP as the catalyst?

(4) What is the interplay between cAMP and Ca^{++}, the latter being, beyond doubt, the final regulator of heart muscle contraction–relaxation?

ACKNOWLEDGEMENTS

I am grateful to Dr P. A. J. Janssen, Director of the Laboratories, for his continuous interest, to my colleagues J. Leysen, P. Laduron, D. de Chaffoy de Courcelles, F. Awouters, J. Van Wauwe, and D. Ashton for helpful comments, to Mrs L. Geentjens for the typewriting, and to H. Vanhove for linguistic assistance.

REFERENCES

Arner, P., and Östman, J. (1975). Methodological aspects of protein-binding assays for cyclic AMP in human adipose tissue. *Scand. J. Clin. Lab. Invest.*, **35**, 691–697.

Benfey, B. G., Kunos, G., and Nickerson, M. (1974). Dissociation of cardiac inotropic and adenylate cyclase activating adrenoceptors. *Brit. J. Pharmacol.*, **51**, 253–257.

Birnbauer, L., and Yang, P. C. (1974). Studies on receptor-mediated activation of adenylyl cyclases. I. Preparation and description of general properties of an adenylyl cyclase system in beef adrenal medullary membranes sensitive to neurohypophyseal hormones. *J. Biol. Chem.*, **249**, 7848–7856.

Brooker, G., Harper, J. P., Terasaki, W. L., and Moylan, R. D. (1979). Radioimmunoassay of cyclic AMP and cyclic GMP. *Advanc. Cyclic Nucleotide Res.*, **10**, 1–33.

Brostrom, C. O., and Wolff, D. J. (1981). Properties and functions of calmodulin. *Biochem. Pharmacol.*, **30**, 1395–1405.

Brown, B. L., Albano, J. D. M., Epkins, R. P., and Sgherzi, A. M. (1971). A simple and sensitive saturation assay method for the measurement of adenosine 3′:5′-cyclic monophosphate. *Biochem. J.*, **121**, 561–562.

Brownlee, A. G., and Polya, G. M. (1980). The ligand specificity of the (adenosine 3′,5′-monosphate)-binding site of yeast glyceraldehyde-3-phosphate dehydrogenase. *Europ. J. Biochem.*, **109**, 51–59.

Butcher, R. W., Ho, R. J., Meng, H. C., and Sutherland, E. W. (1965). Adenosine 3′,5′-monophosphate in biological materials: II. Measurement of cyclic 3′,5′-AMP in tissues and the role of the cyclic nucleotide in the lipolytic response of fat to epinephrine, *J. Biol. Chem.*, **240**, 4515–4523.

Chrisman, T. D., Jordan, J. E., and Exton, J. H. (1981). Rat liver phosphorylase kinase. Stimulation by heparin. *J. Biol. Chem.*, **256**, 12981–12985.

Coffino, P., Gray, J. W., and Tomkins, G. M. (1975). Cyclic AMP, a nonessential regulator of the cell cycle. *Proc. Natl Acad. Sci.*, **72**, 878–882.

Cohen, N. R. (1981). Teaching the logic of biochemical research. *TIBS*, v–vii.

Cook, W. H., Lipkin, D., and Markham, R. (1957). The formation of a cyclic dianhydrodiadenylic acid (I) by the alkaline degradation of adenosine-5′-triphosphoric acid (II). *J. Amer. Chem. Soc.*, **79**, 3607.

Cooper, R. H., McPherson, M., and Schofield, J. G. (1972). The effects of prostaglandins on ox pituitary content of adenosine 3′,5′-cyclic monophosphate and the release of growth hormone. *Biochem. J.*, **127**, 143–154.

Cooper, R. H., Ashcroft, S. J. H., and Randle, P. J. (1973). Concentration of adenosine 3′:5′-cyclic monophosphate in mouse pancreatic islets measured by a protein-binding radioassay. *Biochem. J.*, **134**, 599–605.

Cote, T. E., and Epand, R. M. (1979). N-Trinitrophenyl glucagon, an inhibitor of glucagon-stimulated cyclic AMP production and its effect on glycogenolysis. *Biochem. Biophys. Acta*, **582**, 295–306.

Counis, R., and Mongongu, S. (1978). Adenylate cyclase assay with [α-^{32}P]ATP as substrate. *Analyt. Biochem.*, **84**, 179–185.

Delaage, M. A., Bellon, B. N., and Cailla, H. L. (1974). Rapid assays for adenylate cyclase and 3′,5′ cyclic AMP phosphodiesterase activities. Simultaneous measurements of other pathways of ATP catabolism. *Analyt. Biochem.*, **62**, 417–425.

Diamond, J. (1978). Role of cyclic nucleotides in control of smooth muscle contraction. *Advanc. Cyclic Nucleotide Res.*, **9**, 327–340.

Døskeland, S. O., and Haga, H. J. (1978). Measurement of adenosine 3′:5′-cyclic monophosphate by competitive binding to salt-dissociated protein kinase. *Biochem. J.*, **174**, 363–372.

Dousa, T., and Rychlik, I. (1970). The metabolism of adenosine 3′,5′-cyclic phosphate. I. Method for the determination of adenyl cyclase and some properties of the adenyl cyclase isolated from the rat kidney. *Biochim. Biophys. Acta*, **204**, 1–9.

Ebadi, M. S., Weiss, B., and Costa, E. (1971). Microassay of adenosine-3′,5′-monophosphate (cyclic AMP) in brain and other tissues by the luciferin–luciferase system. *J. Neurochem.*, **18**, 183–192.

Fiszman, M. (1978). Les effets de l'acide butyrique sur les cellules en culture. *Biochimie*, **60**, vii–x.

Gabel, N. W. (1972). Brief proposal: Could those rapidly exchangeable phosphoproteins be polyphosphate–protein complexes? *Perspect. Biol. Med.*, **15**, 640–643.

Gabel, N. W., and Thomas, V. (1971). Evidence for the occurrence and distribution of inorganic polyphosphates in vertebrate tissues. *J. Neurochem.*, **18**, 1229–1242.

Gabel, N. W., and Thomas, V. (1976). Inorganic polyphosphate as an integral part of alkaline phosphatase preparations. *Bioinorg. Chem.*, **5**, 189–197.

Garrison, J. C., and Borland, M. K. (1979). Regulation of mitochondrial pyruvate carboxylation and gluconeogenesis in rat leukocytes via an α-adrenergic, adenosine 3′:5′-monophosphate-independent mechanism. *J. Biol. Chem.*, **254**, 1129–1133.

Gilman, A. G. (1970). A protein binding assay for adenosine 3′,5′-cyclic monophosphate. *Proc. Natl Acad. Sci.*, **67**, 305–312.

Hilfiker, M. L., and Higgins, W. J. (1980). Calcium influx, intracellular cyclic AMP levels and DNA synthesis in *Tetrahymena pyriformis*. *Comp. Biochem. Physiol.*, **67A**, 465–469.

Hirata, M., and Hayashi, O. (1967). Adenyl cyclase of *Brevibacterium liquefaciens*. *Biochim. Biophys. Acta*, **149**, 1–11.

Homcy, C. J., Wrenn, S. M., and Haber, E. (1978). Affinity purification of cardiac adenylate cyclase: dependence or prior hydrophobic resolution. *Proc. Natl Acad. Sci.*, **75**, 59–63.

Horak, I., and Koschel, K. (1977). Does cAMP control protein synthesis? *FEBS Lett.*, **83**, 68–70.

Johnson, R. A. (1980). Stimulatory and inhibitory effects of ATP-regenerating systems on liver adenylate cyclase. *J. Biol. Chem.*, **255**, 8252–8258.

Johnson, R. A., and Welden, J. (1977). Characteristics of the enzymatic hydrolysis of 5′-adenylylimidodiphosphate: implications for the study of adenylate cyclase. *Arch. Biochem. Biophys.*, **183**, 216–227.

Johnson, R. A., Hardman, J. G., Broadus, A. E., and Sutherland, E. W. (1970). Analysis of adenosine 3′,5′-monophosphate with luciferase luminescence. *Analyt. Biochem.*, **35**, 91–97.

Katz, S., and Tenenhouse, A. (1973). The relation of adenyl cyclase to the activity of other ATP utilizing enzymes and phosphodiesterase in preparations of rat brain; mechanism of stimulation of cyclic AMP accumulation by adrenaline, ouabain and Mn^{++}. *Brit. J. Pharmacol.*, **48**, 526.

Kimura, H., and Murad, F. (1974). Nonenzymatic formation of guanosine 3′:5′-monophosphate from guanosine triphosphate. *J. Biol. Chem.*, **249**, 329–331.

Kiss, Z. (1979). A note on the synthesis of 5′-AMP ester of tris (hydroxymethyl)aminomethane by rat liver plasma membrane. *Biochim. Biophys. Acta*, **568**, 485–487.

Kiss, Z. (1980). Stimulatory effect of ATP on the activity of adenylate cyclase. *Biochem. Pharmacol.*, **29**, 3203–3204.

Klee, C. B., Crouch, T. H., and Richman, P. G. (1980). Calmodulin. *Annu. Rev. Biochem.*, **49**, 489–515.

Kramer, G. L., and Wells, J. N. (1980). Effect of xanthines to inhibit phosphodiesterase (PD) and increase contraction in skeletal muscle. *Mol. Pharmacol.*, **17**, 73–78.

Krebs, E. G. (1973). The mechanism of hormonal regulation by cyclic AMP. In *Endocrinology*; *Proceedings of the 4th International Congress* (R. O. Scow, ed.), Excerpta Medica, Amsterdam, pp. 17–29.

Krebs, E. G., and Beavo, J. A. (1979). Phosphorylation–dephosphorylation of enzymes. *Annu. Rev. Biochem.*, **48**, 923–959.

Krishna, G. (1968). Estimation of cyclic 3′,5′-adenosine monophosphate (c-AMP) in subnanomole quantities by gas-liquid chromatography (GLC). *Fed. Proc.*, **27**, 649.

Krishna, G., Weiss, B., and Brodie, B. (1968). A simple sensitive method for the assay of adenyl cyclase. *J. Pharmacol. Exp. Ther.*, **163**, 379–385.

Kuo, J. F., and Greengard, P. (1970). Cyclic nucleotide-dependent protein kinases. VIII. An assay method for the measurement of adenosine 3′.5′-monophosphate in various tissues and a study of agents influencing its level in adipose cells. *J. Biol. Chem.*, **245**, 4067–4073.

Kuo, J. F., Andersson, R. G. G., Wise, B. C., Mackerlova, L., Salomonsson, I., Brackett, N. L., Katoh, N., Shoji, M., and Wrenn, R. W. (1980). Calcium-dependent protein kinase: widespread occurrence in various tissues and phyla of the animal kingdom and comparison of effects of phospholipid, calmodulin, and trifluoperazine. *Proc. Natl Acad. Sci.*, **77**, 7039–7043.

Larner, E. H., and Rutherford, C. (1978). An artefact produced by boiling adenyl cyclase reaction mixtures prior to the cyclic AMP-radioimmunoassay. *Analyt. Biochem.*, **91**, 684–690.

Limbird, L. E. (1981). Activation and attenuation of adenylate cyclase. The role of GTP-binding proteins as macromolecular messengers in receptor–cyclase coupling. *Biochem. J.*, **195**, 1–13.

Lipkin, D., Cook, W. H., and Markham, R. (1959). Adenosine 3′ : 5′-phosphoric acid: a proof of structure *J. Amer. Chem. Soc.*, **81**, 6198–6203.

Londos, C., Salomon, Y., Lin, M. C., Harwood, J. P., Schramm, M., Wolff, J., and Rodbell, M. (1974). 5′-Guanylylimidodiphosphate, a potent activator of adenylate cyclase systems in eukaryotic cells. *Proc. Natl Acad. Sci.* **71**, 3087–3090.

Long, R., Zimmer, R., and Oberdörster, G. (1973). Impairment of cerebrovascular autoregulation by theophylline. *Exp. Neurol.*, **40**, 661–674.

Meurs, H., Kauffman, H. F., Koeter, G., and De Vries, K. (1980). Extraction of cyclic AMP for the determination in the competitive protein binding assay. *Clin. Chim. Acta*, **106**, 91–97.

Michell, R. H. (1975). Inositol phospholipids and cell surface receptor function. *Biochim. Biophys. Acta*, **415**, 81–147.

Mitznegg, P., Schubert, E., and Heim, F. (1974). The influence of low and high doses of theophylline on spontaneous motility and cyclic 3′,5′-AMP content in isolated rat uterus. *Life Sci.*, **14**, 711–717.

McManus, J. P., Whitfield, J. F., and Braceland, B. (1971). The metabolism of exogenous cyclic AMP at low concentrations by thymic lymphocytes. *Biochem. Biophys. Res. Commun.*, **42**, 503–509.

Nahorski, S. R., and Rogers, K. J. (1973). The adenosine 3′,5′-monophosphate content of brain tissue obtained by an ultra-rapid freezing technique. *Brain Res.*, **51**, 332–336.

Neer, E. J., and Salter, R. S. (1981). Reconstituted adenylate cyclase from bovine brain. Functions of the subunits. *J. Biol. Chem.*, **256**, 12102–12107.

Nimmo, H. G., and Cohen, P. (1977). Hormonal control of protein phosphorylation. *Advanc. Cyclic Nucleotide Res.*, **8,** 145–266.

Nishizuka, Y., and Takai, Y. (1981). Calcium and phospholipid turnover in a new receptor function for protein phosphorylation. In *Protein Phosphorylation, Book A* (O. M. Rosen and E. G. Krebs, eds), Cold Spring Harbor Laboratory, Cold Spring Harbor, N.Y., pp. 237–249.

Pearlmutter, A. F., Rapino, E., and Saffran, M. (1973). Comparison of steroidogenic effects of cAMP and dbcAMP in the rat adrenal gland. *Endocrinology*, **92,** 679–686.

Picton, C., Klee, C. B., and Cohen, P. (1981). The regulation of muscle phosphorylase kinase by calcium ions, calmodulin and troponin-C. *Cell Calcium*, **2,** 281–294.

Pike, L. J., and Lefkowitz, R. J. (1980). Activation and desensitization of β-adrenergic receptor-coupled GTPase and adenylate cyclase of frog and turkey erythrocyte membranes. *J. Biol. Chem.*, **255,** 6860–6867.

Rall, T. W., and Sutherland, E. W. (1962). Adenyl cyclase: II. The enzymatically catalyzed formation of adenosine-3′,5′-phosphate and inorganic pyrophosphate from adenosine triphosphate. *J. Biol. Chem.*, **237,** 1228–1232.

Ramachandran, J. (1971). A new simple method for separation of adenosine 3′,5′-cyclic monophosphate from other nucleotides and its use in the assay of adenyl cyclase. *Analyt. Biochem.*, **43,** 227–239.

Rasmussen, H., Goodman, D. B. P., and Tenenhouse, A. (1972). The role of cyclic AMP and calcium in cell activation. *CRC Crit. Rev. Biochem.*, **1,** 95–148.

Richards, J. M., Thierney, J. M., and Swislock, N. I. (1981). ATP-dependent activation of adenylate cyclase. *J. Biol. Chem.*, **256,** 8889–8891.

Ross, E. M., and Gilman, A. G. (1980). Biochemical properties of hormone-sensitive adenylate cyclase. *Annu. Rev. Biochem.*, **49,** 533–564.

Salomon, Y. (1979). Adenylate cyclase assay. *Advanc. Cyclic Nucleotide Res.*, **10,** 35–55.

Salomon, Y., Londos, C., and Rodbell, M. (1974). A highly sensitive adenylate cyclase assay. *Analyt. Biochem.*, **58,** 541–548.

Schorderet, M. (1974). AMP cyclique et système nerveux. *J. Physiol. (Paris)*, **68,** 471–505.

Schwabe, U., Ebert, R., and Schönhöfer, P. S. (1974). Sensitive determination for adenylate cyclase activity by cyclic adenosine 3′,5′-monophosphate protein binding assay. *Naunyn-Schmiedebergs Arch. Pharmacol.*, **286,** 83–94.

Schwabe, U., Puchstein, C., Hanneman, H., and Söchtig, E. (1979). Activation of adenylate cyclase by vanadate. *Nature*, **227,** 143–145.

Sen, K. K., and Menon, K. M. J. (1979). Dissociation of cyclic AMP accumulation from that of luteinizing hormone (LH) release in response to gonadotropin releasing hormone (GnRH) and cholera enterotoxin. *Biochem. Biophys. Res. Commun.*, **87,** 221–228.

Sharif, N. A., and Roberts, P. J. (1981). Regulation of cerebellar L-[³H]glutamate binding: influence of guanine nucleotides and Na⁺ ions. *Biochem. Pharmacol.*, **30,** 3019–3022.

Sinha, A. K., and Colman, R. W. (1981). A new method for separating cyclic AMP from 5′-AMP with application to the assay for cyclic AMP phosphodiesterase. *Analyt. Biochem.*, **113,** 239–245

Stansfield, D. D., and Franks, D. J. (1970). Adenylate cyclase and 'adenosine triphosphate' in corpus luteum. *Biochem. J.*, **120,** 5 P.

Stockton, J. M., and Turner, A. J. (1981). Characterization of adenylate cyclase purified from rat brain by hydrophobic chromatography. *J. Neurochem.*, **36,** 1722–1730.

Stoclet, J. C. (1978). 'A reassessment of the criteria used to involve cyclic nucleotides in hormone and drug mechanisms', in *Advanc. Pharmacol. Therapeut.*, **3**, 181–192.

Stoclet, J. C. (1979). Inhibitors of cyclic nucleotide phosphodiesterase, *TIBS*, **1**, 98–100.

Stoclet, J. C. (1981). Calmodulin: an ubiquitous protein which regulates calcium-dependent cellular functions and calcium movements. *Biochem. Pharmacol.*, **30**, 1723–1729.

Stull, J. T., and Mayer, S. E. (1971). Regulation of phosphorylase activation in skeletal muscle *in vivo. J. Biol. Chem.*, **246**, 5716–5723.

Sutherland, E. W., and Rall, T. W. (1957). The properties of an adenine ribonucleotide produced with cellular particles, ATP, Mg^{2+} and epinephrine or glucagon. *J. Amer. Chem. Soc.*, **79**, 3608.

Sutherland, E. W., Rall, T. W., and Menon, T. (1962). Adenyl cyclase: I. Distribution, preparation and properties. *J. Biol. Chem.*, **237**, 1220–1227.

Sutherland, E. W., Robison, G. A., and Butcher, R. W. (1968). Some aspects of the biological role of adenosine-3',5'-monophosphate. *Circulation*, **37**, 279–306.

Swillens, S., Van Cauter, E., and Dumont, J. E. (1974). Protein kinase and cyclic 3',5'-AMP: significance of binding and activation constants. *Biochim. Biophys. Acta*, **364**, 250–259.

Takai, Y., Kishimoto, A., Iwasa, Y., Kawahara, Y., Mori, T., and Nishizuka, Y. (1979). Calcium-dependent activation of a multifunctional protein kinase by membrane phospholipids. *J. Biol. Chem.*, **254**, 3692–3695.

Tihon, C., Goren, M. B., Spitz, E., and Rickenberg, H. V. (1977). Convenient elimination of trichloroacetic acid prior to radioimmunoassay of cyclic nucleotides. *Analyt. Biochem.*, **80**, 652–653.

Tsien, R. W. (1977). Cyclic AMP and contractile activity in heart. *Advanc. Cyclic Nucleotide Res.* **8**, 363–420.

Van den Berg, G. B., Van Berkel, T. J. C., and Koster, J. F. (1980). The role of Ca^{2+} and cyclic AMP in the phosphorylation of rat-liver soluble proteins by endogenous protein kinases. *Europ. J. Biochem.*, **113**, 131–140.

Verbert, A., and Cacan, R. (1972). Description d'un procédé électrophorétique de séparation de l'AMP cyclique de ses métabolites. Application à la détermination de l'activité adénylcyclasique. *Biochimie*, **54**, 1491–1492.

Villar-Palasi, C., and Wei, S. H. (1970). Conversion of glycogen phosphorylase *b* to *a* by non-activated phosphorylase *b* kinase: an *in vitro* model of the mechanism of increase in phosphorylase *a* activity with muscle contraction. *Proc. Natl Acad. Sci.*, **67**, 345–350.

Walsh, D. A., and Ashby, C. D. (1973). Protein kinases: Aspects of their regulation and diversity. *Recent Prog. Horm. Res.*, **29**, 329–359.

Wattiaux-De Coninck, S., Dubois, F., and Wattiaux, R. (1981). Subcellular distribution of adenylate cyclase in rat-liver tissue. *FEBS Lett.*, **123**, 33–36.

Weinhold, B., and Amrhein, N. (1977). Activation of rabbit skeletal muscle adenosine-3':5'-monophosphate-dependent protein kinase by agitation. *Biochem. Biophys. Res. Commun.*, **76**, 1116–1123.

Wells, J. N., and Hardman, J. G. (1977). Cyclic nucleotide phosphodiesterase. *Advanc. Cyclic Nucleotide Res.*, **8**, 119–143.

Zapf, J., Waldvogel, M., and Froesch, E. R. (1981). Is increased basal lipolysis in adipose tissue of fasted-refed rats related to cyclic-AMP-dependent mechanisms? *Europ. J. Biochem.*, **119**, 453–459.

Cardiac Metabolism
Edited by A. J. Drake-Holland and M. I. M. Noble
© 1983 John Wiley & Sons Ltd

CHAPTER 19

Enzyme Histochemistry of the Myocardium

R. G. Butcher

The Midhurst Medical Research Institute, Midhurst, West Sussex GU29 OBL, UK

INTRODUCTION

The many diverse approaches to the study of enzyme behaviour which hide under the umbrella title of 'histochemistry' make a comprehensive review of the subject in any tissue a difficult one. A review of myocardial enzyme histochemistry by Hecht (1971) discussed well over 200 different investigations and many more than that number of new publications on the subject have appeared during the last decade. Only those studies concerning enzyme localization and metabolism most pertinent to myocardial biochemistry and pathology and which most closely reflect the present trends in histochemistry will be discussed here; the choice is inevitably a personal one. Two major trends, the increasing use of electron microscopy to elucidate intracellular enzyme localization and the development of a precise quantitative biochemical approach to the investigation of enzyme behaviour at the cellular level, will be considered separately, though they are not, of course, mutually exclusive. The decision to include a particular enzyme or group of enzymes in one or other of these two sections has been an arbitrary one. For example, lysosomal enzymes appear in the section on localization simply because the vast majority of the recent histochemical literature on these enzymes in the myocardium has been at the electron microscope level.

LOCALIZATION STUDIES

ATPases

Cytochemical demonstration

The ATPases are a group of enzymes linked only by the fact that they metabolize the same substrate; whenever the terminal phosphate group of ATP is removed by enzymatic hydrolysis, the process is ascribed to ATPase activity. The significance of such activity depends on the use made of the energy liberated by such hydrolysis (Firth, 1978).

Until recently almost all the cytochemical methods for demonstrating ATPase activity were based on the calcium–cobalt method of Padykula and Herman (1955) or the lead capture method of Wachstein and Meisel (1957). Though these methods are relatively simple to use both for light and electron microscope studies, they have a basic disadvantage; namely that ATP and the few other substrates which can be used in these methods are hydrolysed by a wide range of ATPases and the specificity of a reaction can only be elucidated by the use of extensive controls. The interpretation of results using modified Wachstein and Meisel methods are further compli-cated by the fact that many ATPases are seriously inhibited by lead salts and that lead concentrations greater than 1 mM induce the non-enzymatic hyd-rolysis of ATP (Moses *et al.*, 1966).

During the last 10 years there has been considerable clarification of the distribution and function of ATPases in the cell (Firth, 1978, 1980). From these findings there would appear to be four enzymes (or groups of en-zymes) of particular significance in myocardial metabolism.

Myosin-type ATPase

This enzyme is generally assumed to function in relation to contraction events rather than to have any role in transport across membranes. It can be demonstrated easily by many variants of the Wachstein–Meisel and Padykula–Herman methods and has been much used in fibre typing in skeletal muscle. The enzyme is stimulated by Ca^{++} but inhibited by Mg^{++}, is sensitive to sulphydryl reagents such as *p*-chloromercuribenzoate (PCMB) but not to ouabain or to oligomycin.

At the light microcope level the method of Niles *et al.* (1964), using unfixed sections of cardiac muscle, showed that myosin ATPase activity could be precisely located within the myofibril, at sites known to contain myosin, provided that the release of phosphate was sufficiently rapid and that the capture of released phosphate was optimized by the addition of a sufficiently high concentration of Ca^{++} in the medium. Activity was high at pH 9.4 but was not demonstrable at pH 7.0. This method has been used extensively in a series of studies using human myocardial biopsies (see later).

For electron microscopic localization the preferred method uses lead citrate, cysteine, and Ca^{++} at pH 9.0 (Somogyi and Sotonyi, 1969). The myofibrillar reaction shows the appropriate ion dependence and inhibitor responses and no reaction is seen in the sarcolemma, the sarcoplasic reticulum or in mitochondria.

Mitochondrial ATPase

The mitochondrial proton-translocating ATPase, located on the inner mitochondrial membrane, is considered to run in the direction of ATP synthesis driven by the electron transport system and so coupling oxidative metabolism to phosphorylation. For sustained ATP hydrolysis, and hence for the cytochemical demonstration of the enzyme, it is necessary to un-couple oxidative phosphorylation with an agent such as 2,4-dinitrophenol (DNP). The reaction is inhibited by oligomycin and by PCMB, activated by Mg^{++}, but inhibited by a high concentration of Ca^{++}; ouabain has no effect. The enzyme has been localized in cardiac muscle by Ogawa and Mayahara (1969) in a modification of the medium of Wachstein and Meisel in which lead citrate replaced lead nitrate, and which contained DNP, and by Sotonyi *et al.* (1974) with neodymium nitrate replacing the lead salt.

Sarcoplasmic reticular Ca^{++}-transporting ATPases

The sarcoplasmic reticulum has a large role in the contraction–relaxation cycle of muscle fibres by its influence on the sarcoplasmic concentration of Ca^{++}. The re-uptake of Ca^{++} into the lumen of the sarcoplasmic reticulum following fibre contraction is dependent on this specialized ATPase.

Whilst demonstration of this enzyme cytochemically is relatively easy, confirmation of specificity is more difficult. Studies of myocardial tissue by Somogyi *et al.* (1972) showed that the reaction was not dependent on Ca^{++} but only on Mg^{++}. In contrast Khan *et al.* (1972, 1975) demonstrated a Mg^{++}-independent reaction in skeletal muscle which was readily distin-guished from mitochondrial and myofibrillar activity on the basis of ion dependence, the negative response to PCMB and oligomycin, and the pH optimum. However, since the method employed by these workers uses Ca^{++} as the trapping agent it is impossible to test its Ca^{++} dependence.

Cytochemical studies in fixed cardiac muscle tissue showed activities localized throughout the sarcoplasmic reticulum (Somogyi *et al.*, 1972) or mainly over the lateral sacs and/or junctional areas of triads (Sommer and Spach, 1964; Essner *et al.*, 1965; Rostgaard and Behnke, 1965); the reaction shown by Rostgaard and Behnke was independent of Mg^{++}. How-ever, skeletal muscle Mg^{++}-dependent, Ca^{++}-stimulated ATPase is inacti-vated by glutaraldehyde (Sommer and Hasselback, 1967) and by parafomal-dehyde (Malouf and Meissner, 1979); paraformaldehyde also inhibits this enzyme in cardiac muscle (Malouf and Meissner, 1980). Their findings suggest that it is possible to distinguish two Ca^{++}-activated membrane-associated ATPases in the myocardium; Mg^{++}- or Ca^{++}-activated 'basic' ATPase, affected little by fixation, and associated with the surface mem-brane of the cell, and Mg^{++}-dependent Ca^{++}-stimulated ATPase almost completely inhibited by fixation, and localized only in the sarcoplasmic reticulum. The physiological role of the 'basic' surface membrane ATPase is presumably to maintain Ca^{++} homeostasis.

Na^+,K^+-ATPase

This ouabain-sensitive enzyme is of special interest because of its role in the maintenance of both electrical and physical properties of myocardial cells and particularly in the regulation of cell volume. Since it is strongly inhibited by both lead salts and by fixation, interpretation of results using modified Wachstein–Meisel methods are difficult. By keeping the lead concentration below 0.01 mM, Wollenberger and Schulze (1976) were able to localize a Na^+,K^+-ATPase in the plasmalemma of myocardial cells. A more suitable method for the demonstration of this enzyme is the strontium capture technique of Ernst (1972b) which employs p-nitrophenol phosphate as substrate for the K^+-dependent phosphate step of the reaction. With this method Asano *et al.* (1980) localized an ouabain-sensitive, K^+-dependent ATPase in the plasmalemma and the T-tubules. Reactions in the sarcoplasmic reticulum, subsarcolemmal cisternae, and mitochondria were not inhibited by ouabain, suggesting the possibility that enzymes other than Na^+,K^+-ATPase also hydrolyse the p-nitrophenyl phosphate substrate (Ernst, 1972a).

A labelled inhibitor method which localizes the enzyme autoradiographically (Stirling, 1972) and an immunocytochemical method (Kyte, 1974) have recently been described for demonstrating Na^+,K^+-ATPase activity. It is hoped that these methods may be extended for use in clarifying the complex nature of all the ATPases in the myocardium.

Adenylate Cyclase

Adenylate cyclase catalyses the conversion of ATP into cyclic AMP and inorganic phosphate and is thought to play an important role in the events leading to muscle contraction. A knowledge of the localization of adenylate cyclase within the cell is essential to the understanding of the mechanisms of calcium transport across membranes.

Histochemical studies of this enzyme have concentrated on the localization at the electron microscopical level. All methods depend on the formation of an insoluble complex of the inorganic phosphate with a heavy metal ion, usually a lead salt. Reik *et al.* (1970) first reported a cytochemical localization of adenylate cyclase in rat liver using ATP as substrate and this method was used by Schulze *et al.* (1972) to demonstrate the localization in cardiac muscle. Lead precipitate was observed along the plasma membrane of the sarcolemma and membranes of the intercalated disc; staining was also observed in the membranes of the *T*-tubules and the sarcolemmal cisternae. An increase in the amount of reaction product formed on the addition of sodium fluoride, and by catecholamines and glucagon, suggested that this might be the true localization of adenylate cyclase.

However, ATP is also split by the ATPases and other phosphatases. To overcome this problem Howell and Whitfield (1972) and Wagner *et al.* (1972) introduced a substrate specific for adenylate cyclase (adenylylimidodiphosphate (AMP-PNP)). Cutler and Christian (1980) have shown that using this method the lead salt does not inhibit in the presence of 10 mM sodium fluoride and does not cause the non-enzymatic hydrolysis of AMP-PNP. A major problem has been that in order to obtain adequate preservation of structural detail 50–87% of the enzyme activity is inhibited by the fixation procedures. Slezar and Geller (1976) claim an improvement in both tissue preservation and enzymatic integrity of cardiac muscle by including 5% dimethyl sulphoxide in their fixative.

In an attempt to overcome the problems of fixation inhibition Revis (1979) incubated unfixed sections of cardiac muscle in the adenylate cyclase medium and then prepared electron micrographs from post-fixed material. In such sections the enzyme was localized to the sarcotubular system and the sarcolemma. No reaction product was observed in the intercalated disc, in mitochondria, and in the myofibrils; in prefixed sections the reaction product was diffusely localized over the sections.

The specificity of this histochemical reaction and thus its localization in cardiac muscle must remain in doubt. The suggestion that precipitation may be related to the presence and/or release of calcium ions at or near the plasma membrane, rather than to adenylate cyclase activity (Kempen *et al.*, 1978) requires further investigation in myocardial tissue.

Lysosomal Enzymes

Cytochemical demonstration

The study of lysosomal enzymes and their functions in the heart is a relatively recent phenomenon; conclusive biochemical evidence of cardiac lysosomal enzyme activity was not published until 1966 (Romeo *et al.*, 1966). At the same time cytochemical investigations in myocardial tissue localized acid phosphatase (Goldfischer *et al.*, 1966) and lysosomal esterase (Hegab and Ferrans, 1966). These findings were confirmed by Abraham *et al.* (1967) and extended to include B-glucuronidase and aryl sulphatase.

Electron microscopic studies have shown that myocyte lysosomes contribute but little to the total cardiac activity of acid phosphatase; much of the enzyme is localized in interstitial cells. The same is true for other lysosomal enzymes such as B-glucuronidase and aryl sulphatase. There is heterogeneity too within the cell; lysosomes are not uniform organelles with a fixed structure and function but are made up of many bodies of varying characteristics and may be indistinguishably associated with the Golgi complex and the sarcoplasmic reticulum. McCallister *et al.* (1977) found occasional deposits of reaction product in association with residual bodies and primary lysosomes in rat myocardium; reaction was most intense in the perinuclear region of the cell. Decker and Wildenthal (1978a) paid particular attention to interstitial cells as well as to myocytes of rabbit heart muscle. Whilst the intestitial cells stained intensely with large dense bodies containing the reaction products of each of the enzymes studied, acid phosphatase, aryl sulphatase and lysosomal esterase, the myocytes showed relatively little evidence of reaction. Only small deposits of acid phosphatase reaction product were demonstrable in myocyte residual bodies; the Golgi apparatus and the Golgi–endoplasmic reticulum–lysosome complex (GERL (Novikoff, 1976)) showed some reaction and were also occasionally positive for aryl sulphatase. The three enzymes were also detectable, distributed haphazardly, in the sarcoplasmic reticulum. Similar localizations were observed in rat myocardium by Topping and Travis (1974). In contrast, Hoffstein *et al.* (1975) demonstrated a very widespread distribution of acid phosphatase and aryl sulphatase in the sarcoplasmic reticulum of canine myocardium with the reaction product in orderly arrays throughout the myocytes.

Myocardial cells contain much larger amounts of the lysosomal acid proteinase, cathepsin D, and this is the major lysosomal proteinase of the heart (Decker *et al.*, 1980). However, even with this enzyme a single interstitial cell contains more enzyme than a single myocyte, simply because interstitial cells have more lysosomes. Cellular localization of rabbit cathepsin D by specific immunofluorescent staining indicates that this enzyme is normally present in organelles that resemble secondary lysosomes in size and distribution (Wildenthal *et al.*, 1975). Confirmation of this has come with the adaptation of this method for use in the electron microscope (Decker *et al.*, 1980). Reaction product was localized in secondary lysosomes of both cardiac myocytes and interstitial cells; no reaction was seen in components of the Golgi complex or the sarcoplasmic reticulum.

Other lysosomal proteinases have now been demonstrated in cardiac muscle using immunofluorescent techniques; dipeptidyl peptidase I (cathepsin C), dipeptidyl peptidase II and cathepsin B (Stauber and Ong, 1981a,b, 1982).

Lysosomal enzymes in myocardial ischaemia

The process of ischaemia induces structural and metabolic changes in myocytes as they pass from reversible to irreversible damage. In recent years considerable interest has been focused on the behaviour of lysosomes as a possible cause of this change. It has been postulated that during the ischaemic process lysosomal membranes might be labilized, leading to the release of hydrolytic enzymes into the cytosol. This could lead to the degradation of intracellular molecules and ultimately to cell death.

Cytochemical studies have produced evidence both in support of and contrary to this hypothesis. Hoffstein *et al.* (1975) produced ischaemia in dogs by an electrically induced thrombus of the left arterial descending coronary artery. In this model the reaction products of acid phosphatase and aryl sulphatase seen in the sarcoplasmic reticulum of control myocardium diffused into the cytosol after 2 h ischaemia, and hence presumably after the cells had already been irreversibly injured for some time. Similar findings came from Okuda and Lefer (1979) in Langendorff rat heart preparations.

A major contribution has come from the investigations of Decker and his colleagues. Experimentally induced ischaemia in rabbits by coronary artery ligation produced irreversible necrosis after 45–60 min (Decker and Wildenthal, 1978a). However, no evidence of rupture of the lysosomal membrane was detectable after 1 h ligation and loss of acid phosphatase, aryl sulphatase, and lysosomal esterase from lysosomes into the cytosol did not occur until 1–2 h. In contrast, after 30 min ligation there was evidence of hypertrophy of the Golgi apparatus and the appearance of many secondary lysosomes in the interstitial cells. Moreover the Golgi complex and GERL showed considerable deposits of acid phosphatase reaction product in these cells; aryl sulphatase and esterase deposits were also present in lysosomal bodies. Longer periods of ischaemia did not alter the appearance.

The behaviour of cathepsin D in ischaemic myocardium was somewhat different (Decker *et al.*, 1977). After 30–45 min ligation (at or about the time that reversible changes become irreversible) the fine particulate staining seen in control myocytes changed to bright fluorescent particles composed of large granules. Prominent halos of diffuse fluorescence were also present in the neighbouring cytoplasm suggesting leakage of cathepsin D into the cytosol. After 2 h occlusion most of the fluorescent particles had disappeared completely. Similar changes in the activity and distribution of this enzyme were not observed in the interstitial cells. It is tempting to conclude from this that the release of cathepsin D from lysosomes into the cytosol is an important factor in the change from reversible to irreversible cell damage. It has been emphasized by these authors (see, for example, Wildenthal, 1978) that whilst these lysosomal alterations parallel changes that lead to irreversible ischaemic damage, no cause-effect relationship has been conclusively established. Indeed lysosomal alterations may occur as part of the repair process in reversibly injured cells. Thus intervention with steroids, shown by Decker and Wildenthal (1978b) to delay signs of lysosomal damage and leakage of lysosomal enzymes, may not necessarily be beneficial.

Cytochemical investigations of lysosomal enzymes in the myocardium have, almost without exception, been made on fixed tissue. The failure by many workers to show leakage of lysosomal hydrolases into the cytosol of the ischaemic heart until after necrosis has already been produced might be due in part to inhibition of the acid hydrolase activities by the glutaraldehyde fixation, and hence to a decrease in the concentration of precipitable ions (Decker and Wildenthal, 1978a). Studies of the Gomori acid phosphatase reaction in a model system by de Jong *et al.* (1979; reviewed by de Jong, 1982), indicate that the critical phosphate concentration required for precipitation to occur can be dramatically changed by many factors.

The functional state of the lysosomal membrane in unfixed tissue sections can be assessed using the lysosomal fragility test developed by Bitensky (1963; reviewed by Bitensky *et al.*, 1973, and by Bitensky and Chayen, 1979). Three stages of lysosomal function can be observed in this test: (a) an intact membrane which does not permit entry of substrate; (b) entry of substrate after modification of the membrane, for example by pretreatment with acetate buffer of pH 5.0 at 37 °C; and (c) loss of membrane integrity and release of enzyme from the lysosome. This test has proved useful in testing the toxicity of drugs on cultured heart endothelioid cells (Reed and Wenzel, 1975), and dynamic studies of this type in unfixed sections of heart tissue might prove to be of value in the future.

FUNCTIONAL HISTOCHEMISTRY

Introduction

The first attempts to use the techniques of histochemistry as a basis for the development of biochemistry at the cellular level were made during the early 1950s (see, for example, Danielli, 1953). This has been continued in one direction by Glick (reviewed in Glick, 1981) with the development of microchemical techniques using the tissue section, or a microdissected part of that section, as the biochemical sample; such procedures will not be discussed further here. An alternative approach is to incubate the tissue section in a relatively conventional biochemical medium differing only in that final reaction product of the chemical activity is precipitated in the cell in which the activity occurs. Such an approach has several advantages: the biochemistry can be related to the structure by reference to a serial section stained by conventional histological methods; several different enzyme activities can be studied in serial sections from even a small amount of tissue such as is available from a human myocardial biopsy; enzyme activities can be related to other chemical components determined in serial sections and to biophysical parameters measured optically (for reviews see Bitensky *et al,*, 1973; Chayen *et al.*, 1974).

For such a dynamic approach the fixation of sections, causing chemical inactivation and hence inhibition of enzyme activity, is not possible and fresh sections must be used. It is possible to prepare unfixed cryostat sections which show, even at the level of the electron microscope (Altman and Barrnett, 1975), that the processes of chilling and cutting do not cause demonstrable structural damage to the tissue.

Early Studies on Dehydrogenases

The development of this approach is particularly well illustrated by reference to the dehydrogenases. Many of the early histochemical studies on fresh sections of myocardium were concerned with changes in enzyme activity relating to ischaemia. These included investigations on experimentally induced ischaemia by coronary artery ligation in dogs (Kent and Diseker, 1955; Schnitka and Nachlas, 1963; Cox *et al.*, 1968), in rats (Kaufman *et al.*, 1959), and in human biopsies (Wachstein and Meisel, 1955). Amongs many enzymes studied, the only ones to show changes were the dehydrogenases and in particular succinate dehydrogenase. Decrease in activity of this enzyme occurred long after necrosis had arisen, at the earliest at 6 h post ligation, and often changes were not detectable until 15 h post ischaemia. What was noticed by many workers was a change in the nature of the formazan precipitated in the section; in normal myocardium the reaction was a diffuse sarcoplasmic stain whilst in the ischaemic heart a more granular reaction was noted. This granular reaction was particularly evident in the intermediate region of the heart between normal tissue and frankly necrotic cells (Cox *et al.*, 1968).

Human Biopsy Studies

A series of important investigations using functional histochemical techniques to analyse the problems of morbidity and mortality associated with major heart surgery had been reviewed recently by Braimbridge and Cankovic-Darracott (1979). These studies, using full thickness biopsies of approximately 1.5 mm diameter from the apex of the left ventrical (Braimbridge and Niles, 1964) have concentrated on just two enzymes of importance in myocardial contraction: succinate dehydrogenase, demonstrated with nitro blue tetrazolium (NBT) as final electron acceptor, and myosin ATPase (using the method of Niles *et al.*, 1964).

A significant feature of these studies was not so much the alteration in the amount of reaction product as the change in distribution which could occur during open heart surgery. Changes were therefore graded on the basis of appearance rather than on the quantification of the tissue sections. The appearance of the reaction product for succinate dehydrogenase activity in normal myocardium showed the formazan of NBT evenly and strongly distributed along the myofibrils; in contrast in the functionally abnormal myocardium formazan was virtually absent from the myofibrils and occurred in granules which presumably corresponded to mitochondria. Thus these observations paralleled the earlier aspects of change which occurred in experimental ischaemia (see above). What was so significantly different was the ability to detect changes at a sufficiently early stage. The localization of ATPase activity changed too, from a regular cross-striation distribution in the normal to dense contraction bands in the grossly abnormal. These two tests were combined with studies of phospholipid binding demonstrated by the acid haematin reaction (Chayen, 1968) and with quantitative polarizing microscopy from serial sections of the same biopsy. Other enzyme activities, cytochrome oxidase and monoamine oxidase, were the same at the beginning and end of surgery (Cankovic-Darracott *et al.*, 1977).

Using these tests a system of grading from completely normal to grossly dysfunctional was devised (Cankovic-Darracott *et al.*, 1977) and used to determine the myocardial deterioration as shown in a biopsy taken at the end of bypass compared with a biopsy taken from the same heart at the beginning of the operation. From a series of 293 patients impairment of myocardial function was predicted, on the basis of these cytochemical tests, in 77 patients. In all of these, plus three other cases, there was clinical evidence of impaired cardiac function. Thus the combined cytochemical evaluation predicted 96% of the cases that showed post-operative signs of myocardial dysfunction. Of the other 213 patients who had uneventful post-operative recoveries, 33 had positive cytochemical signs of dysfunction. Nor were their findings purely of academic interest. The cytochemical results were usually available to the surgeon on the evening of the operation and so permitted any necessary modification to the post-operative management of the patient (Braimbridge *et al.*, 1973; Braimbridge and Cankovic-Darracott, 1979).

This group of workers has adopted the same cytochemical approach to the analysis of perfusion conditions during bypass, and to the optimal conditions for the maintenance of a functional state of the myocardium during the long periods required for open heart surgery. (Braimbridge *et al.*, 1973, 1977; Cankovic-Darracott *et al.*, 1977). An assessment of five different techniques showed that continuous perfusion at 32 °C with a beating heart or cardioplegic arrest at 4 °C with a perfusate containing Mg^{++}, K^+, and procaine protected the heart best. A comparison of these two methods during aortic valve replacement extended to differences in epi- and endocardial biopsies showed that the epicardium was the region most at risk with cold cardioplegia, whereas the endocardium was more likely to be damaged during continuous perfusion at 32 °C (Braimbridge *et al.*, 1977).

A greater understanding of the mechanisms behind these problems has come with the development of quantitative techniques and the introduction of intermediate acceptors into dehydrogenase methodology.

Quantification by Elution

Quantitative biochemical results have long been obtained easily by spectrophotometry where the end product of the chemical reaction is usually a coloured solution. The first attempts to measure the amount of an enzyme reaction in a tissue section employed the same principle; the final coloured reaction product was eluted from the section into a solvent and the absorbance measured in a spectrophotometer (e.g. Jones *et al.*, 1963). Activity could be related to the unit area of the section (and, by knowing the thickness of the section (Butcher, 1971), to per unit volume of tissue), to the protein nitrogen content (Sloane-Stanley and Jones, 1963), or the nucleic acid content (Butcher, 1968). Although studies using such techniques were able to give only an average measure of the total activity of the section, they nevertheless showed that many of the parameters measured routinely by conventional biochemical homogenization procedures could be measured with equal precision in a single tissue section. Thus, using sections of rat liver, Butcher (1970) was able to determine, by Lineweaver–Burke plots, the Michaelis constant with respect to substrate of succinate dehydrogenase, to show that the inhibition with malonate was competitive, and that the degree of inhibition was the same as was found in a biochemical homogenate.

The use of Phenazine Methosulphate

In dehydrogenase histochemistry, activity is demonstrated by incubating sections in a medium, at the appropriate pH, containing substrate, coenzyme if required, and a tetrazolium salt which on reduction is converted to a coloured insoluble formazan and is deposited in the section at the site of the reduction. However, incubation of, for example, succinate and nitroblue tetrazolium (NBT) in a test tube with purified succinate dehydrogenase would not produce the formazan. The tetrazolium salt alone cannot accept reducing equivalents directly from succinate dehydrogenase but can do so only after the transfer of those equivalents along a number of oxidation–reduction stages in the mitochondrion. Thus all the early studies of succinate dehydrogenase activity in the myocardium were demonstrating, not the activity of succinate dehydrogenase *per se* but, as emphasized in the studies reviewed by Braimbridge and Cankovic-Darracott (1979), the functional capability of the mitochondrial electron transport pathway.

Intermediate acceptors such as phenazine methosulphate (PMS) accept electrons directly from the enzyme complex and transfer them directly to the tetrazole (Farber and Bueding, 1956). In a study of human myocardial biopsies, Niles *et al.* (1966) compared succinate dehydrogenation in the presence and absence of PMS. The addition of PMS changed the appearance of the reaction product in normal myocardium from the intense fibrillar stain to an almost completely particulate reaction, which presumably corresponded to the sarcomeres and thus demonstrated the true localization of succinate dehydrogenase. This study was extended and made quantitative by Chayen *et al.* (1966) in a model system using isolated rat hearts. In the normal heart the appearance of the reaction product with NBT, but in the absence of PMS, was similar to that seen in human material at the beginning of operation. Moreover, experimental anoxia produced the more granular reaction observed after prolonged open heart surgery. Quantitative elution studies using neotetrazolium chloride (NT) as acceptor showed that the total succinate dehydrogenase activity (as measured by the addition of PMS) was not altered by perfusion in anoxia. In contrast, activity in the absence of PMS was reduced by perfusion particularly if prolonged, once again emphasizing that the change resulting from these interventions was associated with a change in the electron transport pathway rather than in the activity of the dehydrogenase *per se*.

Whilst the studies of Butcher *et al.* (1972) failed to show any difference in the pattern of succinate oxidation between control and denervated dog myocardium, they did show that the total activity was the same irrespective of the tetrazolium salt used (NT, NBT or MTT), and that this total activity was approximately three times greater than the rate of transfer of reducing equivalents along the mitochondrial transfer chain.

Considerable confusion has arisen in recent years concerning the use of PMS in dehydrogenase histochemistry and particularly when nitroblue tetrazolium is used as the final acceptor. Hardonk (1965) showed that, with this tetrazole, the addition of PMS dramatically decreased the activity of lactate dehydrogenase in sections of cardiac muscle. In this, and in many other dehydrogenase studies, the sections were incubated under normal atmospheric conditions. The effect of the atmosphere on dehydrogenase reactions in heart muscle is shown in Table 19.1. Whilst oxygen has little or no effect on the reduction of NBT in the absence of PMS it causes considerable inhibition in its presence. Brody and Englel (1964) postulated that PMS facilitates the transfer of electrons directly to cytochrome oxidase since cyanide, but not amytal, reverses inhibition by PMS. In an important, but neglected, paper McMillan (1967) showed that this effect of cyanide can be mimicked by imposing strict anaerobic conditions on the system and concluded that the effect of cyanide was to inhibit the enzyme-catalysed oxidation of reduced PMS by atmospheric oxygen. This has been confirmed in studies by R. G. Butcher (unpublished data), in which the inhibition of succinate dehydrogenase by oxygen in the presence of PMS in different

Table 19.1 The effect of PMS in nitrogen and in oxygen on dehydrogenase activities in rat heart (in nanomoles of H_2 per square centimetre)

Substrate	Coenzyme	−PMS		+PMS	
		N_2	O_2	N_2	O_2
Succinate	—	34.2 ± 2.2	32.0 ± 1.5	83.3 ± 3.2†	4.3 ± 0.3
Glucose 6-phosphate	NADP	5.1 ± 0.6	3.5 ± 0.9	6.7 ± 2.1	1.4 ± 0.1
Lactate	NAD	21.8 ± 1.4	15.6 ± 0.6	50.1 ± 1.6	2.7 ± 0.2
Glutamate	NAD	12.9 ± 1.7	9.0 ± 1.7	14.2 ± 2.2	1.2 ± 0.2
Hydroxybutyrate	NAD	21.4 ± 2.9	20.5 ± 1.9	27.1 ± 3.8	1.8 ± 0.1
—	NAD	11.5 ± 1.5	8.1 ± 0.4	15.9 ± 0.9	1.1 ± 0.1

12% PVA grade G18/140; 50 mmol substrate; 3.7 mmol coenzyme; 5 mmol NBT; 0.65 mmol PMS; 8 μm sections; pH 7.8; 5 min incubation at 37 °C. Quantification by microdensitometry.

† Calculated from 2 min incubation.

tissues was shown to be directly proportional to the cytochrome oxidase activity and could be reversed by the addition of azide. Azide was used since it is less likely to cause the spontaneous reduction of tetrazolium salts than cyanide (van Noorden and Tas, 1982).

Quantification by Microdensitometry

Elution of the final reaction product from a tissue section and subsequent measurement of absorbance by spectrophotometry determines the average activity of that section; yet such a section may contain many different cell types with different chemical activities. In order to quantify the activity of an individual cell or group of cells recourse must be made to microscopical methods. One of the fundamental principles of absorption colourimetry is that the distribution of the absorbing material must be uniform throughout the sample. This is often far from true in a tissue section where the reaction product is likely to be more intense in some cells than in others and heterogeneously distributed within the cell. The true absorbance of such material can only be determined by the measurement of each of the individual and unequal absorbances in that specimen. Failure to do this leads to gross errors in quantification (Gomori, 1952; Bitensky, 1980; Goldstein, 1981).

A successful approach to this problem has come from the development of scanning and integrating microdensitometry. By this method that part of the section to be measured is selected by conventional microscopy and then scanned by a small measuring spot of monochromatic light. The light from each spot scanned is transmitted to a photomultiplier and the absorbance values integrated (Deeley, 1955). In order to convert these observed values into absolute units, it is essential to know the absorption characteristics and extinction coefficients of the final reaction product or products of the enzyme reaction. These have been determined for the formazans of neotetrazolium chloride (Butcher, 1972; Butcher and Altman, 1973), of NBT (Butcher, 1978a), and of 2-(2-benzothiazolyl)-3-(4-phthalhydrazidyl)-5-styryltetrazolium chloride (BPST) (Altman, 1976), and make possible the measurement of the amount of reaction product formed by dehydrogenase activity at both the tissue section level, by elution, and at the cellular level by scanning and integrating microdensitometry.

Continuous Measurement of Enzyme Activity

Microdensitometric methods can be used to evaluate enzyme activities in two ways. The most commonly used method is to assess the total amount of reaction product formed after a given time of incubation. To calculate the *rate* of activity by this method it is necessary to incubate several serial sections for different times and to measure the same types of cell from the same area in each section. The second approach is to follow directly the time course of the reaction by the continuous measurement of the accumulation of coloured end-product in the section (Nolte and Pette, 1971, 1972; Altman, 1978; Butcher, 1978b). Figure 19.1 shows the rate of oxidation of succinate

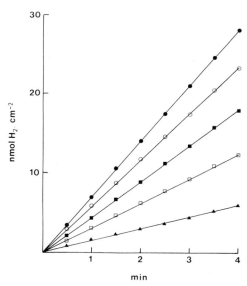

Figure 19.1   The rate of succinate dehydrogenase activity in rat heart sections of different thickness. 12% PVA grade G18/140; 50 mmol succinate; 6 mmol NBT; 2 mmol PMS; 1 mmol sodium azide; 20 °C; pH 7.2. Microtome thickness settings: ▲—▲, 2 μm; □—□, 4 μm; ■—■, 6 μm; ○—○, 8 μm; ●—●, 10 μm

in sections of rat myocardium measured directly by scanning and integrating microdensitometry. The formation of reaction product is proportional both to the time of incubation and to the thickness of the sections, two parameters essential for precise measurement of enzyme activity. Recent developments by Pette *et al.* (1979) allow comparative microphotometric measurements to be made of the initial reaction rates of up to 12 pre-selected areas within the same tissue section, though the use of a non-scanning measuring device in this method casts some doubt on the interpretation of the results (see Pette and Wimmer, 1980; Bitensky, 1980). A comparison of end-point and continuous measurement methods for the assessment of cytochrome oxidase activity in rabbit myocardium has been made recently by Ballantyne and Bright (1979).

Tissue Stabilization

When dry, unfixed tissue sections are incubated in a conventional histochemical medium up to 70% of the nitrogenous material is lost from the section into the surrounding liquid (Jones, 1965). Enzymes, too are lost; whilst tightly bound enzymes such as succinate dehydrogenase may be unaffected, the more soluble ones diffuse from the section during the first few minutes of incubation. In homogenates of cardiac muscle only 6% of the total creatine phosphokinase activity remained after minimal fixation with formaldehyde (Baba *et al.*, 1976). Yet tissue sections fixed in the same way reacted more intensely than unfixed tissue, indicating that the loss of enzyme by diffusion was greater than the inhibition caused by fixation. Three alternative approaches have been used to overcome this problem:

(a) The incorporation into the incubation medium of a chemically inert polymer which stabilizes the tissue section sufficiently to prevent disruption and enzyme loss whilst not interfering with enzyme activity. The most commonly used of these polymers are various grades of polyvinyl alcohol (Altman and Chayen, 1965; Altman, 1980).

(b) The use of an agarose gel film which contains the complete reaction medium (Pette and Brandau, 1962; Pette and Wimmer, 1980). The reaction is started by placing the film over the tissue section.

(c) The interposition of a semipermeable membrane between the incubation medium and the tissue section (McMillan, 1967; Meijer, 1980). Because only molecules with a molecular weight of less than 20 000 daltons can penetrate the membrane, diffusion of enzyme is prevented yet at the same time allowing free flow of substrates, coenzymes, and other components necessary for the formation of the final reaction product.

It might be supposed that the increase in viscosity resulting from the inclusion of polyvinyl alcohol (PVA) or agarose into the medium, or the imposition of a semipermeable membrane, might create a barrier to the penetration of substrates, etc., and so cause inhibition of the enzyme activity. The experimental results do not bear this out and many studies indicate that enzyme activities are higher in the presence of a stabilizer than in its absence (Altman, 1971). Even the tightly bound mitochondrial oxidation of succinate does not appear to be inhibited (Butcher, 1970). Moreover, similar enzyme activities have been recorded for homogenates and for sections from the same tissue which have been incubated with PVA (Altman, 1969; Teutsch and Rieder, 1979) and with gel films (Nolte and Pette, 1972). Kinetic measurement of enzyme activities can be made with these stabilizing systems though not with the gel film technique.

Multistep Reaction Methods

Enzymes of glycolysis and glycogenolysis

Although it is not possible to demonstrate the activity of these enzymes directly in tissue sections, they can be shown by multistep reactions which couple the end-product of the specific activity through exogenous enzymes to the formation of either NADH or NADPH and visualized by the addition of PMS and a tetrazolium salt to produce the coloured insoluble formazan (Sigel and Pette, 1969).

Glucose-6-phosphate is an end-product of the activity of phospho-glucomutase and of glucosephosphate isomerase; glucose-1-phosphate resulting from phosphorylase activity can be converted to glucose-6-phosphate by the addition of exogenous phosphoglucomatase. The activity of these three enzymes can be demonstrated by the addition of NADP and glucose-6-phosphate dehydrogenase, so generating NADPH. The more conventional method for phosphorylase utilizes glucose-1-phosphate as substrate, the reaction proceeding in favour of glycogen synthesis (Takeuchi *et al.*, 1955); activity can be visualized by staining the glycogen formed with iodine or with the periodic acid Schiff reaction, or by converting the phosphate produced to visible lead sulphide. Decreased phosphorylase activity shown in infarcted heart muscle is almost certainly due to the lack, in such tissue, of the glycogen necessary as a primer for the reaction to take place (Martin and Engel, 1972). Whether the improvement in the staining intensity seen in ischaemic cardiac muscle as a result of adding dextran to the medium (Meijer, 1968a,b) is due to its action as a glycosyl acceptor or as a tissue stabilizer is open to question. Factors affecting the phosphorylase reaction and its use as a histochemical marker of specialized tissue of the heart have been investigated by Pathak and Goyal (1978).

Triosphosphate isomerase, aldolase, and phosphofructokinase can be studied in tissue sections by a method involving the formation of NADH from exogenous glyceraldehyde-3-phosphate dehydrogenase and NAD; the methods were developed by Sigel and Pette (1969) for use in skeletal muscle with the agarose gel film technique. The most important of these in glycolytic regulation in the myocardium is phosphofructokinase; it is also the most difficult to demonstrate since it involves the addition also of exogenous aldolase and triosephosphate isomerase to the incubation medium. A quantitative study in rat cardiac muscle using neotetrazolium as the final acceptor and PVA as the tissue stabilizer has been made by Butcher and Papadoyannis (1979); optimal concentrations of each of the reactants were determined by scanning and integrating microdensitometry. A semipermeable membrane method for this enzyme in the heart has been developed by Meijer and Stegehuis (1980).

Non-specific formazan precipitation is likely to be high in these multistep methods and the incorporation of a tissue stabilizer in the medium, preventing diffusion of endogenous substrates, increases the possibility of high control reactions. The use of kinetic microdensitometry has facilitated the quantification of specific enzyme activities with these methods. The reaction kinetics of two serial sections of rat cardiac muscle incubated for phosphofructokinase activity in the presence and absence of substrate are shown in Figure 19.2. At first the rate of formazan production in the control section approaches that of the test section, but declines dramatically as endogenous

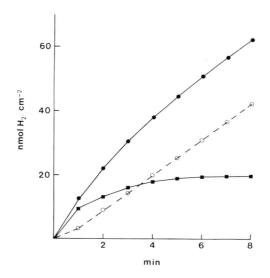

Figure 19.2 The rate of PFK activity in fresh sections of rat heart. ●—●, test; ■—■, control lacking fructose-6-phosphate; ○—○, test–control. 12% PVA grade G18/140; 2 mmol F-6-P; 1 mmol ATP; 2 mmol MgCl; 6 mmol NAD: 3 mmol NT; 0.65 mmol PMS; pH 8.0; 37 C; 8 μm sections

substrates are exhausted. Subtraction of control values from test values gives a measure of the rate of formation of reducing equivalents specifically due to phosphofructokinase activity; after an initial lag phase the reaction is linear with incubation time.

Creatine phosphokinase

A multistep method for the demonstration of creatine phosphokinase was developed by Sjovall (1967) and by Kishino *et al.* (1969). ATP formed by the activity of the enzyme is coupled, via reactions catalysed by exogenous hexokinase and glucose-6-phosphate dehydrogenase, to the reduction of nitroblue tetrazolium. As with all multistep reactions the specificity of the reaction can only be elucidated by the use of extensive controls; in a study of cardiac muscle activity Baba *et al.* (1976) employed no less than 20 different control media. The interpretation of results in fixed sections, in which only 6% of the total activity remains, should therefore be made with caution. The use of tissue stabilization methods in the demonstration of creatine phosphokinase activity warrants investigation in the future.

CONCLUSION

The division of this review into two major sections, one dealing with the localization of enzymes, the other with a totally different quantitative microbiochemical approach, has emphasized the great diversity of enzyme histochemistry in the heart. This increasing specialization should not cloud the possible value of more simple studies; the appearance of the reaction product in the section, even at the light microscope level, might give more information on how the myocyte functions than a complex kinetic study of the reaction rate. What is important in each case, and also in the subcellular localization of enzymes in the electron microscope, is that the underlying mechanisms of each histochemical reaction are fully understood. Nor should enzyme histochemistry be considered exclusive of other disciplines but rather used in conjunction with them to obtain a greater comprehension of the functioning of the myocardium in health and disease.

REFERENCES

Abraham, R., Morris, M., and Smith, J. (1967). Histochemistry of lysosomes in rat heart muscle. *J. Histochem. Cytochem.*, **15,** 596–599.

Altman, F. P. (1969). A comparison of dehydrogenase activities in tissue homogenates and tissue sections. *Biochem. J.*, **144,** 13P.

Altman, F. P. (1971). The use of a new grade of polyvinyl alcohol for stabilising tissue sections during histochemical reactions. *Histochemie*, **28,** 236–242.

Altman, F. P. (1976). The quantification of formazans in tissue sections by microdensitometry II. The use of BPST, a new tetrazolium salt. *Histochem. J.*, **8,** 501–506.

Altman, F. P. (1978). The use of a heated stage for following histochemical reactions under a microdensitometer. *Histochem. J.*, **10,** 611–614.

Altman, F. P. (1980). Tissue stabilizer methods in histochemistry. In *Trends in Histochemistry and Cytochemistry*, CIBA Foundation Symposium No. 73, Excerpta Medica, Oxford, pp. 81–101.

Altman, F. P., and Barrnett, R. J. (1975). The ultrastructural localisation of enzyme activities in unfixed sections. *Histochemie*, **44,** 179–183.

Altman, F. P., and Chayen, J. (1965). Retention of nitrogenous material in unfixed sections during incubation for histochemical demonstration of enzymes. *Nature*, **207,** 1205–1206.

Asano, G., Ashraf, M., and Schwartz, A. (1980). Localization of Na–K-ATPase in guinea-pig myocardium. *J. Mol. Cell. Cardiol.*, **12,** 257–266.

Baba, N., Kim, S., and Farrell, E. C. (1976). Histochemistry of creatine phosphokinase. *J. Mol. Cell. Cardiol.*, **8,** 599–617.

Ballantyne, B., and Bright, J. E. (1979). Comparison of kinetic and end-point microdensitometry for the direct quantitative histochemical assessment of cytochrome oxidase activity. *Histochem. J.*, **11,** 173–186.

Bitensky, L. (1963). The reversible activation of lysosomes in normal cells and the effects of pathological conditions. In CIBA Symposium on Lysosomes (A. V. S. de Reuck and M. P. Cameron, eds), London, Churchill, pp. 362–383.

Bitensky, L. (1980). Microdensitometry. In *Trends in Enzyme Histochemistry and Cytochemistry*, CIBA Foundation Symposium No. 73, Excerpta Medica, Oxford, pp. 181–202.

Bitensky, L., and Chayen, J. (1979). Cytochemical methods for studing lysosomes. In *Quantitative Cytochemistry and its Applictions* (J. R. Pattison, L. Bitensky, and J. Chayen, eds), Academic Press, London, pp. 49–61.

Bitensky, L., Butcher, R. G., and Chayen, J. (1973). Quantitative cytochemistry in the study of lysosomal function. In *Lysosomes in Biology and Pathology*, Vol. 3 (J. T. Dingle, ed.), North Holland, Amsterdam, pp. 465–510.

Braimbridge, M. V., and Cankovic-Darracott, S. (1979). Quantitative polarising microscopy and cytochemistry in assessing myocardial function. In *Quantitative Cytochemistry and its Applications* (J. R. Pattison, L. Bitensky, and J. Chayen, eds), Academic Press, London, pp. 221–230.

Braimbridge, M. V., and Niles, N. R. (1964). Left ventricular drill biopsy. *J. Thorac. Cardiovasc. Surg.*, **47,** 685–687.

Braimbridge, M. V., Darracott, S., Clement, A. J., Bitensky, L., and Chayen, J. (1973). Myocardial deterioration during aortic valve replacement assessed by cellular biological tests. *J. Thorac. Cardiovasc. Surg.*, **66,** 241–254.

Braimbridge, M. V., Chayen, J., Bitensky, L., Hearse, D. J., Jynge, P., and Cankovic-Darracott, S. (1977). Cold cardioplegia or continuous coronary perfusion? *J. Thorac. Cardiovasc. Surg.*, **74,** 900–906

Brody, I. A., and Engel, W. K. (1964). Isozyme histochemistry: the display of selective lactate dehydrogenase isozymes in sections of skeletal muscle. *J. Histochem. Cytochem.*, **12,** 928–929.

Butcher, R. G. (1968). The estimation of the nucleic acids of tissue sections and its use as a unit of comparison for quantitative histochemistry. *Histochemie*, **13,** 263–275.

Butcher, R. G. (1970). Studies on succinate oxidation. I. The use of intact tissue sections. *Exp. Cell. Res.*, **60,** 54–60.

Butcher, R. G. (1971). The chemical determination of section thickness. *Histochemie*, **28,** 131–136.

Butcher, R. G. (1972). Precise cytochemical measurement of neotetrazolium formazan by scanning and integrating microdensitometry. *Histochemie*, **32,** 171–190.

Butcher, R. G. (1978a). The measurement in tissue sections of the two formazans derived from nitroblue tetrazolium in dehydrogenase reactions. *Histochem. J.*, **10,** 739–744.

Butcher, R. G. (1978b). Oxygen and the production of formazan from neotetrazolium chloride. *Histochemistry*, **56,** 329–340.

Butcher, R. G., and Altman, F. P. (1973). Studies on the reduction of tetrazolium salts. II. The measurement of the half reduced and fully reduced formazans of neotetrazolium chloride in tissue sections. *Histochemie*, **37,** 351–363.

Butcher, R. G., Bitensky, L., and Chayen, J. (1972). Histochemical assessment of myocardial function. Appendix to Noble, M.I.M., Stubbs, J., Trenchard, D., Else, W., Eisele, J. H., and Guz, A. Left ventricular performance in the conscious dog with chronically denervated heart. *Cardiovasc. Res.*, **6,** 457–477.

Butcher, R. G., and Papadoyannis, D. E. (1979). Histochemical measurement of myocardial phosphofructokinase activity. *J. Physiol. (Lond.)*, **289,** 18–19P.

Cankovic-Darracott, S., Braimbridge, M. V., Williams, B. T., Bitensky, L., and Chayen, J. (1977). Myocardial preservation during aortic valve surgery. Assessment of five techniques by cellular, chemical and biophysical methods. *J. Thorac. Cardiovasc. Surg.*, **73,** 699–706.

Chayen, J. (1968). The histochemistry of phospholipids and its significance in the interpretation of the structure of cells. In *Cell Structure and its Interpretation* (S. M. McGee-Russell and K. F. A. Ross, eds), Edward Arnold, London, pp. 149–156.

Chayen, J., Altman, F. P., Bitensky, L., Braimbridge, M. V., Kadas, T., and Wells, P. J. (1966). A study of the changes in hydrogen tranport in an isolated rat heart preparation. *J. Roy. Microsc. Soc.*, **86,** 151–158.

Chayen, J., Bitensky, L., Butcher, R. G., and Altman, F. P. (1974). Cellular biochemical assessment of steroid activity. *Advan. Steroid Biochem. Pharmacol.* **4,** 1–60.

Cox, J. L., McLaughlin, V. W., Flowers, N. C., and Horan, L. G. (1968). The ischaemic zone surrounding acute myocardial infarction. Its morphology as detected by dehydrogenase staining. *Amer. Heart J.*, **76,** 650–659.

Cutler, L. S. and Christian, C. P. (1980). Cytochemical localisation of adenylate cyclase. *J. Histochem. Cytochem.*, **28,** 62–65.

Danielli, J. F. (1953). *Cytochemistry, A Critical Approach*, John Wiley, New York.

Decker, R. S., and Wildenthal, K. (1978a). Sequential lysosomal alterations during cardiac ischaemia. II. Ultrastructural and cytochemical changes. *Lab. Invest.*, **38,** 662–673.

Decker, R. S., and Wildenthal, K. (1978b). Influence of methylprednisolone on ultrastructural and cytochemical changes during myocardial ischaemia. *Amer. J. Path.*, **92,** 1–22.

Decker, R. S., Poole, A. R., Griffin, E. E., Dingle, J. T., and Wildenthal, K. (1977). Altered distribution of lysosomal cathepsin D in ischaemic myocardium. *J. Clin. Invest.*, **59,** 911–921.

Decker, R. S., Decker, M. L., and Poole, A. R. (1980). The distribution of lysosomal cathepsin D in cardiac myocytes. *J. Histochem. Cytochem.*, **28,** 231–237.

Deeley, E. M. (1955). An integrating microdensitometer for biological cells. *J. Sci. Instrum.*, **32,** 263–267.

Ernst, S. A. (1972a). Transport adenosine triphosphatase cytochemistry I. Biochemical characterization of a cytochemical medium for the ultrastructural localization of ouabain-sensitive, potassium-dependent phosphatase activity in the avian salt gland. *J. Histochem. Cytochem.*, **20,** 13–22.

Ernst, S. A. (1972b). Transport adenosine triphosphatase cytochemistry II. Cytochemical localization of ouabain-sensitive, potassium-dependent phosphatase activity in the secretory epithelium of the avain salt gland. *J. Histochem. Cytochem.*, **20**, 23–38.

Essner, E., Novikoff, A. B., and Quintana, N. (1965). Nucleoside phosphatase activities in rat cardiac muscle. *J. Cell. Biol.*, **25**, 201–215.

Farber, E., and Bueding, E. (1956). Histochemical localization of specific oxidative enzymes: V. The dissociation of succinic dehydrogenase from carriers by lipase and the specific histochemical localisation of the dehydrogenase with phenazine methosulphate and tetrazolium salts. *J. Histochem. Cytochem.*, **4**, 357–362.

Firth, J. A. (1978). Cytochemical approaches to the localisation of specific adenosine triphosphatases. *Histochem. J.*, **10**, 253–269.

Firth, J. A. (1980). Reliability and specificity of membrane adenosine triphosphatase localisations. *J. Histochem. Cytochem.*, **28**, 69–71.

Glick, D. (1981). Trends in quantification in histochemistry and cytochemistry. *Histochem. J.*, **13**, 227–240.

Goldfischer, S., Villaverde, H., and Furschirm, R. (1966). The demonstration of acid hydrolase, thermostable reduced diphosphopyridine nucleotide tetrazolium reductase and peroxidase activities in human lipofuscin pigment granules. *J. Histochem. Cytochem.*, **14**, 641–652.

Goldstein, D. J. (1981). Errors in microdensitometry. *Histochem. J.*, **13**, 251–267.

Gomori, G. (1952). *Microscopic Histochemistry, Principles and Practice*, University of Chicago Press, Chicago.

Hardonk, M. J. (1965). The use of phenazine methosulphate as an electron carrier in the histochemical demonstration of dehydrogenases. *Histochemie*, **4**, 563–568.

Hecht, E. (1971). Enzyme histochemistry of heart muscle in normal and pathologic conditions. In *Mathematical Achievements in Experimental Pathology*, Vol. 5 (E. Bejusz and G. Jasmin, eds), Karger, Basel, pp. 384–435.

Hegab, El-Sayed H. H., and Ferrans, V. J. (1966). A histochemical study of the esterases of the rat heart. *Amer. J. Anat.* **119**, 235–265.

Hoffstein, S. G., Gennaro, D. E., Weissmann, G., Hirsch, J., Streuli, F., and Fox, A. C. (1975). Cytochemical localization of lysosomal enzyme activity in normal and ischaemic dog myocardium. *Amer. J. Pathol.*, **79**, 716–722.

Howell, S. L., and Whitfield, M. (1972). Cytochemical localisation of adenyl cyclase activity in rat islets of Langerhans. *J. Histochem. Cytochem.*, **20**, 873–879.

Jones, G. R. N. (1965). Losses of nitrogenous material occurring from frozen sections of rat liver during incubation in an aqueous medium. *Biochem. J.*, **96**, 10P.

Jones, G. R. N., Maple, A. J., Aves, E. K., Chayen, J., and Cunningham, G. J. (1963). Quantitative histochemistry of succinate dehydrogenase in tissue sections. *Nature*, **197**, 568–570.

de Jong, A. S. H. (1982). Mechanics of metal-salt methods in enzyme cytochemistry with special reference to acid phosphatase. *Histochem. J.*, **14**, 1–34.

de Jong, A. S. H., Hak, T. J., van Duijn, P., and Daems, W. Th. (1979). A new dynamic model system for the study of capture reactions for diffusable compounds in cytochemistry II. Effect of the composition of the incubation medium on the trapping of phosphate ions in acid phosphatase cytochemistry. *Histochem. J.*, **11**, 145–161.

Kaufman, N., Gavan, T. L., and Hill, R. W. (1959). Experimental myocardial infarction in the rat. *Arch. Pathol.*, **67**, 482–488.

Kempen, H. J. M., de Pont, J. J., Bonting, S. L., and Stadhouders, A. M. (1978). The cytochemical localisation of adenylate cyclase: fact or artefact? *J. Histochem. Cytochem.*, **26**, 298–312.

Kent, S. P., and Diseker, M. (1955). Early myocardial ischaemia. Study of histochemical changes in dogs. *Lab. Invest.* **4**, 398–405.

Khan, M. A., Papadimitriou, J. M., Holt, P. G., and Kakulas, B. A. (1972). A
modified histochemical technique for sarcoplasmic reticular ATPase. *Histochemie*,
30, 329–333.

Khan, M. A., Papadimitriou, J. M., and Kakulas, B. A. (1975). On the specificity of
the histochemical technique for sarcoplasmic reticular adenosine triphosphatase: a
light and electron microscopic study. *Histochemistry*, **43**, 101–111.

Kishino, Y., Katsne, R., and Hizawa, K. (1969). Histochemical detection of creatine
kinase and its distribution in tissue. *Med. Biol.* (*Tokyo*) **78**, 113–118.

Kyte, J. (1974). The reaction of sodium and potassium ion-activated adenosine
triphosphatase with specific antibodies. *J. Biol. Chem.*, **249**, 3652–3660.

McCallister, L. P., Munger, B. L., and Neeley, J. R. (1977). Electron microscopic
observations and acid phosphatase activity in the ischaemic rat heart. *J. Mol. Cell.
Cardiol.*, **9**, 353–364.

McMillan, P. J. (1967). Differential demonstration of muscle and heart type lactic
dehydrogenase of rat muscle and kidney. *J. Histochem. Cytochem.*, **15**, 21–31.

Malouf, N. N., and Meissner, G. (1979). Localization of a Mg^{2+} or Ca^{2+} activated
'basic' ATPase in skeletal muscle. *Exp. Cell Res.*, **122**, 233–250.

Malouf, N. N., and Meissner, G. (1980). Cytochemical localization of a 'basic'
ATPase to canine myocardial surface membrane. *J. Histochem. Cytochem.*, **28**,
1286–1294.

Martin, L., and Engel, W. K. (1972). Dependency of histochemical phosphorylase
staining on amount of cellular glycogen. *J. Histochem. Cytochem.*, **20**, 476–479.

Meijer, A. E. F. H. (1968a). Improved histochemical method for the demonstration
of the activity of α-glucan phosphorylase I. The use of glucosyl acceptor dextran.
Histochemie, **12**, 244–252.

Meijer, A. E. F. H. (1968b). Improved histochemical method for the demonstration
of the activity of α-glucan phosphorylase II. Relation of molecular weight of
glucosyl acceptor dextran to activation of phosphorylase. *Histochemie*, **16**, 134–
143.

Meijer, A. E. F. H. (1980). Semipermeable membrane techniques in quantitative
enzyme histochemistry. In *Trends in Histochemistry and Cytochemistry*, CIBA
Foundation Symposium No. 73, Excerpta Medica, Oxford, pp. 103–120.

Meijer, A. E., and Stegehuis, F. (1980). Histochemical technique for the demonstration of phosphofructokinase activity. *Histochemie*, **66**, 75–81.

Moses, H. L., Rosenthal, A. S., Beaver, D. L., and Schuffman, S. S. (1966). Lead ion
and phosphatase histochemistry II. Effects of adenosine triphosphate hydrolysis by
lead ion on the histochemical localization of adenosine triphosphatase activity. *J.
Histochem. Cytochem.*, **14**, 702–710.

Niles, N. R., Chayen, J., Cunningham, G. J., and Bitensky, L. (1964). The histochemical demonstration of adenosine triphosphatase activity in myocardium. *J.
Histochem. Cytochem.*, **12**, 704–743.

Niles, N. R., Bitensky, L., Braimbridge, M. V., and Chayen, J. (1966). Histochemical
changes related to oxidation and phosphorylation in human heart muscle. *J. Roy.
Microsc. Soc.*, **86**, 159–166.

Nolte, J., and Pette, D. (1971). Quantitative microscope photometric determination
of enzyme activities in cryostat sections. In *Recent Advances in Quantitative Histo-
and Cytochemistry*, Hans Huber, Berne, pp. 54–62.

Nolte, J., and Pette, D. (1972). Microphotometric determination of enzyme activity
in single cells in cryostat sections. I. Application of the gel film technique to

microphotometry and studies on the intralobular distribution of succinate dehydrogenase and lactate dehydrogenase activities in rat liver. *J. Histochem. Cytochem.,* **20,** 567–576.

van Noorden, C. J. F., and Tas, J. (1982). The role of exogeneous electron carriers in NAD(P)-dependent dehydrogenase cytochemistry studied *in vitro* and with a model system of polyacrylamide films. *J. Histochem. Cytochem.,* **30,** 12–20.

Novikoff, A. B. (1976). The endoplasmic reticulum. A cytochemist's view (A review). *Proc. Natl Acad. Sci.,* **73,** 2781–2787.

Ogawa, K., and Mayahara, H. (1969). Intramitochondrial localisation of adenosine triphosphatase activity. *J. Histochem. Cytochem.,* **17,** 487–490.

Okuda, M., and Lefer, A. M. (1979). Lysosomal hypothesis in evolution of myocardial infarction. Subcellular fractionation and electron microscopic cytochemistry study. *Jpn. Heart J.,* **20,** 643–656.

Padykula, H. A., and Herman, E. (1955). Factors affecting the activity of adenosine triphosphatase and other phosphatases as measured by histochemical techniques. *J. Histochem. Cytochem.,* **3,** 161–167.

Pathak, C. L., and Goyal, S. (1978). Phosphorylase activity as a histochemical marker of specialized tissue of heart. *Histochem. J.,* **10,** 633–640.

Pette, D., and Brandau, H. (1962). Intracellular localization of glycolytic enzymes in cross-striated muscles of *Locusta migratoria. Biochem. Biophys. Res. Commun.,* **9,** 367–370.

Pette, D., and Wimmer, M. (1980). Microphotometric determination of enzyme activities in cryostat sections by the gel film technique. In *Trends in Enzyme Histochemistry and Cytochemistry,* CIBA Foundation Symposium No. 73, Excerpta Medica, Oxford, pp. 121–134.

Pette, D., Wasmund, H., and Wimmer, M. (1979). Principle and method of microphotometric enzyme activity determination. *Histochemistry,* **64,** 1–10.

Reed, B. L., and Wenzel, D. G. (1975). The lysosomal permeability test modified for toxicity testing with cultured heart endothelioid cells. *Histochem. J.,* **7,** 115–126.

Reik, L., Petzold, G. L., Higgins, J. A., Greengard, P., and Barrnett, R. J. (1970). Hormone sensitive adenyl cyclase: cytochemical localization in rat liver. *Science,* **168,** 382–384.

Revis, N. W. (1979). Localisation of adenylate cyclase in unfixed sections of cardiac muscle. *J. Histochem. Cytochem.,* **27,** 1322–1326.

Romeo, D., Stagni, N., Sotlocesa, G. L., Pugllianello, M. C., de Bernard, B., and Vittur, F. (1966). Lysosomes in heart tissue. *Biochim. Biophys. Acta,* **130,** 64–80.

Rostgaard, J., and Behnke, O. (1965). Fine structure localisation of adenosine nucleoside phosphatase activity in the sarcoplasmic reticulum and the T system of rat myocardium. *J. Ultrastruct. Res.* **12,** 579–591.

Schulze, W., Krause, E.-G., and Wollenberger, A. (1972). Cytochemical demonstration and localization of adenyl cyclase in skeletal and cardiac muscle. *Advanc. Cyclic Nucleotide Res.,* **1,** 249–260.

Shnitka, T. K., and Nachlas, M. M. (1963). Histochemical alterations in ischaemic heart muscle and early myocardial infarction. *Amer. J. Pathol.,* **42,** 507–527.

Sigel, P., and Pette, D. (1969). Intracellular localization of glycogenolytic and glycolytic enzymes in white and red rabbit skeletal muscle. A gel film method for coupled enzyme reactions in histochemistry. *J. Histochem. Cytochem.,* **17,** 225–237.

Sjovall, K. (1967). A tetrazolium technique for the histochemical localisation of ATP creatine phosphotransferase. *Histochemie,* **10,** 336–340.

Slezak, J., and Geller, S. A. (1979). Cytochemical demonstration of adenylate cyclase in cardiac muscle: effect of dimethyl sulfoxide. *J. Histochem. Cytochem.*, **27,** 774–781.

Sloane-Stanley, G. H., and Jones, G. R. N. (1963). A simple method for the determination of very small amounts of nitrogen in organic matter. *Biochem. J.*, **86,** 16P.

Sommer, J. R., and Hasselbach, W. (1967). The effect of glutaraldehyde and formaldehyde on the calcium pump of the sarcoplasmic reticulum. *J. Cell Biol.*, **34,** 902–905.

Sommer, J. R., and Spach, M. S. (1964). Electron microscopic demonstration of adenosine triphosphate in myofibrils and sarcoplasmic membranes of cardiac muscle of normal and abnormal dogs. *Amer. J. Path.*, **44,** 491–505.

Somogyi, E., and Sotonyi, P. (1969). Data relevant to the electron microscopic demonstration of ATPase. *Acta Histochim.*, **34,** 70–85.

Somogyi, E., Sotonyi, P., and Bujdoso, G. (1972). Electron-microscopic histochemical demonstration of sarcotubular ATPase in the myocardium. *Acta Histochim*, **43,** 302–308.

Sotonyi, P., Somogyi, E., and Kerenyi, N. A. (1974). Use of neodymium nitrate in electron microscopic histochemical demonstration of ATPase. *Histochemistry*, **42,** 265–269.

Stauber, W. T., and Ong, S.-H. (1981a). Fluorescence demonstration of dipeptidyl peptidase II in skeletal, cardiac and vascular smooth muscles. *J. Histochem. Cytochem.*, **29,** 675–677.

Stauber, W. T., and Ong, S.-H. (1981b). Fluorescence demonstration of cathepsin B activity in skeletal, cardiac and vascular smooth muscle. *J. Histochem.*, **29,** 866–869.

Stauber, W. T., and Ong, S.-H. (1982). Fluorescence demonstration of dipeptidyl peptidase I (cathepsin C) in skeletal, cardiac and vascular smooth muscles. *J. Histochem. Cytochem.*, **30,** 162–164.

Stirling, C. E. (1972). Radioautographic localization of sodium pump sites in rabbit intestine. *J. Cell Biol.*, **53,** 704–714.

Takeuchi, T. K., Higashi, K., and Watanuki, S. (1955). Distribution of amylophosphorylase in various tissues of human and mammalian organs. *J. Histochem. Cytochem.*, **3,** 485–491.

Teutsch, H. F., and Rieder, H. (1979). NADP dependent dehydrogenases in rat liver parenchyma, II. Comparision of quantitative G-6-P distribution patterns with particular reference to sex differences. *Histochemistry*, **60,** 43–52.

Topping, T. M., and Travis, D. F. (1974). An electron cytochemical study of mechanisms of lysosomal activity in the rat left ventricular mural myocardium. *J. Ultrastruct. Res.*, **46,** 1–22.

Wachstein, M., and Meisel, E. (1955). Succinic dehydrogenase activity in myocardial infarction and in induced myocardial necrosis. *Amer. J. Pathol.*, **31,** 353–365.

Wachstein, M., and Meisel, E. (1957). Histochemistry of hepatic phosphatases at a physiologic pH with a special reference to the demonstration of bile canaliculi. *Amer. J. Path.*, **27,** 13–23.

Wagner, R. C., Kreiner, P., Barrnett, R. J., and Bitensky, M. W. (1972). Biochemical characterization and cytochemical localization of a catecholamine-sensitive adenylate cyclase in isolated capillary endothelium. *Proc. Natl Acad. Sci.*, **69,** 3157–3179.

Wildenthal, K. (1978). Lysosomal alterations in ischaemic myocardium. Result or cause of myocellular damage? *J. Mol. Cell. Cardiol.*, **10,** 595–603.

Wildenthal, K., Poole, A. R., and Dingle, J. T. (1975). Influence of starvation on the activities and localization of cathepsin D and other lysosomal enzymes in hearts of rabbits and mice. *J. Mol. Cell. Cardiol.* **7**, 841–855.

Wollenberger, A. and Schulze, W. (1976). Cytochemical studies on sarcolemma: Na–K adenosine triphosphatase and adenylate cyclase. *Recent Advanc. Stud. Cardiac Struct. Metab.*, **9**, 101–115.

Cardiac Metabolism
Edited by A. J. Drake-Holland and M. I. M. Noble
© 1983 John Wiley & Sons Ltd

CHAPTER 20

Catecholamines and Sympathetic Innervation

Marianne Fillenz

University Laboratory of Physiology, Oxford OX1 3PT, UK

INTRODUCTION

Myocardial function is modulated by catecholamines derived from two sources: noradrenaline released from the sympathetic nerve terminals innervating the heart and the catecholamines in the circulation reaching the myocardium by way of its blood supply.

Sympathetic Innervation of the Heart

The development of the histochemical fluorescence technique for catecholamines has revealed the distribution of sympathetic noradrenergic fibres in the different regions of the heart (Jacobowitz *et al.*, 1967; Nielsen and Owman, 1968; Dolezel *et al.*, 1978). The myocardium has a three-dimensional network of preterminal and terminal fibres, which are clearly distinguishable from the perivascular fibres surrounding branches of the coronary vessels; the myocardial fibres are finer and more dimly fluorescent than the perivascular fibres. In addition to the myocardial fibres, the inner and outer surfaces of the heart have a distinct monoaminergic innervation which consists of a subepicardial and an endocardial plexus. Occasionally in the atria intensely fluorescent cells with short non-varicose processes are seen: these look like solitary chromaffin-type cells, and may be part of the chemoreceptor system. The innervation density of the auricles is about twice that of the ventricles. Innervation density can also be assessed by measuring the noradrenaline content of the various parts of the heart; such studies have confirmed the results of the fluorescence histochemical studies in that they show that the noradrenaline content of the atria is about twice that of the ventricles (Shore *et al.*, 1958). Electron microscopy of cardiac innervation shows bundles of axons contained in Schwann cells (Winckler, 1969; Ehinger *et al.*, 1970; van der Zypen, 1974). The axons are of two kinds, containing either clear vesicles (cholinergic terminals) or dense-cored vesicles (noradrenergic terminals). Vesicle-filled synaptic terminals are always

471

found opposite the middle of the sarcomere. Both pacemaker cells and myocardial cells receive a dual innervation consisting of cholinergic and noradrenergic terminals.

Plasma Catecholamines

Circulating blood contains adrenaline, noradrenaline, and dopamine (Callingham, 1975). Adrenaline is derived exclusively from chromaffin cells: most of these are in the adrenal medulla and this is the main, if not the only, source of circulating adrenaline. There are additional small groups of chromaffin cells, such as those seen in the heart: their contribution to either local or circulating adrenaline is at present unknown. However, in addition to chromaffin cells which secrete adrenaline, there are those which secrete noradrenaline. The enzyme phenylethanolamine *N*-methyltransferase (PNMT) is regulated by glucocortocoids secreted by cells of the adrenal cortex (Pohorecky and Wurtman, 1971) and in mammals there is a correlation between the intimacy of contact of chromaffin cells with adrenal cortical cells and the relative proportion of adrenaline and noradrenaline in the adrenal medulla (Coupland, 1965). Thus the high percentage of adrenaline in adrenal catecholamines of guinea-pig and rabbit compared to that of cat, dog, and man can be explained in terms of the anatomical relationship of adrenal medulla and cortex. The activity of the adrenal medullary cells is controlled by the splanchnic nerve and there is evidence that the nerve supply to adrenaline- and noradrenaline-secreting cells is under separate control and can be selectively activated. All the circulating adrenaline therefore will come from the adrenal medulla, which will in addition make a contribution to circulating noradrenaline. The size of the contribution of the two types of cell will vary with the species of the animal and with its physiological state.

A contribution to circulating noradrenaline is also made by sympathetic nerve terminals: this is the fraction of noradrenaline released from the nerve terminals which has escaped neuronal and extraneuronal uptake and has overflowed into the circulation. There is a considerable difference in the contribution made by different organs to circulating noradrenaline, as shown by the amine content of the venous effluent from different organs. The overflow of noradrenaline from a given organ will depend on a number of factors: density of innervation (on which will depend both release and re-uptake), degree of vascularization, and width of synaptic cleft. Thus the vas deferens, one of the organs with the richest sympathetic innervation, would be expected to make only a minimal contribution to normal plasma noradrenaline: there is little tonic activity, the geometry of the innervation favours maximal neuronal re-uptake, and the vascularization is poor. Estimations of the arteriovenous differences in catecholamines suggest that the heart, on the other hand, does release catecholamines into the circulation (Callingham, 1975).

It is difficult to establish the normal plasma concentrations of adrenaline and noradrenaline, since the sampling procedure itself tends to elevate levels. As experimental techniques have improved the concentrations measured have shown a progressive fall. The figures for man (0.05 ng ml^{-1} and 0.3 ng ml^{-1} for venous adrenaline and noradrenaline respectively) are the lowest so far, probably because of better control of sampling. The very short half-life of noradrenaline in the circulation (Ferreira and Vane, 1967) suggests that there could be rapid fluctuations, which would be very difficult to detect without a method of continuous monitoring. Various physiological stimuli can produce very large changes both in absolute and in relative concentrations of the two amines. Thus hypoglycaemia, hypoxia, and hypercapnia, as well as emotional and mental stress, can increase plasma adrenaline by a factor of up to 50, leaving noradrenaline relatively unchanged; on the other hand, temperature changes and muscular exercise produce large increases in plasma noradrenaline with little change in adrenaline; haemorrhage and hypotension lead to an increase in both catecholamines (Callingham, 1975). Finally there have been reports of concentrations of dopamine in peripheral blood considerably in excess of both noradrenaline and adrenaline; it is not clear whether these values, obtained in chloralose-anaesthetized cats (Street and Roberts, 1969) represent normal concentrations, since the concentrations found in conscious sheep and goats were much lower (Kelly *et al.*, 1970).

MYOCARDIAL ADRENERGIC RECEPTORS

Loewi (1921) showed that stimulation of the sympathetic innervation of the frog heart produced an increase in heart rate and the release into the incubation medium of a chemical mediator, since increase in heart rate of a second heart could be produced simply by exposure to the incubation medium from the first stimulated heart. He thus demonstrated the chemical mediation of the sympathetic control of the heart and identified the mediator as adrenaline. Von Euler (1948) later showed that in mammals the transmitter released by sympathetic nerve terminals is noradrenaline. Clark (1933) was the first to suggest that chemical mediators acted on specialized receptors on the surface of effector cells.

The various peripheral sympathetic effects could be mimicked by both noradrenaline and adrenaline, although there were quantitative differences in the sensitivity of various responses to the two catecholamines. However, the use of catecholamine analogues revealed qualitative differences: thus there were two classes of effects which could be mimicked and blocked by two classes of substances. To explain these observations Ahlquist, in 1948, proposed that there were two kinds of adrenergic receptors which he called alpha and beta. In the heart, both adrenaline and noradrenaline have arrhythmic, inotropic, and chronotropic effects. These effects were also produced by isoprenaline, were not blocked by the alpha antagonists, but were blocked by beta antagonists (Moran and Perkins, 1961; Nickerson and Chan, 1961). This led to the conclusion that the heart had only beta- and no alpha-receptors. The criteria for alpha-receptors were activation by phenylephrine but not isoprenaline and they were blocked by phentolamine and phenoxybenzamine. Wenzel and Su (1966), using the rat, and Govier (1968), using guinea-pig atria, found a positive inotropic effect which fulfilled these criteria, thus proving that alpha- as well as beta-receptors are present in the heart. In most other organs which have both kinds of receptors, alpha- and beta-receptor activation produce antagonistic effects, whereas in the heart activation of alpha- and beta-receptors produced similar although not identical effects; thus selective activation of alpha-receptors by phenylephrine or adrenaline plus propranalol causes increased contractility, increased functional refractory period, increased duration of the action potential, and a decrease in the phase 4 repolarization; there is no positive chronotropic effect. Isoprenaline, on the other hand, has a positive inotropic and a positive chronotropic effect. The positive inotropic effect therefore is common to both receptors, although it is thought to be brought about by different mechanisms (for further discussion, see Drake-Holland and Noble, Chapter 17 in this volume). Robison *et al.* (1965) were the first to suggest that the beta-receptor effect was mediated through adenylate cyclase as receptor activation led to an accumulation of cAMP. The lack of correlation between the inotropic effect and cAMP accumulation observed in the early experiments was later explained by the presence of alpha-receptors and is abolished in the presence of the blocking agents (Osnes and Oye, 1975). Alpha-receptor activation does not stimulate adenyl cyclase: it opens Ca^{++} channels and possibly inhibits adenylate cyclase (see Van Belle, Chapter 18 in this volume). In 1967 Lands *et al.* showed that the rank order of potency of a series of catecholamines for a variety of beta-receptor-midiated responses could be divided into two major groups: they postulated that this corresponded to the existence of two subtypes of beta-receptors which they called β_1 and β_2. The receptors responsible for cardiac stimulation were β_1 receptors. The development of selective agonists and antagonists led to a further analysis of the receptors involved in cardiac stimulation. Thus it appears that only β_1 receptors mediate the positive inotropic effects, while both β_1 and β_2 receptors mediate the positive chronotropic effect (Carlsson *et al.*, 1977). The evidence is similar for cat, dog, and human atria (Bonelli, 1978).

The discovery of presynaptic alpha-receptors (see next section) with pharmacological properties different from those of postsynaptic alpha-receptors led to the distinction between α_1 and α_2 receptors. This has now become a distinction based on relative affinities for catecholamines and their synthetic analogues and does not necessarily correspond to pre- and post-synaptic localization. The myocardial alpha-receptors belong to the α_1 category. Various attempts have been made to map the distribution of the receptors in the heart. Wagner and Brodde (1978) carried out a pharmacological mapping of myocardial alpha-receptors in a number of different species. They found that alpha-receptors were present in all parts of the heart. The affinity of the cardiac alpha-receptors for blocking agents was higher than in other tissues, and they suggested that this could mean that cardiac alpha-receptors were different from other alpha-receptors. The question whether agonist and antagonist binding sites represent different forms of the receptor or two different receptors is at present under debate: Lefkowitz has reported that the agonist and antagonist forms have different molecular weights and suggests that binding of the agonist leads to allosteric changes in the receptor which may involve the binding of additional molecules and so an increase in molecular weight (Limbird and Lefkowitz, 1978).

The introduction of radioligands has led to mapping of receptors by *in vitro* binding studies. Williams and Lefkowitz (1978) measured the number and affinity of alpha- and beta-receptors in rat heart. They obtained very similar values for the two receptors: thus the B_{max} for alpha-receptors was 41 fmol per milligram of protein and for beta-receptors 46 fmol per milligram of protein, whereas the K_d was 2.9 nM for alpha- and 2.5 nM for beta-receptors using [^{3}H]dihydroergocryptine and [^{3}H]dihydroalprenolol respectively in rat ventricle. The number for both receptors was slightly smaller in the atria. The left ventricle had more beta-receptors than the right ventricle. A study of the distribution of β_1 and β_2 receptors in right atrium and left ventricle of cat and guinea-pig was carried out by Hedberg *et al.* (1980). In both species the ventricle had only β_1 receptors and the atria contained both β_1 and β_2 receptors in a $3:1$ ratio.

Regulation of Receptors

Radioligand binding studies have shown that a variety of mechanisms produce changes in both affinity and number of adrenergic receptors. They have also revealed the presence of spare receptors. The evidence for spare receptors (Stephenson, 1956) is the finding that catecholamines can elicit nearly maximum inotropic effects with only fractional receptor occupancy. The functional consequences of a change in receptor number will depend on the presence of spare receptors. In the absence of spare receptors a change in receptor number will produce a corresponding change in the maximal physiological response; if there are spare receptors there will be a change in the *sensitivity* to catecholamine but no change in the maximal response. Kaumann (1981a) carried out a study of a series of sympathomimetic drugs and found that in general their inotropic potencies were higher than their affinity for beta-receptors, which implies the presence of spare receptors. He suggested that the degree of dissociation between inotropic potency and receptor affinity was proportional to the intrinsic activity of adenylate cyclase activation and this in turn might be explained by the size of receptor conformational change produced by the different agonists. In all cases there was evidence for spare receptors (Kaumann, 1981b). However, in a recent series of papers, Cousineau *et al.* (1981), using an *in vivo* method for measuring receptor number, found a close parallelism between physiological effect and receptor occupancy and rejected the hypothesis of spare myocardial receptors in the intact animal.

The change in the number of receptors in response to changes in the concentration of their own transmitter has been called homologous regulation. This phenomenon has been demonstrated both *in vitro* and *in vivo*. Thus denervation leads to an increase and incubation with noradrenaline to a decrease in the number of receptors. The important factor appears to be receptor activation since chronic administration of receptor blocking agents will lead to an increase in receptor number similar to that resulting from denervation. Changes in adrenergic receptors in the heart have been reported as a result of chronic administration of beta blocking drugs (Glaubiger and Lefkowitz, 1977), and of the tricyclic antidepressant desmethylimipramine (DMI) (Crews and Smith, 1978). The latter blocks neuronal re-uptake of noradrenaline and so increases its concentration in the synaptic cleft. Chronic DMI administration caused a shift to the left of the frequency–response curve for field stimulation of isolated atrial strips and an enhanced overflow of [^{3}H]noradrenaline. This was attributed to a decrease in the number of presynaptic alpha-receptors and thus to a reduction in the inhibition of release by presynaptic autoreceptors (see next section). Changes in the number of postsynaptic beta-receptors following chronic DMI administration have been reported for cerebral cortex but not for myocardium.

In addition to homologous regulation of receptors there is heterologous regulation which is mediated by mechanisms other than the concentration of the adrenergic transmitter. One of these mechanisms is pH (Camillon de Hurtado *et al.*, 1981): lowering of pH causes a shift to the right of the dose–response curve for the chronotropic response to catecholamines of the atrium. The effect of isoprenaline on cAMP formation was similarly shifted to the right and the change was greater than that for the chronotropic response. In addition, a decrease in the maximum increment of cAMP but not of heart rate was seen. Thus changes in sensitivity induced by changes in pH probably involve properties of receptors, membrane characteristics, and intracellular events. Changes in temperature also have an effect on adrenergic receptors which is different for alpha- and beta-receptors; a lowering of temperature increases the sensitivity of cardiac alpha-receptors but not of beta-receptors (Wagner and Brodde, 1978). The suggestion that temperature leads to an interconversion of receptors (Kunos and Szentivanyi, 1968) is not generally accepted for the mammalian myocardium.

Another heterologous mechanism is the effect of thyroid hormone on myocardial adrenergic receptors. Propylthiouracil administration or thyroidectomy (Banerjee and Kung, 1977; Ciaraldi and Marinetti, 1977) increases the positive inotropic effect of phenylephrine (a selective alpha-agonist), but decreases that of isoprenaline (a selective beta-agonist). Administration of tri-iodothyronine or thyroxine has the reverse effect: the chronotropic effect of phenylephrine is decreased and that of isoprenaline is increased. It appears therefore that thyroxine decreases the sensitivity of alpha-receptors and enhances that of beta-receptors. This has been confirmed by receptor binding studies: tri-iodothyronine administration leads to a decrease in the number of alpha-receptors (Sharma and Banerjee, 1978) and in hyperthyroidism the number of beta-receptors is increased (Lefkowitz, 1979). The nature of the receptor change is at present unknown: it may be a covalent change, a change in receptor turnover, or a change in the rate of internalization.

REGULATION OF NORADRENALINE RELEASE

Noradrenaline in sympathetic nerve terminals is stored in specialized subcellular organelles, the noradrenaline storage vesicles; the axon terminal is a length of axon characterized by vesicle-filled varicosities which are the release sites. The arrival of the nerve impulse leads to an increase in the calcium conductance of the nerve terminal membrane and this triggers the release of noradrenaline by exocytosis. In addition to release, the arrival of the nerve impulse also initiates an acceleration in the rate of synthesis which enables the nerve terminal to replace the transmitter lost by release and so maintain its store of noradrenaline for release by subsequent nerve impulses. The nerve impulse acts as the trigger for noradrenaline release, but there are a number of regulatory mechanisms, operating over both short and long term periods, which control the amount of transmitter released by the nerve impulse. These mechanisms include activation of presynaptic receptors on sympathetic nerve terminals and changes in the two transmitter specific enzymes, tyrosine hydroxylase (TH), which catalyses the rate-limiting step in noradrenaline synthesis, and dopamine β-hydroxylase (DBH), which is the marker for noradrenaline storage vesicles (Fillenz, 1982).

Presynaptic Receptors

The first indication of the existence of presynaptic autoreceptors came from the experiments of Brown and Gillespie on the cat spleen (Brown,

1965); they found that phenoxybenzamine, which was known to block both neuronal and extraneuronal uptake of noradrenaline, as well as adrenergic alpha-receptors, caused a larger overflow of noradrenaline than a combination of neuronal and extraneuronal uptake blockers. The excess overflow was first attributed to the blockage of the postsynaptic receptors. But when it was found that phentolamine enhanced the effect of sympathetic stimulation in atria (which were thought at this stage to have only beta-receptors) the presence of presynaptic autoreceptors controlling noradrenaline release was suggested. This was confirmed when De Potter *et al.* (1971) showed that phenoxybenzamine caused an enhancement of release of dopamine β-hydroxylase, a soluble vesicle marker, as well as noradrenaline. A number of different groups studying the properties of the presynaptic autoreceptor found that although they resembled the postsynaptic alpha-receptors, there were important pharmacological differences. For this reason the presynaptic receptors were designated α_2 receptors.

Three main approaches have been used to identify presynaptic autoreceptors in the heart: (1) the action of sympathetic agonists and antagonists on the chronotropic and inotropic effect of sympathetic stimulation; (2) the effect of these same drugs on the overflow of endogenous and ^{3}H-labelled noradrenaline; and (3) radioligand receptor binding before and after denervation.

Drew (1976), using stimulation of the sympathetic outflow in the pithed rat, compared the effect on the chronotropic response of the heart of a series of sympathomimetic agents in order to characterize the presynaptic receptors on the cardiac sympathetic nerves. He found that these differed in a number of respects from postsynaptic alpha-receptors which mediated the sympathetic control of diastolic blood pressure.

In experiments measuring [3H]noradrenaline overflow in isolated guinea-pig atria, phentolamine caused an increase and propranolol a decrease in overflow; conversely the agonists clonidine and isoprenaline led to a decrease and increase respectively. This provided evidence for two presynaptic autoreceptors with antagonistic effects: the beta-receptors, which have a lower threshold, enhance impulse-evoked release, whereas the α_2 receptors inhibit release. Although it is not yet firmly established whether the presynaptic receptors are β_1 or β_2, pharmacological evidence (Stjärne and Brundin, 1976) suggests that they are β_2 receptors. Recent receptor-binding studies have confirmed the presence of α_2 receptors in the heart and their reduction by 60% after sympathetic denervation (Schümann, 1981).

Although the existence of these receptors is well established, their physiological role is still unclear: selective blockade of presynaptic beta-receptors is not possible. The α_2 receptors come into action at higher concentrations of noradrenaline than the beta-receptors; since they inhibit release they constitute a negative feedback mechanism. In *in vitro* experiments the inhibition of release is much more effective at low than at high frequencies of stimulation and at low rather than high concentrations of calcium; this suggests that they may regulate the availability of calcium for release. In experiments with isolated hearts the effect of presynaptic alpha-receptors is only demonstrable if the heart rate is high and in these preparations their role remains controversial (Langer, 1981). In the intact animal, however, it is likely that their regulation depends less on noradrenaline released by nerve terminals than on circulating adrenaline released by the adrenal medulla. Strictly speaking therefore they are acting as hormonal receptors rather than presynaptic autoreceptors. This is emphasized by the fact that α_2 receptors show a greater sensitivity to adrenaline than to noradrenaline.

In addition to receptors responding to transmitter from their own nerve terminals, there is evidence for a number of other receptors activated by transmitters of other neurones, or substances circulating in the blood (Lokhandwala, 1979).

Probably the most important of these is the cholinergic receptor. Burn and Rand in 1965 put forward the hypothesis that acetylcholine regulated the release of noradrenaline. In spite of the very close anatomical relationship of sympathetic and parasympathetic terminal fibres seen in electron micrographs, there was great resistance to this theory. However, the idea became acceptable when Levy (1971) demonstrated this interaction in the heart where he showed that negative chronotropic and inotropic effects of vagal stimulation were greatly enhanced in the presence of sympathetic activity. He suggested that acetylcholine, in addition to its effect on the myocardium, was reducing the release of noradrenaline from sympathetic nerve terminals. This was confirmed for the atrium by Lindmar et al. (1968) and for the ventricle by Levy and Blattberg (1976) by measuring changes in overflow of noradrenaline resulting from vagal stimulation. Since the effect was blocked by atropine they postulated inhibitory muscarinic presynaptic receptors on cardiac sympathetic nerve terminals. The fact that there is evidence of interaction between acetylcholine and noradrenaline even when these substances are infused suggests that in addition to presynaptic interaction there is postsynaptic interaction. Nicotinic agents (Lindmar et al., 1968) were found to enhance noradrenaline overflow.

The source for the cholinergic agonist are the parasympathetic cardiac nerves. There are, however, other receptors for which the source of the agonist and therefore the physiological role are less clear. Thus 5-hydroxytryptamine (5-HT) has a sympathomimetic effect, which in the isolated rabbit heart has been shown to be reduced by reserpine or 6-hydroxydopamine pretreatment and must, therefore, be an indirect effect, presumably acting through presynaptic 5-HT receptors (Fozard and Mwaluko, 1976). 5-HT, probably derived from platelets, is found in circulating blood.

The cardioaccelerator effect of sympathetic nerve stimulation in the cat is inhibited by apomorphine and dopamine; these effects are blocked by haloperiodol and chlorpromazine; the existence of presynaptic dopamine receptors have been inferred from these observations (Long *et al.*, 1975).

Prostaglandins of the E_1 and E_2 series have little effect on the isolated heart but inhibit the inotropic and chronotropic effects of sympathetic nerve stimulation as well as the overflow of noradrenaline.

Effect of Transmitter Store Size on Noradrenaline Release

Release of noradrenaline from sympathetic nerve terminals, in addition to being regulated by presynaptic receptors, is also influenced by the size of the releasable store. Since noradrenaline is released by exocytosis, the releasable store consists of noradrenaline-filled vesicles. Noradrenaline is stored in two populations of vesicles, the small and large vesicles. The relative proportions of these two vesicles show species variation, in the rat 90% of vesicles in noradrenergic terminals are small and only 4% large, but in other species, including man, the percentage of large vesicles is considerably higher. The large vesicles besides noradrenaline also contain soluble proteins, such as the enzyme dopamine β-hydroxylase and opioid peptides. On exocytosis these substances are released together with noradrenaline. The significance of this is not clear at present. The only substances identified in the core of the small vesicles are noradrenaline and ATP, the enzyme dopamine β-hydroxylase being confined to the inner aspect of the vesicle membrane (Fried, 1980). The noradrenaline content of the small vesicles is normally well below the maximum storage capacity: the degree of saturation (ratio of content to storage capacity) varies between nerve terminals in different organs. It represents the balance between the rate of tyrosine hydroxylation, the rate-limiting step in noradrenaline synthesis, intraneuronal deamination by monoamine oxidase, and release by exocytosis (Fillenz, 1982). Thus the vesicles in the sympathetic nerve terminals in the rat heart normally have a saturation of about 50%; a brief cold stress (Fillenz and West, 1974), which accelerates synthesis rate, or administration of tranylcypromine (Fillenz and Stanford, 1981), which inhibits monoamine oxidase, both increase the degree of vesicular saturation. However, cold exposure for periods between 6 and 24 h results in a decrease of vesicular saturation (Fillenz and West, 1976; Fillenz *et al.*, 1979). The changes in vesicular saturation in the above examples all result from a relatively greater change in vesicular noradrenaline content than in storage capacity, although changes in the latter can also occur. The size of the storage capacity is a reflection of the number of vesicles; prolonged stimulation of release results in a reduction of storage capacity, of the number of small vesicles, and of particulate dopamine β-hydroxylase, the marker enzyme for vesicles. Storage capacity in sympathetic nerve terminals in the heart has been found to be increased after tranylcypromine administration and moderate cold exposure and reduced after prolonged cold exposure (Fillenz *et al.*, 1979; Fillenz and Stanford, 1981).

The significance of changes in vesicular content and storage capacity is that they parallel, and may be responsible for, fluctuations in noradrenaline release. Thus potassium evoked release of noradrenaline from synaptosomes is proportional to the size of the vesicular store (West and Fillenz, 1981) which in turn is determined by the number of vesicles and their degree of saturation. In the intact animal parallel changes in noradrenaline release from sympathetic nerve terminals (as measured by plasma noradrenaline) and vesicular noradrenaline content, saturation, and storage capacity in sympathetic nerve terminals of the heart occur during a 6 h cold exposure (Fillenz *et al.*, 1979).

Trans-synaptic Enzyme Induction

The phenomenon of trans-synaptic enzyme induction is well documented in the adrenal medulla and in noradrenergic neurones (Thoenen, 1975); it involves the regulation of the synthesis of the two transmitter-specific enzymes, TH and DBH, by acetylcholine, which is the excitatory transmitter at the ganglionic synapse. Thus an increase in the preganglionic impulse traffic leads to an increase in the activity of TH and DBH isolated from the superior cervical and stellate ganglia. It has been established that this increase in activity represents an increase in the amounts of enzyme and not a change in enzyme kinetics; the increase is due to an increase in enzyme synthesis, not a decrease in breakdown. This trans-synaptic induction is mediated by nicotinic cholinergic receptors; the second messenger is at present unknown.

Trans-synaptic induction is most easily demonstrated after the administration of drugs which decrease the activation of post-synaptic receptors, and so lead to reflex activation of the preganglionic sympathetic outflow. Examples of such drugs are phenoxybenzamine and reserpine. But it also occurs after activation of the sympathetic nervous system by stressors such as cold exposure or swim-stress. The increase in enzyme activity in the ganglion is demonstrable 16–18 h after a single dose of reserpine or 2 h of intermittent swim-stress. The increase persists for periods up to 3 weeks. The increase in enzyme activity is not confined to the cell body, but appears in the nerve terminals after a delay which is attributed to the time required for the axoplasmic transport of the enzyme to the nerve terminals. Thus the maximum increase in TH and DBH in the stellate ganglion occurred 3 days after a single dose of 5 mg of reserpine per kilogram body weight; in the heart the maximum increase in DBH occurred 4 days and in TH 7 days after the reserpine injection (Thoenen and Oesch, 1973).

The functional implications of enzyme induction are at present not clear. It has been shown that induction of TH by phenoxybenzamine is accompanied by an increase in the *in vivo* synthesis rate of noradrenaline in the heart (Dairman and Udenfriend, 1970). It would be valuable to know whether such an increase in synthesis rate produces an increase in release. Results discussed in the previous section suggests that this might be so.

There is evidence that changes in preganglionic transmitter can also lead to a reduction in enzyme. Thus both preganglionic nerve section and chronic administration of propranolol lead to a reduction of TH isolated from the superior cervical ganglion (Raine and Chubb, 1977). The latter effect is attributed to a reduction of preganglionic impulse frequency resulting from a central action of propranolol; the propranolol effect on TH is abolished by deafferentation of the ganglion.

CONCLUSION

Two aspects of myocardial function are regulated by catecholamines: heart rate and the force of contraction. Catecholamines increase both these parameters. The myocardium has three kinds of adrenergic receptor: α_1, β_1, and β_2. Force of contraction is regulated by α_1 and β_1 receptors, and heart rate by β_1 and β_2 receptors. The cellular mechanisms activated by the various receptors are discussed in other chapters in this volume.

Two catecholamines act on the myocardial receptors: adrenaline from the adrenal and noradrenaline from cardiac sympathetic nerves. These two systems are under separate control and this activation occurs under different circumstances: furthermore the two catecholamines have different potencies for the various myocardial receptors.

In addition to the myocardial adrenergic receptors, there are two kinds of adrenergic receptors on the cardiac sympathetic nerve terminals; these are the α_2 and β_2 presynaptic receptors, which respectively decrease and increase the release of noradrenaline from these nerve terminals. These receptors can be activated either by noradrenaline released from these nerve terminals, and so act as autoreceptors, or by circulating catecholamines, in which case they are acting as hormonal receptors. The receptors differ in their sensitivity to the two catecholamines. For α_1 receptors noradrenaline has a greater potency than adrenaline, for α_2 and β_2 receptors adrenaline is more potent and for β_1 receptors the two catecholamines have equal potencies.

This means that selective activation of the sympathetic, as occurs in exercise, will activate mainly α_1 and β_1 receptors and so lead primarily to an increase in the force of contraction; whereas stress, which increases the release of adrenaline from the adrenal, will primarily increase heart rate, by activating β_2 myocardial receptors and by reducing noradrenaline release through activation of α_2 presynaptic receptors.

However, these responses to physiological stimuli may be considerably altered by changes in sympathetic nerve terminals and in the receptors. Thus, a fall in pH or a fall in thyroid hormone concentration reduces the sensitivity of β receptors relative to α receptors; this will enhance the potency of noradrenaline over that of adrenaline. Prolonged activation of sympathetic nerve terminals leads to an initial reduction in noradrenaline release due to a reduction in the size of the releasable store; this is followed by a delayed and long-lasting increase in functional capacity brought about by trans-synaptic induction. Similar delayed, long-lasting changes occur in the receptors, as a result of prolonged changes in receptor activation.

Most of these slow changes in both nerve terminals and receptors have so far been produced by drug administration, when the changes produced are quite substantial, and have to be taken into account in trying to understand the effects of drug therapy. It is not clear at present whether similar changes occur under normal physiological conditions and if so what their role is: this could either be homeostatic, thus ensuring a constant level of control, or it could involve plasticity in the system, leading to altered levels of control of myocardial function.

ACKNOWLEDGEMENTS

I wish to thank Dr Clare Stanford for useful discussion and Miss Christine Lake for typing the manuscript.

REFERENCES

Ahlquist, R. P. (1948). A study of adrenotropic receptors. *Amer. J. Physiol.,* **153,** 586–600.

Banerjee, S. P. and Kung, L. S. (1977). β-Adrenergic receptors in rat heart: effects of thyroidectomy. *Europ. J. Pharmacol.,* **43,** 207–208.

Bonelli, J. (1978). Demonstration of two different types of β_1-receptors in man. *Internat. J. Clin. Pharmacol.,* **16,** 313–319.

Brown, G. L. (1965). The release and fate of the transmitter liberated by adrenergic nerves. *Proc. Roy. Soc. Lond. B,* **162,** 1–19.

Burn, J. H., and Rand, M. J. (1965). Acetylcholine in adrenergic transmission. *Annu. Rev. Pharmacol.,* **5,** 163–182.

Callingham, B. A. (1975). Catecholamines in blood. In *Handbook of Physiology,* Section 7, Vol. 6. (H. Blaschko, G. Sayer, and A. D. Smith, eds), American Physiological Society, Bethesda, Md, pp. 427–446.

Camilion de Hurtado, M. C., Argel, M. I., and Ciangolani, H. E. (1981). Influence of acid–base alterations on myocardial sensitivity to catecholamines. *Naunyn-Schmiedebergs Arch. Pharmacol.,* **317,** 219–224.

Carlsson, E., Dahlof, C. G., Hedberg, A., Persson, H., and Tangstrand, B. (1977). Differentiation of cardiac chronotropic and inotropic effects of B-adrenoceptor agonists. *Naunyn-Schmiedebergs Arch. Pharmacol.,* **300,** 101–105.

Ciaraldi, T., and Marinetti, G. V. (1977). Thyroxine and propylthiuracil effects *in vivo* on α and β-adrenergic receptors in rat heart. *Biochem. Biophys. Res. Commun.*, **74**, 984–991.

Clark, A. J. (1933). *The Mode of Action on Drugs on Cells*, Edward Arnold, London.

Coupland, R. E. (1965). *The Natural History of the Chromaffin Cell*, Longmans, Green, London.

Cousineau, D., Rose, C. P., and Goresky, C. A. (1981). *In vivo* characterization of the adrenergic receptors in the working canine heart. *Circulation Res.*, **49**, 501–510.

Crews, F. T., and Smith, C. B. (1978). Presynaptic alpha-receptor subsensitivity after long-term antidepressant treatment. *Science*, **202**, 322–324.

Dairman, W., and Udenfriend, S. (1970). Increased conversion of tyrosine to catecholamines in the intact rat following elevation of tissue tyrosine hydroxylase levels by administered phenoxybenzamine. *Mol. Pharmacol.*, **6**, 350–356.

De Potter, W. P., Chubb, I. W., Put, A., and De Schaepdryver, A. F. (1971). Facilitation of the release of noradrenaline and dopamine-β-hydroxylase at low stimulation frequencies by α-blocking agents. *Arch. Internat. Pharmacodyn. Ther.*, **193**, 191–197.

Dolezel, S., Gerova, M., Gero, J., Sladek, T., and Vasku, J. (1978). Adrenergic innervation of the coronary arteries and the myocardium. *Acta Anat.*, **100**, 306–316.

Drew, G. M. (1976). Effects of α-adrenoceptor agonists and antagonists on pre and post-synaptically located α-adrenoceptors. *Europ. J. Pharmacol.*, **36**, 313–320.

Ehinger, B., Falck, B., Sporrong, B. (1970). Possible axo-axonal synapses between peripheral adrenergic and cholinergic nerve terminals. *Z. Zellforsch. Mikrosk. Anat.*, **107**, 508–521.

von Euler, U.S. (1948). Identification of the sympathometic ergone in adrenergic nerves of cattle (sympathia N) with noradrenaline. *Acta. Physiol. Scand.*, **16**, 63–74.

Ferreira, S. H., and Vane, J. R. (1967). Half-lives of peptides and amines in the circulation. *Nature*, **215**, 1237–1240.

Fillenz, M. (1982). Noradrenaline. In *Handbook of Neurochemistry*, Vol. 6 (A. Lajtha, ed.), Plenum, New York, in press.

Fillenz, M., and Stanford, S. C. (1981). Vesicular noradrenaline stores in peripheral nerves of the rat and their modification by tranylcypromine. *Brit. J. Pharmacol.*, **73**, 404–404.

Fillenz, M., and West, D. P. (1974). Changes in vesicular dopamine-β-hydroxylase resulting from transmitter release. *J. Neurochem.*, **23**, 411–416.

Fillenz, M., and West, D. P. (1976). Fate of noradrenaline storage vesicles after release. *Neurosci. Lett.*, **2**, 285–287.

Fillenz, M., Stanford, S. C., and Benedict, C. R. (1979). Changes in noradrenaline release rate and noradrenaline storage vesicles during prolonged activity of sympathetic neurones. In *Catecholamines: Basic and Clinical Frontiers* (E. Usdin, I. Kopin, and J. D. Barchas, eds.), Pergamon Press, Oxford, pp. 936–938.

Fozard, J. R., and Mwaluko, G. M. P. (1976). Mechanism of the indirect sympathomimetic effect of 5-hydroxytryptamine on the isolated heart of the rabbit. *Brit. J. Pharmacol.*, **57**, 115–215.

Fried, G. (1980). Small noradrenergic storage vesicles isolated from rat vas deferens – biochemical and morphological characterization. *Acta. Physiol. Scand.*, Suppl. 493.

Glaubiger, G., and Lefkowitz, R. J. (1977). Elevated beta-adrenergic receptor number after chronic propranalol treatment. *Biochem. Biophys. Res. Commun.,* **78,** 720–725.

Govier, W. C. (1968). Myocardial alpha adrenergic receptors and their role in the production of a positive inotropic effect by sympathomimetic agents. *J. Pharmacol. Exp. Ther.,* **159,** 82–90.

Hedberg, A., Minneman, K. P., and Molinoff, P. B. (1980). Differential distribution of beta-1 and beta-2 adrenergic receptors in cat and guinea pig heart. *J. Pharmacol. Exp. Ther.,* **212,** 503–508.

Hedqvist, P., and Wennmalm, A. (1971). Comparison of the effects of prostaglandins E_1, E_2 and F_2 on the sympathetically stimulated rabbit heart. *Acta Physiol. Scand.,* **83,** 156–162.

Jacobowitz, D., Cooper, T., and Barner, H. B. (1967). Histochemical and chemical studies of the localisation of adrenergic and cholinergic nerves in normal and denervated cat hearts. *Circulation Res.,* **20,** 289–298.

Kaumann, A. J. (1981a). In kitten ventricular myocardium the inotropic potency of an agonist is determined by both its intrinsic activity for the adenylyl cyclase and its affinity for the β-adrenoceptors. *Naunyn-Schmiedebergs Arch. Pharmacol.,* **17,** 13–18.

Kaumann, A. J. (1981b). On the relationship between stimulation of the adenylyl cyclase (AC) β-adrenoceptor occupancy and positive chronotropic effects of catecholamines. *Naunyn-Schmiedebergs Arch. Pharmacol.,* **317,** 371.

Kelly, M., Sharman, D. J., and Tegerdine, P. (1970). Dopamine in the blood of the ruminant. *J. Physiol. (Lond.),* **210,** 130P.

Kunos, G., and Szentivanyi, M. (1968). Evidence favouring the existence of a single adrenergic receptor. *Nature,* **217,** 1077–1078.

Lands, A. M., Arnold, A., McAuliff, J. R., Luduena, F. P., and Brown, T. G. (1967). Differentiation of receptor system activated by sympathomimetic amines. *Nature,* **214,** 597–598.

Langer, S. Z. (1981). Presence and physiological role of presynaptic inhibitory α_2-adrenoceptors in guinea pig atria. *Nature,* **294,** 671.

Lefkowitz, R. J. (1979). Direct binding studies of adrenergic receptors: biochemical, physiologic and chemical implications. *Ann. Intern. Med.,* **91,** 450–458.

Levy, M. N. (1971). Sympathetic–parasympathetic interactions in the heart. *Circulation Res.,* **29,** 437–445.

Levy, M. N., and Blattberg, B. (1976). Effect of vagal stimulation on the overflow of norepinephrine into the coronary sinus during cardiac sympathetic nerve stimulation in the dog. *Circulation Res.,* **38,** 81–85.

Limbird, L. E., and Lefkowitz, R. J. (1978). Agonist-induced increase in apparent β-adrenergic receptor size. *Proc. Natl. Acad. Sci.,* **75,** 228–232.

Lindmar, R., Loffelholz, K., and Muscholl, E. (1968). Muscarinic mechanism inhibiting the release of noradrenaline from peripheral adrenergic nerve fibres of nicotinic agents. *Brit. J. Pharmacol.,* **32,** 280–294.

Lokhandwala, M. F. (1979). Presynaptic receptor systems on cardiac sympathetic nerves. *Life Sci.,* **24,** 1823–1832.

Loewi, O. (1921). Ueber humorale Uebertragbarkeit der Herznerven wirkung. *Pflügers Arch. Ges. Physiol.,* **189,** 239–242.

Long, J. P., Heintz, F. G. S., Cannon, J. G., and Kim, J. (1975). Inhibition of the sympathetic nervous system by 5,6-dihydro-2-dimethylaminetetraline (MZ), apomorphine and dopamine. *J. Pharmacol. Exp. Ther.,* **192,** 336–342.

Moran, N. C., and Perkins, M. E. (1961). An evaluation of adrenergic blockade of the mammalian heart. *J. Pharmacol. Exp. Ther.,* **133,** 192–201.

Nickerson, M. and Chan, G. C.-M. (1961). Blockage of responses of isolated myocardium to epinephrine. *J. Pharmacol. Exp. Ther.*, **133**, 186–191.

Nielsen, K. C., and Owman, Ch. (1968). Difference in cardiac adrenergic innervation between hibernators and non-hibernating animals. *Acta. Physiol. Scand.*, Suppl. 316, 1–16.

Osnes, J.-B., and Oye, I. (1975). Relationship betwen cyclic AMP metabolism and inotropic response of perfused rat hearts to phenylephrine and other adrenergic amines. *Advanc. Cyclic Nucleotide Res.*, **5**, 415–433.

Pohorecky, L. A., and Wurtman, R. J. (1971). Adrenocortical control of epinephrine synthesis. *Phamacol. Rev.*, **23**, 1–35.

Raine, A. E. G., and Chubb, I. W. (1977). Long-term β-adrenergic blockade reduces tyrosine hydroxylase and dopamine-β-hydroxylase activities in sympathetic ganglia. *Nature*, **267**, 265–267.

Robison, G. A., Butcher, R. W., Oye, I., Morgan, H. E., and Sutherland, E. W. (1965). The effect of epinephrine on adenosine 3′,5′-phosphate levels in the isolated perfused rat heart. *Mol. Pharmacol.*, **1**, 168–177.

Schümann, H. J. (1981). Myocardial α-adrenoceptors: results of radioligand binding studies and functional experiments. *Naunyn-Schmiedebergs Arch. Pharmacol.*, **317**, 371.

Sharma, V. K., and Banerjee, S. P. (1978). α-Adrenergic receptor in rat heart: effects of thyroidectomy. *J. Biol. Chem.*, **253**, 5277–5279.

Shore, P. A., Cohn, V. H., Higman, B., and Maling, H. M. (1958). Distribution of norepinephrine in the heart. *Nature*, **181**, 848–849.

Stephenson, R. P. (1956). A modification of receptor theory. *Brit. J. Pharmacol.*, **11**, 379–386.

Stjarne, L., and Brundin, J. (1976). β₂-Adrenoceptors facilitating noradrenaline secretion from human vasoconstrictor nerves. *Acta Physiol. Scand.*, **97**, 88–93.

Street, D. M., and Roberts, D. J. (1969). The presence of dopamine in cat spleen and blood. *J. Pharm. Pharmacol.*, **21**, 199–201.

Thoenen, M. (1975). Transynaptic regulation of neuronal enzyme synthesis. In *Handbook of Psychopharmacology*, Vol. 3 (L. L. Iverson, S. D. Iverson, and S. H. Snyder, eds), Plenum, New York.

Thoenen, H., and Oesch, F. (1973). New enzyme synthesis as a long-term adaptation to increased transmitter utilization. In *New Concepts in Neurotransmitter Regulation* (A. J. Mandell, ed.), Plenum, New York.

Wagner, J., and Brodde, O.-E. (1978). On the presence and distribution of α-adrenoceptors in the heart of various mammalian species. *Naunyn-Schmiedebergs Arch. Pharmacol.*, **302**, 239–253.

Wenzel, D. G., and Su, J. L. (1966). Interaction between sympathomimetic amines and blocking agents on the rat ventricle strip. *Arch. Internat. Pharmacodyn. Ther.*, **160**, 379–389.

West, D. P., and Fillenz, M. (1981). Control of noradrenaline release from hippocampal synaptosomes. *J. Neurochem.*, **37**, 1052–1053.

Williams, R. S., and Lefkowitz, R. J. (1978). Alpha-adrenergic receptors in rat myocardium: identification by binding of ³H-dihydroergoeryptine. *Circulation Res.*, **43**, 721–727.

Winckler, J. (1969). Uber die adrenergen Herznerven bei Ratte und Meerschweinchen. *Z. Zellforsch. Mikrosk. Anat.*, **98**, 106–121.

van der Zypen, E. (1974). Uber die Ausbreitung des vegetativen Nervensystems in den Vorhofen des Herzeus. *Acta Anat.*, **88**, 363–384.

Cardiac Metabolism
Edited by A. J. Drake-Holland and M. I. M. Noble
© 1983 John Wiley & Sons Ltd

CHAPTER 21

The Influence of Innervation on Cardiac Metabolism

Angela J. Drake-Holland

Department of Medicine 1, St George's Hospital Medical School, London SW17 0RE, UK

INTRODUCTION

The heart beats spontaneously, so nervous activity is only required to modify the force and the frequency of contraction. For this the heart is innervated by both sympathetic (adrenergic) and parasympathetic (cholinergic) fibres. The sympathetic innervation arises from the second to the fourth thoracic segments. These nerves synapse mainly in the stellate ganglion. The post-ganglionic fibres are distributed in the cardiac plexuses. The sympathetic fibres innervate both the atria and ventricles. Sensory pain fibres ascend along the same nerve trunks. No specialized nerve endings have been identified in heart muscle; the nerves terminate in depressions in the sarcolemma of the cells they innervate. The parasympathetic innervation of the heart arises in the medulla oblongata from the vagal nuclei. The parasympathetic nerves synapse in the heart, primarily in the pacemaker region, atrioventricular node, and the atria. There is some functional evidence for limited parasympathetic innervation of the ventricles (DeGeest *et al.*, 1964; Buccino *et al.*, 1966; Kent *et al.*, 1975). Both the sympathetic and parasympathetic fibres are closely associated with the coronary arteries down to the precapillary arterioles. The nerve terminals lie adjacent to the coronary arterial smooth muscle, without penetration into the muscle coat. The large arteries are not closely innervated. Though light microscopy has revealed extensive nerve plexuses within the myocardium (Hirsch, 1971), the resolution is inadequate to define accurately the neuromuscular relationships. The evidence from electron miscroscopy on this point is contradictory. There is some evidence for direct terminations (Hayashi, 1962) in the conducting tissue, whilst other workers have failed to confirm this (Phillips, 1963; Napolitano *et al.*, 1965). If the latter is the case, then the neurotransmitters have to cross relatively wide spaces. More information on the innervation of the mammalian myocardium is given in the review by Yamuchi (1973).

EFFECT OF STIMULATION ON CARDIAC
AUTONOMIC NERVES

In the intact preparation differences in results are sometimes obtained when the autonomic nerves are stimulated. The differences are largely due to the complicated effects of cardiac nerve stimulation on myocardial vasculature and/or metabolism. If the autonomic nerves are activated the response will be a change in heart rate and contractility which in turn will change metabolism, and thus the coronary blood flow.

Vagal stimulation (parasympathetic) causes bradycardia, systemic hypotension, and a decrease in metabolism. It was originally thought that vagal activity caused a decrease in coronary blood flow; this is secondary to the bradycardia, hypotension, and the concomitant decrease in metabolism, rather than the direct effect on coronary vessel tone. If the heart is paced at a constant rate during vagal stimulation, the coronary vessels dilate (Feigl, 1969).

Activation of the sympathetic nerves by stimulation of the stellate ganglia causes a tachycardia, a rise in arterial pressure, and an increase in myocardial contractility with an increase in coronary blood flow (Gollwitzer-Meier and Kruger, 1938; Shipley and Gegg, 1945; Berne *et al.*, 1965), the rise in coronary blood flow following the increase in metabolic demand. The question arises: 'Is there a direct effect of sympathetic stimulation on the coronary vessels?' The positive inotropic and chronotropic effects of sympathetic stimulation can be prevented by beta-blockade. If the sympathetic nerves are stimulated in the presence of beta-blockade, a vasoconstriction is seen (Fiegl, 1967; Ross and Mulder, 1969; McRaven *et al.*, 1971). The vasoconstriction is due to alpha-receptors as the response is abolished by alpha-blockade (Feigl, 1967). These results indicate that sympathetic vasoconstriction is mediated through alpha-receptors (Feigl, 1967; Pitt *et al.*, 1967; McRaven *et al.*, 1971; Mark *et al.*, 1972). Later studies showed that the coronary alpha-receptor mechanism competes with metabolic vasodilation during sympathetic stimulation, even in the presence of large increase in myocardial metabolism (Mohrman and Feigl, 1978). It is therefore difficult to evaluate the importance of alpha-adrenergic vasoconstrictor effects in response to changes in myocardial metabolism.

The matter is further complicated by the fact that the response of the smooth muscle in the coronary artery wall to catecholamine stimulation appears to be dependent on the size of the vessel (Zuberbuhler and Bohr, 1965). In small coronary arteries (250–500 μm diameter) and at low concentrations, noradrenaline was a more potent vasodilator than adrenaline. This response could be blocked by beta-adrenergic blockade. In larger vessels (1.5–2.4 mm) constriction was produced by low doses of both adrenaline and noradrenaline, but at high doses relaxation was produced in these vessels, adrenaline being more potent than noradrenaline. In some coronary artery strips there was a transient contraction followed by a relaxation.

Reflex control over myocardial activity is exerted by reciprocal activation and inhibition, e.g. an inhibition of the sympathetic activity accompanies the activation of the vagus in the response to baroreceptor stimulation.

Neurotransmitters

Acetylcholine is the mediator of the parasympathetic influences. The general effect of acetylcholine is to increase the potassium conductance, thus causing hyperpolarization, together with a decrease in the action potential duration. Noradrenaline is the neurotransmitter released from the sympathetic nerve terminals. Adrenaline, released from the adrenal medulla, has a similar action on the myocardium. The effects of both catecholamines on the heart are more complex than those of acetylcholine and include such reactions as enhanced contractility, increased heart rate, accelerated conduction, and a decrease in the action potential duration. Noradrenaline has both alpha and beta effects, the mechanism by which the latter effect is mediated is thought to be cyclic AMP (cAMP). However, the role of cAMP (with the subsequent increase in membrane phosphorylation) in producing the electrophysiological responses to catecholamines is unclear (see Drake-Holland and Noble, Chapter 17, and Van Belle, Chapter 18, in this volume).

The main innervation of the ventricle is sympathetic, thus noradrenaline may be expected to have the largest influence on myocardial metabolism. It is possible to look at the effect of noradrenaline (i.e. the sympathetic nerves) on metabolism by stimulation of the nerves. However, the physiological role of the nerves is more simply analysed by removal of the nerves (denervation) or by pharmacological blockade. Unfortunately the latter studies have invariably used beta-adrenergic blockade which only blocks noradrenaline partially (see below).

IS SURGICAL DENERVATION EQUIVALENT TO CHRONIC BETA-BLOCKADE?

This question has not been systematically investigated. With chronic beta-blockade the noradrenaline content of the tissue will be relatively unchanged, whereas with denervation the noradrenaline content of myocardial tissue drops to between 1 and 0% of the control level (Donald, 1974; Drake *et al.*, 1978). If noradrenaline is still present in the myocardial tissue it will exert an alpha effect, causing for example changes in Ca^{++} conductance. There are also some reports of different effects of chronic noradrenaline depletion (see section below on glucose oxidation). A danger in using synthetic pharmacological agents to intervene in sympathetic neuro-transmission is that the possibility arises of separation of only some, and not all, of the physiological effects of the natural neurotransmitter.

Methods of Denervation

Though it is technically possible to denervate the heart chemically, this method is unsatisfactory as the drugs have to be administered to the whole animal, and thus are not specific to the myocardium. Various chemicals have been used in the past, such as reserpine (Paasonen and Krayer, 1958), 6-hydroxydopamine and immunosympathectomy (Steiner and Schonbaum, 1972). These methods produce an effect on the *whole* animal, which may thus in turn affect myocardial metabolism. More recently chronic administ-ration of high doses of guanethidine have been used to produce chemical sympathectomy in rats (Burnstock *et al.*, 1971; Östman-Smith, 1980). Though this method permanently destroys at least 97% of the sympathetic ganglion cells, with no effect on the central nervous system or adrenal medulla, the maintenance of normal blood pressure is due to increased secretion of adrenal catecholamines (Östman-Smith, 1976), which may also have an unknown effect on metabolism.

Surgical Techniques of Cardiac Denervation

Though early physiologists in the latter half of the nineteenth century spent some time looking at the effect of cutting the accelerator or inhibitory cardiac nerves (reviewed by Hunt in 1899), no techniques for complete cardiac denervation were forthcoming. In 1914 an attempt was made by Gasser and Meake to remove the parasympathetic and sympathetic nerves using a double operation. This technique was used for many years (Asker and Hamilton, 1963) in spite of the problems that occurred during the recovery phase of the animals. In the first procedure the stellate ganglia and thoracic paravertebral sympathetic chains are bilaterally excised from the first to the fourth thoracic segment, and the right vagus nerve is sectioned distal to the right recurrent laryngeal. In the second operation (left side) the left vagus nerve is sectioned in the neck. With this double procedure some cardiac sympathetic fibres remain, but have been decentralized. The degree of cardiac denervation is variable, as not only does the myocardial norad-renaline content decrease by varying amounts, but supersensitivity to norad-renaline does not develop. In addition there are altered respiratory dynamics and gastrointestinal disturbances (with consequent loss in body weight) due to the fact that the lungs and viscera are vagally denervated.

Geis *et al.* (1971) have described a modification of the technique of excision and re-implantation, using a two-stage technique (with double thoracotomy). In the first stage the entire free wall of the atrium is transected and re-anastamosed. The adventitia of the main pulmonary artery and aorta are then transected circumferentially. During the second stage, the free wall of the right atrium, the interarterial septum, and the superior vena cava are all transected and re-anastomosed. The pulmonary afferent fibres are preserved. Heart denervated using this technique becomes depleted of catecholamines and develops noradrenaline sensitivity. It has been reported that it is possible to perform the above denervation procedure in a single stage through a median sternotomy (Kaye and Isobe, 1973), though this can lead to post-operative complications.

With cardiac autotransplantation or transplantation there is complete denervation. The surgery is more complex as the technique requires cardiac bypass and with transplantation there is the complication of rejection. The sympathetic denervation using this procedure is postganglionic, and the heart becomes depleted of catecholamines. These also show supersensitivity to noradrenaline. The afferent pulmonary fibres remain intact; those afferents which course along the aorta, main pulmonary artery, and superior vena cava are removed. The afferent fibres from receptors in the pulmonary veins, posterior wall, and ostia of the vena cava may or may not be preserved, depending on the technique used. Sometimes after transplantation there is variability in the function of the donor sinus node.

Cooper *et al.* (1961) introduced the technique of regional neural ablation for cardiac denervation. This was based on Cooper's studies of the neuroanatomy of the dog. This method was modified by Donald and Shepherd (1963) who used a double thoracotomy, but in one operation, instead of a median sternotomy. The technique of regional neural ablation involves the stripping of adventitia from the aorta, the main, right, and left pulmonary arteries, the pulmonary veins, and the atria and vena cava. The pericardium is removed. Both the efferent and afferent fibres in the aforementioned regions are removed. There are sufficient pulmonary afferent fibres to maintain normal respiration both at rest and during exercise. The sympathetic denervation is postganglionic, and the heart becomes supersensitive to noradrenaline, as well as becoming depleted of catecholamines. In the past there was some mortality due to pulmonary complications, but the present survival rate, with no implanted transducers, is over 85% (A. J. Drake-Holland, M. I. M. Noble, and J. Stubbs, unpublished data).

In any discussion on the functional results of total cardiac denervation it should be emphasized that any data presented should be evaluated in terms of the technique used, the time from denervation to the time of study, and the anaesthetics used. Completeness of denervation can be tested for in several different ways. The most conclusive method is that of measurement of tissue catecholamine content. The noradrenaline content should be below

5 μg per gram wet weight, if denervation is complete. However, this measurement can only be made *post mortem*. In the intact animal tests for completeness of denervation can be made by intravenous injection of the following drugs:

(a) *Atropine*   There should be no effect after denervation on heart rate, or the maximum rate of rise of the left ventricular pressure, i.e. no vagal tone.

(b) *Adrenaline and noradrenaline*   After denervation the response of the heart is greater to noradrenaline than to adrenaline; the opposite is the case prior to denervation.

(c) *Tyramine*   This drug causes release of adrenaline from sympathetic postganglionic nerve terminals. At a dose of $0.1\,mg\,kg^{-1}$ in normal dogs there is simultaneous tachycardia, increased contractility, and hypertension. In the denervated dog the hypertension precedes any tachycardia. This occurs later when noradrenaline released from the periphery reaches the heart via the circulation.

It has also been suggested that vago-sympathetic stimulation (using the stellate ganglion) can be used as a test of completeness of denervation (Peiss *et al.*, 1966). However, such a stimulation would release catecholamines from the adrenal medulla and non-sympathetic nerve endings, thus producing a humoral effect on the heart. This is not an immediate response; there is a time lag of about 10 s. Because of this lag adequate paper speeds must be used when recording the response, so that the time course can be analysed critically.

Evidence of Re-innervation

In the autotransplanted heart (in the dog) there is evidence of re-innervation (Beck *et al.*, 1969; Kontos *et al.*, 1970), though not in humans (Stinson *et al.*, 1972). The problems as to the testing for evidence of re-innervation are similar to those outlined for testing for the completeness of denervation. Stimulation of the stellate ganglion involves further surgery and gives rise to an increase in circulating catecholamines. The Bezold–Jarisch reflex can re-occur 6–9 months post denervation but this may not be true evidence of ventricular re-innervation as it may only be recovery of that afferent pathway. There is a decrease in the noradrenaline hypersensitivity with re-innervation, but the catecholamine content takes a long time to return towards normal even after 1–2 years (Kaye and Isobe, 1973).

It is perhaps here that a note should be introduced concerning partial denervation techniques. It may be possible to remove the sympathetic supply to the left ventricle alone, but not to remove the parasympathetics alone. There is a marked degree of intermingling of nerve fibres at the caudal cervical ganglion, so it is impossible to preserve all the sympathetic nerves whilst performing parasympathectomy. Any attempt to do so will result in both pulmonary and oesphagogastric dysfunction.

Intraeardiac Nerves

These are those nerves which remain after total extrinsic denervation. They presumably originate from cell bodies within the heart itself (Napolitano *et al.*, 1965). Between the myocardial cells are bundles of collagen fibres which contain small blood vessels and neural elements. These neural elements are C-fibres which are embedded in Schwann cells (known as Remak bundles) and are more numerous in the atria than the ventricles.

CHANGES IN TISSUE CATECHOLAMINE CONTENT WITH CARDIAC DENERVATION

Depletion of Adrenaline and Noradrenaline

After cardiac denervation the catecholamine content of the tissue decreases. This is true both for adrenaline and for noradrenaline. The adrenaline content depletes to about 10% of the control value, whilst the noradrenaline content falls to 1–2% of control, or to zero. The values of adrenaline and noradrenaline for 13 dogs measured by fluorescent techniques (trihydroxyindole reaction) after column separation are shown in Table 21.1. This depletion of catecholamines has been found by many workers using the technique of regional neural ablation (Cooper *et al.*, 1961; Donald and Shepherd, 1963; Noble *et al.*, 1972; Drake *et al.* 1978; Drake and Stanford, 1982), autotransplantation (Lower and Shumway, 1960; Willman *et al.*, 1962), excision, and re-implantation (Geis *et al.*, 1971; Kaye and Isobe, 1973).

Table 21.1 Adrenaline and nonadrenaline levels (in nanograms per gram wet weight) measured by fluorescent techniques after Bio-rex separation

	Innervated	Denervated
Adrenaline	91.8 ± 20.0 (6)	13.1 ± 4.2 (7)
Noradrenaline	581.0 ± 65.7 (6)	17.1 ± 17.4 (7)

All values are means ± s.D. Values in parentheses indicate numbers of samples.

Dr E. Maruchin (Warsaw) is thanked for some of the measurements.

Metabolism of Noradrenaline

Noradrenaline is synthesized from tyrosine in the postganglionic neurones (Figure 21.1). The noradrenaline is stored in vesicles at the neuromuscular junctions, as well as in varicosities formed by the unmyelinated neurones as it passes between the muscle cells. Though there is some migration of vesicles from the cell body to the terminals, the rate of turnover of the transmitter is so fast that there must be local synthesis. The enzyme for the last step, dopamine β-hydroxylase is apparently confined to the vesicles. The vesicles also remove dopamine from the cytoplasm for synthesis of noradrenaline. Normal hearts can synthesize noradrenaline from dopamine in both the atria and the ventricles (Potter *et al.*, 1965). Vesicular turnover is slow, but that of noradrenaline is rapid. It is reasonable to postulate, therefore, that the emptying of the vesicle during transmission is not 'all-or-none', but that after losing some noradrenaline the vesicle accumulates dopamine and resynthesizes noradrenaline. However, as proteins will be lost during exocytosis the vesicle will eventually become exhausted, and will then be replaced.

The breakdown of noradrenaline is complex. In the adrenergic sytem chemical inactivation of noradrenaline is not so important as the uptake of the liberated transmitter by the neurone or the effector tissue. The enzymes that convert noradrenaline to inactive compounds are catechol-O-methyl transferase (COMT) and monoamine oxidase (MAO), the former being responsible for catabolism of extracellular and the latter for intracellular noradrenaline.

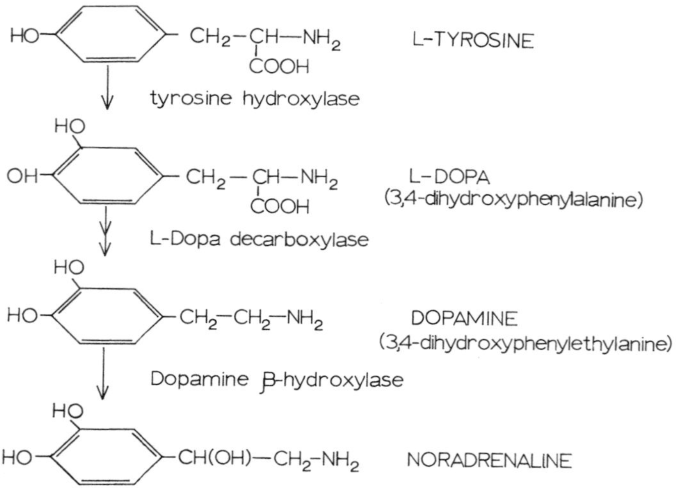

Figure 21.1 Conversion of L-tyrosine to noradrenaline. The enzyme tyrosine hydroxylase is the rate-limiting step

The synthesis of noradrenaline is a continuous process. Within the vesicle the bulk is stored as a complex with protein–chromogranin–ATP and calcium. In this form it has little osmotic activity. This store is in equilibrium with a mobilized form of noradrenaline with the vesicle, which is in dynamic equilibrium with the cytoplasmic store of noradrenaline. The rate-limiting enzyme in noradrenaline synthesis is tyrosine hydroxylase, and is itself inhibited by noradrenaline. Thus uptake of noradrenaline by the neurone after transmission will act as a negative feedback mechanism. Storage within the granules is specific, so a noradrenaline-containing neurone will not store precursors such as dopamine or 5-hydroxytryptamine (Geffen and Livett, 1971). In contrast, the active pump mechanisms that transport the transmitter across the neuronal or granular membrane are not selective. Thus, it seems that the storage function rather than the transport function is the determining factor where accumulation of a transmitter is concerned.

In the denervated heart the ability to synthesize noradrenaline and the uptake of dopamine are very much reduced (Potter *et al.*, 1965). The denervated heart is still able to inactivate noradrenaline, as shown by [^{3}H]noradrenaline binding studies (Potter *et al.*, 1965). Thus an intact adrenergic system is essential for the normal synthesis, storage, and inactivation of noradrenaline.

The denervated myocardium is supersensitive to its neurotransmitter noradrenaline. It has been known for some time that denervated organs become supersensitive to their neurotransmitters (Canon, 1939). As mentioned earlier, with the techniques of regional neural ablation and autotransplantation noradrenaline supersensitivity always develops. This increase in supersensitivity cannot be explained only on an increase in receptor number with denervation, as the denervated heart does not become supersensitive to adrenaline as well (Noble *et al.*, 1972). Nor is there much residual humoral effect of circulating adrenaline as the spontaneous post-denervation heart rate is very little affected after adminstration of a pure beta-adrenergic blocking agent (Drake, 1980). The supersensitivity to noradrenaline could, however, be due to an increase in the ratio of alpha- to beta-adrenergic receptors, with no net increase in total adrenergic receptor number (see Fillenz, Chapter 20 in this volume).

Dopamine

Dopamine can be measured fluorometrically in myocardial tissue after differential separation on Dowex or alumina columns. It is present in innervated hearts at levels very similar to those of noradrenaline (approximately 200 μg per gram of tissue wet weight). There is no depletion of dopamine in the denervated heart and the levels are unchanged from the innervated condition; values are shown in Table 21.2. The precise location

Table 21.2 Dopamine levels (in nanograms per gram of wet weight of tissue)
measured by fluorescent techniques at
two different centres (A and B)

	Innervated	Denervated
A	82.0 ± 17.2 (6)	116.0 ± 60.8 (7)
B	190.1 ± 59.0 (9)	200.0 ± 69.0 (5)

All values are means $\pm$ s.d. Values in
parentheses indicate numbers of samples.
I am indebted to Dr E. Maruchin (Warsaw)
and Mr M. Bloomfield (Oxford) for the measurements.

of this dopamine is at present unknown. Preliminary results have shown that
60% of the retained dopamine is located in the vesicular pellet. The
noradrenaline content of such a pellet is zero. Tyrosine hydroxylase activity
of the denervated heart is nearly normal. The presence of dopaminergic
ligand binding sites in both the innervated and denervated heart has been
shown (Drake *et al.*, 1982), the physiological significance of which remains
uncertain. The location of these sites, vascular or cellular, remains to be
ascertained. The failure of dopamine levels to fall following total cardiac
denervation, with the presence of dopamine receptor-like activity and a
capacity for dopamine synthesis, are compatible with the hypothesis that
there is a peripheral dopaminergic system in the heart.

The action of dopamine on the myocardium is dose-dependent.
Dopamine can cause an increase or a decrease in the resistance of the
coronary circulation. Vasodilatation is predominant when dopamine is given
intravenously (Brooks *et al.*, 1969); vasoconstriction is apparent when
dopamine is given directly into the coronary arteries or as a large single dose
(Cobb *et al.*, 1972). The vasoconstriction is due to the stimulation of the
alpha-receptors. Each effect (alpha- and beta-adrenergic) of dopamine can
be abolished by administration of the appropriate receptor antagonist
(Scheulke *et al.*, 1971; Tada and Goldberg, 1975). These cardiovascular
actions of dopamine could be caused by reflex or neurogenic mechanisms. If
the cardiac output or contractility is increased, then there will be an increase
in coronary blood flow, presumably because of the increase in oxygen
demand.

There is much less information available on the cardiovascular metabolic
effects of dopamine. In studies in anaesthetized dogs, Hall *et al.* (1979)
showed that there were no major changes in lactate or potassium arterio-
coronary sinus differences, but there was a change in both the glucose and
glycerol uptakes. As the authors pointed out, at the doses given (10 or 30 μg

kg^{-1} min^{-1}), in the absence of beta-adrenergic blockade, the effects seen were alpha- and beta-adrenergic. From studies in man it has been proposed that dopamine increases 'volume' work, but not pressure work for the same oxygen consumption, i.e. an increase in efficiency (Crexells *et al.*, 1973). Further studies on the metabolic effect of dopamine on the myocardium under conditions of adequate alpha- and beta-adrenergic blockade would be interesting in order to determine the effect of stimulating the dopaminergic receptors.

THE EFFECT OF DENERVATION ON MYOCARDIAL METABOLISM

There have been only a few studies on the metabolism of the denervated heart, and the findings are controversial. These variations are probably due to differing techniques of cardiac denervation, species studied, and the lack of constancy of the time between surgery and study. The preparations studied have ranged from isolated papillary muscles to conscious dogs.

From the studies on isolated papillary muscle (cat) it was concluded that the denervated heart has a normal basal metabolism with no impairment of the conservation of energy into mechanical work (Colman *et al.*, 1970). Unpaired studies in autotransplanted hearts led to the suggestion that the autotransplanted heart was less efficient (Daggett *et al.*, 1967). Gregg *et al.* (1972) suggested that the denervated dog heart functions at a lower metabolic rate (i.e. increased efficiency). These findings were opposite to those described by Barta *et al.* (1966, 1967) who found large decreases in coronary blood flow, and myocardial efficiency. These authors thought that the denervated myocardium becomes hypoxic and showed a decreased ability to convert chemical to mechanical energy. However, it was shown by Noble *et al.* (1972) that the heart denervated by regional neural ablation contains normal levels of intracellular enzymes, lipid, and glycogen, i.e. the nerves do not have a trophic effect in maintaining tissue composition. Recently it has been shown in a paired study (Drake *et al.*, 1978) that the heart denervated by the same technique and studied at constant heart rate shows no change in external work, but an increase in oxygen consumption, i.e. the denervated heart is inefficient in terms of mechanical output. This is further supported by measurement of myocardial oxygen consumption *in vitro*, before and after denervation in small biopsies taken from the same dog. There is an increase in the oxygen consumption post denervation (A. J. Drake-Holland and R. Wanless, unpublished observations). In the intact preparation there was always a parallel increase in left ventricular blood flow, but with no evidence for a change in vasomotor tone. The increase in coronary blood flow is presumably due to the higher myocardial metabolic rate; this is presumably due to the lack of myocardial tissue noradrenaline.

This means that the nerves have a primary effect on myocardial metabolism which could then determine myocardial blood flow secondarily through local tissue metabolic autoregulation (Donald, 1974).

The major difference between the denervated and the innervated heart is the lack of noradrenaline from the former. The release of noradrenaline from the sympathetic nerve terminals might influence the balance of aerobic to anaerobic metabolism. Information in the published literature on any direct effect of noradrenaline on myocardial glycolytic metabolism is small. A mechanism of action is thought to be via cyclic adenosine 3,5'-monophosphate (cAMP), which could then influence the activity of certain regulatory enzymes such as phosphofructokinase (Newsholme and Start, 1973). Inhibition of phosphofructokinase activity in the denervated heart has been indicated by the findings of Drake *et al.* (1980). In these hearts the oxidation of glucose to carbon dioxide was inhibited, and there was an increase in the level of fructose-6-phosphate, the substrate for phosphofructokinase. There were no changes in the amount of phosphofructokinase present in these hearts (Papadoyannis, 1980), but it was impossible to measure the *in vivo* activity of the enzyme. The mechanism of this change of activity remains obscure as factors known to control phosphofructokinase activity did not change. There were no changes in ATP or CP levels (Drake, 1980), though other high energy phosphate levels such as ADP and AMP were not measured. The effect of cAMP on phosphofructokinase activity is to remove the ATP inhibition (Mansour, 1972), thus enhancing the enzyme's activity. It is possible that a decreased level of noradrenaline could lead to a decreased level of cAMP activation, though the receptors are supersensitive to noradrenaline. If cAMP levels are affected this may have an effect on calcium uptake by the sarcolemma and/or sarcoplasmic reticulum (see Chapters 2 and 18 in this volume). Preliminary results show no change in cyclic AMP in denervated hearts (A. J. Drake-Holland, unpublished data). However, the chronically denervated heart has a metabolic abnormality with a minimal effect on contractility (Drake *et al.*, 1980; Noble *et al.*, 1972).

It would appear that the sympathetic nerves, with the constant uptake and release of noradrenaline, are necessary for the normal metabolism of the myocardium. The effect of noradrenaline may be complex, perhaps affecting the intracellular concentration of regulatory metabolites rather than having a direct action on a specific regulatory enzyme.

INVOLVEMENT OF CARDIAC SYMPATHETIC NERVES IN ADAPTIVE CARDIAC HYPERTROPHY

If the myocardium has to cope with an increased workload, some degree of mild to moderate hypertrophy may be beneficial. However, when the hypertrophy develops to such an extent that myocardial performance deteriorates, it is pathological (Span *et al.*, 1967). The normal growth of the heart after the early post-natal period is achieved by an increase in cell size, with no increase in cell number. Compensatory hypertrophy may be generalized, or involve one chamber only, depending on the cause. Neither growth hormone nor thyroxine is necessary for the adaptive hypertrophy, as it can occur in hyposectomized rats (Tipton and Tcheng, 1971).

There are three successive steps in adaptive cardiac hypertrophy: (1) a condition which places a greater workload on the heart; (2) an intermediate link through which extra work triggers events at the cellular level; which leads to (3) the biochemical changes in the cell leading to cell growth. The biochemical changes have been extensively studied (Alpert, 1971; Rabinowitz, 1974; Wilkman-Coffelt *et al.*, 1979). These changes lead to a sustained increase in myofibrils resulting in an increase in the myofibrillar : mitochondrial ratio. There is also an increase in cell diameter and length. The 'trigger factor' which initiates the biochemical factors must be distinguished from other factors that may be necessary (though not in themselves sufficient) for hypertrophy to occur.

An essential criterion for the triggering factor is that it must be capable of influencing only one side of the heart as cardiac hypertrophy can be restricted to one chamber only. This then excludes all circulating agents from a causative role. The cardiac sympathetic nerves may be the physiological signal, having both inotropic and chronotropic influences. In other organs, such as the salivary gland, the hypertrophy caused by the sympathetic stimulation can be blocked by beta-adrenoreceptor blockade (Wells *et al.*, 1961; Brenner and Stanton, 1970; Muir *et al.*, 1975). However, there are at least two conditions which have to be fulfilled before a role for the sympathetic nervous system in the development of cardiac hypertrophy can be accepted:

(1) There should be an anatomical basis for selective innervation to each chamber, which is mainly the case. The central pathways involved in cardiovascular control can be selectively activated on the right and left sides (Calaresu *et al.*, 1975).

(2) There should be increased cardiac nerve activity in conditions that lead to compensatory cardiac hypertrophy. This has been shown to be so in experimental preparations leading to both generalized and localized cardiac hypertrophy (Downing and Siegel, 1963; Fischer *et al.*, 1965; de Champlain *et al.*, 1969; Goldman and Harrison, 1970; Whitehorn, 1971).

Evidence to support the involvement of the sympathetic nerves in adaptive cardiac hypertrophy has been obtained in rats treated with guanethidine. Though guanethidine destroys approximately 97% of the sympathetic ganglion cells without affecting the central nervous system nor the adrenal medulla, all organs receiving sympathetic innervation will be affected. In these guanethidine-treated rats, no adaptive cardiac hypertrophy developed after a strenous daily swimming programme that lasted 3 months (Östman-Smith, 1980), whereas the control group developed hypertrophy. In animals in which the circulating catecholamines were moderately elevated, there was no evidence of cardiac hypertrophy (Östman-Smith, 1976). This suggests that it is the high local concentrations of noradrenaline, such as occur at the sympathetic nerve terminals, that are required for the triggering of the hypertrophic response in the myocardial cell. Thus, with increased sympathetic activity, compensatory growth of cardiac cells is induced, and the trophic action is mediated by noradrenaline. If this hypothesis is true it might be beneficial to limit hypertrophy in the presence of a continuing stimulus by using a therapy which would decrease in some way the activity of the cardiac sympathetic nervous system, i.e. selective cardiac adrenegic receptor antagonists, or surgical denervation.

REFERENCES

Alpert, N. R. (ed.) (1971). *Cardiac Hypertrophy*, Academic Press, New York.

Askar, E., and Hamilton, W. F. (1963). Cardiovascular response to graded exercise in the sympathectomized-vagotomized dog. *Amer. J. Physiol.*, **204**, 291–296.

Barta, E., Breuer, E., Pappova, E., and Zlatos, L. (1966). Influence of surgical denervation of the heart on the energetic metabolism and cardiac efficiency. *Exp. Med. Surg.*, **24**, 319–333.

Barta, E., Fizelova, A., Breuer, E., and Fizela, A. (1967). Participation of the nervous system in the control of protein and nucleic acid metabolism and cardiac efficiency. *Cor Vasa*, **9**, 282–287.

Beck, W., Barnard, C. N., and Schire, V. (1969). Heart rate after cardiac transplantation. *Circulation*, **40**, 437–444.

Berne, R. M., DeGeest, H., and Levy, M. N. (1965). Influence of the cardiac nerves on coronary resistance. *Amer. J. Physiol.*, **208**, 763–769.

Brenner, G. M., and Stanton, H. C. (1970). Adrenergic mechanisms responsible for submandibular salivary gland hypertrophy in the rat. *J. Pharmacol. Exp. Ther.*, **173**, 166–175.

Brooks, H. L., Stein, P. D., Matson, J. L., and Hyland, J. W. (1969). Dopamine induced alterations in coronary haemodynamics in dogs. *Circulation Res.*, **24**, 699–704.

Buccino, R. A., Sonnenblick, E. H., Cooper, T., and Braunwald, E. (1966). Direct positive effect of acetylcholine on myocardium. Evidence for multiple cholinergic receptors in the heart. *Circulation Res.*, **19**, 1097–1108.

Burnstock, G., Evans, B., Gannon, B. J., Heath, J. W., and James, V. (1971). A new method for destroying adrenergic nerves in adult animals using guanethidine. *Brit. J. Pharmacol.*, **43**, 295–301.

Calaresu, F. R., Fraiers, A. A., and Morgenson, G. J. (1975). Central neural regulation of heart and blood vessels in mammals. *Prog. Neurobiol.*, **5**, 1–35.

Canon, W. B. (1939). A law of denervation. *Amer. J. Med. Sci.*, **198**, 737–750.

de Champlain, E., Meuller, R, A., and Axelrod, J. (1969). Turnover and synthesis of norepinephrine in experimental hypertension in rats. *Circulation Res.*, **25**, 285–291.

Cobb, F. R., McHale, P. A., Bach, R. J., and Greenfield, J. C. (1972). Coronary and systemic hemodynamic effects of dopamine in the awake dog. *Amer. J. Physiol.*, **222**, 1355–1360.

Coleman, H. N., Dempsey, P. J., and Cooper, T. (1970). Myocardial oxygen consumption following chronic cardiac denervation. *Amer. J. Physiol.*, **218**, 475–478.

Cooper, T., Gilbert, J. W., Bloodwell, R. D., and Crout, J. R. (1961). Chronic extrinsic cardiac denervation by regional neural ablation: description of the operation, verification of the denervation and its effects on myocardial catecholamines. *Circulation Res.*, **9**, 275–281.

Crexells, C., Bourassa, M. G., and Biron, P. (1973) Effects of dopamine on myocardial metabolism in patients with ischaemic heart disease. *Cardiovasc. Res.*, **7**, 438–445.

Daggett, Wm, Wilman, V. L., Cooper, T., and Hanlon, C. R. (1967). Work capacity and efficiency of the autotransplanted heart. *Circulation*, **35**, Supp. I, I-96–I-104.

DeGeest, H., Levy, M. N., and Ziezke, H. (1964). Relative inotropic effect of the vagus nerves on the canine ventricle. *Science*, **144**, 1223–1225.

Donald, D. E. (1974). Myocardial performance after excision of the extrinsic cardiac nerves in the dog. *Circulation Res.*, **34**, 417–424.

Donald, D. E., and Shepherd, T. (1963). Response to exercise in dogs with cardiac denervation. *Amer. J. Physiol.*, **205**, 393–400.

Downing, S. E., and Siegel, J. H. (1963). Baroreceptor and chemoreceptor influences on sympathetic discharge to the heart. *Amer. J. Physiol.*, **204**, 471–479.

Drake, A. J. (1980). The effect of intracellular pH, substrates and innervation on myocardial oxygen consumption and metabolism. PhD thesis, University of London.

Drake, A. J., and Stanford, C. (1982). Effect of cardiac denervation on catecholamine levels in dog heart. *J. Physiol. (Lond.)*, **324**, 14P.

Drake, A. J., Stubbs, J., and Noble, M. I. M. (1978) Dependence of myocardial blood flow and metabolism on cardiac innervation. *Cardiovasc. Res.*, **12**, 69–80.

Drake, A. J., Papadoyannis, D. E., Butcher, R. G., Stubbs, J., and Noble, M. I. M. (1980). Inhibition of glycolysis in the denervated dog heart. *Circulation Res.*, **47**, 338–345.

Drake, A. J., Stanford, S. C., and Templeton, W. W. (1982). Evidence for a role of dopamine in cardiac function. *Neurochem. Internat.*, (1982) **4**, 435–439.

Feigl, E. O. (1967). Sympathetic control of coronary circulation. *Circulation Res.*, **20**, 262–271.

Feigl, E. O. (1969). Parasympathetic control of coronary blood flow. *Circulation Res.*, **25**, 509–519.

Fischer, J. E., Horst, W. D., and Kopin, I. J. (1965). Norepinephrine metabolism in hypertrophied hearts. *Nature*, **207**, 951–953.

Gasser, H. S., and Meeke, W. J. (1914). A study of the mechanisms by which muscular exercise produces acceleration of the heart. *Amer. J. Physiol.*, **34**, 48–71.

Geffen, L. B., and Livett, B. G. (1971). Synaptic vesicles in sympathetic neurones. *Physiol. Rev.*, **51**, 98–157.

Geis, W. P., Tatooles, J., Kaye, M. P., and Randall, C. (1971). Complete cardiac denervation without transplantation: a simple and reliable technique. *J. Appl. Physiol.*, **30**, 289–293.

Goldman, R. H., and Harrison, D. C. (1970). The effects of hypoxia and hypercapnia on myocardial catecholamines. *J. Pharmacol. Exp. Ther.*, **174**, 307–314.

Gollwitzer-Meier, K., and Kruger, E. (1938). Einfluss der Herzen auf den Gaswescehl des Wärmbluterherzens. *Pflügers Arch. Ges. Physiol.*, **240**, 89–110.

Gregg, D. E., Khuori, E. M., Donald, E. E., Lowensohn, H. S., and Pasyk, S. (1972) Coronary circulation in the conscious dog with cardiac neural ablation. *Circulation Res.*, **32**, 129–144.

Hall, G. M., Young, C., and Scott, A. (1979). Metabolic changes during dopamine infusion on dogs. *Brit. J. Anaesthes.* **51**, 1021–1025.

Hayashi, K. (1962). An electron microscope study on the conduction system of the cow heart. *Jpn Circulation J.*, **26**, 765–842.

Hirsch, E. F. (ed.) (1971). *The Innervation of the Vertebrate Heart*, C. C. Thomas, Springfield, Ill.

Hunt, R. (1899). Direct reflex acceleration of the mammalian heart with some observations on the relations of the inhibitory and accelerator nerves. *Amer. J. Physiol.*, **2**, 395–470.

Kaye, M. P., and Isobe, J. (1973). One stage cardiac denervation without transplantation. *J. Surg. Res.*, **15**, 357–362.

Kent, K. M., Epstein, S. E., Cooper, T., and Jacobowitz, D. C. (1975). Cholinergic innervation of the canine and human conducting system, autonomic and electrophysiologic correlations. *Circulation*, **50**, 948–975.

Kontos, H. A., Thames, M. D., and Lower, R. R. (1970). Responses to electrical and reflex autonomic stimulation on dogs with cardiac transplantation before and after reinnervation. *J. Thorac. Surg.*, **59**, 382–392.

Lower, R. R., and Shumway, N. E. (1960). Studies on orthotopic homotransplantation of the canine heart. *Surg. Forum*, **11**, 18–19.

Jonsson, G., and Sach, C. (1972). Degenerative and nondegenerative effects of 6-hydroxydopamine on adrenergic nerves. *J. Pharmacol. Exp. Ther.*, **180**, 625–635.

McRaven D. R., Mark, A. L., Abboud, F. M., and Mayer, H. E. (1971). Responses of coronary vessels to adrenergic stimuli. *J. Clin. Invest.*, **50**, 773–778.

Mansour, T. E. (1972). Phosphofructokinase. *Curr. Topics Cell Regulation*, **5**, 2–46.

Mark, A. L., Abboud, F. M., Schmid, P. G., Heistad, D. D., and Mayer, H. E. (1972). Differences in direct effects of adrenergic stimuli on coronary, cutaneous and muscular vessels. *J. Clin. Invest.*, **51**, 279–287.

Mohrman, D. E., and Feigl, E. O. (1978). Competition between sympathetic vasoconstriction and metabolic vasodilation in the canine coronary circulation. *Circulation Res.*, **42**, 79–91.

Muir, T. C., Pollock, D., and Turner, C. J. (1975). The effects of electrical stimulation of the autonomic nerves and of drugs on the salivary glands and their rate of cell division. *J. Pharmacol. Exp. Ther.*, **195**, 372–381.

Napolitano, L. M., Willman, V. L., Hanlon, C. R., and Cooper, T. (1965). Intrinsic innervation of the heart. *Amer. J. Physiol.*, **208**, 455–458.

Newsholme, R. A., and Start, C. (1973). In *Regulation of Metabolism*, John Wiley, London.

Noble, M. I. M., Stubbs, J., Trenchard, D., Else, W., Eisele, J. H., and Guz, A. (1972). Left ventricular performance in the conscious dog with chronically denervated heart. *Cardiovasc. Res.*, **6**, 457–477.

Östman-Smith, I. (1976). Prevention of exercise induced cardiac hypertrophy in rats by chemical sympathectomy (guanethedine treatment). *Neuroscience*, **1**, 497–507.

Östman-Smith, I. (1980). Adaptive changes in the sympathetic nervous system and some effector organs of the rat following long-term exercise or cold acclimation, and the role of cardiac sympathetic nerves in the genesis of compensatory cardiac hypertrophy. *Acta Physiol. Scand.*, Suppl. **477**, 1–118.

Paasonen, M. K., and Krayer, O. (1958). The release of norepinephrine from the mammalian heart by reserpine. *J. Pharmacol. Exp. Ther.*, **123**, 153–160.

Papadoyannis, D. E. (1980). The influence of calcium ion availability on cardiac contraction. A study of energy requirements and factors affecting glycolysis. PhD thesis, University of London.

Parratt, J. R. (1965). Blockade of sympathetic β-receptors in the myocardial circulation. *Brit. J. Pharmacol.*, **24**, 601–611.

Peiss, C. N., Cooper, T., Willman, V. L., and Randall, W. C. (1966). Circulatory responses to electrical and reflex activation of the nervous system after cardiac denervation. *Circulation Res.*, **19**, 153–166.

Phillips, S. J. (1963). Preliminary observations of the fine structure of myocardial innervation in monkey and man. *Anat. Rec.*, **145**, 272 (Abstr.).

Pitt, B., Elliot, E. C., and Gregg, D. E. (1967). Adrenergic receptor activity in the coronary arteries of the anaesthetized dog. *Circulation Res.*, **21**, 75–84.

Potter, L. T., Cooper, T., Willman, V. L., and Wolfe, D. E. (1965). Synthesis, binding, release and metabolism of norepinephrine in normal and transplanted dog hearts. *Circulation Res.*, **16**, 468–481.

Rabinowitz, M. (1974). Overview on pathogenesis of cardiac hypertrophy. *Circulation Res.*, **35**, Suppl. II, 3–11.

Ross, G., and Mulder, D. G. (1969). Effects of left and right cardiosympathetic nerve stimulation on blood flow in the major coronary arteries of the anaesthetized dog. *Cardiovasc. Res.*, **3**, 22–29.

Scheulke, D. M., Mark, A. L., Schmid, P. G., and Eckstein, J. W. (1971). Coronary vasodilation produced by dopamine after adrenergic blockade. *J. Pharmacol. Exp. Ther.*, **176**, 320–327.

Shipley, R. E., and Gregg, D. E. (1945). The cardiac response to stimulation of the stellate ganglia and cardiac nerves. *Amer. J. Physiol.*, **143**, 396–401.

Span, J. R., Bussino, R. A., Sonnenblick, E. H., and Braunwald, E. (1967). Contractile state of cardiac muscle obtained from cats with experimentally produced ventricular hypertrophy and heart failure. *Circulation Res.*, **21**, 341–354.

Steiner, G., and Schonbaum, E. (1972). *Immunosympathectomy*, Elsevier, New York.

Stinson, E. B., Griepp, R. B., Schroder, J. S., Dong, E., and Shumway, N. E. (1972). Hemodynamic observations one and two years after cardiac transplantation in man. *Circulation*, **45**, 1183–1194.

Tada, N., and Goldberg, L. I. (1975). Effects of dopamine on isolated coronary arteries. *Cardiovasc. Res.*, **9**, 384–389.

Tipton, C. M., and Tcheng, T.-K. (1971). Influence on physical training, aortic constriction and exogeneous pituitary hormones on heart weight of hypophysectomized rats. *Pflügers Arch. Ges. Physiol.*, **325**, 103–112.

Wells, H., Handleman, C., and Milgram, E. (1961). Regulation by sympathetic nervous system on accelerated growth of salivary glands in rats. *Amer. J. Physiol.*, **301**, 707–710.

Whitehorn, W. V. (1971). Effects of hypophyseal hormones on cardiac growth and function. In *Cardiac Hypertrophy* (N. R. Alpert, ed.), Academic Press, New York, pp. 27–37.

Wikman-Coffelt, J., Parmley, W. W., and Mason, D. T. (1979). The cardiac hypertrophy process. Analyses of factors determining pathological vs. physiological development. *Circulation Res.*, **45**, 697–707.

Willman, V. L., Cooper, T., Cian, L. G., and Hanlon, C. R. (1962). Autotransplata-
tion of the canine heart. *Surg. Gynecol Obstet.*, **115,** 299–302.
Yamuchi, A. (1973). Ultrastructure of the innervation of the mammalian heart. In
Ultrastructure of the Mammalian Heart (C. E., Challise and S. Viragh, eds),
Academic Press, New York.
Zuberbuhler, R. C., and Bohr, D. F. (1965). Responses of coronary smooth muscle
to catecholamines. *Circulation Res.*, **16,** 431–440.

CHAPTER 22

Thyroid Hormones

J. Nauman

Medical Centre for Postgraduate Education, Marymoncka 99, 01-813 Warsaw, Poland

INTRODUCTION

This chapter reviews those data and hypotheses which might be pertinent to possible thyroid hormone involvement in some aspects of heart metabolism, in both physiological and pathological conditions.

THYROID HORMONE BIOSYNTHESIS, TRANSPORT IN BLOOD, AND TISSUE DISTRIBUTION

Thyroid glands synthesize and secrete 1-thyroxine (T_4), 3,5,3'-1-triiodo-thyronine (T_3), and 3,3',5'-1-triiodothyronine (reverse triiodothyronine, rT_3), but only T_4 is at present considered a principal secretory product of the thyroid. In normal humans, the total production rates for T_4, T_3, and rT_3 amount to approximately 115, 45, and 30 nmol per day, respectively, while thyroidal secretion accounts for 100, 20, and 6% respectively (Chopra *et al.*, 1978). In relative values 80% of T_3 and 94% of rT_3 are produced peripherally by intracellular enzymatic monodeiodination.

The iodide present in blood is actively transported and cellular integrity and adequate energy supply are prerequisities for normal function of the thyroid iodide pump. A ouabain-sensitive Na^+,K^+-ATPase, and a membrane carrier of phospholipid nature, are of key importance. Active transport of iodide follows Michaelis – Menten kinetics with a K_m value for human thyroid of magnitude 10^{-5} (Gluzman and Niepomiszcze, 1980). Extensive reviews on iodide transport are available elsewhere (Werner and Nauman, 1968; Medeiros-Neto, 1980).

Thyroglobulin synthesis has been described in detail (Robbins *et al.*, 1974). Oxidation of iodide is a rapid process appearing in the thyroid cell in the presence of thyroid peroxidase and hydrogen peroxide (H_2O_2). The possible sources of the H_2O_2 generating system, the nature of thyroid peroxidase, and possible mechanisms involved in iodotyrosine formation and the coupling reaction are discussed in detail by DeGroot and Niepomiszcze

(1977). Major factors in thyroglobulin proteolysis within thyroid cells include cathepsin D, reduced glutathione, and exopeptidases (Dunn *et al.*, 1980). Droplets of colloid are moved from the lumen to the cell by pinocytosis, thus permitting an interaction between thyroglobulin, lysosomes, and other enzyme-rich subcellular structures (Werner and Nauman, 1968). More than 99% of the liberated iodothyronines present in blood are bound to protein carriers and only minute amounts of T_4, T_3, and rT_3 are in free forms. Two specific carriers – thyroxine or triiodothyronine, binding globulin and thyroxine, or triiodothyronine, binding prealbumin – have been isolated and purified, and their binding properties have been described in detail (Robbins *et al.*, 1978). The concentration of the globulin in blood is about $0.1 \, mg \, l^{-1}$ in middle age, and the protein shows an age dependency, having highest concentration in early childhood and during ageing (Hesch *et al.*, 1977). Several factors, including pregnancy, starvation, liver and kidney diseases, and some drugs, influence the globulins' capacity for thyroid hormone (Moreira-Andreas *et al.*, 1980). A number of non-thyroidal pathological states, including acute stress, surgery, and myocardial infarction, markedly decrease the concentration of the prealbumin (Surks and Oppenheimer, 1964; Prince *et al.*, 1976).

Do thyroid hormones enter the intracellular pool as free hormones or bound to a particular carrier? Since the relationship of thyroid hormones bound to all protein carriers can be described in terms of multiple equilibria obeying the law of mass action (Oppenheimer and Surks, 1971), it could be suspected that binding proteins would, in part, regulate free hormone concentration. Studies relevant to this problem include those of Irvine and Simpson-Morgan (1974), Robbins *et al.* (1978), Hesch (1981), Pardridge and Mietus (1980), Pardridge (1979), Krenning *et al.* (1978), and Holm and Jacquemin (1979).

PERIPHERAL METABOLISM OF THYROID HORMONES

Thyroid hormones are peripherally metabolized through oxidative deamination, conjugation, ether-bond cleavage, and deiodination. The first three pathways account for 20–40% of T_4 and T_3 turnover in humans and lead to deactivation of hormones (Burger *et al.*, 1981). Deiodination is the most important pathway to T_4 metabolism, accounting for 60–80% of hormone turnover (Gavin *et al.*, 1977).

The reaction often called 'conversion' of T_4 or T_4-'biotransformation' (Hesch, 1981) is enzymatically catalysed and it is strongly suggested (Visser, 1978) that two enzymes are involved, both localized in the microsomal fraction. T_4-5'-deiodinase (T_4-5'-D) catalyses the formation of T_3 while T_4-5-deiodinase (T_4-5-D) leads to the formation of reverse T_3 (rT_3). The production of both iodothyronines may vary independently. However, in the majority of physiopathological states, a decrease of T_3 formation is accompanied by an increase of rT_3. The T_3 and rT_3 formed undergo further deiodination (Visser, 1978) which is sequential in its nature and leads to the formation of diiodothyronines, monoiodothyronines, and finally thyronine. The monodeiodination of T_4 is a most crucial peripheral phenomenon since there is growing evidence that T_4 might be a prohormone and T_3 possesses the strongest thyromimetic activity (Morreale de Escobar *et al.*, 1981). Oppenheimer *et al.* (1979) concluded that the biological effects in liver and kidney are due 85% to T_3 and 15% to T_4, but T_4 has little activity in the anterior pitutary (Obregon *et al.*, 1980).

The physiological role of rT_3 is unclear. In biological tests rT_3 proved to be almost inactive (Jorgensen, 1976) but was shown to be a regulatory factor limiting T_4 to T_3 conversion (Kohrle, 1981) and to accelerate oxidative deamination of T_4, and may act through high affinity nuclear binding sites for rT_3 (Smith *et al.*, 1980a; Dozin-Van Roye *et al.*, 1981). Conversion of T_4 is significantly changed in several non-thyroidal pathological states, and, among others, in acute heart diseases (Wiersinga *et al.*, 1981; Nauman *et al.*, 1982a,b).

Several regulatory factors of enzymatic T_4 monodeiodination are presently recognized, including thyroid state (Nauman *et al.*, 1979), nutritional state (Kaplan *et al.*, 1979), intracellular reduced glutathione concentration (Visser, 1978), and the pH of the intracellular medium (Kohrle, 1981); there are also tissue variations (Kaplan, 1980). The role of catecholamines in acute situations was recently stressed (Nauman *et al.*, 1980). The serum levels of iodothyronines do not necessarily reflect intracellular thyroid hormone metabolism in a particular tissue (Morreale de Escobar *et al.*, 1981).

MECHANISM OF THYROID HORMONE ACTION

Thyroid hormones regulate growth, development, and differentiation of virtually all cells. They have profound effects on protein (Tata and Widnell, 1966), lipid (Fain, 1973; Laker and Mayes, 1981), and carbohydrate metabolism (Muller and Seitz, 1980; Huang and Lardy, 1981), as well as being major factors in the regulation of oxygen consumption and thermogenesis (Ismail-Beigi *et al.*, 1979) and oxidative phosphorylation (Chen and Hoch, 1976; Evans and Hoch, 1976; Nishiki *et al.*, 1978). The majority of these diverse biological effects are a consequence of thyroid hormone interaction with putative receptors in the cell membrane, nucleus, and mitochondria. Other effects seen might have an indirect character and be due to thyroid hormone-dependent changes in the cell sensitivity of such metabolically active hormones as catecholamines (Williams and Lefkowitz, 1979; Tse *et al.*, 1980) or cortisol (Shapiro *et al.*, 1978).

Thyroid hormones can also activate some enzymes already present within the cell of an inactive state (Kaminski, 1982). The nuclear receptor for thyroid hormones was originally demonstrated by Oppenheimer *et al.* (1972) and its presence in other tissues and different species including humans was soon described (for a review see Oppenheimer *et al.*, 1973). The nuclear receptor proved to be a non-histone protein which binds to DNA and is randomly distributed in chromatin both in transcriptionally active and inactive DNA (Levy and Baxter, 1976). Hormones bound to the nuclear receptor exchange relatively rapidly with those bound to cytosolic binding proteins. However, the movement of T_3 or T_4 from the cytosol to the nucleus does not require the participation of the cytosolic receptor. The binding affinity to different iodothyronines correlated with their biological activity; the sensitivity of a given tissue is reflected by the number of receptor binding sites, and the saturation of receptor binding sites correlates, not necessarily linearly, with the intensity of the organ response (Oppenheimer and Dillman, 1978). T_3 and T_4 can be bound by different binding sites within the nucleus (Knopp and Brtko, 1981) and that the affinity of rT_3 nuclear binding can be high (Dozin-Van Roye *et al.*, 1981). The degree of nuclear occupancy of T_3 is not always sufficient to predict the cellular responses (Mariash *et al.*, 1981); several post-receptor regulatory factors might be important to determine the final end effect of hormone. The nuclear receptor shows a certain degree of autoregulation in prolonged excess or deficiency of thyroid hormone (Samuels *et al.*, 1977) and can also be rapidly regulated by catecholamines (Dung *et al.*, 1982). Therefore Oppenheimer's hypothesis (Oppenheimer *et al.*, 1979) that the thyroid hormone signal can be modulated, amplified, or attenuated within the receptor or in post-receptor events seems more and more justified. Oppenheimer *et al.* (1979) describe events that could lead to synthesis of proteins but it is impossible at present to connect them in causal relationship.

The cell machinery seems to determine final response. While in the pituitary, T_3 augments synthesis of only few proteins (Oppenheimer and Dillman, 1978; in hepatocytes, the effect of hormone is pleiotypic in its nature (Bernal and Refetoff, 1977)). The importance of mitochondria as the site of initiation of thyroid hormone action was neglected, as direct effects on oxygen consumption or structural protein synthesis required pharmacological rather than physiological doses of hormones (for a review see Werner and Nauman, 1968). In 1975, Sterling and Milch discovered specific low capacity binding sites on the inner membrane of mitochondria possessing even higher affinity for T_3 than that found within the cell nucleus. The binding properties of the mitochondrial receptor (which is a lipoprotein) for different iodothyronines reflect their biological potency, and the coupling of T_3 with hormone rapidly increases oxygen consumption and ATP formation

(Sterling *et al.*, 1980; Goglia *et al.*, 1981). Several other effects of thyroid hormone on mitochondria were also recently reported. T_4 was shown to affect mitochondrial synthesis of phosphatidylcholine (Pasquini *et al.*, 1980) as well as to modify fatty acid and phospholipid composition in the inner mitochondrial membrane (Clejan *et al.*, 1980); the resulting change in membrane fluidity could be correlated with the respiratory control ratio. A similar mechanism of thyroid control over oxidative phosphorylation was also previously demonstrated (Shaw and Hoch, 1977). Tobin *et al.* (1980) demonstrated that thyroidectomy in rats decreases the activity of α-glycerophosphate, malate–asparte, and malate–citrate shuttles known to affect high energy bond formation directly, or indirectly. Whether these effects are initiated through T_3 and T_4 coupling with the mitochondrial receptor remains to be seen.

The influence of thyroid hormones on transport of amino acids and carbohydrates across cell membranes was first reported by Adamson and Ingbar (1967) and recently confirmed. Using rat thymocytes, Segal and Ingbar (1979) demonstrated that T_3, in a dose close to physiological, accelerated glucose accumulation, and this effect could not be attenuated during profound inhibition of protein synthesis, thus excluding mediation of a nuclear-dependent mechanism. The study by Segal and Ingbar (1980) revealed the sequential character of this T_3 action. The hormone produced an immediate increase in membrane calcium accumulation, followed by calcium-dependent enhancement in cyclic AMP concentration, which in turn led to an increase of carbohydrate uptake. It was suggested (Segal and Ingbar, 1980) that this effect is mediated through high affinity, low capacity membrane binding sites, since the ability of various iodothyronines to displace T_3 from the putative receptor in the membrane correlated with their potency in stimulating amino acids or carbohydrate uptake. The majority of thyroid hormone effects are probably a consequence of their simultaneous coupling with different receptors rather than a single receptor.

THE EFFECTS OF THYROID HORMONES ON HEART

Initiation of Thyroid Hormone Action in Heart

Among the different specific receptors described so far in subcellular fractions, only the nuclear receptor isolated from rat heart possessed similar properties to those found in liver and kidney (Oppenheimer *et al.*, 1973, 1974). The nuclear receptor was also demonstrated in dog heart and it was shown that approximately 50% of the binding sites are occupied by T_3 under physiological conditions (Nauman *et al.*, 1976). Although ^{125}I-labelled T_3 was found to be present in other subcellular fractions of dog heart

(Nauman *et al.*, 1976), specificity of binding was not demonstrated. There is growing evidence that besides coupling with specific receptors, thyroid hormones might also initiate the metabolic response indirectly by augmentation of tissue responsivenes to catecholamines, and that such a mode of action might be of special importance in heart.

The Thyroid Hormone–Catecholamine Interrelationship in Heart

It is well established that several manifestations of hyperthyroidism, including hypermetabolism, tachycardia, and the altered electrophysiological and contractile response, are similar to those seen in sympathetic hyperactivity. However, no significant effects of thyroid hormone excess or deficiency on the release or peripheral metabolism of catecholamines could be demonstrated (Coulombe, 1977). Scarpace and Abrass (1981) demonstrated that excess of thyroid hormone increases the number of beta-adrenergic receptors and decreases the number of alpha-adrenergic receptors (Kunos, 1977; Williams and Lefkowitz, 1979). The affinity of the beta-receptors was not affected (Tse *et al.*, 1980), whereas the affinity of alpha-receptors to catecholamines was decreased (Williams and Lefkowitz, 1979).

Thyroid hormone deficiency produced opposite effects, increasing the number of alpha-adrenergic receptors and decreasing the number of beta-receptors (Williams and Lefkowitz, 1979). Kunos (1977) suggested that thyroid hormone might mediate an allosteric transition between two forms of a single adrenergic receptor, but this hypothesis could not be supported by any firm data. Potentation of beta-adrenergic influences can also be produced by altering adenylate cyclase or the activity of intracellular processes which are stimulated by catecholamines. Basal myocardial adenylate cyclase activity was found to be high in hypotyhroidism (Brockhuysen and Ghislain, 1972) and unaltered in hyperthyroidism (McNeill *et al.*, 1969), while T_4 in pharmacological and T_3 in supraphysiological doses increased adenylate cyclase activity in isolated heart membranes (Adler *et al.*, 1976). The magnitude of the adenylate cyclase response to isoproterenol stimulation and the resultant cyclic AMP (cAMP) formation were augmented by thyroid hormone in the heart in the presence of exogenous ATP (Tse *et al.*, 1980).

On the other hand, in minced heart obtained from hyperthyroid rats, the formation of cAMP either in the presence or absence of isoproterenol was diminished, as well as subsequent activation of cAMP-dependent protein kinase (Tse *et al.*, 1980); these unexpected effects were most probably due to a significantly depressed level of endogenous ATP observed by these investigators. As cAMP concentration depends not only on the accessibility of substrate (ATP) and adenylate cyclase activity, but also on the activity of phosphodiesterase, the possible thyroid hormone influence on this enzyme was also investigated. Levey and Epstein (1968) found that regardless of thyroid state, phosphodiesterase activity was unaffected.

Contrary to this, Tse *et al.* (1980) demonstrated that prolonged administration of T_4 decreases the activity of the enzyme in a particulate fraction and that this alteration disappeared upon regression of hyperthyroidism. Tse *et al.* (1980) showed that an excess of thyroid hormone depresses cyclic GMP (cGMP) and, in consequence, decreases cGMP-dependent kinase. Finally it was suggested that catecholamine supersensitivity of the heart in hyperthyroidism can be, at least in part, a result of an enhanced expression of overall cAMP effects, with depressed expression of overall cGMP effects. Catecholamine supersensitivity of the heart might be further enhanced by the influence of thyroid hormone on the parasympathetic nervous system. It has been shown that an excess of thyroid hormone decreases the number of cholinergic receptors (Sharma and Banerjee, 1977) and desensitizes the heart to the action of acetylcholine (Frazer and Hess, 1969). Extensive reviews on different aspects of the thyroid hormone–catecholamine interaction (Fein, 1981) and the importance of cardiac beta-adrenergic receptors (Kaumann *et al.*, 1978) are available.

Direct Effects of Thyroid Hormones on Myocardial Contractility

Positive inotropic effects of thyroid hormones have been demonstrated in intact experimental animals (Strauer and Schulze, 1976) and in humans by non-invasive evaluation (Chakravarty *et al.*, 1978; Cohen *et al.*, 1981). Positive chronotropic effects were also documented when thyroid hormones were added to myocardial cells in tissue culture (Schwartz and Gordon, 1975) and by electrocardiographic voltage changes in humans with disturbed thyroid state (Wong *et al.*, 1979). The pre-ejection period is shortened in hyperthyroidism and prolonged in hypothyroidism (Chakraarty *et al.*, 1978). The left ventricular ejection period gave contradictory results; no significant changes were reported in one study (Chakravarty *et al.*, 1978) while others showed changes similar to those of the pre-ejection period. The latter regressed as hypothyroidism returned to euthyroidism due to replacement therapy (Chakravarty *et al.*, 1978), correlating well with serum levels of T_3, T_4, and TSH. The velocity of circumferential fibre shortening was increased in hyperthyroidism and decreased in hypothyroidism, the values correlating with serum T_3 (Cohen *et al.*, 1981). The mechanism of the direct inotopic effects of thyroid hormone was extensively studied (for a review see Morkin, 1979) and is mostly dependent on altered cardiac myosin ATPase activity or the transcription of additional isozymes. In hypothyroidism, or after hypophysectomy in rats, Ca^{++}- or Mg^{++}-stimulated myosin ATPase activity was decreased and could be restored by T_3 administration but not by growth hormone.

In contrast an excess of thyroid hormone increases myosin ATPase activity. Since thyroid hormones rapidly augment contractile performance it was suggested (Fink *et al.*, 1977) that independent of the known T_3 effect on the nucleus (gene expression and *de novo* synthesis of myosin and isozymes) the hormone might increase or decrease enzyme activity through allosteric effects, leading to a modification of SH_1-thiols which are located at or near the active site of myosin ATPase. The possibility of conformational changes around thiol groups of the enzyme was further supported by Banerjee and Morkin (1977). The hypothesis that thyroid hormone stimulates *de novo* synthesis of myosin ATPase was experimentally confirmed. It was also pointed out that an excess of thyroid hormone leads to the production of more active isozymes. An abnormality of the amino acid composition of myosin from thyrotoxic heart was presented by Thyrum *et al.* (1970) but could not be confirmed by others (Banerjee *et al.*, 1976). The problem was re-examined by using more accurate methods (Fink and Morkin, 1977), showing that augmented contractile properties of the heart in hyperthyroidism can be partly explained by the appearance of new myosin species having greater actin-activated ATPase activity. As the inotropic state of the heart might also be dependent on alterations in myofibrillar protein phosphorylation, the effects of thyroid hormones on the covalent phosphate content of troponin-I and of the P-light chain of myosin was recently studied (Litten *et al.*, 1981). This study revealed, however, that the increased myofibrillar ATPase of thyrotoxic myofibrils occurred with no changes in covalent phosphorylation of either troponin-I or myosin P-light chain. Litten *et al.* (1981) have also shown that the calcium sensitivities of the myofibrillar ATPase from normal and thyrotoxic myofibrils are similar.

As phosphocreatine is an essential high energy donor for muscle contraction, the effect of thyroid hormone on creatine phosphokinase (CPK) activity was also investigated. Reduced levels of total serum CPK in hyperthyroidism and elevated levels in hypothyroidism were reported (Smith, 1976) but a direct effect of thyroid state upon the activity of the enzyme in heart could not be presented.

Direct Effects of Thyroid Hormone on Na^+,K^+-dependent ATPase in Heart

The maintainance by the Na^+ pump of transmembrane gradients for Na^+ and K^+ is especially important for heart muscle that depolarizes in order to propagate or produce an action potential. The mechanism for setting and maintaining the resting membrane potential is believed to reside in part in the plasma membrane enzyme complex, Na^+,K^+-ATPase.

It has been postulated for a long time (Asano *et al.*, 1976) that increased energy utilization by the Na^+ pump mediates the majority of thyroid hormone-induced increase in the resting oxygen consumption in muscles. However, such a degree of thermogenic effect was recently questioned (Biron *et al.*, 1979). Administration of a physiological dose of T_3 to hypothyroid rats (Philipson and Edelman, 1977) lowered cardiac Na^+ and increased cardiac K^+, and this effect correlated with Na^+,K^+-ATPase activity. The fact that T_3 does not alter the K_m for ATP and the $K_{1/2}$ for Na^+ and K^+ excludes both the formation of Na^+,K^+-ATPase isozymes and conformational modification of the enzyme (Phillipson and Edelman, 1977). Thus, under physiological conditions, T_3 induces the synthesis of Na^+ transport enzymes with the same properties as those present in the hypothyroid state.

The effect of T_3 on this enzyme is nuclear receptor mediated, as it was shown that the degree of response correlates with the affinity of thyroid hormones and their analogues to receptor binding sites (Phillipson and Edelman, 1977). The problem whether Na^+,K^+-ATPase is solely responsible for the transmembrane gradient of Na^+ and K^+ was recently re-evaluated (Smith *et al.*, 1980b) and the effect of T_3 in heart confirmed. However, in other muscles the Na^+–K^+ transmembrane gradient was not tightly coupled to thyroid hormone-dependent Na^+,K^+-ATPase, but also to a significant increase in non-plasma Ca^{++}. Although calcium plays a critical role in catalysing muscle contraction, the effect of thyroid hormone on calcium cell transport was demonstrated only in hepatocytes (Wallach *et al.*, 1972). Since delivery of Ca^{++} to the appropriate intracellular site is related to the flux of Na^+ into and out of the muscle cell (Van Winkle and Schwartz, 1976), and since the thyroid hormone control of Na^+ pump number cannot be questioned, indirect control of intracellular calcium metabolism should be considered. The fact that the number of calcium channels might be reflected by the number of beta-adrenergic receptors (Reuter, 1974) further stresses such indirect thyroid hormone action.

Direct Effects of Thyroid Hormone on Oxidative Phosphorylation in Heart

The possible thyroid hormone regulation of the energy conservation system in mitochondria was suggested some time ago (for a review see Werner and Nauman, 1968) and is still a subject of speculation and controversy (Chen and Hoch, 1976.) Evaluation of oxidative phosphorylation in the heart of hypothyroid rats revealed (Nishiki *et al.*, 1978) a lower content of both cytochromes and mitochondrial proteins per wet weight of heart, while in hyperthyroidism both contents were increased.

The rapid effect of thyroid hormone in mitochondrial protein synthesis was previously reported (Buchanann *et al.*, 1971) and recently confirmed (Nelson *et al.*, 1980); T_3 significantly augmented translation on mitochondrial ribosomes, leading to the formation of four major mitochondrially translated peptides. At the same time it had little or no effect on the general synthesis of cytoplasmically translated mitochondrial proteins (Nelson *et al.*, 1980). As cytochromes and mitochondrial protein content decreased in hypothyroidism and increased in hyperthyroidism the ratio of cytochrome *c* to cytochrome aa_3 remained unchanged (Nishiki *et al.*, 1978). From the free energy relationship between the mitochondrial redox reaction and ATP synthesis it could be calculated that the two first sites of oxidative phosphorylation remain at near equilibrium both in hypothyroidism and hyperthyroidism, thus excluding the possible uncoupling action of thyroid hormone (Nishiki *et al.*, 1978) in heart mitochondria. There are many data pointing out that regulation of mitochondrial oxidative phosphorylation is a consequence of the interplay of three variables: mitochondrial $NAD^+/NADH$, cytosolic ATP/ADP, P_i, and oxidation–reduction turnover for cytochrome oxidase or cytochrome *c* (Wilson *et al.*, 1977). The transition from the hypothyroid state to the hyperthyroid state and the increased demand for ATP in heart is met by changes in all metabolic parameters. The amount of enzymes forming the respiratory chain is increased, the cytosolic ATP/ADP–P_i is lowered and activation of metabolic pathways involved in the intramitochondrial rate of NADH production is increased in hyperthyroidism (Nishiki *et al.*, 1978); the time course of these effects is uncertain.

A different mechanism of thyroid hormone regulation of oxidative phosphorylation was stressed by Chen and Hoch (1976). As these authors were unable to find changes in cytochrome content of the inner membrane vesicles of mitochondria obtained from normal, hypothyroid, and T_4-injected hypothyroid rats, the effect of thyroid hormone on alteration of unsaturated mitochondrial membrane fatty acids was strongly pointed out. Chen and Hoch (1976) postulated that acceleration in oxidative phosphorylation is a consequence of membrane modification, an activation of microsomal enzymes which modifies mitochondrial unsaturated fatty acyl and cholesterol content, and activation of the nuclear receptor which promotes synthesis of respiratory assemblies. A decrease of efficiency of oxidative phosphorylation seen in hypothyroidism was also proposed to be a result of increased activity of mitochondrial transhydrogenase (Evans and Hoch, 1976). In consequence, available energy was redistributed, favouring transhydrogenation over phosphorylation.

These findings led to the suggestion that thyroid state controls the use rather than the supply of energy potential. As the latter mechanisms and hypotheses came from experiments with liver mitochondria, their relevance for heart must be carefully evaluated. It seems obvious that heart function and metabolism is also affected by thyroid hormone-mediated changes in whole body metabolism.

THYROID HORMONE METABOLISM AND ACTION IN HEART DISEASE

Reduced serum T_3, augmented serum rT_3 levels, and unchanged serum T_4 and TSH constitutes the 'low T_3 syndrome' (Nauman *et al.*, 1974). 'Low T_3 syndrome' then became the target for intensive studies (for reviews see Hesch, 1981, and Werner, 1981). The low T_3 syndrome was described in myocarditis, cardiomyopathy, cardiac cachexia, and congestive cardiac failure (Bermudes *et al.*, 1975), in compensated cardiac insufficiency (Burger, 1976), and in subacute bacerial endocarditis (Chopra *et al.*, 1979). It was suggested (Westergren *et al.*, 1977), that 'low T_3 syndrome' might reflect a favourable adaptive response. Such an assumption seemed reasonable in chronic disease but it can hardly be accepted for acute myocardial infarction. The degree of fall in serum T_3 was found to correlate with the severity of the clinical course of infarction (Nauman *et al.*, 1974) and with the severity and infarct size (Wiersinga *et al.*, 1981), and both total serum T_3 and free T_3 decreased to almost undetectable levels prior to the patient's death (Nauman *et al.*, 1979). Moreover, the majority of patients with significantly decreased T_3 demonstrated several clinical symptoms seen in hyperthyroidism, and had prolonged negative nitrogen balance. Several questions seemed important:

(1) Which mechanisms are mainly responsible for low T_3 syndrome in acute myocardial infarction?

(2) Is decreased serum T_3 accompanied by low T_3 concentration in intracellular compartments?

(3) Is the intracellular compartmentalization of T_3 changed and what proportion of the nuclear receptor binding sites are occupied?

(4) Are receptor properties changed by the general humoral and metabolic responses seen in acute myocardial infarction?

(5) Are the effects of thyroid hormone augmented or diminished?

As could be expected, dogs with experimental myocardial infarction demonstrated a typical fall in serum T_3 (Nauman *et al.*, 1975); when T_4 monodeiodination was studied in heart and liver homogenates, T_3 production rate was diminished in experimental as compared with control dogs, but to a lesser degree than could be evaluated from serum T_3 values. As it was clearly shown (Ceremużyński *et al.*, 1978) that the majority of humoral, metabolic, and ultrastructural changes in heart muscle seen in experimental myocardial infarction can be produced by infusion of adrenaline to healthy dogs, the effect of such infusions on monodeiodination of T_4 in liver and heart homogenates were studied (Nauman *et al.*, 1980).

This study revealed that adrenaline infused *in vivo* or added *in vitro* significantly diminished conversion of T_4 to T_3 and has only a slight effect on conversion of T_4 to rT_3. Chopra (1976) and Pittman *et al.* (1979) concluded that while the decreased serum level of T_3 is caused by diminished extra-thyroidal conversion of T_4 to T_3, the increased serum rT_3 values are due to reduced metabolic clearance rate of rT_3, rather than to an increased conversion rate of T_4 to rT_3. Most recently, the effect of adrenaline on T_4 conversion was further examined by Nauman *et al.* (1982a) who showed that the 'low T_3 syndrome' produced in adrenaline-treated animals was a consequence of diminished activity of T_4-5'-deiodinase. Adrenaline had no effect on the cytosolic coenzyme for this reaction. Insulin and cortisol are both also involved in the humoural changes evoked by acute myocardial infarction (Ceremużyński, 1981) and these hormones also affect T_4 to T_3 conversion (for references see Werner, 1981). The diminished T_3 peripheral production seen in acute myocardial infarction could therefore be a result of the simultaneous action of adrenaline, diminished insulin, and augmented cortisol, although it is suggested that the adrenergic response is a main factor in the rapid decrease of T_3, as suggested by the high negative correlation between adrenaline and T_3 in patients with severe myocardial infarction (Ceremużyński *et al.*, 1978).

To answer questions (2) and (3), another series of experiments was conducted (Nauman *et al.*, 1976). Both experimental and control animals were injected intravenously with ^{125}I-labelled T_3 of high specific activity and were killed 30 min later. The hearts and livers were rapidly removed and the radioactivity per milligram of wet weight in the homogenates measured. Radioactivity per milligram of protein was also estimated in mitochondrial, cytosolic, and nuclear fractions, being in the last case expressed as counts per minute per milligram of DNA. To find whether radioactivity is due to T_3 or iodide, each cellular subfraction was extracted and chromatographed. The validity of the chromatographic studies were later re-examined using an immunoprecipitation procedure with highly specific T_3 antiserum. It was shown that both heart and liver homogenates from dogs with myocardial infarction have more ^{125}I-labelled T_3 than homogenates from controls. It was also demonstrated that while in controls the majority of labelled T_3 was localized in the cytosol fraction and the cytosol:nucleus radioactivity ratio was close to 4, in myocardial infarction this ratio was reversed and was close to 0.5. Finally, while in controls about 50% of nuclear receptor binding sites were occupied, in infarct dogs or dogs infused with adrenaline occupancy of heart nuclear receptors was increased by approximately 10% (while in liver by about 20%). As serum T_3 was low, these highly unexpected results can be explained by several findings. Hiller (1968) showed that lipids augment significantly the uptake of T_4 by the perfused rat heart. Since blood non-esterified fatty acid levels in the blood of dogs with experimental infarction was found to be very high (Wasilewska-Dziubińska *et al.*, 1981) it is possible to suggest that not only T_4 but also T_3 uptake by the heart could be augmented.

T_3 resin uptake reflecting thyroid hormone binding globulin was normal in acute myocardial infarction (Farber *et al.*, 1981), but a decrease of the binding prealbumin in acute myocardial infarction was reported (Berstein and Oppenheimer, 1966). As already pointed out in this chapter, unchanged binding globulin and diminished binding prealbumin can lead to a redistribution of T_3 and T_4 to albumin. Since the T_3 and T_4–albumin complex is of significance for the transport of thyroid hormone to some tissues (Pardridge and Mietus, 1980), it can be suggested that this mechanism plays at least some role in increased uptake of T_3 in liver in experimental infarction. Finally, as increased uptake of ^{125}I-labelled T_3 with low serum T_3 is a typical 'uphill' phenomenon, active T_3 transport must be involved, and the presence of high affinity, low capacity membrane binding sites for T_3 was recently reported (Krenning *et al.*, 1978). At present, all these arguments are speculative and more firm data must be obtained to explain the T_3 tissue uptake and intracellular hormone distribution in experimental and clinical myocardial infarction.

There are only fragmentary and indirect data available which might in part answer questions (4) and (5). Adrenaline was found to increase the affinity of nuclear receptors to T_3 in a dose-dependent manner in rat liver (Dung *et al.*, 1982) and the blood adrenaline level is high both in clinical and experimental infarction (Valori *et al.*, 1967; Ceremużyński, 1981). Fasting in obese humans led to both a decrease of serum T_3 and an increase of maximal binding capacity of nuclear receptors in mononuclear blood cells (Wartofsky *et al.*, 1981). In contrast, fasting in diabetic patients decreases both the serum T_3 level and the maximal binding capacity of nuclear receptors in blood cells (Wartofsky *et al.*, 1981). As the results of these studies do not give any direct answer to the question whether heart nuclear receptor properties are changed in infarction, they are compatible with the assumption that it can be so. The activity of cytosolic malic enzymes and mitochondrial α-glycerophosphate dehydrogenase is a generally recognized response to T_3 and hormone nuclear receptor occupancy (Oppenheimer *et al.*, 1979). It was demonstrated (Nauman *et al.*, 1982b) that in the liver of rats implanted with adrenaline tablets the activities of both enzymes were augmented in a dose-dependent manner.

To summarize, it is suggested that thyroid hormone metabolism is deeply disturbed in acute myocardial infarction and that these disturbances might be either favourable or unfavourable for the course of disease. Since there is good evidence that thyroid hormone metabolism is triggered by adrenaline, the degree of change in the intracellular metabolism of thyroid hormone might depend on adrenaline augmentation. If adrenaline is only moderately increased, as seen in infarction with a moderate course and in chronic heart diseases, the changes produced in the peripheral metabolism of thyroid hormones are limited to relatively small inhibition of T_4-5′-deiodinase activity, with a resultant decrease in the level of T_3 in serum. The effect of a low serum T_3 level is followed by diminished saturation of receptor binding sites and decreased cell metabolism and oxygen consumption. Contrariwise, a high rise of adrenaline, and possibly other catecholamines, although further decreasing T_4-5′-deiodinase activity, at the same time produces a cascade of unfavourable responses. Tissue uptake of thyroid hormones becomes increased due to 'uphill' transport, increased affinity of the receptor binding sites to T_3 and possibly to T_4, changed hormone intracellular distribution, and increased receptor occupancy. These events lead to cellular hypermetabolism and increased oxygen consumption. As one of the effects of cellular hyperthroidism is an increased adrenergic responsiveness, thyroid hormones can potentiate indirectly those mechanisms which lead in turn to cellular superexpression of thyroid hormone. It is once more stressed that this hypothesis of cellular hyperthyroidism in severe acute myocardial infarction is based on circumstantial evidence and has a speculatory character. Nevertheless, the symptoms seen in severe infarction resemble more those observed in a hypermetabolic than a hypometabolic state. Although a deleterious influence of hypothroidism on experimental infarction was recently reported (Karlsberg *et al.*, 1981), the possibility that the response to severe infarction is due to overexpressed hypometabolism is unlikely. It should be remembered that in cases where the serum T_3 level was almost undetectable, T_4 was normal. About 15% of thyroid hormone metabolic action is produced by T_4 (Oppenheimer *et al.*, 1979). It seems most probable that, in the cellular absence of T_3, much more T_4 could couple with putative receptors and initiate a metabolic response.

REFERENCES

Adamson, L. F., and Ingbar, S. H. (1967). Some properties of the stimulatory effect of thyroid hormones on amino-acid transport by embryonic chick bone. *Endocrinology*, **81**, 1372–1378.

Adler, G., Czarnocka, B., and Nauman, J. (1976). Thyroid hormones stimulation of adenyl-cyclase activity in rat heart. In *Proceedings of the 20th Conference of the Polish Thyroid Association*, Warsaw, pp. 9–10.

Asano, Y., Liverman, I. A., and Edelman, I. S. (1976). Thyroid thermogenesis. Relationship between Na^+-dependent respiration and Na^+,K^+-ATPase activity in rat skeletal muscle. *J. Clin. Invest.*, **57**, 368–379.

Banerjee, S. K., and Morkin, E. (1977). Actin-activated adenosine-triphosphatase activity of native and N-ethylmaleimide-modified cardiac myosin from normal and thyrotoxic rabbits. *Clin. Res.*, **41**, 630–634.

Banerjee, S. K., Flink, I. L., and Morkin, E. (1976). Enzymatic properties of native and N-ethylmaleimide-modified cardiac myosine from normal and thyrotoxic rabbits. *Circulation Res.*, **39**, 319–326.

Bermudes, F., Surks, M. I., and Oppenheimer, J. H. (1975). High incidence of decreased serum triiodothyronine concentration in patients with non-thyroidal disease. *J. Clin. Endocrinol. Metab.*, **41**, 27–40.

Bernal, J., and Refetoff, S. (1977). The action of thyroid hormones. *Clin. Endocrinol.*, **6**, 227–249.

Berstein, G., and Oppenheimer, J. H. (1966). Factors influencing the concentration of free and total thyroxine in patients with non-thyroidal disease. *J. Clin. Endocrinol. Metab.*, **26**, 227–249.

Biron, R., Burger, A., Chinet, A., Clausen, T., and Dubois-Ferriere, R. (1979). Thyroid hormones and the energetics of active sodium–potassium transport in mammalian skeletal muscles. *J. Physiol. (Lond.)*, **297**, 47–60.

Brockhuyesen, J., and Ghislain, M. (1972). Increased heart adenyl-cyclase in the hypothyroid rat. *Biochem. Pharmacol.*, **21**, 1493–1497.

Buchanan, J. L., Primack, M. P., and Tapley, D. F. (1971). Effect of inhibition of mitochondrial protein synthesis *in vitro* upon thyroxine stimulation of oxygen consumption. *Endocrinology*, **89**, 534–537.

Burger, A., Nicod, P., Suter, P., Valloton, M. B., Vagenakis, A., and Braverman, L. E. (1976). Reduced activity of thyroid hormones levels in acute illness. *Lancet, i*, 653–655.

Burger, A., Merhelbach, U., and Burgi, U. (1981). Pathways of thyroxine metabolism excluding monodeiodination. In *The Low T3 Syndrome* (R. D. Hesch, ed.), Academic Press, London, pp. 49–54.

Ceremużyński, L., Herbaczyńska-Cedro, K., Broniszewska-Adelt, B., Nauman, J., Nauman, A., Woźniewicz, B., and Ławecki, J. (1978). Evidence for detrimental effects of adrenaline infused to healthy dogs in doses imitating spontaneous secretion after coronary occlusion. *Cardiovasc. Res.*, **12**, 179–189.

Ceremużyński, L. (1981). Hormonal and metabolic reactions evoked by acute myocardial infarctions. *Circulation Res.*, **48**, 767–776.

Chakravarty, J., Guansing, A. R., Chakravarty, S., and Hughes, C. V. (1978). Systolic time intervals (STI) as indicators of myocardial thyroid hormone effect. *Acta Endocrinol.*, **87**, 507–515.

Chen, D. J., and Hoch, F. L. (1976). Mitochondrial inner membrane in hypothyroidism. *Arch. Biochem. Biophys.*, **172**, 741–744.

Chopra, I. J. (1976). An assessment of daily production and significance of thyroidal secretion of 3,3′,5′-triiododothyronine (rT3) in man. *J. Clin. Invest.*, **58**, 32–40.

Chopra, I. J., Solomon, D. H., Chopra, U., Wu, S. Y., Fisher, D. A., and Nakamura, Y. (1978). Pathways of metabolism of thyroid hormones. *Rec. Prog. Horm. Res.*, **34**, 521–567.

Chopra, I. J., Chopra, U., Smith, S. R., Reza, M., and Solomon, D. H. (1979). Misleadingly low free thyroxine index and usefulness of reverse triiodothyronine measurement in non-thyroidal illnesses. *Ann. Intern. Med.*, **90**, 905–909.

Clejan, S., Collipp, P. J., and Maddaiah, V. T. (1980). Hormones and liver mitochondria: influence of growth hormone, thyroxine, testosterone, and insulin on thermotropic effects of respiration and fatty acid composition of membranes. *Arch. Biochem. Biophys.*, **203**, 744–752.

Cohen, M. V., Schulman, J. C., Spenillo, A., and Surks, M. J. (1981). Effects of thyroid hormone on left ventricular function in patients treated for thyrotoxicosis. *Amer. J. Cardiol.*, **48**, 33–38.

Coulombe, P., Dussault, J. H., and Walker, P. (1977). Catecholamine metabolism in thyroid disease. II. Norepinephrine secretion rate in hyperthyroidism and hypothyroidism. *J. Clin. Endocrinol. Metab.*, **44**, 1185–1189.

DeGroot, L. J., and Niepomnieszcze, H. (1977). Biosynthesis of thyroid hormone: basic and clinical aspects. *Metabolism*, **26**, 665–718.

Dozin-Van Roye, B., Renotte, B., Place, M., De Nayer, Ph. (1981). Nuclear binding of T3 and T4 interaction with rT3: evidence for an additional binding site for thyroid hormone. In *The Low T3 Syndrome* (R. D. Hesch, ed.), Academic Press, London, pp. 101–104.

Dung, N. T., Nauman, J., and Porta, J. (1982). Dose- and time-dependent effect of epinephrine on affinity and maximal binding capacity of T3 nuclear receptor in rat liver. *Endokrynologia Polska*, in press.

Dunn, A. D., Dunn, J. T., and Heppner, D. G. (1980). The role of cathepsin D in the proteolysis of thyroglobulin. In *Thyroid Research*, Vol. VIII (J. R. Stockigt and S. Nagataki, eds), Australian Academy of Sciences, Canberra, pp. 164–167.

Evans, T. C., and Hoch, F. L. (1976). Energy-linked reactions in hypothyroid rat liver submitochondrial vesicles. *Biochem. Biophys. Res. Commun.*, **69**, 635–640.

Faber, J., Kirkeegaard, C., Lubholtz, J. B., Sierback-Nielsen, K., and Friis, T. (1980). Variation in serum T3, rT3, 3,3'-diiodothyronine and 3',5'-diiodothyronine induced by acute myocardial infarction and propranolol. *Acta Endocrinol.*, **94**, 341–345.

Fain, J. N. (1973). Aspects of drug and hormone action on adipose tissue. *Pharmacol. Rev.*, **25**, 67–118.

Fein, G. N. (1981). Catecholamine–thyroid hormone interaction in liver and adipose tissue. *Life Sci.*, **28**, 1745–1754.

Fink, I. L., and Morkin, E. (1977). Evidence for a new cardiac myosin species in thyrotoxic rabbits. *FEBS Lett.*, **81**, 391–394.

Fink, I. L., Morkin, E., and Elzinga, M. (1977). Cyanogen bromide peptide from bovine cardiac myosin containing two essential thiols. Evidence for sequence homology with skeletal myosin in the region of the active site. *FEBS Lett.*, **84**, 261–265.

Frazer, A., and Hess, M. E. (1969). Parasympathetic response in hypertyroid rats. *J. Pharmacol. Exp. Ther.*, **170**, 1–8.

Gavin, L., Casttle, J., McMahon, F., Martin, P., Hammond, M., and Cavallieri, R. R. (1977). Extrathyroidal conversion of thyroxine to 3,3',5'-triiodothyronine and 3,5,3'-triiodothyronine in humans. *J. Clin. Endocrin. Metab.*, **44**, 733–742.

Gluzman, B. E., and Niepomniszcze, H. (1980). Kinetics of the iodide trapping mechanism in normal and pathological human thyroid slices. In *Thyroid Research*, Vol. VIII (J. R. Stockigt and S. Nagataki, eds), Australian Academy of Sciences, Canberra, pp. 109–112.

Goglia, F., Torresani, J., Bugli, P., Barletta, A., and Levirini, G. (1981). *In vitro* binding of triiodothyronine to rat liver mitochondria. *Pflügers Arch. Europ. J. Physiol.*, **390**, 120–124.

Goslings, B., Schwartz, H. L., Dillman, W. H., Surks, M. I., and Oppenheimer, J. H. (1976). Comparison of the metabolism and the distribution of triiodothyronine and triiodothyroacetic acid in the rat. *Endocrinology*, **98**, 666–675.

Hesch, R. D. (1981). Conversion of thyroxine: the central process for thyroid hormone action. In *The Low T3 Syndrome* (R. D. Hesch, ed.), Academic Press, London, pp. 1–12.

Hesch, R. D., Gatz, J., and Juppner, H. (1977). TBG dependency of age-related variation of thyroxine and triiodothyronine. *Hormone Metab. Res.*, **9**, 141–146.

Hillier, A. P. (1968). The effect of fatty acid on the uptake of thyroxine by the perfused rat heart. *J. Physiol. (Lond.)*, **199**, 169–175.

Holm, A. G., and Jacquemin, C. (1979). Membrane transport of triiodothyronine by human red cell ghosts. *Biochem. Biophys. Res. Commun.*, **89**, 1006–1017.

Huang, M. T., and Lardy, H. A. (1981). Effects of thyroid states on the Cori cycle, glucose–alanine cycle and futile cycling of glucose metabolism in rats. *Arch. Biochem. Biophys.*, **209**, 41–51.

Irvine, C. H. G., and Simpson-Morgan, M. W. (1974). Relative rates of transcapillary movement of free thyroxine, protein-bound thyroxine, thyroxine-binding proteins and albumin. *J. Clin. Invest.*, **54**, 156–164.

Ismail-Beigi, F., Bisell, D. M., and Edelman, I. S. (1979). Thyroid thermogenesis in adult rat hepatocytes in primary monolayer culture. *J. Gen. Physiol.*, **73**, 369–383.

Jorgensen, E. C. (1976). Structure–activity relation of thyroxine analogs. *Pharmacol. Ther.*, **2**, 661–682.

Kamiński, T., Nauman, J., and Hesch, R. D. (1982). The effect of thyroid hormones on gluconeogenesis in isolated rat liver cells. *Life Sci.*, in press.

Kaplan, M. M., Tatro, J. B., Breibart, R., and Larsen, R. P. (1979). Comparison of thyroxine and 3,3',5'-triiodothyronine metabolism in rat kidney and liver homogenates. *Metabolism*, **28**, 1139–1148.

Kaplan, M. M. (1980). Thyroxine 5'-monodeiodination in rat pituitary homogenates. *Endocrinology*, **106**, 567–576.

Karlsberg, R. P., Friscia, D. A., Aronow, W. S., and Sekhorn, S. S. (1981). Deleterious influence of hypothyroidism on evolving myocardial infarction in conscious dogs. *J. Clin. Invest.*, **67**, 1024–1034.

Kaumann, A. J., Birnbaumer, L., and Wittmann, R. (1978). Heart beta-adrenoceptors. In *Receptors and Hormone Action*, Vol. III (L. Birnbaumer and B. O'Malley, eds), Academic Press, New York, pp. 134–175.

Knopp, J., and Brtko, K. (1981). Effects of thiol blocking agents on the binding of T3 and T4 in rat liver nuclear extract. *Acta Endocrinol.*, **98**, 68–72.

Kohrle, J. (1981). Biochemistry of iodothyronine deiodination. Importance of pH and regulatory iodothyronines. In *The Low T3 Syndrome* (R. D. Hesch, ed.), Academic Press, London, pp. 27–40.

Krenning, E. P., Docter, R., Bernard, F., Visser, T. J., and Hennemann, G. (1978). Active transport of triiodothyronine into isolated rat liver cells. *FEBS Lett.*, **91**, 113–116.

Kunos, G. (1977). Thyroid hormone-dependent interconversion of myocardial alpha and beta adrenoceptors in the rat. *Brit. J. Pharmacol.*, **59**, 177–189.

Laker, M. E., and Mayes, P. A. (1981). Effect of hyperthyroidism and hypothyroidism on lipid and carbohydrate metabolism of the perfused rat liver. *Biochem. J.*, **196**, 247–255.

Levy, B., and Baxter, J. D. (1976). Distribution of thyroid and glucocorticoid hormorne receptors in transcriptionally active and inactive chromatin. *Biochem. Biophys. Res. Commun.*, **68**, 1045–1051.

Levey, G. S., and Epstein, S. E. (1968). Activation of cardiac adenyl-cyclase by thyroid hormone. *Biochem. Biophys. Res. Commun.*, **33**, 990–996.

Litten, R. Z., Martin, B. J., Hove, E. R., Alpert, N. R., and Solaro, R. J. (1981). Phosphorylation and adenosine triphosphatase activity of myofibrils from thyrotoxic rabbit hearts. *Circulation Res.*, **48**, 498–501.

MacLeod, J. M., and Baxter, J. D. (1976). Chromatin receptors for thyroid hormones: interaction of solubilized proteins with DNA. *J. Biol. Chem.*, **251**, 3780–3787.

Mariash, C. N., Kaiser, F. E., and Oppenheimer, J. H. (1981). Comparison of the response characteristics of four lipogenic enzymes to triiodothyronine administration. Evidence for variable degrees of amplification of the nuclear signal. *Endocrinology*, **106**, 22–27.

McNeill, J. H., Muschek, L. D., and Brody, T. M. (1969). The effect of triiodothyronine on cyclic AMP phosphorylase, and adenyl-cyclase in rat heart. *Canad. J. Physiol. Pharmacol.*, **47**, 913–916.

Medeiros-Neto, H. (1980). Inherited disorders of intrathyroidal metabolism. In *Thyroid Research*, Vol. VIII (J. R. Stockigt and S. Nagataki, eds.), Australian Academy of Sciences, Canberra, pp. 101–109.

Moreira-Andreas, M. D., Black, E. G., Ramsden, D. B., and Hoffenberg, R. (1980).

The effects of caloric restriction on serum thyroid hormone binding proteins and free hromones in obese patients. *Clin. Endocrinol.*, **12**, 249–257.

Morkin, E. (1979). Stimulation of cardiac myosin adenosine triphosphatase in thyrotoxicosis. *Circulation Res.*, **44**, 1–7.

Morreale de Escobar, G., Obregon, M. J., and Escobar del Rey, F. (1981). Relative *in vivo* activities of iodothyronines. In *The Low T3 Syndrome* (R. D. Hesch, ed.), Academic Press, London, pp. 55–70.

Muller, M. J., and Seitz, H. J. (1980). Rapid and direct stimulation of hepatic gluconeogenesis by triiodothyronone in the isolated perfused rat liver. *Life Sci.*, **27**, 827–835.

Nauman, A., Lewartowski, B., Nauman, J., Kamiński, T., Michałowski, J., and Sędek, G. (1975). Thyroid hormones in experimental myocardial infarction in dog. *Europ. J. Clin. Invest.*, **5**, 338 (Abstr.).

Nauman, A., Kamiński, T., and Herbaczyńska-Cedro, K. (1980). *In vivo* and *in vitro* effects of adrenaline on conversion of thyroxine to triiodothyronine and to reverse triiodothyronine in dog liver and heart. *Europ. J. Clin. Invest.*, **10**, 189–192.

Nauman, A., Porta, J., Bardowska, U., Fiedorowicz, K., and Kamiński, T. (1982a). Dose- and time-dependent effects of epinephrine on T4-5′-deiodinase and T4-5-deiodinase activity. *Endokrynologia Polska*, in press.

Nauman, J., Ceremużyński, L., Nauman, A., and Gunther-Krawczyńska, E. (1974). Serum triiodothyronine and thyroxine in relation to clinical course of recent myocardial infarction. In *Nuclear Medicine*, Schaftener Verlag, Stuttgart, pp. 461–466.

Nauman, J., Nauman, A., Kubica, A., Kamiński, T., Lewartowski, B., Ceremużyński, L., and Herbaczyńska-Cedro, K. (1976). Specific nuclear receptor for T3 in experimental myocardial infarction and after adrenaline infusion. *Europ. J. Clin. Invest.*, **6**, 339 (Abstr.).

Nauman, J., Ceremużyński, L., and Nauman, A. (1979). Total and free thyroid hormones and TSH in acute myocardial infarction. *Materia Med. Pol.*, **3**, 212–217.

Nauman, J., Porta, J., Nauman, A., and Fiedorowicz, K. (1982b). Dose- and time-dependent effect of epinephrine on mitochondrial alpha-glycerophosphate dehydrogenase and cytosolic malic enzyme activity in rat liver. *Endokrynologia Polska*, in press.

Nelson, B. D., Joste, V., Wielburski, A., and Rosenquist, U. (1980). The effects of triiodothyronine on the synthesis of mitochondrial proteins in isolated rat hepatocytes. *Biochem. Biophys. Acta*, **608**, 422–426.

Nishiki, K., Erecińska, M., Wilson, D. F., and Cooper, S. (1978). Evolution of oxidative phosphorylation in hearts from euthyroid, hypothyroid, and hyperthyroid rats. *Amer. J. Physiol.*, **235**, C212–C219.

Obregon, M. J., Pascual, A., Mallof, J., Morreale de Escobar, G., Escobar del Rey, F. (1980). Evidence against a major role of 1-thyroxine at the pituitary level: studies in rats treated with iopanoic acid. *Endocrinology*, **106**, 1827–1836.

Oppenheimer, J. H., and Dillmann, W. H. (1978). Nuclear receptors for triiodothyronine: a physiological perspective. In *Receptors and Hormone Action*, Vol. III (L. Birnbaumer and B. H. O'Malley, eds), Academic Press, New York, pp. 1–32.

Oppenheimer, J. H., and Surks, M. I. (1971). Nature, transport in plasma and metabolism of thyroid hormones. In *The Thyroid*, 3rd edn (S. C. Werner and S. H. Ingbar, eds), Harper and Row, New York, pp. 52–65.

Oppenheimer, J. H., Koerner, D., Schwartz, H. L., and Surks, M. I. (1972). Specific nuclear triiodothyronine binding sites in rat liver and kidney. *J. Clin. Endocrinol. Metab.*, **35**, 330–333.

Oppenheimer, J. H., Schwartz, H. L., and Surks, M. I. (1973). Effects of thyroid hormone analogs on the displacement of ^{125}I-triiodothyronine from hepatic and heart nuclei *in vivo*: possible relationship to hormonal activity. *Biochem. Biophys. Res. Commun.*, **55**, 544–550.

Oppenheimer, J. H., Schwartz, H. L., and Surks, M. I. (1974). Tissue differences in the concentration of triiodothyronine nuclear binding sites in the rat liver, kidney, pituitary, heart, brain, spleen and testis. *Endocrinology*, **95**, 897–903.

Oppenheimer, J. H., Dillman, W. H., Schwartz, H. L., and Howle, H. C. (1979). Nuclear receptors and thyroid hormone action: a progress report. *Fed. Proc.*, **38**, 2154–2161.

Pardridge, W. M. (1979). Carrier-mediated transport of thyroid hormones through the rat blood–brain barrier: primary role of albumin-bound hormone. *Endocrinology*, **105**, 605–612.

Pardridge, W. M., and Mietus, L. J. (1980). Influx of thyroid hormones into rat liver *in vivo*. *J. Clin. Invest.*, **66**, 367–374.

Pasquini, J. M., De Reveglia, F., Capitman, N., and Sota, E. F. (1980). Differential effect of 1-thyroxine on phospholipid biosynthesis in mitochondria and microsomal fraction. *Biochem. J.*, **186**, 127–133.

Philipson, K. D., and Edelman, I. S. (1977). Thyroid hormone control of Na^+,K^+-ATPase and K^+-dependent phosphatase in rat heart. *Amer. J. Physiol.*, **232**, C196–C206.

Pittman, G. S., Suda, A. K., Chambers, J. B., Ray, G. Y. (1979). Impaired 3,5,3'-triiodothyronine production in diabetic patients. *Metabolism*, **28**, 333–338.

Prince, H. P., Burr, W. A., Ramsden, D. B., Black, E. G., Griffiths, R. S., and Bradwell, A. R. (1976). The interaction of thyroid hormones, vitamin A and their binding proteins following surgical stress. *Clin. Sci. Mol. Med.*, **51**, 20–26.

Reuter, H. (1974). Localization of beta-adrenergic receptors and effects of noradrenaline and cyclic nucleotides on action potentials, ionic currents and tension in mammalian cardiac muscle. *J. Physiol. (Lond.)*, **242**, 429–451.

Robbins, J., Rall, J. E., and Gordon, P. (1974). The thyroid and iodine metabolism. In *Duncan's Diseases of Metabolism* (P. K. Bondy and L. E. Rosenberg, eds), W. B. Saunders, Philadelphia, pp. 1009–1104.

Robbins, J., Cheng, S. Y., Gershogorn, M. C., Glinoer, D., Cahmann, H. J., and Edelnoch, H. I. (1978). Thyroxine proteins' transport of plasma. Molecular properties and biosynthesis. *Rec. Prog. Hormone Res.*, **34**, 477–519.

Samuels, H. H., Stanley, F., and Shapiro, L. H. (1977). Modulation of thyroid hormone nuclear receptor levels by triiodothyronine in GH_1 cells. *J. Biol. Chem.*, **252**, 6052–6060.

Scarpace, P. J., and Abrass, J. B. (1981). Thyroid hormone regulation of heart, lymphocyte and lung beta adrenergic receptors. *Endocrinology*, **108**, 1007–1011.

Schwartz, H., and Gordon, A. (1975). Effect of triiodothyronine on chick embryo heart cell in tissue culture. *Israel J. Med. Sci.*, **11**, 877–883.

Segal, J., and Ingbar, S. H. (1979). Stimulation by triiodothyronine of the *in vitro* uptake of sugars in rat thymocytes. *J. Clin. Invest.*, **63**, 507–515.

Segal, J., and Ingbar, S. H. (1980). Plasma membrane-mediated effects of thyroid hormones. In *Thyroid Research*, Vol. VIII (J. R. Stockigt and S. Nagataki, eds), Australian Academy of Sciences, Canberra, pp. 405–408.

Shapiro, L. E., Samuels, H. H., and Yaffe, B. M. (1978). Thyroid and glucocorticoid hormones synergistically control growth hormone mRNA in cultured GH_1 cells. *Proc. natl Acad. Sci.*, **75**, 45–49.

Sharma, V. K., and Banerjee, S. P. (1977). Muscarinic cholinergic receptors in rat hearts. Effect of thyroidectomy. *J. Biol. Chem.*, **252,** 7444–7449.

Shaw, M. J., and Hoch, F. L. (1977). Thyroid control over membranes. Rat heart muscle mitochondria. *J. Mol. Cell Cardiol.*, **9,** 749–761.

Smith, D. P. (1976). The relationship betwen serum creatine kinase and thyroid hormones *in vivo* and *in vitro*. *Clin. Chim. Acta*, **68,** 333–338.

Smith, H. C., Robinson, S. E., and Eastman, C. J. (1980a). Evidence for a second nuclear binding site for thyroid hormones. Binding of reverse T3 to hepatic nuclear protein and regulation by thiol active agents. In *Thyroid Research*, Vol. VIII (J. R. Stockigt and S. Nagataki, eds), Australian Academy of Sciences, Canberra, pp. 283–286.

Smith, R. M., King, R. A., and Buckley, R. A. (1980b). Intracellular sodium and potassium concentration in heart and skeletal muscles from chronically hypothyroid sheep. In *Thyroid Research*, Vol. VIII (J. R. Stockigt and S. Nagataki, eds), Australian Academy of Sciences, Canberra, pp. 298–301.

Sterling, K., and Milch, P. O. (1975). Thyroid hormone binding by a component of mitochondrial membrane. *Proc. Natl Acad. Sci.*, **72,** 3225–3229.

Sterling, K., Brenner, M. A., and Sakurada, T. (1980). Rapid effect of triiodothyronine on the mitochondrial pathway in rat liver *in vivo*. *Science*, **210,** 340–342.

Strauer, B. E., and Schulze, W. (1976). Experimental hyperthyroidism: depression of muscle contraction function and hemodynamics and their reversibility by substitution with thyroid hormones. *Basic Res. Cardiol.*, **71,** 624–644.

Surks, M. I., and Oppenheimer, J. H. (1964). Postoperative changes in the concentration of TBPA and serum-free thyroxine. *J. Clin. Endocrinol. Metab.*, **24,** 794–802.

Tata, J. R., and Widnell, C. C. (1966). Ribonucleic acid synthesis during the early action of thyroid hormones. *Biochem. J.*, **98,** 604–609.

Thyrum, P. T., Kritcher, E. M., and Luchi, R. J. (1970). Effect of 1-thyroxine on the primary structure of cardiac myosin. *Biochim. Biophys. Acta*, **197,** 335–336.

Tobin, R. B., Berdaniew, C. D., and Ecklund, R. E. (1980). Effect of thyroidectomy upon activity of three mitochondrial schuttles in rat. *J. Environ. Pathol. Toxicol.*, **3,** 307–314.

Tse, J., Wrenn, R. W., and Kuo, J. E. (1980). Thyroxine-induced changes in characteristics and activities of beta-adrenergic receptors and 3′,5′-adenosine monophosphate and guanosine 3′,5′-monophosphate in the heart may be related to reputed catecholamine supersensitivity in hyperthyroidism. *Endocrinology*, **107,** 6–16.

Valori, C., Thomas, M., and Schillingford, J. (1967). Free adrenaline and adrenaline in relation to syndromes following myocardial infarction. *Amer. J. Cardiol.*, **5,** 605–617.

Van Winkle, W. B., and Schwartz, A. (1976). Ions and inotropy. *Annu. Rev. Physiol.*, **38,** 247–272.

Visser, T. J. (1978). A tentative review of recent *in vitro* observation of the enzymatic deiodination of iodothyronines and its possible physiological implications. *Mol. Cell. Endocrinol.*, **10,** 241–249.

Wallach, S., Bellavia, J. V., Gamponia, P. J., and Bristrim, P. (1972). Thyroxine induced stimulation of hepatic cell transport of calcium and magnesium. *J. Clin. Invest.*, **51,** 1572–1578.

Wartofsky, L., Latham, K. R., Diuh, Y. Y., and Burman, K. D. (1981). Alterations in T3 and T4 receptor binding in fasting and diabetes mellitus. *Life Sci.*, **28,** 1683–1691.

Wasilewska-Dziubińska, E., Nauman, A., Lewartowski, B., Nauman, J., Michałowski, J., and Sędek, G. (1981). Influence of surgery and experimental myocardial infarction on blood levels of free fatty acids and triiodothyronine in dogs. *Acta. Physiol. Pol.*, **32**, 283–291.

Westergren, V., Burger, A., Levin, K., Melander, A., Nilsson, G., and Peterson, V. (1977). Divergent changes in serum triiodothyronine and reverse triiodothyronine in patients with acute myocardial infarction. *Acta Med. Scand.*, **201**, 269–272.

Wiersinga, W. M., Lie, K. I., and Touber, J. L. (1981). Thyroid hormones in acute myocardial infarction. *Clin. Endocrinol.*, **14**, 367–374.

Williams, R. S., and Lefkowitz, R. J. (1979). Thyroid hormones regulation of alpha adrenergic receptors: studies in rat myocardium. *J. Cardiovasc. Pharmacol.*, **1**, 181–189.

Wilson, D. F., Owen, C. S., and Holian, A. (1977). Control of mitochondrial respiration: a quantitative evaluation of a role of cytochrome c and oxygen. *Arch. Biochem. Biophys.*, **182**, 749–762.

Wong, T. C. T., Barzila, D. C., Smith, D. C., Smith, R. E., and McConahey, W. M. (1979). Electrocardiographic voltage changes during hyperthyroidism. *Mayo Clinic Proc.*, **54**, 763–768.

Werner, S. C., Nauman, J. (1968). The thyroid. *Ann. Rev. Physiol.*, **30**, 213–244.

Werner, S. C., (1981). The thyroid in diabetes mellitus, obesity and fasting. Research Workshop of the Thyroid Foundation. *Life Sci.*, **28**, Nr 15–16.

Cardiac Metabolism
Edited by A. J. Drake-Holland and M. I. M. Noble
© 1983 John Wiley & Sons Ltd

CHAPTER 23

Adenosine

R. A. Olsson

Suncoast Cardiovascular Research Laboratory, Department of Internal Medicine, University of South Florida College of Medicine, Tampa, Florida 33612, USA

INTRODUCTION

It has now been 50 years since Lindner and Rigler (1931) crystallized adenosine from heart muscle extracts, confirmed its coronary vasoactivity in mammalian hearts, and proposed the hypothesis that it is a physiological regulatory of coronary flow. Largely through the work of Berne, Gerlach, and their colleagues, this hypothesis has received intense scrutiny over the past 20 years. Overall, support for this hypothesis is strong, but in some areas the experimental evidence is weak and in others it is contradictory.

Figure 23.1 is a general model describing coronary flow regulations by adenosine, presented here as a point of departure for the discussion which follows. This model, which has been synthesized from two recent reviews (Berne and Rubio, 1979; Berne, 1980), incorporates the widely held beliefs that myocardial oxygen consumption rate ($M\dot{V}O_2$) is proportional to cardiac effort and, in turn, is the primary determinant of coronary flow rate (CBF). I have added myocardial P_{O_2} as the error signal and mitochondrial cytochrome aa_3 as the sensor which actuates a negative feedback control system.

Current thinking holds that effort-linked changes in the extramitochondrial adenylate system, e.g. the ATP:ADP ratio, may play an important role in the regulation of $M\dot{V}O_2$ (Williamson, 1979). Extramitochondrial ADP can also furnish, via myokinase, the substrate for adenosine production. ATP hydrolysis releases Mg^{++} and concomitantly stimulates creatine phosphate hydrolysis, two events which tend allosterically to deinhibit 5'-nucleotidase, the sarcolemmal enzyme which catalyses adenosine formation. The stimulation of AMP formation, Mg^{++} release, and creatine phosphate hydrolysis implies a fall in ATP and a rise in ADP concentration. These are thought to be too small to be detected experimentally. Since oxygen delivery seems just to meet the demand of $M\dot{V}O_2$ at any level of cardiac effort, the transition to a higher level of effort must create a temporary imbalance between supply and demand which is restored only when the events just

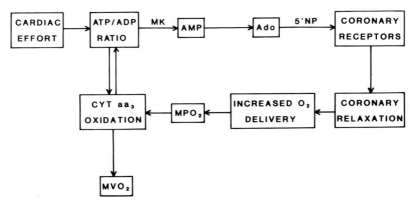

Figure 23.1 A general model for the regulation of coronary flow by adenosine, based on the recent reviews of Berne and Rubio (1979) and Berne (1980). See text for details

described result in coronary vasodilation. At the molecular level, this imbalance would be expected to reduce cytochrome aa_3 until enhanced oxygen delivery restores this enzyme to its usual oxidation state. Adenosine formed by the hydrolysis of AMP at the cell margins and released into the interstitial space appears to initiate coronary relaxation by interacting with specific receptors on the coronary myocyte surface. Although the mechanism of relaxation is incompletely understood, the resulting increase in CBF enhances oxygen availability, thus permitting cytochrome aa_3 oxidation, ADP concentration, and $M\dot{V}O_2$ to assume new steady state levels.

Such a 'micro-hypoxia' model is consistent with several characteristics of heart muscle and the coronary circulation. Owing to its constant activity, cardiac muscle has a high energy requirement which requires oxidative metabolism to sustain performance. Despite a high $M\dot{V}O_2$, basal coronary tone is high. This combination of circumstances causes a high degree of oxygen extraction and low tissue p_{O_2}. Another consequence of high basal tone – which appears to be non-metabolic in origin – is that coronary flow regulation is essentially graded vasodilatation in response to increases in cardiac effort. Apparently cardiac cells do not produce endogenous vasoconstrictors.

This chapter examines critically the premise that the relationships between cardiac effort, $M\dot{V}O_2$, and CBF are strictly proportional and unique, i.e. that they hold under all experimental conditions and for all chambers of the heart. It continues with reviews of three areas in which recent experiments have modified the adenosine hypothesis significantly. These are (1) the compartmentation of the cardiac adenosine pool; (2) control of the adenosine concentration in the vicinity of the coronary resistance vessels; and (3) the mechanism by which adenosine initiates coronary relaxation.

The chapter concludes by considering evidence that adenosine mediates cardiac performance in addition to its role in coronary regulation.

DEPENDENCE OF MV̇O₂ AND CBF ON CARDIAC EFFORT

Most models of metabolic coronary vasoregulation assume a chain of causality linking cardiac effort, $M\dot{V}O_2$, and CBF. Because of the fundamental importance of this idea, it is worth examining the limitations of its experimental support. The task is to discriminate between coincidence and causality. Of necessity, the need to control conditions makes the results of an experiment a special case, which in the strictest sense applies only to the particular circumstances of that experiment. Thus, one stringent test of causality is to determine the extent to which one may generalize from a special case.

Experiments from many laboratories which show that cardiac work, $M\dot{V}O_2$, and CBF are highly covariant (Berne and Rubio, 1979; Suga *et al.*, 1981) support the hypothesis that these variables are causally related. However, these experiments concern mainly the dog left ventricle. While available evidence suggests that this covariance is generalizable to other species, relationships which describe the left ventricle under one set of conditions may not predict the effects of changing experimental conditions or the behaviour of other cardiac chambers. For example, the type of substrate supporting the heart may alter the relationship between cardiac effort and $M\dot{V}O_2$. Calculations of oxygen requirements for and the energy yield from the combustion of oleic acid and glucose are, respectively 52.0 and 45.3 ml O_2 kJ^{-1}. This predicts that, at a constant workload, hearts supported by glucose will require 15–20% less oxygen than hearts supported by fatty acids (see Drake-Holland, Chapter 9 in this volume). The relationship of $M\dot{V}O_2$ to cardiac effort is discussed by Elzinga (Chapter 8 in this volume). Whether coronary flow rate also depends on the type of substrate supporting cardiac work is unknown, but see Chapter 9 in this volume.

One may similarly question the apparently close correlation between CBF and $M\dot{V}O_2$. All experiments examining this relationship estimate $M\dot{V}O_2$ by calculating the product CBF and arteriovenous oxygen difference, then test the covariance of $M\dot{V}O_2$ and CBF. This, of course, is the comparison of CBF with a multiple of itself – a spurious correlation. Moreover, the Fick equation used to calculate $M\dot{V}O_2$ implies that CBF is directly proportional to $M\dot{V}O_2$ only if oxygen extraction is absolutely invariant. This is clearly not the case; left ventricular oxygen extraction changes substantially during physiological responses such as exercise (Khouri *et al.*, 1965; VonRestorff *et al.*, 1977). Moreover, recent work (S. Kusachi, personal communication) suggests that the relationship between CBF and $M\dot{V}O_2$ in the left ventricle is not applicable to the right ventricle. Simultaneous comparisons of the responses of these chambers to interventions which changed MVO_2 show that changes in oxygen extraction are much more important in the right than in the left ventricle.

Thus, it appears that the dependence of $M\dot{V}O_2$ on cardiac effort and the dependence of CBF on $M\dot{V}O_2$ may not be exact and are not generally applicable. What are the consequences of this imperfection? Just as the $M\dot{V}O_2$ response to cardiac effort may vary according to circumstances, so the CBF response to a change in $M\dot{V}O_2$ may depend on undefined factors which simultaneously modify oxygen extraction. Secondly, if $M\dot{V}O_2$ is not the only link between cardiac effort and CBF, it is possible that the heart may elaborate more than one vasodilator metabolite, depending on the stimulus which modifies cardiac effort. In the case of adenosine, removing the constraint of a precise relationship between CBF and $M\dot{V}O_2$ obviates the need to link adenosine production directly to $M\dot{V}O_2$. Thus, there may be alternatives to the 'classical' model of adenosine production.

COMPARTMENTALIZATION OF THE CARDIAC ADENOSINE POOL

Recent experiments show that the cardiac adenosine pool consists of a major intracellular compartment of adenosine bound to S-adenosyl-homocysteine hydrolase and a much smaller interstitial compartment of free adenosine which participates in coronary vasomotion (Schrader *et al.*, 1981; Schütz *et al.*, 1981; Olsson *et al.*, 1982). This model departs significantly from the earlier view that adenosine in heart muscle is exclusively extracellular. The older one-compartment model was based on estimates that placed the size of the cardiac adenosine pool at $0.2–0.3$ nmol g^{-1} (Rubio and Berne, 1969; Olsson, 1970). This amount of adenosine, if distributed in the interstitial space, would achieve concentrations within the vasoactive range of exogenous adensine. This model drew additional support from the likelihood that the high adenosine deaminase and adenosine kinase activities in heart muscle would preclude an intracellular compartment of free adenosine (Olsson *et al.*, 1972), and from experiments showing that [^{14}C]adenosine entering cardiac cells is rapidly and completely incorporated in the adenine nucleotide pool (Jacob and Berne, 1960); Liu and Feinberg, 1971; Namm, 1973).

Improved analytical techniques subsequently showed that normally oxygenated dog and guinea-pig hearts contained 1–2 nmol adenosine per gram (Schrader and Gerlach, 1976; Olsson *et al.*, 1978). If distributed only in the interstitial space, which has a volume of 0.2 ml g^{-1} (Frank and Langer, 1974; Polimeni, 1974), this much adenosine is equivalent to concentrations between 5 and 10 μM. However, intracoronary infusions of adenosine cause half-maximum coronary vasodilation at concentrations at or below 1 μM and maximum coronary vasodilation at concentrations between 3 and 5 μM (Schrader *et al.*, 1977c; Olsson *et al.*, 1978, 1979). Thus, the notion that adenosine exists in a single extracellular compartment fails to account for the high basal tone characteristic of the coronary circulation.

This crucial inconsistency in the one-compartment model stimulated the search for more direct evidence of an intracellular adenosine compartment. Work in a number of laboratories (Hershfield and Kredich, 1978; Ueland and Sabeø, 1979; Schrader *et al.*, 1981; Schütz *et al.*, 1981; Olsson *et al.*, 1981) shows that adenosine exists intracellularly in many tissues as a complex with the enzyme *S*-adenosylhomocysteine hydrolase. Although the adenosine bound to this enzyme can serve as a substrate for the synthesis of *S*-adenosylhomocysteine when the second substrate, L-homocysteine, is supplied (Schrader *et al.*, 1981), it appears to be insensitive to hydrolysis by the high adenosine deaminase activity present in dog heart muscle. In dog heart the intracellular compartment accounts for over 90% of the cardiac adenosine pool (Olsson *et al.*, 1981). Concentrations in the extracellular compartment, about 0.2 μM, are at or below the threshold of adenosine's coronary vasoactivity, which probably explains why sustained intracoronary infusions of adenosine deaminase and/or the adenosine receptor antagonist theophylline do not affect basal coronary resistance (Saito *et al.*, 1981). Thus, it appears that adenosine contributes little to setting basal coronary tone.

The discovery that only a minor fraction of the cardiac adenosine pool participates in coronary vasomotion has another extremely important consequence. Many tests of the adenosine hypothesis in the past 10 years have compared coronary resistance with *total* cardiac adenosine content. The conclusions drawn from these experiments may be invalid, because it is not yet known whether the sizes of the two compartments change concordantly.

CONTROL OF INTERSTITIAL ADENOSINE CONCENTRATION

The balance between the rates at which adenosine enters and departs from the interstitial compartment determines its concentration in the vicinity of the coronary resistance vessels. The discussion which follows first disposes of the mechanisms by which adenosine is dissipated, which are fairly well understood, then takes up the uncertain issue of the mechanisms of adenosine production.

In the open-chest dog, total purine loss (adenosine + inosine + hypoxanthine) is about 0.8 nmol min^{-1} per gram of left ventricle (Wiedmeier *et al.*, 1972; Snow *et al.*, 1973). In dog and man, arterial plasma adenosine concentrations are low, typically 50–90 nM, and estimates of the coronary arteriovenous difference under basal conditions range between 5 nM (uptake) and -30 nM (release) (Schrader *et al.*, 1979; Manfredi and Sparks, 1982; R. A. Olsson, unpublished). This small arteriovenous difference is consistent with the notion that interstitial adenosine concentration is low, but may additionally reflect a diffusion barrier at the capillary wall and uptake by endothelial cells (Nees *et al.*, 1981). It does not necessarily imply that adenosine is extensively degraded *in situ* after its release from the cardiac cell, for alternative pathways such as the hydrolysis of 5'-IMP by 5'-nucleotidase, do exist. Indeed, tracer studies showing that specific activity of [^{14}C]adenosine released from guinea-pig hearts is many times higher than that of either inosine or hypoxanthine minimizes the importance of *in situ* degradation (Schrader and Gerlach, 1976). Thus, adenosine accounts for only a small fraction of the purines lost from heart muscle, perhaps no more than 0.01 nmol min^{-1} g^{-1} (Manfredi and Sparks, 1981).

Abundant evidence from many types of cells support the generalization that adenosine and other nucleosides penetrate cells by a combination of passive diffusion and carrier-mediated, non-concentrative, facilitated diffusion (Paterson, 1979). Cardiac muscle is no exception (Olsson *et al.*, 1972, 1973a); adenosine uptake by blood-perfused dog hearts is half-maximum at about 10 μM and has a maximum rate of about 5 nmol min^{-1} g^{-1}.

The most recent information about fluxes into and out of the cardiac interstitial adenosine compartment comes from a model developed by Manfredi and Sparks (1981). This model employs their estimate of the rate of adenosine release, and others' estimates of the rates of cardiocyte and endothelial cell uptake, capillary pore size, and the diffusion coefficient of sucrose, whose hydrodynamic radius is similar to that of adenosine. This model predicts an adenosine production rate of about 7.5 nmol min^{-1} per 100 g, with disposition as follows: cardiocyte uptake, 87%; endothelial uptake, 3%; and loss by washout, 20%. The model predicts an interstitial adenosine concentration of 0.15 μM, not greatly different from that estimated from pericardial superfusates, 0.24 μM (Olsson *et al.*, 1982). This model also predicts a compartment turnover rate of 325 min^{-1}, two orders of magnitude faster than older estimates. The many assumptions underlying this extrapolation are a weakness. However, if further experiments independently validate the use of adenosine release rates to estimate interstitial concentrations, this technique could be a powerful tool for estimating the concentration of adenosine in the vicinity of the coronary resistance vessels.

Control of Adenosine Production

Until about 5 years ago much of the evidence supporting the adenosine hypothesis came from experiments in which hypoxia served as a stimulus to adenosine production. Recent experiments demonstrating directionally similar changes in adenosine production, $M\dot{V}O_2$, and CBF in response to physiological, i.e. non-hypoxic, stimuli show that overt hypoxia is not required for adenosine production (Watkinson *et al.*, 1979; Foley *et al.*, 1979; Miller *et al.*, 1979; McKenzie *et al.*, 1980; Saito *et al.*, 1980, Manfredi and Sparks, 1980). However, there are important obstacles between these qualitative results and the conclusion that $M\dot{V}O_2$ determines adenosine production. Foremost is that each of these studies employed indirect methods to estimate the interstitial concentration of adenosine, and each of these methods has significant drawbacks. Because of the large intracellular adenosine compartment in cardiac muscle, total adenosine content might not accurately reflect changes in the 5 or 10% actually involved in coronary vasomotion. Estimates of adenosine concentration in pericardial superfusion fluids obtained under non-equilibrium conditions likewise have an undefined relationship to the concentration of adenosine in the interstitial space. Estimates based on adenosine release rates depend on accurately estimating small arteriovenous differences.

Two experiments suggest that changes in $M\dot{V}O_2$ may not invariably produce proportional changes in the rate of adenosine production. Modifying $M\dot{V}O_2$ by atrial pacing, paired ventricular pacing, aortic constriction, or beta-adrenergic blockade changes cardiac adenosine content in proportion to the change in $M\dot{V}O_2$, but raising $M\dot{V}O_2$ by beta-adrenergic stimulation (isoproterenol) produces a disproportionately large increase in adenosine content (Saito *et al.*, 1980). Similarly, stimulating $M\dot{V}O_2$ by noradrenaline infusion leads to the release of adenosine into coronary venous blood, but atrial pacing to comparable levels of $M\dot{V}O_2$ does not elicit adenosine release (Manfredi and Sparks, 1980). These experiments suggest that the rate of adenosine production depends on the stimulus used to alter $M\dot{V}O_2$ rather than on $M\dot{V}O_2$ itself.

The hydrolysis of 5'-AMP by 5'-nucleotidase is historically the first hypothesis advanced to explain cardiac adenosine production (Gerlach *et al.*, 1963; Burger and Lowenstein, 1967). In essentially all mammalian cells, 5'-nucleotidase is an *ecto*enzyme, i.e. its catalytic site is located on the external surface of the plasma membrane, where it has access to extracellular substrate (DePierre and Karnovsky, 1974). In normoxic dog heart, adenosine production accounts for far less than 1% of the potential catalytic rate of 5'-nucleotidase (about 0.5 μmol min^{-1} per gram of left ventricle) and rises about 10-fold during ischaemia (Olsson, 1970). Why the catalytic rate of 5'-nucleotidase is so low is uncertain, but of great importance, since this suppression of activity may be a manifestation of the mechanism which controls adenosine production.

Previous investigations into the mechanism controlling adenosine production have examined two hypotheses, that 5'-nucleotidase is a substrate-limited enzyme or, alternatively, that cardiac metabolites regulate the catalytic properties of this enzyme.

Two experiments provide evidence that only a small compartment of the total cardiac 5'-AMP pool subserves adenosine production. Schrader and Gerlach (1976) labelled the adenine nucleotides of isolated guinea-pig hearts with [^{14}C]adenine and then estimated the specific activities of the purines in these hearts and also of purines released into the coronary venous effluent. Under normoxic conditions the specific activities of [^{14}C]cyclic AMP and [^{14}C]adenosine were 32–38 times higher than the specific activities of cardiac [^{14}C]ATP and [^{14}C]AMP. Hypoxic perfusion enhanced adenosine release several-fold but significantly reduced its specific activity. One interpretation of these results is that, under these experimental conditions, adenine labels only a small compartment of the total 5'-AMP pool, presumably via the adenine phosphoribosyltransferase pathway, and that this 5'-AMP compartment communicates with a similarly restricted 5-ATP compartment supporting cyclic AMP synthesis. This interpretation resembles that of radiolabelling studies of cyclic AMP production in brain slices (Schultz and Daly, 1973). These results further suggest that hypoxia evokes the participation of additional 5'-AMP derived from nucleotide compartments which are poorly labelled under these conditions.

A different experimental approach additionally supports the notion that a small AMP compartment supports adenosine production (Sobell and Bunger, 1981; R. Bunger, personal communication). Homogenization of guinea-pig hearts in mixtures of non-polar solvents followed by density gradient centrifugation separated mitochrondria from cytosolic organelles. Analysis of the adenine nucleotide content of each fraction showed that most of the cardiac 5'-AMP pool is intramitochondrial, a result in accord with previous work (Illingworth *et al.*, 1975). Applying the myokinase equilibrium to estimates of free cytosolic ATP and ADP predicts that in oxygenated hearts the cytosolic AMP concentration is only about 1 µM. While this estimate of substrate concentration is far smaller than that based on the assumption that the cardiac AMP pool consists of a single cytosolic compartment, it still predicts implausibly large rates of adenosine production. The 5'-nucleotidase activity of guinea-pig hearts is 33 µmol min^{-1} g^{-1} (Baer *et al.*, 1966) and has a K_m of about 15 µM (Baer *et al.*, 1966; Edwards and Maguire, 1970; Sullivan and Alpers, 1971; Olsson *et al.*, 1973b). Michaelis–Menten kinetics predict that at a substrate concentration of 1 µM, adenosine production will be about 2 µmol min^{-1} per gram of heart weight, a rate equivalent to the turnover of one-third of the entire adenine nucleotide pool each minute. This incongruence suggests that, in addition to a low substrate concentration, other factors must limit AMP hydrolysis by this enzyme.

Since AMP in the cytosol is separated from the catalytic site of 5'-nucleotidase by a plasma membrane which is impermeable to nucleotides, it is necessary to postulate some sort of permeation process which moves this nucleotide across the plasma membrane in order for hydrolysis to occur.

Frick and Lowenstein (1978) offer evidence that adenosine production is vectorial; in other words either 5′-nucleotidase itself or an associated permease accomplishes this translocation. This evidence consists of the observation that the incorporation of the adenosine moiety of radioactively labelled exogenous AMP appears to enter the cardiac adenine nucleotide pool more rapidly than exogenous adenosine labelled with a different radioisotope. However, if one corrects the apparent relative specific activity of each species of radiolabelled adenosine for the presence of the other species, the rates of incorporation are essentially equal (J. Schrader, personal communication).

Although the Schrader and Bunger experiments support the idea that substrate restriction controls adenosine production, the experiments are both complicated and sensitive to the validity of the assumptions underlying the experimental approaches which were used. Even though they fall short of an unambiguous description of cardiac adenosine metabolism, it seems likely then only through demanding experiments such as these will we ever understand the control of adenosine production.

Support is generally weak for the hypothesis that regulating the catalytic properties of 5′-nucleotidase controls adenosine production. Frick and Lowenstein (1976) report that the catalytic properties of this enzyme in isolated hearts perfused with AMP are markedly different from those found *in vitro*. Their experiment shows that at high perfusate AMP concentrations, the rate of AMP hydrolysis equals the maximum rate attainable in heart homogenates, but the perfusate concentration needed to produce half-maximum hydrolysis is 2 mM, or about two orders of magnitude greater than that of detergent-solubilized 5′-nucleotidase. Frick and Lowenstein (1976) suggest that this difference may reflect the influence of the membrane in which 5′-nucleotidase is embedded. However, the conditions of the experiment do not exclude the possibility that a barrier to diffusion at the capillary wall may have significantly lowered the concentration of substrate available to the enzyme. Thus, the difference between this estimate of K_m and that of the enzyme *in vitro* may reflect the difference between the AMP concentration in the perfusate and that at the cardiocyte surface. The K_m of 5′-nucleotidase in cardiac membrane fragments not exposed to detergents is similar to that of detergent-treated enzyme (Olsson *et al.*, 1973a), which argues against the 'membrane environment' hypothesis.

Adenine nucleotides have long been known to inhibit 5′-nucleotidase (Baer *et al.*, 1966) and could thus account for the low rate of adenosine formation, relative to 5′-nucleotidase activity, seen in the beating heart. This sort of control seems unlikely for two reasons. ATP and ADP inhibit the enzyme *competitively* (Burger and Lowenstein, 1975), which means they inhibit at the catalytic site. Since this site is external and these nucleotides are confined to the cell interior, their influence on catalytic activity seems improbable. As described above, Frick and Lowenstein (1976) have shown that at high substrate concentrations the 5′-nucleotidase of beating hearts is fully active. This further argues against the possibility of allosteric (non-competitive) inhibition by nucleotides, creatine phosphate, or Mg^{++} (Sullivan and Alpers, 1971; Rubio and Berne, 1979).

Recently Schütz et al. (1981) proposed that the intracellular pool of adenosine bound to S-adenosylhomocysteine hydrolase is the source of adenosine released by hypoxic hearts. Perfusion of guinea-pig hearts with the 5′-nucleotidase inhibitor adenosine-α,β-methylenediphosphonate (AOPCP) reduced the hydrolysis of exogenous 5′-AMP by 85%, yet had no effect on the release of adenosine during hypoxia. Conversely, the adenosine transport inhibitor 6-(4-nitrobenzylthio)purine riboside (NBTPR) reduced adenosine release during hypoxia. L-Homocysteine also reduced hypoxic adenosine release, presumably by promoting the synthesis of S-adenosylhomocysteine and thus depleting the intracellular adenosine pool. Work from the same laboratory has described a 'soluble', presumably cytosolic, 5′-nucleotidase, which is thought to generate adenosine intracellularly (Schrader et al., 1981). Presumably this enzyme, rather than the *ecto* 5′-nucleotidase, catalyses accelerated adenosine production during hypoxia.

Experiments with polymorphonuclear leukocytes corroborate the importance of adenosine formation by pathways independent of 5′-nucleotidase. Treating these cells with 2-deoxyglucose causes ATP depletion and greatly stimulates the accumulation of intracellular adenosine. A combination of β-glycerophosphate and antibodies against 5′-nucleotidase inhibited *ecto* phosphatase activity by 98% but had no effect on the rate of adenosine accumulation. Unlike heart muscle, S-adenosylhomocysteine levels did not change (Newby and Holmquist, 1981).

Several inconsistencies prevent immediate acceptance of the S-adenosylhomocysteine hydrolase hypothesis. The conflicting observation that AOPCP inhibits adenosine release from hypoxic rat hearts (Frick and Lowenstein, 1978) perhaps reflects differences in the ways the hearts of these two species handle purines (Hopkins and Goldie, 1971) and, in any event precludes generalizing the results of either experiment. Further, the Schütz study does not provide direct evidence that the adenosine released during hypoxia had previously been bound to S-adenosylhomocysteine hydrolase. Work to date has not identified the stimulus for adenosine release from this enzyme nor does it explain how subsequent metabolism by adenosine deaminase or adenosine kinase is avoided. Indeed, the dissociation of adenosine from S-adenosylhomocysteine hydrolase *in vitro*, $t_{1/2} > 2$ h (Olsson et al., 1981), is too slow to account for the exuberant release of adenosine from hypoxic hearts. The cytosolic 5′-nucleotidase identified by these workers is only partially characterized; additional work is needed to confirm its identity and to explain how catalytic activity accelerates under hypoxic conditions in which the concentration of ADP, a powerful 5'-nucleotidase inhibitor, is rising. Thus, further experiments are necessary to consolidate this attractive, new hypothesis which aims at explaining hypoxic adenosine release.

ADENOSINE ACTIONS ON CORONARY SMOOTH MUSCLE

Adenosine appears to initiate coronary relaxation by binding to a specific receptor on the surface of the coronary myocyte (Olsson *et al.*, 1976; Schrader *et al.*, 1977b). In isolated guinea-pig hearts and in the conscious dog, exogenous adenosine produces half-maximum coronary vasodilation at concentrations (ED_{50}) of about 0.5 μM: open-chest dogs are one to several times less responsive. The vasoactive range, i.e. the difference between the threshold and maximally active doses, extends over two orders of magnitude in the guinea-pig and over at least one order of magnitude in the dog (Schrader *et al.*, 1977a; Olsson *et al.*, 1979). Owing to some metabolism of adenosine by blood and endothelial cells and to the diffusion barrier at the capillary wall, these experiments overestimate the true ED_{50} by an unknown amount. Because the true ED_{50} is probably lower than the apparent ED_{50} and because the vasodilatory range is fairly wide, it is possible that under basal conditions adenosine participates in setting coronary tone. This seems not to be the case, however, since neither destroying interstitial adenosine by intracoronary infusions of adenosine deaminase catalytic subunits nor administration of the coronary adenosine receptor antagonist theophylline has any effect on coronary flow (Saito *et al.*, 1981).

The adenosine sensitivity of resistance vessels is greater in the subendocardium than in the subepicardium. In conscious dogs, intracoronary adenosine infusions which fully dilate the coronary bed do not alter transmural flow distribution, but submaximal doses greatly increase the subendocardial:subepicardial flow ratio. The adenosine transport inhibitor dipyridamole mimics this effect, suggesting that the subendocardial vessels are also more sensitive to endogenous adenosine (Rembert *et al.*, 1980). Other work shows that adenosine concentration is uniform across the ventricular wall (Foley *et al.*, 1979), so the difference in sensitivity could reflect either differences in receptor number, ligand affinity, and/or how tightly these receptors are coupled to the mechanism of relaxation. Alternatively, either the participation of other vasodilatory metabolites or the existence of a transmural gradient in the intensity of non-metabolic factors which oppose adenosine vasodilation, e.g. myogenic tone, could account for this observation.

Two hypotheses seek to describe the events linking coronary relaxation to adenosine receptor occupancy. The first, that adenosine is a Ca^{++} channel blocker, is supported by electrophysiological studies showing that adenosine and certain of its analogues suppress phase 2 (slow inward current) of the action potential of atrial muscle (Schrader *et al.*, 1975, 1977b) and of cultured vasocular myocytes (Harder *et al.*, 1979). As work on this hypothesis proceeds it will be interesting to learn whether endogenous adenosine in physiological concentrations reproduces these results and whether adenosine blockade with drugs such as theophylline or the destruction of adenosine with exogenous adenosine deaminase prevents these effects. Studies of $^{45}Ca^{++}$ flux in cultured aortic smooth muscle cells appear to confirm the electrophysiological inference that Ca^{++} influx is indeed blocked by adenosine (Fenton *et al.*, 1982). Recently Young and Merrill (1981), reported that the Ca^{++} transport blocker nifedipine antagonizes the coronary vasoactivity of adenosine. One possible explanation for this paradoxical result is that nifedipine is a partial agonist; that is, it is able to occupy an adenosine receptor (and thus block occupancy by adenosine) at concentrations sufficient to materially effect Ca^{++} influx. Whether this antagonism is a specific effect of nifedipine on the Ca^{++} channel is an important uncertainty which can only be clarified by examining other Ca^{++} agonists. Since the several Ca^{++} blockers now available have no obvious chemical features in common, the hypothesis that nifedipine acts via a specific adenosine receptor on the Ca^{++} channel predicts that its antagonism of adenosine is unique. Thus, adenosine antagonism by other Ca^{++} agonists would be evidence that the effect is non-specific.

The second hypothesis, that adenylate cyclase activation mediates adenosine relaxation, is supported by experiments which show that washed coronary artery membranes contain an adenosine-stimulated adenylate cyclase and that adenosine produces dose-dependent increases of cyclic AMP levels parallel with relaxation of bovine coronary artery rings (Kukovetz *et al.*, 1979). Evidence that adenylate cyclase-associated adenosine receptors occur in many types of cells (Sattin and Rall, 1970; Braun and Levitzki, 1979; Daly *et al.*, 1981; Wolff *et al.*, 1981) further support this hypothesis indirectly. These studies have identified three types of adenosine receptors, stimulatory and inhibitory surface receptors designated 'R_a' and 'R_i', respectively, and an intracellular inhibitory 'P' site which may be part of the GTP-binding regulatory subunit (Wolff *et al.*, 1981). Each receptor exhibits a rather well defined specificity for activation by adenosine analogues. Study of the coronary vasoactivity of adenosine and its analogues in conscious, instrumented dogs (Olsson *et al.*, 1979) show a spectrum of activity remarkably similar to that of required for 'R_a' receptor activation. Dialkylxanthines antagonize the activation of the coronary artery adenosine receptor (Afonso, 1970), just as they inhibit adenosine activation of 'R' receptors. Finally, studies employing adenosine analogues and also theophylline covalently coupled to molecules too large to penetrate cells show that like the cyclase

'R' receptors, the coronary adenosine receptor is located on the coronary myocyte surface (Olsson *et al.*, 1976; Schrader *et al.*, 1977b). Thus, it is possible that adenosine and beta-adrenergic coronary vasodilation share a common pathway which begins with the activation of adenylate cyclase.

The 'Ca^{++} channel blocker' and 'adenylate cyclase activator' hypotheses need not be mutually exclusive, for membrane phosphorylation by cyclic AMP-dependent protein kinase(s) could effect Ca^{++} permeability. This may be the case in cardiac muscle (Walsh *et al.*, 1979; Drake-Holland and Noble, Chapter 17 in this volume), but whether this mechanism operates in the coronary myocyte is, at this time, unknown.

EFFECTS OF ADENOSINE ON CARDIAC FUNCTION

The initial description of adenosine's cardiovascular effects reports coronary vasodilation but emphasizes its species-specific extracoronary action on cardiac performance and blood pressure (Drury and Szent-Gyorgyi, 1929). These effects include slowing of atrial rate and attenuation of atrial (but not ventricular) contractile force, atrioventricular block, and systemic hypotension. These effects are prominent in the guinea-pig and dog. Recent experiments have begun to identify the mechanisms which underlie these actions.

Chronotropic and dromotropic effects have been described by Szentmiklósi *et al.* (1980) and Bellardinelli *et al.* (1980, 1981). Inotropic effects of adenosine have been described by Lammerant and Becsei, 1973, Szentmiklósi *et al.*, 1980 and Endoh and Yamashita, 1980. However, adenosine stimulates adenylate cyclase activity in guinea-pig ventricular slices (Huang and Drummond, 1976) and, at low Mg^{++} concentration, in dog left ventricular membranes (Webster and Olsson, 1981). Additionally, intracoronary adenosine infusions stimulate cyclic AMP release into the left ventricular venous drainage (Huynh-Tho and Lammerant, 1978, 1980). In view of the widely held hypothesis that the positive inotropic effects of hormones such as noradrenaline and glucagon are mediated through adenylate cyclase stimulation, the lack of an inotopic effect of adenosine in the face of evidence for enhanced cyclic AMP production, is paradoxical; similar dissociations between positive inotropic effects and cyclic AMP are discussed by Drake-Holland and Noble (Chapter 17 in this volume).

Although adenosine has no inotropic effect on ventricular muscle, in guinea-pig and rat hearts it strongly antagonizes the positive inotropic and metabolic consequences of beta-adrenergic activation by noradrenaline, adrenaline, or isoproterenol (Schrader *et al.*, 1977a; Dobson, 1978). Adenosine and P site-specific ligands inhibit 'basal' cyclase activity and also antagonize activation by catecholamines, dopamine and histamine. The two R$_i$ receptor-specific ligands had no effect on catalytic activity. What seems to be a contradiction of the observations in beating hearts seems traceable to the conditions of cyclase assay, which employed a medium containing 15 mM Mg^{++}. This concentration of Mg^{++} should simultaneously elicit P-site effects and suppress R_i receptor antagonism (Wolff *et al.*, 1981). The high ligand concentrations needed to inhibit catalytic activity (10^{-4} M) are also characteristic of a P-site effect. Thus, these membrane experiments neither support nor refute what appears to be R_i receptor-mediated antagonism of hormonal stimulation in beating hearts.

The effect of adenosine on catecholamine-stimulated adenylate cyclase activity in guinea-pig heart slices differs from that in beating hearts (Huang and Drummond, 1978). In slice preparations adenosine and isoproterenol both stimulate cyclic AMP accumulation, and their effects are more than additive. However, these experiments employed a single concentration of adenosine and relatively high concentrations of catecholamine, conditions which might have obscured adenosine antagonism. Additionally, damage to R_i receptors during tissue preparation cannot be excluded.

Available evidence (Angus *et al.*, 1971) and our unpublished observations indicate that R_a receptor-specific adenosine analogues such as 2-chloroadenosine and adenosine-5'-uronic acid carboxamides have powerful negative chronotropic, dromotropic, and atrial inotropic effects whereas R_i receptor-specific analogues appear to have none. Pharmacological evidence such as this suggests that there is a heirarchy of cardiac adenosine receptors, the R_a type predominating in supraventricular tissue and the R_i type of receptor in ventricular muscle.

CLINICAL IMPLICATIONS

Schrader's demonstration that adenosine antagonizes the inotropic effects of hormones such as noradrenaline suggests that the release of this nucleoside might contribute to the depressed performance of ischaemic myocardium. Adenosine is a powerful antagonist of platelet aggregation and thereby could modify the extent of thrombosis and antagonize the effects of the several injurious substances released from platelets within an infarct. Bellardinelli's work on the role of adenosine in the genesis of conduction defects (Bellardinelli *et al.*, 1981) provides new insights about the mechanism and treatment of the sinus node dysfunction and atrioventricular block which occur in ischaemic heart disease. Further, this new initiative has stimulated inquiry into the possible role of adenosine in the genesis of tachyarrythmias (Rosen *et al.*, 1981).

ACKNOWLEDGEMENTS

I am deeply indebted to Drs Rolf Bunger, Michael R. Rosen, Jürgen Schrader, Harvey V. Sparks, Jr, C. I. Thompson, and J. R. Wiggins for critical reviews and thoughtful suggestions for improving this manuscript. Drs Luis Bellardinelli, Rolf Bunger, and Showzo Kusachi very generously made available the results of experiments which have not yet been published. Mrs Eunice Oliver assisted greatly in the preparation of the manuscript. The writing of this paper was supported in part by the Suncoast Chapter, Florida American Heart Association Affiliate, Inc.

REFERENCES

Afonso, S. (1970). Inhibition of coronary vasodilating action of dipyridamole and adenosine by aminophylline in the dog. *Circulation Res.*, **26**, 743–752.

Angus, J. A., Cobbin, L. B., Einstein, R., and Maguire, M. H. (1971). Cardiovascular actions of substituted adenosine analogs. *Brit. J. Pharmacol.*, **41**, 592–599.

Baer, H. P., Drummond, G. I., and Duncan, E. L. (1966). Formation and deamination of adenosine by cardiac muscle enzymes. *Mol. Pharmacol.*, **2**, 67–76.

Bellardinelli, L., Belloni, F. L., Rubio, R., and Berne, R. M. (1980). Atrioventricular conduction disturbances during hypoxia; possible role of adenosine in rabbit and guinea pig heart. *Circulation Res.*, **47**, 684–691.

Bellardinelli, L., Mattos, E. C., and Berne, R. M. (1981). Evidence for adenosine mediation of atrioventricular block in the ischemic myocardium. *J. Clin. Invest.*, **68**, 195–205.

Berne, R. M., and Rubio, R. (1979). Coronary circulation. In *Handbook of Physiology*, Vol. 1, American Physiological Society, Bethesda, Md, pp. 873–952.

Berne, R. M. (1980). The role of adenosine in the regulation of coronary flow. *Circulation Res.*, **47**, 807–813.

Braun, S., and Levitzki, A. (1979). The attenuation of epinephrine-dependent adenylate cyclase by adenosine and the characteristics of the adenosine stimulatory and inhibitory sites. *Mol. Pharmacol.*, **16**, 737–748.

Burger, R., and Lowenstein, J. M. (1967). Adenylate deaminase III. Regulation of deamination pathways in extracts of rat heart and lung. *J. Biol. Chem.*, **242**, 5281–5288.

Burger, R. M., and Lowenstein, J. M. (1975). 5′-Nucleotidase from smooth muscle of small intestine and from brain. Inhibition by nucleotides. *Biochemistry*, **14**, 2362–2366.

Daly, J. W., Bruns, R. F., and Snyder, S. H. (1981). Adenosine receptors in the central nervous system: relationship to the central actions of methylxanthines. *Life Sci.*, **28**, 2083–2097.

DePierre, J. W., and Karnovsky, M. L. (1974). Ecto-enzymes of the guinea pig polymorphonuclear leukocyte. *J. Biol. Chem.*, **249**, 7121–7129.

Dobson, J. G., Jr (1978). Reduction by adenosine of the isoproterenol-induced increase in cyclic adenosine 3′,5′-monophosphate formation and glycogen phosphorylase activity in rat heart muscle. *Circulation Res.*, **43**, 785–792.

Drury, A. N., and Szent-Gyorgyi, A. (1929). The physiological activity of adenine compounds with especial reference to their action upon the mammalian heart. *J. Physiol. (Lond.)*, **68**, 213–237.

Edwards, M. T., and Maguire, M. H. (1970). Purification and properties of rat heart 5′-nucleotidase. *Mol. Pharmacol.*, **6**, 641–648.

Endoh, M., and Yamashita, S. (1980). Adenosine antagonizes the positive inotropic action mediated by β- but not α-adrenoreceptors in the rabbit papillary muscle. *Europ. J. Pharmacol.*, **65**, 445–448.

Fenton, R. A., Bruttig, S. P., Rubio, R., and Berne, K. M. (1982). Effect of adenosine uptake by intact and cultured smooth muscle. *Am. J. Physiol.*, **242**, H797–H804.

Foley, D. H., Miller, W. L., Rubio, R., and Berne, R. M. (1979). Transmural distribution of myocardial adenosine content during coronary constriction. *Amer. J. Physiol.*, **236**, H833–H838.

Frank, J. S., and Langer, G. A. (1974). The myocardial interstitium: its structure and its role in ionic exchange. *J. Cell Biol.*, **60**, 586–601.

Frick, G. P., and Lowenstein, J. M. (1976). Studies of 5′-nucleotidase in the perfused rat heart including measurements of the enzyme in perfused skeletal muscle and liver. *J. Biol. Chem.*, **251**, 6372–6378.

Frick, G. P., and Lowenstein, J. M. (1978). Vectorial production of adenosine by 5′-nucleotidase in the perfused rat heart. *J. Biol. Chem.*, **253**, 1240–1244.

Gerlach, E., Deuticke, B., and Dreisbach, R. H. (1963). Der Nucleotid-Abbau im Herzmuskel bei Sauerstoffmangel und seine mögliche Bedeutung für die Coronardurchblutung. *Naturwissenschaften*, **50**, 228–229.

Harder, D. R., Bellardinelli, L., Sperelakis, N., Rubio, R., and Berne, R. M. (1979). Differential effects of adenosine and nitroglycerin on the action potentials of large and small coronary arteries. *Circulation Res.*, **44**, 176–182.

Hershfield, M. S., and Kredich, N. M. (1978). S-Adenosylhomocysteine hydrolase is an adenosine-binding protein: a target for adenosine toxicity. *Science*, **202**, 757–760.

Hopkins, S. V., and Goldie, R. V. (1971). A species difference in the uptake of adenosine by heart. *Biochem. Pharmacol.*, **20**, 3359–3365.

Huang, M., and Drummond, G. I. (1976). Effect of adenosine on cyclic AMP accumulation in ventricular myocardium. *Biochem. Pharmacol.*, **25**, 2713–2719.

Huang, M., and Drummond, G. I. (1978). Interaction between adenosine and catecholamines on cyclic AMP accumulation in guinea pig ventricular myocardium. *Biochem. Pharmacol.*, **27**, 187–191.

Huynh-Thu, T., and Lammerant, J. (1978). Adenosine-induced release of cyclic adenosine 3′,5′-monophosphate from the left ventricle in the anesthetized intact dog. *J. Physiol. (Lond.)*, **279**, 641–654.

Huynh-Thu, T., and Lammerant, J. (1980). Release of cyclic adenosine 3′,5′-monophosphate in the coronary venous blood during an intracoronary infusion of adenosine. *Arch. Internat. Phamacodyn. Ther.*, **243**, 74–85.

Illingworth, J. A., Ford, W. C. L., Kobayashi, K., and Williamson, J. R. (1975). Regulation of myocardial energy metabolism, *Recent Advanc. Cardiac Struct. Metab.*, **8**, 271–290.

Jacob, M. I., and Berne, R. M. (1960). Metabolism of purine derivatives by isolated cat heart. *Amer. J. Physiol.*, **198**, 332–326.

Khouri, E. M., Gregg, D. E., and Rayford, C. R. (1965). Effect of exercise on cardiac output, left coronary flow and myocardial metabolism in the unanesthetized dog. *Circulation Res.*, **17**, 427–437.

Kukovetz, W. R., Pöch, G., Holzmann, S., Wurm, A., and Rinner, A. (1978). Role of cyclic nucleotides in adenosine-mediated regulation of coronary flow, *Advanc. Cyclic Nucleotide Res.*, **9**, 397–409.

Lammerant, J., and Becsei, I. (1973). Left ventricular contractility and developed tension in the intact dog submitted to an intracoronary infusion of adenosine. *J. Physiol. (Lond.)*, **229**, 41–49.

Lindner, E., and Rigler, R. (1931). Über die Beeinflussung der Weite der Herzkrankgefässe durch Produkte des Zellkernstoffwechsels. *Pflügers Arch. Ges. Physiol.*, **226**, 697–708.

Liu, M. S., and Feinberg, H. (1971). Incorporation of adenosine-8-^{14}C and inosine-8-^{14}C into rabbit heart adenine nucleotides. *Amer. J. Physiol.*, **220,** 1242–1248.

McKenzie, J. E., McCoy, F. P., and Bockman, E. L. (1980). Myocardial adenosine and coronary resistance during increased cardiac performance. *Amer. J. Physiol.*, **239,** H509–H515.

Manfredi, J. P., and Sparks, H. V., Jr (1982). Adenosine's role in coronary vasodilation induced by atrial pacing and norepinephrine. *Am. J. Physiol.*, **243,** H536–545.

Manfredi, J. P., and Sparks, H. V., Jr (1981). Model of adenosine transport across myocardial capillary wall. *Physiologist*, **24,** 82 (Abstr.).

Miller, W. L., Bellardinelli, L., Bacchus, A., Foley, D. H., Rubio, R., and Berne, R. M. (1979). Canine myocardial adenosine and lactate production, oxygen consumption and coronary blood flow during stellate ganglion stimulation. *Circulation Res.*, **45,** 708–718.

Namm, D. H. (1973). Myocardial nucleotide synthesis from purine bases and nucleosides. Comparison of the rates of formation of purine nucleotides from various precursors and identification of the enzymatic routes for nucleotide formation in the isolated rat heart. *Circulation Res.*, **33,** 686–695.

Nees, S., Gerbes, A. L., Gerlach, E., and Staubesand, J. (1981). Isolation, identification, and continuous culture of coronary endothelial cells from guinea pig hearts. *Europ. J. Cell Biol.*, **24,** 287–297.

Newby, A. C., and Holmquist (1981). Adenosine production inside rat polymorphonuclear leucocytes. *Biochem. J.*, **200,** 399–403.

Olsson, R. A. (1970). Changes in content of purine nucleoside in canine myocardium during coronary occlusion. *Circulation Res.*, **26,** 301–306.

Olsson, R. A., Snow, J. A., Gentry, M. K., and Frick, G. P. (1972). Adenosine uptake by canine heart. *Circulation Res.*, **31,** 767–778.

Olsson, R. A., Snow, J. A., and Gentry, M. K. (1973a). Steric requirements for binding of adenosine to a membrane carrier in canine heart. *Biochem. Biophys. Acta*, **311,** 242–250.

Olsson, R. A., Gentry, M. K., and Townsend, R. S. (1973b). Adenosine metabolism: properties of dog heart microsomal 5'-nucleotidase. *Advanc. Exp. Med. Biol.*, **39,** 27–39.

Olsson, R. A., Davis, C. J., Khouri, E. M., and Patterson, R. E. (1976). Evidence for an adenosine receptor on the surface of dog coronary myocytes. *Circulation Res.*, **39,** 93–98.

Olsson, R. A., Snow, J. A., and Gentry, M. K. (1978). Adenosine metabolism in canine myocardial reactive hyperemia. *Circulation Res.*, **42,** 358–362.

Olsson, R. A., Khouri, E. M., Bedynek, J. L., Jr., and McLean, J. (1979). Coronary vasoactivity of adenosine in the conscious dog. *Circulation Res.*, **45,** 468–478.

Olsson, R. A., Daito, D., and Steinhart, C. R. (1982). Compartmentalization of the adenosine pool of dog and rat hearts. *Circ. Res.*, **50,** 617–626.

Paterson, A. R. P. (1979). Adenosine transport. In *Physiological and Regulatory Functions of Adenosine and Adenine Nucleotides* (H. P. Baer and G. I. Drummond, eds), Raven Press, New York, pp. 305–313.

Polimeni, P. I. (1974). Extracellular space and ionic distribution in rat ventricle. *Amer. J. Physiol.*, **227,** 676–683.

Rembert, J. C., Boyd, L. M., Watkinson, W. P., and Greenfield, J. C., Jr (1980). Effects of adenosine on transmural myocardial blood flow distribution in the awake dog. *Amer. J. Physiol.*, **239,** H7–H13.

Rosen, M. R., Weiss, R. M., and Danilo, P., Jr. (1981). The actions of adenosine on normal and abnormal cardiac impulse initiation. *Circulation,* **64,** Suppl. II, IV-50 (Abstr.).

Rubio, R., and Berne, R. M. (1969). Release of adenosine by the normal myocardium in dogs and its relationship to the regulation of coronary resistance, *Circulation Res.,* **25,** 407–415.

Rubio, R., and Berne, R. M. (1979). Inhibition of 5'-nucleotidase (5'-Nuc) by high energy phosphates (~P): a possible mechanism in coupling adenosine (Ado) release to metabolism. *Fed. Proc.,* **38,** 1037 (Abstr.).

Saito, D., Nixon, D. G., Vomacka, R. B., and Olsson, R. A. (1980). Relationship of cardiac oxygen usage, adenosine content and coronary resistance in dogs. *Circulation Res.,* **47,** 875–882.

Saito, D., Steinhart, C. R., Nixon, D. G., and Olsson, R. A. (1981). Intracoronary adenosine deaminase reduces canine myocardial reactive hyperemia. *Circulation Res.,* **49,** 1262–1267.

Sattin, A., and Rall, T. W. (1970). The effect of adenosine and adenosine nucleotides on the cyclic adenosine 3',5'-phosphate content of guinea pig cerebral cortex slices. *Mol. Pharmacol.,* **6,** 13–23.

Schrader, J., and Gerlach, E. (1976). Compartmentation of cardiac adenine nucleotides and formation of adenosine. *Pflügers Arch. Europ. J. Physiol.,* **367,** 129–135.

Schrader, J., Baumann, G., and Gerlach, E. (1977a). Adenosine as inhibitor of myocardial effects of catecholamines. *Pflügers Arch. Europ. J. Physiol.,* **372,** 29–35.

Schrader, J., Nees, S., and Gerlach, E. (1977b). Evidence for a cell surface adenosine receptor on coronary myocytes and atrial muscle cells. Studies with an adenosine derivative of high molecular weight. *Pflügers Arch., Europ. J. Physiol.,* **369,** 251–257.

Schrader, J., Haddy, F. J., and Gerlach, E. (1977c). Release of adenosine, inosine and hypoxanthine from the isolated guinea pig heart during hypoxia, flow-autoregulation and reactive hyperemia. *Pflügers Arch. Europ. J. Physiol.,* **369,** 1–6.

Schrader, J., Strauer, B. E., and Bürger, S. (1979). Release of adenosine from the human heart before and after digoxin. *Pflügers Arch. Europ. J. Physiol.,* **382,** R2 (Abstr.).

Schrader, J., Schütz, W., and Bardenheuer, H. (1981). Role of S-adenosylhomocysteine hydrolase in adenosine metabolism in mammalian heart. *Biochem. J.,* **196,** 65–70.

Schultz, J., and Daly, J. W. (1973). Cyclic adenosine 3',5'-monophosphate in guinea pig cerebral cortical slices. *J. Biol Chem.,* **248,** 843–852.

Schütz, W., Schrader, J., and Gerlach, E. (1981). Different sites of adenosine formation in the heart. *Amer. J. Physiol.,* **240,** H963–H970.

Snow, J. A., Olsson, R. A., and Gentry, M. K. (1973). Myocardial: blood purine nucleoside concentration ratios in canine myocardium. *Advanc. Exp. Med. Biol.,* **39,** 41–54.

Sobell, S., and Bunger, R. (1981). Compartmentation of adenine nucleotides in the isolated working guinea pig heart stimulated by noradrenaline. *Hoppe-Seyler's Z. Physiol. Chem.,* **362,** 125–132.

Suga, H., Hayashi, T., Suehiro, S., Hisano, R., Shirahata, M., and Ninomiya, I. (1981). Equal oxygen consumption rates of isovolumic and ejecting contractions with equal systolic pressure–volume area in canine ventricle. *Circulation Res.,* **49,** 1082–1091.

Sullivan, J. M., and Alpers, J. B. (1971). *In vitro* regulation of rat heart 5'-

nucleotidase by adenine nucleotides and magnesium. *J. Biol. Chem.*, **246**, 3057–3063.

Szentmiklósi, A. J., Nemeth, M., Szegi, M., Papp, j. Gyl, and Szekeres, L. (1980). Effect of adenosine on sinoatrial and ventricular automaticity of the guinea pig. *Naunyn-Schmiedeberg's Arch. Pharmacol.*, **311**, 147–149.

Ueland, P. m., and Saebø, J. (1979). Sequestration of adenosine in crude extract from mouse liver and other tissues. *Biochem. Biophys. Acta*, **587**, 341–352.

VonRestorff, W., Holtz, H., and Bassenge, E. (1977). Exercise induced augmentation of myocardial oxygen extraction in spite of normal coronary dilatory capacity in dogs. *Pflügers Arch. Europ. J. Physiol.*, **372**, 181–185.

Walsh, D. A., Clippinger, M. S., Sivaramakrishnan, S., and McCullough, T. E. (1979). Cyclic adenosine monophosphate dependent and independent phosphorylation of sarcolemma membrane proteins in perfused rat heart. *Biochemistry*, **18**, 871–877.

Watkinson, W. P., Foley, D. H., Rubio, R., and Berne, R. M. (1979). Myocardial adenosine formation with increased cardiac performance in the dog. *Amer. J. Physiol.*, **236**, H13–H21.

Webster, S., and Olsson, R. A. (1981). Adenosine regulation of canine cardiac adenylate cyclase. *Biochem. Pharmacol.*, **30**, 369–373.

Wiedmeier, V. T., Rubio, R., and Berne, R. M. (1972). Incorporation and turnover of adenosine-U-^{14}C in perfused guinea pig myocardium. *Amer. J. Physiol.*, **223**, 51–54.

Williamson, J. R. (1979). Mitochondrial function in the heart. *Annu. Rev. Physiol.*, **41**, 485–506.

Wolff, J., Londos, C., and Cooper, D. M. F. (1981). Adenosine receptors and the regulation of adenylate cyclase. *Advanc. Cyclic Nucleotide Res.*, **14**, 199–214.

Young, M. A., and Merrill, G. F. (1981). Nifedipine inhibition of adenosine dilation and reactive hyperemia in the coronary vasculature of dogs. *Fed. Proc.*, **40**, 691.

Index